Christensen's

Introduction to the Physics
of Diagnostic Radiology

Christensen's

Introduction to the Physics of Diagnostic Radiology

THOMAS S. CURRY III, M.D.

*Professor of Radiology, University of Texas
Health Science Center at Dallas
and Parkland Memorial Hospital*

JAMES E. DOWDEY, Ph.D.

*Associate Professor of Radiology (Physics)
University of Texas Health Science Center
at Dallas and Parkland Memorial Hospital*

ROBERT C. MURRY, Jr., Ph.D.

*Assistant Professor of Radiology (Physics)
University of Texas Health Science Center
at Dallas and Parkland Memorial Hospital*

3rd Edition

Lea & Febiger • Philadelphia

Lea & Febiger
600 Washington Square
Philadelphia, PA 19106-4198
U.S.A.
215-922-1330

Library of Congress Cataloging in Publication Data
Christensen, Edward E., 1929–
  Christensen's Introduction to the physics of diagnostic radiology.

  Bibliography: p.
  Includes Index.
  1. Diagnosis, Radioscopic. 2. Medical physics.
I. Curry, Thomas S., 1935–   . II. Dowdey, James E.
III. Murry, Robert C. IV. Title. V. Introduction to the physics of diagnostic radiology. [DNLM: 1. Physics.
2. Radiography. 3. Radiology. WN 110 C554i]
RC78.C467   1984   616.07'57   84-3951
ISBN 0-8121-0918-X

1st Edition, 1972
  Reprinted 1973, 1975, 1976, 1977
2nd Edition, 1978
  Reprinted 1979, 1981, 1982, 1983
3rd Edition, 1984

PRINTED IN THE UNITED STATES OF AMERICA

Print Number: 6 5 4 3 2

Dedicated to: _____

MISS WINN

VAUDA

BARBARA

PREFACE

The senior author of this textbook, Edward E. Christensen, M.D. died of an acute myocardial infarction on December 21, 1980 at the age of 51. He joined the faculty of the Department of Radiology of the University of Texas Southwestern Medical School in Dallas during the summer of 1965. Ed's teaching career was characterized by an ability to combine the unbridled exuberance of new residents with the disciplined experience of the "old professor" into an amalgam compatible with a harmonious learning and teaching atmosphere. He soon recognized that residents' frantic efforts at studying radiological physics were producing little more than frantic residents. Thus began a modest series of informal conferences dealing with physics. Soon "handouts" began to appear, and by 1968 an in-service quiz tested both the teacher and his students. Ed was, but should not have been, surprised to find that this written material he had so painfully produced was finding its way about the country as friend traded with friend. In this manner was born the framework for the first edition of *Christensen's Introduction to the Physics of Diagnostic Radiology*. This text was the direct result of a teacher's effort to teach where he was most needed. A few of us knew Ed Christensen as teacher, colleague, and friend. We are grateful for the opportunity. Most will remember Ed as a remarkable teacher, for he was certainly one of the best. But his love for his family and his skills as a craftsman and photographer showed his zest for a full life. It is appropriate that future editions of this textbook will preserve the memory of this extraordinary man.

With this third edition we welcome Robert C. Murry, Jr., Ph.D., as a co-author. It is a sad but unavoidable fact that physicists now outnumber physicians as authors of this text. Technology no longer threatens to overwhelm radiologists and technologists; it has done so. This edition introduces digital fluoroscopy, with its awesome array of statistics and computers. At least digital fluoroscopy uses x rays to generate the basic image, so the topic is not entirely foreign. That brings us to the other new chapter, "Nuclear Magnetic Resonance." No longer do our old friends, the x rays, create the image. Instead, we are forced to crawl inside an atom and consider classical and quantum physics. The words and concepts are unfamiliar to many of us. We have tried to present the basics of NMR in a manner that will allow the student to follow developments in this exciting new imaging technique. The chapter on ultrasound has been expanded to explore new ideas in transducers, and real-time and Doppler techniques.

Our purpose remains firm: to present the new material in an understandable format. The compromises among clarity, completeness, and accuracy involved many painful decisions.

Now we say our final good-bye to our great friend Ed, who provided much of the work for the first two editions of this book and the inspiration for the current one.

Dallas, Texas

T.S. Curry III, M.D.
J.E. Dowdey, Ph.D.
R.C. Murry, Jr., Ph.D.

ACKNOWLEDGMENTS _____

As we begin to relax after spending many months struggling with this third edition, our thoughts and gratitude turn toward the many people who have offered help and encouragment.

Over the years the E.I. du Pont de Nemours and Company (Inc.) has continued to support our efforts. Several individuals in the Photo Products Department of Du Pont have given us many hours of their time. To these valuable friends we again offer a warm thank you. In Dallas, Jerry Jones has been the liaison between ourselves and the Du Pont headquarters in Wilmington, Delaware. At the Du Pont Photo Products Department Chestnut Run Laboratory in Wilmington we have been hosted by Reid Kellogg, Ph.D., Russell Holland, Ph.D., Ronald Schwenker, and Charles Hall, Ph.D. The entire Du Pont effort on our behalf has been orchestrated by our old friend, Robert E. Wayrynen, Ph.D., who is technical manager of X-Ray Markets. Bob is the type of friend everyone should have, and his wife Edna makes a great crab dip.

The Eastman Kodak Company has provided significant technical advice. Special thanks go to our local representative Hoye Underwood for arranging a visit with Leland Erickson (now retired).

Marty Burgin was the talent behind all the new illustrations. Two photographers, Dorothy Gutekunst and Jerry Cheek, reproduced the new illustrations and refrained from complaining too much when we made changes after they had prepared what they thought was the final print.

John Moore built the third edition, just like he did the first and second. John does everything the rest of us cannot or will not do; he holds the team together and insists that the work get done. Curtis Chaney also assisted with many construction chores.

A task such as this requires the support and understanding of our colleagues in the Radiology Department. In the Radiological Physics Section, graduate students Sherye Horner, Geoff Clarke, and Sarah Haynes were often available to research articles and to answer questions. Ray Nunnally, Ph.D., was a great help in the NMR section, and supplied some of the material you will study. An unexpected vacancy in the clinical staff threatened to delay this edition beyond the 6 months by which we missed our initial deadline. But some of our senior residents took up much of the slack and allowed T.S.C. to be free for many all-day work sessions necessary. Special plaudits go to Drs. Bill Henry, Mike Knox, Val Phillips, Fred Walters, and Fernando Bazan. To Dr. Joe Franklin we say thanks for sticking so many kidneys for us. Chief Residents Bill Schmid, Jim Buck, David Kilgore, and Gary Webb rewrote the schedule many times to be sure that senior residents were covering critical areas while the old professor was away. Almost every other resident in our department contributed to the effort by tolerating delays and loss of teaching conferences. We will not name them all, but we will always remember these fine men and women with warmth and affection. Our colleagues on the teaching staff remained as understanding as ever, particularly Drs. Robert Parkey, George Curry, Bill Kilman, Geral Dietz, Mike Landay, Bob Epstein, Jan Diehl, and Ken Maravilla. And our reliable colleague Dr. Jack Reynolds once again read the new manuscripts and offered appropriate suggestions. Jack is the sort of fellow all departments need but few find.

Cathy Starnes and Scherri Fugitt helped with the typing and organization. Our chief typist, organizer, critic, and slave driver was Dianna Hallford. She was given free rein to edit any part of the entire manuscript except this paragraph. Thanks, Dianna; we could have done it without you, but we could not have done it as well.

Finally, a simple thanks for the support of our wives and families, the most important people behind the whole project.

T.S.C.
J.E.D.
R.C.M.

CONTENTS

1

Radiation

Wilhelm Conrad Roentgen, a German physicist, discovered x rays on November 8, 1895. Several fortunate coincidences set the stage for the discovery. Roentgen was investigating the behavior of cathode rays (electrons) in high-energy cathode ray tubes, which consisted of a glass envelope from which as much air as possible had been evacuated. A short platinum electrode was fitted into each end and when a high-voltage discharge was passed through this tube, ionization of the remaining gas produced a faint light. Roentgen had enclosed his cathode ray tube in black cardboard to prevent this light from escaping to block any effect the light might have on experiments he was conducting. He then darkened his laboratory room to be sure there were no light leaks in the cardboard cover. On passing a high-tension discharge through the tube, he noticed a faint light glowing on a work bench about 3 ft away. He discovered that the source of the light was the fluorescence of a small piece of paper coated with barium platinocyanide. Because electrons could not escape the glass envelope of the tube to produce fluorescence, and because the cardboard permitted no light to escape from the tube, he concluded that some unknown type of ray was produced when the tube was energized. We can imagine his excitement as he investigated the mysterious new ray. He began placing objects between the tube and the fluorescent screen: a book, a block of wood, and a sheet of aluminum. The brightness of the fluorescence differed with each, indicating that the ray penetrated some objects more easily than others. Then he held his hand between the tube and the screen and, to his surprise, the outline of his skeleton appeared on the screen. By December 28, 1895, he had thoroughly investigated the properties of the rays and had prepared a manuscript describing his experiments. In recognition of his outstanding contribution to science, Wilhelm Conrad Roentgen was awarded the first Nobel Prize for Physics in 1901.

ELECTROMAGNETIC SPECTRUM

X rays belong to a group of radiations called electromagnetic radiation. **Electromagnetic radiation is the transport of energy through space as a combination of electric and magnetic fields** (hence the name electromagnetic). Familiar members of the family of electromagnetic radiation include radio waves, radiant heat, visible light, and gamma radiation.

Electromagnetic (EM) radiation is produced by a charge (usually a charged particle) being accelerated. The converse is also true; that is, a charge being accelerated will emit EM radiation. Right here at the beginning we run into our first problem. Physics, our beloved exact science, presents a contradiction. The problem is just this: in our discussion of atomic structure (see Chap. 2) we will discuss electrons (charged particles) revolving around the nucleus in circular orbits while maintaining a precise energy. (This is a result of the Bohr theory of the hydrogen atom.) This picture of

1

atomic structure violates the converse statement above. First, if an electron moves in a circular orbit, it must have centripetal acceleration (an acceleration toward the center of the circular path); therefore, it should emit EM radiation. The loss of energy would require the electron to change its orbit and energy. As a matter of fact, there was some heated discussion when Bohr first introduced his theory that electrons could not possibly be in circular orbits because, being accelerated, they would emit energy and spiral into the nucleus. Shifty-eyed physicists easily get around this argument by saying that electrons, after all, are standing waves about the nucleus and therefore do not represent accelerating charges. It is fair to say, however, that outside the atom a charge being accelerated will emit EM radiation. The energy that charged particles obtain in circular particle accelerators is limited by the energy loss to EM radiation as the particles move about the accelerator. A cyclotron is a good example of an accelerator type that is EM radiation-limited.

But we haven't finished. In the same atomic structure discussion, we allow electronic transitions from one energy state to another with emission of EM radiation energy, but with no mention of acceleration. In fact, we really think of instantaneous transitions across regions in which electrons cannot possibly exist. This concept of energy level transitions seems to contradict the first statement that EM radiation is produced by an accelerated charge.

There are a couple of observations that must be made. First, the world of quantum physics (represented here by Bohr's theory) does not always behave as we, living in a somewhat larger world, might expect. Because x rays are produced in the quantum physics world, we must understand some of the laws governing that world. Second, in this book we have endeavored to be as physically accurate as possible while emphasizing those points that we feel clinicians should understand.

Perhaps we should then rephrase the statement: EM radiation, except for that produced in energy level transitions (including nuclear transitions), is produced by accelerating charge. Any accelerating charge not bound to an atom (including the nucleus) will emit EM radiation.

Some time should be spent here discussing the production and structure of EM radiation. To do that, we will start with a single small charged ball. (Because we recognize the electron as a charged particle, we can put a charge on a ball by adding or taking away electrons. If we add electrons, we will charge the ball negatively. Subtraction of electrons results in a positively charged ball.) We can only determine if we are successful in placing a charge on the ball by observing its interactions with the world around it. Coulomb studied the forces that exist between two charged balls, and today we call the forces between charged objects Coulomb forces. The force between two small balls having charges q_1 and q_2 is

$$F = \frac{kq_1q_2}{r^2}$$

F = force (a vector)
k = a constant whose value depends on the system of units
q_1 and q_2 = charge on balls
r = distance between balls.

This force is always along the line joining the two balls. (More accurately, it is the line joining the centers of the two charge distributions. If we use "point" charges we don't have to worry about the charge distribution.) If q_1 and q_2 are like charges (same sign; positive and positive or negative and negative), the force is a repelling force. If q_1 and q_2 are unlike charges, the force is attractive. Gravity force also has this mathematical form, but it is always attractive.

We nearly always introduce the electric field (E) to describe the possible interactive forces. We define the electric field for a charge distribution (q_1) as the force that q_1

would exert on a positive unit charge (q_2 equals 1). Note that E has a unique value and direction at each point surrounding a charge. Figure 1–1 shows the E field surrounding a point positive charge. Note that E is radially directed and falls off (decreases in size) as $1/r^2$. The electric field for more complicated charge distributions could be more or even less complicated. (The electric field for an infinite plane uniformly charged is constant everywhere.) This electric field is sometimes called the static (electric is implied) field because the charge is at rest.

If the charge moves with a constant velocity, we not only see an electric field (E) moving with the charge, but also a magnetic field (H) surrounding the line (path) along which the charge is moving. (A more detailed discussion of magnetic fields will be found in Chapter 28.) Figure 1–2 shows the electric field radially directed and the circular magnetic field (H). Here E and H (both vectors) are perpendicular at any one point.

The next thing to do is to let the charge accelerate. Here we have conceptual problems. At constant velocity, the electric field moves along with the charge. But, with acceleration, the charge moves to a new location before the outer regions of the elec-

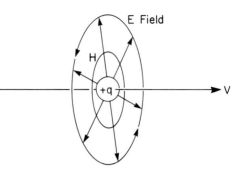

Figure 1–2 Electric and magnetic fields surrounding a positive charge moving with constant velocity

tric field realize that the charge is at a different place than it should be. The electric field lags behind the charge, as does the magnetic field. The lagging behind produces a "kink" in the electric field lines that moves outward from the charge with a finite (but large) velocity. We can think of this kink as being the EM radiation. We don't know any better way to describe this rather complex concept.

EM radiation is made up of an electric field and a magnetic field that mutually support each other. Figure 1–3 shows the E and H fields and the direction of propagation of the EM radiation. Note that E and H are perpendicular, that they reverse together, and that both E and H are perpendicular to the direction of propagation. The concept to be visualized is that E and H interact to build each other up to some value, then collapse together and build each other up in the opposite direction. Energy is transmitted through space by the EM radiation.

The radiation depicted in Figure 1–3 was produced by a charge oscillating back and forth. Suppose we consider a radio transmission tower. The purpose of the tower is to transmit radio signals that, as you might have guessed, are EM radiation. The transmission is accomplished by accelerating charge up and down a conductor in the tower. As the charge is accelerated up the tower, we might get one section of

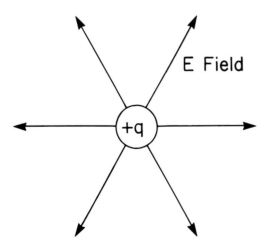

Figure 1–1 Electric field surrounding a positive charge at rest

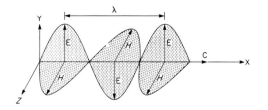

Figure 1–3 Representation of electromagnetic radiation

the EM radiation shown in Figure 1–3. As the charge moves down the tower, the following section of the EM radiation is produced. When the charge changes direction, so do the E and H fields. Thus, a radio wave can be produced by forcing charge to move up and down the tower by applying an alternating voltage to the tower. The frequency of the radio wave is just how many times per second the charge changes direction. Of course, we tune our radios at home to a given frequency to find a particular station. The information we obtain from the radio, perhaps music, is superimposed on the EM radiation generated by the tower. How that is done is another story.

We would be in excellent shape if EM radiation didn't interact with the particles of our old world. Obviously, without such interaction we wouldn't be here to wonder about EM radiation anyway. Life-giving energy from the sun gets here by EM radiation.

Maybe it would be instructive to see how radio waves interact with your radio. Just a little while ago we talked about EM radiation in the form of radio waves being emitted from a radio tower. (We didn't say there that the energy emitted was emitted outward from the tower in something of a doughnut-shaped pattern. The maximum intensity is emitted perpendicularly to the tower, while there is no intensity directly above the tower. That pattern is best for us, because most of us don't listen to a radio while directly above the tower.) What we need to detect the radio wave is some antenna (an electrical conductor) in the radio

radiation pattern. When the radio wave (the E and H fields) passes the antenna, the E-field part of the EM radio wave exerts a force on the electrons in the antenna, which makes the electrons oscillate back and forth in the antenna at the frequency of the radio wave. Consequently, the antenna detects the EM radiation by the electrons moving under the influence of the E field in the EM radiation. In this type of detection, the EM radiation looks and behaves as a wave. As the frequency of the EM radiation increases, however, a point is reached in the frequency range (not a single precise frequency) at which the electron can no longer follow the electric field. At frequencies in this range and higher, the electrons interact with the EM radiation as if the EM radiation were an energy bundle, rather than made up of waves. Later, we will see that coherent scattering of x rays is by an interaction of the wave type, while photoelectric absorption is an interaction of the energy bundle (called a photon) type. To stay away from exotic physics, it is necessary to discuss EM radiation as if it were comprised of both particles (photons) and waves. Let us hasten to add that EM radiation will behave as only one of the two, and that this behavior is always the same for a given interaction (or experimental measurement).

To finish the radio detection, we note one problem: there are a number of radio stations broadcasting at the same time. We must pick one frequency (the station we want to listen to) and discard the rest. This selection is done by a "tank" circuit on the end of the antenna. We tune the tank circuit (by the station selection knob) to keep only one frequency. What we hear on the radio is the second part of the other story introduced in the paragraph on radio transmission.

In the first chapters in this text, we will be interested in how the E part of the EM radiation reacts with electrons. Later, when discussing nuclear magnetic resonance, we will consider reactions with the H (magnetic) part of the field that are produced by oscillating electrons.

The interactions of different kinds of EM radiation are difficult to understand. Some are explained only if they are assumed to be particles, while others are explained only by theories of wave propagation. **It is necessary to discuss electromagnetic radiation as if it were comprised of both particles and waves.**

Wave Concept of Electromagnetic Radiation

Electromagnetic radiation is propagated through space in the form of waves. They may be compared to waves traveling down a stretched rope when one end is moved up and down in a rhythmic motion. While the waves with which we are familiar must be propagated in a medium (such as the example of the rope, waves traveling in water, or sound waves traveling in air), electromagnetic waves need no such medium; that is, they can be propagated through a vacuum. Waves of all types have an associated wavelength and frequency. The distance between two successive crests, or troughs, is the wavelength of the wave, and is given the symbol λ (the Greek letter *lambda*, the initial for length). The number of waves passing a particular point in a unit of time is called the frequency, and is given the symbol ν (the Greek letter *nu*, the initial for number). If each wave has a length λ, and ν waves pass a given point in unit time, the velocity of the wave is given by

$$V = \lambda \times \nu$$

For example, if the wavelength is 4 ft and the frequency is 60 waves/min, then

$$V = 4 \text{ ft} \times 60/\text{min}$$
$$V = 240 \text{ ft/min}$$

EM radiation always travels at the same velocity in a vacuum. This velocity is 186,000 miles per second (3×10^8 meters per second), which is usually referred to as the velocity of light and given the symbol c.

Therefore, we may express the relationship between velocity, wavelength, and frequency as

$$c = \lambda \nu$$

c = velocity of light (m/sec)
λ = wavelength (meters)
ν = frequency (per second).

Because all types of electromagnetic radiation have the same velocity, the frequency of the radiation must be inversely proportional to its wavelength. All types of radiation in the electromagnetic spectrum differ basically only in wavelength. The wavelength of a radio wave may be 5 miles long, while a typical x ray is only 1 billionth of an inch. The wavelength of diagnostic x rays is extremely short and it is usually expressed in Angstrom units (Å). An Angstrom is 10^{-10} meters. The wavelength of most diagnostic x rays is between 1 and 0.1 Å. The wavelength of an electromagnetic wave determines how it interacts with matter. For example, an electromagnetic wave 7000 Å long can be seen by the human eye as red light, and a wavelength of 4000 Å is seen as blue light. The frequency of blue light may be calculated by knowing its wavelength (4000 Å = 4×10^{-7} m):

$$c = \lambda \nu \text{ or } \nu = \frac{c}{\lambda}$$
$$\nu = \frac{3 \times 10^8 \text{ m/sec}}{4 \times 10^{-7} \text{ m}}$$
$$\nu = 7.5 \times 10^{14}/\text{sec}$$

Blue light, with a wavelength of 4000 Å, has a frequency of 7.5×10^{14} vibrations per second. Similarly calculated, the frequency of an x ray of wavelength 0.1 Å is 3×10^{19} vibrations per second.

The complete spectrum of electromagnetic radiation covers a wide range of wavelengths and frequencies. The various parts of the spectrum are named according to the manner in which the type of radiation is generated or detected. Some members of the group, listed in order of decreasing wavelength, are

Radio, television, radar:	3×10^5 to 1 cm
Infrared radiation:	0.01 to 0.00008 cm (8000 Å)
Visible light:	7500 (0.000075 cm) to 3900 Å
Ultraviolet radiation:	3900 to 20 Å
Soft x rays:	100 to 1 Å
Diagnostic x rays:	1 to 0.1 Å
Therapeutic x ray and gamma rays:	0.1 to 10^{-4} Å

There is considerable overlap in the wavelengths of the various members of the electromagnetic spectrum; the numbers listed are rough guides. It is again stressed that the great differences in properties of these different types of radiation are attributable to their differences in wavelength (or frequency).

The wave concept of electromagnetic radiation explains why it may be reflected, refracted, diffracted, and polarized. There are some phenomena, however, that cannot be explained by the wave concept.

Particle Concept of Electromagnetic Radiation

Short electromagnetic waves, such as x rays, may react with matter as if they were particles rather than waves. These particles are actually discrete bundles of energy, and each of these bundles of energy is called a **quantum,** or a **photon.** Photons travel at the speed of light. The amount of energy carried by each quantum, or photon, depends on the frequency (v) of the radiation. If the frequency (number of vibrations per second) is doubled, the energy of the photon is doubled. The actual amount of energy of the photon may be calculated by multiplying its frequency by a constant. The constant has been determined experimentally to be 4.13×10^{-18} keV sec, and is called Planck's constant. The mathematical expression is written as follows:

$$E = hv$$

E = photon energy
h = Planck's constant
v = frequency.

The ability to visualize the dual characteristics of electromagnetic radiation presents a true challenge. But we must unavoidably reach the conclusion that EM radiation sometimes behaves as a wave and other times as a particle. The particle concept is used to describe the interactions between radiation and matter. Because we will be concerned principally with interactions, such as the photoelectric effect and Compton scatter, we will use the photon (or quantum) concept in this text.

The unit used to measure the energy of photons is the electron volt (eV). An electron volt is the amount of energy that an electron gains as it is accelerated by a potential difference of 1 volt. Because the electron volt is a small unit, x ray energies are usually measured in terms of the kiloelectron volt (keV), which is 1000 electron volts. We will usually discuss x rays in terms of their energy rather than their wavelengths, but the two are related as follows:

$$c = \lambda v \text{ or } v = \frac{c}{\lambda}$$

and

$$E = hv$$

Substituting $\frac{c}{\lambda}$ for v,

$$E = \frac{hc}{\lambda}$$

The product of the velocity of light (c) and Planck's constant (h) is 12.4 when the unit of energy is keV and the wavelength is in Angstroms. The final equation showing the relationship between energy and wavelength is

$$E = \frac{12.4}{\lambda}$$

E = energy (in keV)
λ = wavelength (in Å).

Table 1–1 shows the relationship between energy and wavelength for various photons.

If a photon has 15 eV or more of energy

Table 1–1. Correlation Between Wavelength and Energy

WAVELENGTH (Å)	ENERGY (keV)
0.0005	24,800
0.08	155
0.1	124
1.24	10

it is capable of ionizing atoms and molecules, and it is called ionizing radiation. An atom is ionized when it loses an electron. Gamma rays, x rays, and some ultraviolet rays are all types of ionizing radiation.

UNITS

While writing this text we encountered a problem regarding the units used to measure various quantities. Whenever possible we have tried to use SI units. Sometimes this resulted in very large or very small numbers, and often in such cases we used cgs system units. A brief description of units will help you to follow the various units used in this text. In the future, it is probable that SI units will predominate.

The SI system (Systéme Internationale d'Unités) is a modernized metric system based on the MKS (meter-kilogram-second) system. The SI system was originally defined and given official status by the Eleventh General Conference on Weights and Measures in 1960. (A complete listing of SI units can be found in the National Bureau of Standards Special Publication 330, 1977 edition.) There are only seven base units and two supplementary units. All others are derived from these nine units, although some are given special names. Table 1–2 gives the seven fundamental quantities to which the seven base SI units refer. The MKS units for these seven quantities are identical to the SI units. For comparison, Table 1–2 also lists those common cgs (centimeter-gram-second) units that have been used elsewhere in this book. A blank entry does not mean that there is no cgs equivalent, but that we have not used those units elsewhere and do not wish to add complications. Note that the two supplementary units at the bottom of Table 1–2 (radians and steradians) merely formalize the use of radians for angular measurements. There are 2π radians in 360° (i.e., in a complete circle), so one radian is about 57.3°; there are 4π steradians in a sphere.

Units for any physically known quantity can be derived from these nine SI units. Table 1–3 lists some quantities mentioned in this book, and all but one also have a name in SI units. Again, those common units used elsewhere are also listed. Of course, each unit in the table can be expressed in SI base units only, and a column is included to show this. Sometimes expressing one derived SI unit in terms of other derived SI units reveals some underlying principles of physics. For instance, we note that the SI unit of power is the Watt, which in base SI units equals $1 \frac{m^2 kg}{s^3}$. The meaning of the base SI units might be immediately apparent to a physicist, but J/s (Joules per second) is a little easier to comprehend. This is just energy per unit time, or power. Electrical power would be even harder to understand in base SI units, but $V \cdot A$ (volts times amps) is our comfortable definition.

The SI unit of radionuclide activity is the Becquerel (Becquerel has finally made the big time, after discovering radioactivity in 1896, the same year that Roentgen discovered x rays). The fact that one Bq is the decay of one nucleus per second may be a little inconvenient, but even simplicity has its price. The SI unit of radiation absorbed dose is the Gray, which again refers to the quantity of ionizing radiation energy absorbed per unit of mass. There is no special SI unit corresponding to the familiar radiation exposure unit of the Roentgen. The Roentgen was originally defined as the charge produced in a given mass of air, and comparable SI units are C/kg (C = Coulomb).

A good table is needed to convert from

Table 1–2. SI Base and Supplementary Units

QUANTITY	SI UNIT NAME	SI SYMBOL	FAMILIAR cgs UNIT	cgs SYMBOL
SI base units:				
Length	meter	m	centimeter	cm
Mass	kilogram	kg	gram	g
Time	second	s	second	s
Electric current	ampere	A		
Temperature	kelvin	K		
Amount of substance	mole	mol		
Luminous intensity	candela	cd		
SI supplementary units:				
Plane angle	radian	rad		
Solid angle	steradian	sr		

Table 1–3. SI Derived Units with Special Names

QUANTITY	SI UNIT NAME	SI SYMBOL	EXPRESSED IN SI BASE UNITS	EXPRESSED IN OTHER SI UNITS	MORE FAMILIAR UNIT
Frequency	Hertz	Hz	$\dfrac{1}{s}$		
Force	Newton	N	$\dfrac{m \cdot kg}{s^2}$		
Energy	Joule	J	$\dfrac{m^2 kg}{s^2}$	$N \cdot m$	erg (cgs)
Power	Watt	W	$\dfrac{m^2 kg}{s^3}$	$\dfrac{J}{s}$ or $V \cdot A$	
Charge	Coulomb	C	$A \cdot s$		
Radioactivity	Becquerel	Bq	$\dfrac{1}{s}$		Curie
Absorbed dose	Gray	Gy	$\dfrac{m^2}{s^2}$	$\dfrac{J}{kg}$	rad
			$\dfrac{A \cdot s}{kg}$	$\dfrac{C}{kg}$	Roentgen
Electric potential	Volt	V	$\dfrac{m^2 \cdot kg}{s^3 \cdot A}$	$\dfrac{W}{A}$	
Capacitance	Farad	F	$\dfrac{A^2 s^4}{m^2 kg}$	$\dfrac{C}{V}$	
Magnetic flux	Weber	Wb	$\dfrac{m^2 kg}{s^2 \cdot A}$	$V \cdot s$	
Magnetic flux density (magnetic induction)	Tesla	T	$\dfrac{kg}{s^2 \cdot A}$	$\dfrac{Wb}{m^2}$	Gauss

the older units and from United States units (based on the British engineering system) to SI units. A foot is about 0.305 meters, a Joule is 10 million ergs, and so forth. We will undoubtedly continue to use a combination of units from different systems for some time. For instance, we purchase electric power in kilowatts (SI units), potatoes in pounds (British engineering unit), and heat energy in BTUs (British thermal units), all different systems. An increasingly complex world should uniformly use something like SI units. A sixteenth-century English peasant may not have needed to convert a speed of furlongs per fortnight into inches per second, and we should not have to either.

SUMMARY

Wilhelm Conrad Roentgen discovered x rays on November 8, 1895. X rays are members of a group of radiations known as electromagnetic radiations, of which light is the best-known member. They have a dual nature, behaving in some circumstances as waves and under different conditions as particles. Therefore, two concepts have been postulated to explain their characteristics. A single particle of radiation is called a photon, and we will discuss x rays in terms of photons.

REFERENCE

1. Glasser, O.: Wilhelm Conrad Roentgen and the Early History of the Roentgen Rays. Springfield, IL, Charles C Thomas, 1934.

2

Production of X Rays

DIAGNOSTIC X-RAY TUBES

X rays are produced by **energy conversion** when a fast-moving stream of electrons is suddenly decelerated in the "target" anode of an x-ray tube. The x-ray tube is made of Pyrex glass that encloses a vacuum containing two electrodes (this is a diode tube). The electrodes are designed so that electrons produced at the cathode (negative electrode or filament) can be accelerated by a high potential difference toward the anode (positive or target electrode). The basic elements of an x-ray tube are shown in Figure 2–1, a diagram of a stationary anode x-ray tube. Electrons are produced by the heated tungsten filament and accelerated across the tube to hit the tungsten target, where x rays are produced. This section will describe the design of the x-ray tube and will review the way in which x rays are produced.

Glass Enclosure

It is necessary to seal the two electrodes of the x-ray tube in a vacuum. If gas were present inside the tube, the electrons that were being accelerated toward the anode (target) would collide with the gas molecules, lose energy, and cause secondary electrons to be ejected from the gas molecules. By this process (ionization) additional electrons would be available for acceleration toward the anode. Obviously, this production of secondary electrons could not be satisfactorily controlled. Their presence would result in variation in the number and, more strikingly, in the reduced speed of the electrons impinging on the target. This would cause a wide variation in tube current and in the energy of the x rays produced. Actually, this principle was used in the design of the early so called "gas" x-ray tubes, which contained

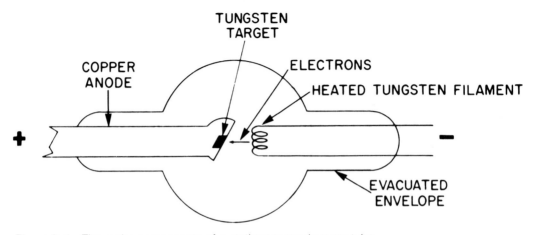

Figure 2–1 The major components of a stationary anode x-ray tube

small amounts of gas to serve as a source of secondary electrons. The purpose of the vacuum in the modern x-ray tube is to allow the number and speed of the accelerated electrons to be controlled independently. The shape and size of these x-ray tubes are specifically designed to prevent electric discharge between the electrodes.

The connecting wires must be sealed into the glass wall of the x-ray tube. During operation of the x-ray tube, both the glass and the connecting wires are heated to high temperatures. Because of differences in their coefficients of expansion, most metals expand more than glass when heated. This difference in expansion would cause the glass-metal seal to break and would destroy the vacuum in the tube if special precautions were not taken. Because of this problem, special alloys, having approximately the same coefficients of linear expansion as borosilicate glass, are generally used in x-ray tubes.

Cathode

The negative terminal of the x-ray tube is called the cathode. In referring to an x-ray tube, the terms **cathode** and **filament** may be used interchangeably, a statement that is not true for other types of diode tubes. In addition to the **filament, which is the source of electrons** for the x-ray tube, the cathode has two other elements. These are the connecting wires, which supply the source of voltage (average about 10 volts) and amperage (average about 3 to 5 amperes) that heat the filament, and a metallic focusing cup. The number (quantity) of x rays produced depends entirely on the number of electrons that flow from the filament to the target (anode) of the tube. **The x-ray tube current, measured in milliamperes** (1 mA = 0.001 ampere), **refers to the number of electrons flowing per second from the filament to the target.** It is important to understand where these electrons come from, and to remember that the number of electrons determines x-ray tube current. For example, in a given unit of time, a tube current of 200 mA is produced by twice as many electrons as a current of 100 mA, and 200 mA produces twice as many x rays as 100 mA.

The filament is made of tungsten wire, about 0.2 mm in diameter, that is coiled to form a vertical spiral about 0.2 cm in diameter and 1 cm or less in length. When current flows through this fine tungsten wire, it becomes heated. When a metal is heated its atoms absorb thermal energy, and some of the electrons in the metal acquire enough energy to allow them to move a small distance from the surface of the metal (normally, electrons can move within a metal, but cannot escape from the metal). Their escape is referred to as the process of **thermionic emission,** which may be defined as the emission of electrons resulting from the absorption of thermal energy. A pure tungsten filament must be heated to a temperature of at least 2200° C to emit a useful number of electrons (thermions). Tungsten is not as efficient an emitting material as other materials (such as alloys of tungsten) used in some electron tubes. It is chosen for use in x-ray tubes, however, because it can be drawn into a thin wire that is quite strong, has a high melting point (3370° C), and has little tendency to vaporize; thus, such a filament has a reasonably long life expectancy.

Electrons emitted from the tungsten filament form a small cloud in the immediate vicinity of the filament. This collection of negatively charged electrons forms what is called the **space charge.** This cloud of negative charges tends to prevent other electrons from being emitted from the filament until they have acquired sufficient thermal energy to overcome the force caused by the space charge. The tendency of the space charge to limit the emission of more electrons from the filament is called the **space charge effect.** When electrons leave the filament, the loss of negative charges causes the filament to acquire a positive charge. The filament then attracts some emitted electrons back to itself. When a filament is heated to its emission temperature, a state of equilibrium is quickly reached. In equilibrium the number of electrons returning to the filament is equal to the number of electrons being emitted. As a result, the number of electrons in the space charge remains constant, with the actual number depending on filament temperature.

The high currents that can be produced by the use of thermionic emission are possible because large numbers of electrons can be accelerated from the cathode (negative electrode) to the anode (positive electrode) of the x-ray tube. The number of electrons involved is enormous. The unit of electric current is the Ampere, which may be defined as the rate of "flow" when 1 Cou of electricity flows through a conductor in 1 sec. The Coulomb may be defined as the amount of electric charge carried by 6.25×10^{18} electrons. Therefore, an x-ray tube current of 100 milliamperes (0.1 Ampere) may be considered as the "flow" of 6.25×10^{17} electrons from the cathode to the anode in 1 second. **Electron current across an x-ray tube is in one direction only** (always cathode to anode). Because of the forces of mutual repulsion and the large number of electrons, this electron stream would tend to spread itself out and result in bombardment of an unacceptably large area on the anode of the x-ray tube. This is prevented by a structure called the cathode **focusing cup,** which surrounds the filament (Figs. 2–2 and 2–4). When the x-ray tube is conducting, the focusing cup is maintained at the same negative potential as the filament. The focusing cup is designed so that its electrical forces cause the electron stream to converge onto the target anode in the required size and shape. The focusing cup is usually made of molybdenum. Modern x-ray tubes may be supplied with a single or, more commonly, a double filament. Each filament consists of a spiral of wire, and they are mounted side by side or one above the other, with one being longer than the other (Fig. 2–2). It

is important to understand that only one filament is used for any given x-ray exposure; the larger filament is generally used for larger exposures. The heated filament glows and can be easily observed by looking into the beam exit port of an x-ray tube housing (do not forget to remove the filter).

Vaporization of the filament when it is heated acts to shorten the life of an x-ray tube, because the filament will break if it becomes too thin. The filament should never be heated for longer periods than necessary. Many modern x-ray circuits contain an automatic filament-boosting circuit. When the x-ray circuit is turned on, but no exposure is being made, a "standby" current heats the filament to a value corresponding to low current, commonly about 5 mA. This amount of filament heating is all that is required for fluoroscopy. When exposures requiring larger tube currents are desired, an automatic filament-boosting circuit will raise the filament current from the standby value to the required value before the exposure is made, and lower it to the standby value immediately after the exposure.

Tungsten that is vaporized from the filament (and occasionally from the anode) is deposited as an extremely thin coating on the inner surface of the glass wall of the x-ray tube. It produces a color that becomes deeper as the tube ages. Old tubes acquire a bronze-colored "sunburn." This tungsten coat has two effects: it tends to filter the x-ray beam, gradually changing the quality

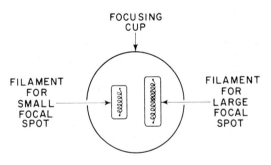

Figure 2–2 A double filament contained in the focusing cup

of the beam, and, in addition, the presence of the metal on the glass increases the possibility of arcing between the glass and the electrodes at higher peak kilovoltage (kVp) values, which may result in puncture of the tube.

Line Focus Principle

The focal spot is the area of the tungsten target (anode) that is bombarded by electrons from the cathode. **Most of the energy of the electrons is converted into heat,** with less than 1% being converted into x rays. Because the heat is uniformly distributed over the focal spot, a large focal spot allows the accumulation of larger amounts of heat before damage to the tungsten target occurs. The melting point of tungsten is about 3370° C, but it is best to keep the temperature below 3000° C. The problems posed by the need for a large focal spot to allow greater heat loading, and the conflicting need for a small focal area to produce good radiographic detail, were resolved in 1918 with the development of the **line focus principle.** The theory of line focus is illustrated in Figure 2–3. The size and shape of the focal spot are determined by the size and shape of the electron stream when it hits the anode. The size and shape of the electron stream are determined by the dimensions of the filament tungsten wire coil, the construction of the focusing cup, and the position of the filament in the focusing cup. The electron stream bombards the target, the surface of which is inclined so that it forms an angle with the plane perpendicular to the incident beam. The anode angle differs according to individual tube design and may vary from 6 to 20°. Because of this angulation, when the slanted surface of the focal spot is viewed from the direction in which x rays emerge from the x-ray tube, it is foreshortened and appears small. It is evident, therefore, that the size of the effective, or apparent, focal spot is considerably smaller than that of the actual focal spot. If the decrease in projected focal spot size is calculated, it is found that the size of the projected focal spot is directly related to the sine of the angle of the anode. Because sine 20° = 0.342 and sine 16.5° = 0.284, an anode angle of 16.5° will produce a smaller focal spot size than an angle of 20°. Thus, as the angle of the anode is made smaller, the apparent focal spot also becomes smaller.

Some newer 0.3 mm focal spot tubes may use an anode angle of only 6°. Such small angles permit the use of larger areas of the target for electron bombardment (and heat dissipation), and yet achieve a small apparent focal spot size. For practical purposes, however, there is a limit to which the anode angle can be decreased as dictated by the heel effect (the point of anode cutoff). For general diagnostic radiography done at a 40-in. focus-film distance, the anode angle is usually no smaller than 15°.

Focal spot size is expressed in terms of the apparent or projected focal spot; sizes of 0.3, 0.6, 1.0, 1.2, and 2.0 mm are commonly employed.

Anode

Anodes (positive electrodes) of x-ray tubes are of two types, **stationary** or **rotating.** The stationary anode will be discussed first because many of its basic principles also apply to the rotating anode.

Stationary Anode

The anode of a stationary anode x-ray tube consists of a small plate of tungsten, 2 or 3 mm thick, that is embedded in a

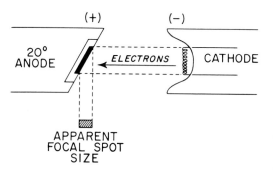

Figure 2–3   The line focus principle

large mass of copper. The tungsten plate is square or rectangular in shape, with each dimension usually being greater than 1 cm. The anode angle is usually 15 to 20°, as discussed above.

Tungsten is chosen as the target material for several reasons. It has a **high atomic number** (74), which makes it more efficient for the production of x rays. In addition, because of its **high melting point,** it is able to withstand the high temperature produced. Most metals melt between 300 and 1500° C, while tungsten melts at 3370° C. Tungsten provides a reasonably good material for the absorption of heat and for the rapid dissipation of the heat away from the target area.

The rather small tungsten target must be bonded to the much larger copper portion of the anode to facilitate heat dissipation. In spite of its rather good thermal characteristics, tungsten cannot withstand the heat of repeated exposures. Copper is a better conductor of heat than tungsten, so the massive copper anode acts to increase the total thermal capacity of the anode and to speed its rate of cooling.

The actual size of the tungsten target is considerably larger than the area bombarded by the electron stream (Fig. 2–4). This is necessary because of the relatively low melting point of copper (1070° C). A single x-ray exposure may raise the temperature of the bombarded area of the

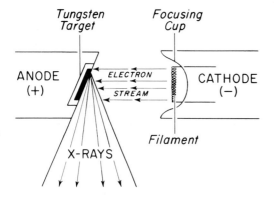

Figure 2–4 Lateral view of the cathode and anode of a stationary anode x-ray tube

tungsten target by 1000° C or more. This high temperature is reached by any metal in the immediate vicinity of the focal spot. If the tungsten target were not sufficiently large to allow for some cooling around the edges of the focal spot, the heat produced would melt the copper in the immediate vicinity of the target.

All the metals expand when heated, but they expand at different rates. The bonding between the tungsten target and the copper anode provides technical problems because tungsten and copper have different coefficients of expansion. If the bond between the tungsten and the copper were not satisfactorily produced, the tungsten target would tend to peel away from the copper anode.

Rotating Anode

With the development of x-ray generators capable of delivering large amounts of power, the limiting factor in the output of an x-ray circuit became the x-ray tube itself. The ability of the x-ray tube to achieve high x-ray outputs is limited by the heat generated at the anode. The rotating anode principle is used to produce x-ray tubes capable of withstanding the heat generated by large exposures.

The anode of a rotating anode tube consists of a large disc of tungsten, or an alloy of tungsten, which theoretically rotates at a speed of about 3600 revolutions per minute (rpm) when an exposure is being made. In practice, the anode never reaches a speed of 3600 rpm because of mechanical factors such as slipping between the rotor and bearings so, to calculate the ability of a tube to withstand high loads, a speed of 3000 rpm is usually assumed. Although the actual speed of anode rotation varies even between new tubes of identical design, it is safe to assume that anode rotation of any functioning rotating anode will never drop below 3000 rpm, and will usually be greater than 3000 rpm, if 60 cycles/sec current is used.

The tungsten disc has a beveled edge.

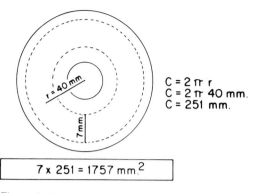

C = 2 π r
C = 2 π 40 mm.
C = 251 mm.

7 x 251 = 1757 mm.²

Figure 2–5 A rotating anode increases the total target area

The angle of the bevel may vary from 6 to 20°. The bevel is used to take advantage of the line focus principle previously described. **The purpose of the rotating anode is to spread the heat produced during an exposure over a large area of the anode.** Figure 2–5 illustrates this principle. (The dimensions are not drawn to scale.) If we assume that the filament and focusing cup of the x-ray tube produce an electron beam that covers an area of the anode 7 mm high and 2 mm wide, the area of the anode bombarded by electrons is represented by a 14-mm² rectangle. If the bevel of the target is 16.5°, the effective or apparent focal spot size in our illustration will be about 2 × 2 mm. If the anode were stationary, the entire heat load would be delivered to this one small 14-mm² area of the target. If the target is made to rotate at a speed of 3600 rpm, however, the electrons will bombard a constantly changing area of the target. The total bombarded area of tungsten is represented by a track 7 mm wide that extends around the periphery of the beveled rotating tungsten disc. The effective focal spot will, of course, appear to remain stationary. At a speed of 3600 rpm, any given area on the tungsten disc is found opposite the electron stream only once every 1/60 sec, and the remainder of the time heat generated during the exposure can be dissipated. During a 1/60-sec exposure, the

entire circumference of the tungsten disc will be exposed to the electron beam.

A comparison between the total and instantaneous target areas will illustrate the tremendous advantage offered by the rotating anode tube (Fig. 2–5). At any instant an area of 14 mm² is bombarded by the electron beam in our example. If we assume the average radius of the bombarded area of the tungsten disc to be 40 mm, which is a typical value, the circumference of the disc at a radius equal to 40 mm will be 251 mm. The total target area will then be represented by the height of the electron stream (7 mm) times the average circumference of the disc (251 mm), or a total of 1757 mm². Even though there has been an increase in the total loading area by a factor of about 125 (14 versus 1757 mm²), the apparent or effective focal spot size has remained the same.

The diameter of the tungsten disc determines the total length of the target track, and obviously affects the maximum permissible loading of the anode. Typical disc diameters will be found to vary from 75 to 100 mm (3 to 4 in.), although a tube with high capacity may have an anode 5 in. in diameter.

To make the anode rotate some mechanical problems must be overcome, because the anode is contained within the vacuum of the glass tube. The power to effect rotation is provided by a magnetic field

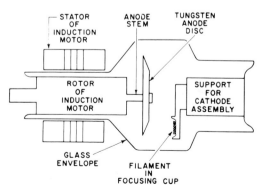

Figure 2–6 The major components of a rotating anode x-ray tube

produced by stator coils that surround the neck of the x-ray tube outside the glass envelope (Fig. 2–6). The magnetic field produced by the stator coils induces a current in the copper rotor of the induction motor, and this induced current provides the power to rotate the anode assembly. The clearance between the rotor and the glass neck of the tube is made as small as possible to ensure maximum efficiency in utilization of the magnetic force supplied by the stator core and windings. Early in the development of rotating anode x-ray tubes, the life of the tube was quite short because of the lack of durable bearings on which the anode assumbly could rotate. Because of the friction produced it was necessary to lubricate the bearings, but commonly available lubricants could not be used. Lubricants such as oil would vaporize when heated and destroy the vacuum in the tube; dry lubricants such as graphite would wear off as a powder and destroy the vacuum. This problem was solved by the use of metallic lubricants (especially silver), which are suitable for use in a high vacuum. In modern rotating anode tubes, bearing wear has become a negligible factor in overall tube life.

Heat dissipation in a rotating anode tube presents an additional problem. Heat generated in a solid tungsten disc is dissipated by radiation through the vacuum to the wall of the glass tube, and then into the surrounding oil and tube housing. Recall that heat is dissipated in a stationary anode by absorption and conductivity is provided by the massive copper anode. In the rotating anode tube, absorption of heat by the anode assembly is undesirable because heat absorbed by the bearings of the anode assembly would cause them to expand and bind. Because of this problem the stem (Fig. 2–6), which connects the tungsten target to the remainder of the anode assembly, is made of molybdenum. Molybdenum has a high melting point (2600° C) and is a poor heat conductor. Thus, the molybdenum stem provides a partial heat barrier between the tungsten disc and the bearings of the anode assembly.

The length of the molybdenum stem is another important consideration. As the length of the stem is increased, the inertia of the tungsten disc increases; this increases the load on the bearings of the anode assembly. It is desirable to keep the stem as short as possible.

Even if all the factors that affect rotation of the relatively heavy anode assembly are optimally controlled, inertia is still a problem. Because of this inertia there is a short delay between application of force to the anode assembly and the time at which the rotor reaches its full angular velocity. This period usually varies from 0.5 to 1 sec, and can be several seconds long when large (5-in.) anodes are used. A safety circuit is incorporated into the x-ray circuit that prevents an x-ray exposure from being made until the rotor has reached its full speed.

The life of a rotating anode x-ray tube is usually limited by roughening and pitting of the surface of the anode exposed to the electron beam. These physical changes are the result of thermal stress, and they act to diminish the x-ray output of the tube. The decreased output of x radiation from a rough target surface results from excessive scattering of the x rays (more radiation is directed away from the exit window of the tube) and increased absorption of x rays by the target itself. The combination of short exposure time and fast anode rotation causes very rapid heating and cooling of the surface of the anode disc. The loss of heat by radiation from the disc surface occurs before there is time for any significant amount of heat to be conducted into the main mass of the tungsten disc. Therefore, thermal expansion of the metal on the surface is much greater than expansion of metal immediately beneath the surface. This condition causes stresses to develop that distort the target surface of the anode disc. It has been found that an alloy of about **90% tungsten and 10% rhenium** (a heavy metal with good thermal capacity) produces an anode that is more resistant to surface roughening and has a higher thermal capacity than an anode of pure tungsten.

The usual speed of anode rotation using 60-cycle current varies between 3000 and 3600 rpm. If the speed of rotation is increased, the ability of the anode to withstand heat will become greater because any given area of the target is exposed to the electron beam for a shorter period of time during each revolution of the anode. By use of proper circuits, the speed of anode rotation can be increased to about 10,000 rpm. Three modifications of the tube help to overcome the problem associated with this increased velocity: the length of the anode stem is made as short as possible to decrease the inertia of the anode; the anode assembly rotates on two sets of bearings, which are placed as far apart as is possible; finally, the inertia of the anode is reduced by decreasing the weight of the anode itself. This is achieved by employing a compound anode disc in which the largest part of the disc is made of molybdenum (specific gravity 10.2), which is considerably lighter than tungsten (specific gravity 19.3). A relatively thin layer of tungsten-rhenium alloy attached to the molybdenum disc serves as the actual target for the electron beam. A high-speed anode should be used whenever large tube currents must be used, such as during serial exposures in angiography.

Grid-Controlled X-ray Tubes

Conventional x-ray tubes contain two electrodes (cathode and anode). The switches used to initiate and to stop an exposure with these tubes must be able to withstand the large changes in voltage applied between the cathode and anode. The rather involved topic dealing with the timers and switches used in the x-ray circuit will be considered in Chapter 3. A **grid-controlled x-ray tube** contains its own "switch," which allows the x-ray tube to be turned on and off rapidly, as is required with cinefluorography (see Chap. 16).

A third electrode is used in the grid-controlled tube to control the flow of electrons from the filament to the target. **The third electrode is the focusing cup that surrounds the filament.** In conventional x-ray tubes there is a focusing cup that is electrically connected to the filament. This focusing cup helps to focus the electrons on the target. Because each electron is negatively charged, the electrons repel one another as they travel to the target. As a result, the electron beam (tube current) spreads out. The focusing cup is designed to counteract the spread of the electron beam, which can be accomplished even with the cup and filament electrically connected.

In the grid-controlled tube, the focusing cup can be electrically negative relative to the filament. The voltage across the filament-grid produces an electric field along the path of the electron beam that pushes the electrons even closer together. If the voltage is made large enough, the tube current may be completely pinched off, a condition in which no electrons go from the filament to the target. The voltage applied between the focusing cup and filament may therefore act like a switch to turn the tube current on and off. Because the cup and filament are close together, the voltage necessary to cut off the tube current is not extremely large. For example, to pulse (turn the tube current on and off with the focusing cup), a 0.3-mm focal spot tube operating at 150 kVp requires about -1500 V between the filament and the cup.

Saturation Voltage

When the filament of an x-ray tube is heated, a space charge is produced, as previously discussed. When a potential difference is applied between the cathode and anode, electrons flow from the filament to the anode to produce the tube current. If the potential applied across the tube is insufficient to cause almost all electrons to be

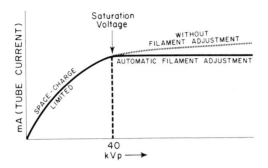

Figure 2–7   Saturation voltage

pulled away from the filament the instant they are emitted, a **residual space charge** will exist about the filament. As we described earlier in this chapter, this residual space charge acts to limit the number of electrons available, and thus it limits the current flowing in the x-ray tube. From the chart shown in Figure 2–7 it can be seen that, up to about 40 kVp, an increase in kilovoltage produces a significant increase in x-ray tube current even though filament heating remains the same. Above 40 kVp, however, further increases in kilovoltage produce very little change in tube current. In our example, 40 kVp defines the location of the saturation point of this x-ray tube. Below 40 kVp, the current flowing in the tube is limited by the space charge effect (space charge-limited). Above 40 kVp (the **saturation voltage**) the space charge effect, theoretically, has no influence on current flowing in the x-ray tube. In this region the current is determined by the number of electrons made available by the heated filament and is said to be emission-limited or temperature-limited. Reference to Figure 2–7 will show that, in actual practice, a continued increase of kilovoltage above 40 kVp will produce a slight increase in tube current because of a small residual space charge effect. In modern x-ray circuits this slight increase in milliamperes accompanying increased kilovoltage is undesirable, because, as a result, the tube current could not be precisely controlled. By the use of resistors the circuit automat-

ically compensates for this change by producing a slight decrease in filament heating as kilovoltage is increased. Note that different x-ray tubes have different saturation voltages and require different amounts of space charge compensation.

Heel Effect

The intensity of the x-ray beam that leaves the x-ray tube is not uniform throughout all portions of the beam. The intensity of the beam depends on the angle at which the x rays are emitted from the focal spot. This variation is termed the heel effect.

Figure 2–8 shows that the intensity of the beam toward the anode side of the tube is less than that which angles toward the cathode. The lessened intensity of the x-ray beam that is emitted more nearly parallel to the surface of the angled target is caused by the absorption of some of the x-ray photons by the target itself. Beam intensity, as related to the angle of emission, varies depending on the physical characteristics of individual x-ray tubes. Figure 2–8 contains average values taken from charts published in several textbooks and is used for purposes of illustration only. If, for example, a 14- × 17-in. film is oriented so that its long axis corresponds with that

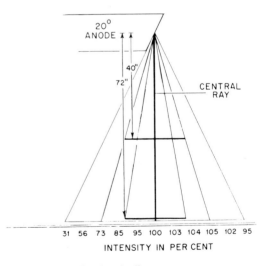

Figure 2–8   The heel effect

of the tube, the heel effect can be studied. At a 40-in. target-film distance, the anode end of the film will receive a relative exposure of 73% and the cathode end will receive a relative exposure of 105%. Thus, there is about a 30% difference in the intensity of exposure between the two ends of the film. If the target-film distance is increased to 72 in., it can be determined from the chart that the difference in exposure intensities will be considerably less, roughly 87 to 104%.

Three clinically important aspects of the heel effect are illustrated with this example. First, **the intensity of film exposure on the anode side of the x-ray tube is significantly less than that on the cathode side of the tube.** This factor can be used in obtaining balanced densities in radiographs of body parts of different thicknesses. The thicker parts should be placed toward the cathode (filament) side of the x-ray tube. This is usually illustrated by pointing out that an anteroposterior (AP) film of the thoracic spine should be made with the tube oriented so that its anode end is over the upper thoracic spine where the body is less thick; the cathode end of the tube is over the lower thoracic spine where thicker body structures will receive the increased exposure, which they require. Second, it can be seen that **the heel effect is less noticeable when larger focus-film distances are used.** Third, for equal target-film distances, the **heel effect will be less for smaller films.** This is because the intensity of the x-ray beam nearest the central ray is more uniform than that toward the periphery of the beam.

Tube Shielding and High-Voltage Cables

Although we usually think of x rays as being confined to the beam emerging from the tube they are, in fact, emitted with more or less equal intensity in every direction from the target. In addition, the x rays are scattered in all directions following collisions with various structures in and around the tube. The tube housing serves to absorb primary and secondary x rays that would otherwise produce a high intensity of radiation around the tube, resulting in needless exposure of patients and personnel and in excessive film fogging. The effectiveness of the tube housing in limiting leakage radiation must meet the specifications listed in the National Council on Radiation Protection and Measurements Report No. 49, stating that: "The leakage radiation measured at a distance of 1 meter from the source shall not exceed 100 mR (milliroentgens) in 1 hour when the tube is operated at its maximum continuous rated current for the maximum rated tube potential."

Another function of the tube housing is to provide shielding from the high voltages required to produce x rays. The high-voltage cables, which are connected to the tube through appropriate receptacles in the tube housing, contain a grounding sheath of wires to provide proper grounding of the tube to earth. To prevent short-circuiting between the grounding wires and the tube, the space between them is filled with extremly thin mineral oil. Thus, the x-ray tube is contained within the tube housing and oil, inside the housing, surrounds the tube. The housing is then carefully sealed to exclude all air, because air would expand excessively when heated and rupture the housing. This oil has good electrical insulating and thermal cooling properties. Because of its insulating properties, the use of oil allows more compact tubes and shields to be used because it permits points of high potential difference to be placed closer to each other. In addition, convection currents set up in the oil help to carry heat away from the tube. Heat from the oil is absorbed through the metal of the tube shield to be dissipated into the atmosphere.

As the oil in the tube housing is heated it will, of course, expand. A metal bellows within the tube shield allows the oil to expand without increasing pressures on the tube and shield, thus averting possible damage. In addition, the expanded bellows can be made to operate a microswitch, which will automatically prevent further exposures if maximum heating of the oil has occurred.

Tube Rating Charts

It is customary to speak of the total load that can be applied to an x-ray tube in terms of kilovoltage, milliamperes, and exposure time. The limit on the load that can be safely accepted by an x-ray tube is a function of the heat generated during the exposure. The maximum temperature to which tungsten can be safely raised is generally considered to be 3000° C. Above this level considerable vaporization of the tungsten target occurs. The rate at which heat is generated by an electric current is proportional to the product of the voltage (kV) and the current (mA). Thus, the total heat produced is a product of voltge and current and exposure time. This total energy is expressed in terms of heat units. The amount of heat produced differs according to whether the power source is single phase or three phase (see Chap. 3). By convention, the peak kilovoltage (kVp) is used in the definition of the heat unit. **The heat unit (HU) is defined as the product of current × kVp × seconds,** for single-phase power supplies. For three-phase supplies, this expression must be multiplied by a factor of approximately 1.35 to obtain the number of HU in an exposure. For example, the HU developed in an x-ray tube during an exposure of 75 kVp, 100 mA, and 2 sec for a single-phase power supply would be $75 \times 100 \times 2 = 15{,}000$ heat units.

The amount of heat that can be applied to an x-ray tube is primarily determined by three factors: the type of rectification and type of power supply (see Chap. 3); the surface area of tungsten bombarded by electrons (focal spot size); and the length of the exposure. The ability of the tube to withstand heating when used with a single-

phase generator is expressed in terms of heat units per second. When a tube is used with high-speed anode rotation and a three-phase generator, it is common to speak of its power rating, or the kilowatt (kW) rating. By convention, **the kilowatt rating of an x-ray tube is 0.001 of the kVp × mA maximum for a 0.1-sec exposure.** For example, a tube capable of withstanding an exposure of 125 kVp at 800 mA for 0.1 sec would be rated at 100 kW $\left(\dfrac{125 \times 800}{1000} = 100 \right)$. When reference is made to the kilowatt rating of an x-ray tube, it is assumed that it is the high-speed three-phase rating, unless otherwise specified. The kilowatt rating refers to the average power (in kilowatts) rather than to heat units, which depend on peak kilovoltage (thus peak power).

The basic principles controlling permissible heat loads for stationary and rotating anode tubes are the same, but it is obvious that the rating of the stationary anode tube will be much lower. Recall that the means of heat dissipation are different in stationary and rotating anode tubes. The stationary anode tube depends on the ability of a large copper anode to transfer heat. The rotating anode tube dissipates heat by radiation from the tungsten disc through the vacuum to the glass enclosure and the surrounding oil and, eventually, to the tube housing.

In considering tube rating, three characteristics are encountered: the ability of the tube to withstand a single exposure; the ability of the tube to function despite multiple rapid exposures (as in angiography); and the ability of the tube to withstand multiple exposures during several hours of heavy use.

The safe limit within which an x-ray tube can be operated for a single exposure can be easily determined by the tube rating chart supplied with all x-ray tubes. An example of such a chart is given in Figure 2–9. For example, if it is determined that

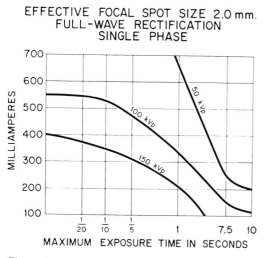

EFFECTIVE FOCAL SPOT SIZE 2.0 mm.
FULL-WAVE RECTIFICATION
SINGLE PHASE

Figure 2–9   An x-ray tube rating chart

an exposure will require 50 mAs (500 mA at 0.1 second), reference to the rating chart will show that the lines signifying 500 mA and 0.1 second cross at a point that limits maximum kilovoltage to about 100 kVp. In similar fashion, the safe loading for any combination of exposure factors can be determined from the tube rating chart. This chart is used as an example only. The manufacturer of the x-ray tube used in any diagnostic installation always supplies tube rating charts for the specific circumstances under which the tube will be used. For instance, tube rating charts for a single-phase power supply are not valid for a three-phase power supply. Tube rating charts contain information for many different kilovoltages, usually ranging from 50 kVp to the maximum operating kilovoltage of the tube in steps of 10 kVp.

Angiographic techniques requiring multiple exposures during a short period of time produce large amounts of heat. For any tube used for angiography, appropriate ratings will be made available in the form of graphs or charts. Several special considerations must be kept in mind when a tube is subjected to the stresses of rapid sequence radiography:

1. The surface of the target can be over-heated by repeating exposures before the surface heat has had time to dissipate into the body of the anode.
2. The entire anode can be overheated by repeating exposures before the heat in the anode has had time to radiate into the surrounding oil and tube housing.
3. The tube housing can be overheated by making too many exposures before the housing has had time to lose its heat to the surrounding air.
4. The total HU of a series of exposures made in rapid-sequence must not exceed the HU permissible for a single exposure of a duration equal to the total elapsed time required to complete the series of exposures.

The chart used to calculate the maximum loading of the x-ray tube for a single exposure can also be used to determine the ability of the tube to withstand multiple rapid exposures (Fig. 2–9). For example, assume exposure factors of 500 mA, 0.1 second, 100 kVp, with ten exposures to be made in 10 seconds. Incidentally, this technique would not produce good quality films, but it will provide easy figures to use for calculating this example. First, reference to the chart will show that the single exposure is within the capability of the tube. Each exposure will produce 500 × 100 × 0.1 = 5000 HU. Ten exposures will produce 50,000 HU in the 10-second interval. The maximum number of heat units the x-ray tube can accept during a 10-second period can be calculated from the chart. Actually, for an exposure time as long as 10 seconds, the number of heat units produced is relatively independent of the kilovoltage used, and the permissible loading of the tube during the 10-second period can be calculated from any convenient kilovoltage curve. On our chart, this calculation could be made using 50 kVp or 100 kVp. For example, 50 kVp applied for 10 seconds could be used with a maximum milliamperage of 200 mA, and 50 × 200

× 10 would allow 100,000 heat units input in 10 seconds. The same calculation for 100 kVp for 10 seconds at approximately 125 mA would allow 125,000 heat units input. In our example, the input of 50,000 heat units in 10 seconds is well within the capability of the tube.

Angiographic rating charts are now frequently available. Such a chart is illustrated in Table 2–1 (this is the angiographic rating chart of a Machlett Dynamax 69 tube used with three-phase rectification, high-speed anode rotation, and 1.2-mm focal spot). Notice the asterisk, which reminds you to correlate this chart with the graph for single-exposure ratings. Let us assume we wish to make 20 exposures at a rate of two exposures per second; the chart indicates we can use 8800 HU per exposure. This results in heat input of 176,000 HU in 10 seconds. Reference to the single-exposure graph for this tube (not illustrated) would show that the tube could accept a 10-second continuous exposure at 70 kVp and 250 mA, or an input of 175,000 HU (10 × 70 × 250) in 10 seconds. The single-exposure graph would also be checked to ensure that the tube could accept each individual exposure in the series. Both the angiographic rating chart and the single-exposure rating graph must be used to cnsure that planned exposure factors will not damage the tube.

The ability of an x-ray tube to withstand heat loading over a period of several hours depends on the anode heat storage characteristics. Figure 2–10 illustrates an anode capable of storing 110,000 HU. Note that anode cooling is much more rapid when the anode has accumulated large amounts of heat. This is a practical application of the physical law stating that **heat loss by radiation is proportional to the fourth power of the temperature.** The rate at which an anode heats during a period of constant exposure is important in fluoroscopy. For example, Figure 2–10 shows that a continuous heat input of 500 units per second will produce an accumulation of the maximum number of heat units in the anode in about 7 min. Therefore, if the tube is used during fluoroscopy at 100 kVp and 5 mA (100 × 5 × 1 = 500 HU/second), continuous fluoroscopy beginning with a cold tube will be limited to 7 minutes. On the other hand, if fluoroscopy is carried out at 90 kVp and 3.8 mA (about 340 HU/second), fluoroscopy can be continued indefinitely without causing excessive anode heating.

One of the most important uses of this anode heat storage chart is to determine the length of time the tube must be allowed

Table 2–1. Dynamax 69 Angiographic Rating Chart†

EXPOSURE(S) PER SEC	TOTAL NUMBER OF EXPOSURES							
	2	5	10	20	30	40	50	60
	MAXIMUM LOAD IN kVp × mA × SEC PER EXPOSURE*							
1	45,000	27,000	17,500	10,800	7,400	5,500	4,400	3,700
2	30,000	20,000	13,600	8,800	6,600	5,400	4,400	3,700
3	24,000	16,500	11,600	7,600	5,800	4,700	4,100	3,600
4	19,500	14,000	10,000	6,800	5,200	4,300	3,700	3,300
5	17,000	12,200	9,000	6,200	4,800	4,000	3,400	3,000
6	14,800	11,000	8,200	5,700	4,500	3,700	3,200	2,900
8	11,800	9,200	7,000	5,000	4,000	3,400	2,950	2,650
10	10,000	7,800	6,200	4,500	3,600	3,100	2,700	2,400
12	8,600	7,000	5,500	4,000	3,300	2,900	2,550	2,250

(Used with permission of the Machlett Laboratories, Inc., Stamford, CT 06907.)
†Effective focal spot size 1.20 mm; stator frequency 180 Hz.

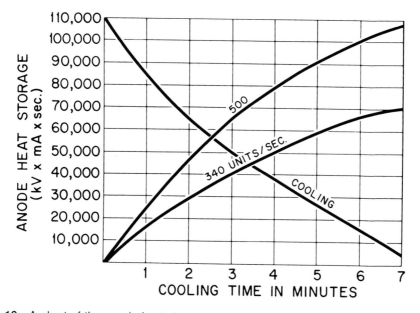

Figure 2–10 A chart of the anode heat storage capacity of an x-ray tube

to cool before additional exposures can be made. For example, assume that an angiographic procedure produces 5000 HU/exposure. If a rapid filming procedure required 20 exposures, the total anode heating would be 100,000 HU. If Figure 2–10 represented the anode heat storage chart for the tube in question, it could be determined from the chart that it would require approximately 6 minutes for the tube to cool from 100,000 to 10,000 HU. Thus, if repeat rapid filming were necessary, a delay of 6 minutes would be needed because of the limitation imposed by the ability of the anode to store heat.

Additional consideration must be given to the ability of the entire tube housing to withstand heat. The tube housing can absorb an enormous amount of heat (a figure of 1,500,000 HU is not unreasonable). Although the tube housing can absorb large amounts of heat, it also requires considerable time for cooling. Reference to some typical charts will show that it takes, in general, about 30 minutes for a tube housing to dissipate 600,000 HU. If more rapid cooling of a tube housing is required, the use of air circulators will usually double the

cooling rate. Cooling rates exceeding 96,000 heat units per minute are possible.

INTERACTION OF ELECTRON BEAM WITH X-RAY TUBE TARGET
Atomic Structure

Before attempting to describe the phenomena that occur when fast-moving electrons encounter the tungsten target in an x-ray tube, we must briefly examine the structure of an atom. In 1897, J.J. Thomson discovered a negatively charged particle much smaller than any atom, which came to be called the electron. Based on the work of Rutherford and Bohr, a simple model of an atom may be visualized as a massive positively charged nucleus surrounded by electrons in orbits of specific diameters. The solar system is organized in similar fashion.

Nucleus

The nucleus of an atom is made up of several types of elementary particles, termed **nucleons.** Of the nucleons, only **protons** and **neutrons** will be considered in this discussion, because they are the only ones of importance outside the field of nuclear physics. The proton has a positive electric charge numerically equal to the charge of the electron, while the neutron has zero electrical charge. The neutron and proton have about the same mass (1.66×10^{-24} g), which is approximately 1836 times greater than the mass of an electron. The number of protons in the nucleus is called the **atomic number** of the atom, and is given the symbol **Z.** The total number of protons and neutrons in the nucleus of an atom is called the **mass number** and is symbolized by the letter **A.** For example, stable gold (Au) has a nucleus with 79 protons (Z = 79) and 118 neutrons (A = 197). All atoms of an element have the same atomic number (Z), but an element may have several isotopes. All the isotopes of an element have the same number of protons in the nucleus; that is, they have the same atomic number but have different numbers of neutrons and therefore different atomic masses.

In summary, the nucleus of an atom contains protons and neutrons, has a positive electrical charge, and contains almost all the mass of an atom.

Electron Orbits and Energy Levels

The electrons are negative charges revolving around the nucleus. Because an atom is always electrically neutral in its normal state, it must contain an equal number of protons and electrons. The simplest way to describe an atom is to visualize a central positive nucleus with electrons in circular orbits about the nucleus. In this description, the atom resembles a tiny planetary system, with the nucleus as the sun and the electrons as the orbiting planets. Unlike the solar system, with one planet in each orbit, the atomic system allows 2 electrons in the first orbit, up to 8 in the second, up to 18 in the third, up to 32 in the fourth, and up to 50 in the fifth. The electron orbits are designated by letters: K, L, M, N, O, and so on.

The planets of the solar system are all nearly in the same plane, whereas the electrons move about the nucleus in spherical shells. An electron in the shell closest to the nucleus is in the K shell and the electron is called a K electron. L electrons are in the L shell, the second nearest shell to the nucleus. As in the planets, the diameters of the electronic shells are determined by the nuclear force on the electron, and by the angular momentum and energy of the electron. Angular momentum simply indicates that the electron is moving in a curved path. The attractive force between the positively charge nucleus and the negatively charged electron is the force that keeps the electrons in the atom. This force is called the binding force of the electron, and is inversely proportional to the square of the distance between the nucleus and electron. Therefore, a K electron has a larger binding force than an L electron. Of course, the binding force of the electron is directed toward the nucleus, and the electron would move toward the nucleus if it were not moving in a curved path. The attractive force caused by the nucleus keeps the electrons moving in a circular path. The earth has a gravitational force toward the sun, but it continues to move around the sun in a stable orbit. Similarly, electrons are in stable orbital shells.

The earth has energy that is the sum of its potential and kinetic energies. The earth's potential energy is a result of the gravitational effect of the sun; its kinetic energy is a result of its motion. By definition, kinetic energy must be positive, but potential energy can be either positive or negative. Thus, the total energy may be positive or negative. **Bound particles always have negative energy.** The earth is in a negative energy state, and electrons in an atom are also in negative energy states. To free an electron from an atom, the energy must be raised to zero or to a positive value. The energy that an electron in a shell must be given to raise the energy value to zero is called the binding energy of the electron. This is also the energy value designated for the atomic shell that houses the electron. The atomic shells are also called **energy shells.** Tungsten has a K-shell energy of 70 keV and an L-shell energy of 11 keV. Remember, these are negative energy values. To free a K electron from tungsten, the electron must be given 70 keV of energy, while only 11 KeV are required to free an L electron. The L electron has 59 keV more energy than the K electron. The binding energy of the electron shells varies from one element to another. For example, tungsten, with an atomic number of 74, has a K-shell binding energy of 70 keV, while copper, with an atomic number of 29, has a K-shell binding energy of only 9 keV.

If a small amount of energy were taken from the earth, it would move a bit closer to the sun. Atomic structural laws, however, prohibit small additions or subtractions of energy from the bound electrons. An electron cannot have any more, or less, energy than that associated with its energy shell but an electron may jump from one energy shell to another if the shell to which it jumps is not already filled. An electron can move to either a higher or lower energy shell. Electron movement to a lower energy shell, for example from an L to a K shell, results in the emission of energy. The amount of energy is equal to the difference in the binding energy between the two shells. The energy may take the form of a photon. If the quantity of energy is sufficient, the photon may be called an x ray. Electron movement to a higher energy (for example from a K to an L shell, or from the K shell to a free electron) requires the addition of energy to the electron. One source of this addition may be the absorption of an x-ray photon.

Each of the atomic energy shells, except the K shell, has subshells of slightly different energies. For example, the L shell has three subshells and an electron in the L shell may have one of three energy values. Of course, a single electron will have only one energy value, but the eight electrons needed to fill the L shell will be divided with two electrons in the lowest, three in the middle, and three in the highest subshells. In a transition from the L shell to the K shell, an electron will emit energy precisely equal to the difference in the energy of the shells. If an L electron leaves the highest subshell and goes to the K shell, it will emit some value of energy. If it leaves the middle shell and goes to the K shell, however, it will emit a slightly different value. An L electron in the lowest subshell may not go to the K shell. This is called a forbidden transition.

There are more elaborate models of atomic structure that suggest that the orbits are elliptic (so are the orbits of the solar system) or that the electron is just a standing wave about the nucleus. For diagnostic radiology the circular orbit model is sufficiently accurate.

The diameter of the nucleus of an atom is about 5×10^{-15} meters and the diameter of the entire atom is about 5×10^{-10} meters. This means that the diameter of the atom is about 100,000 times larger than the diameter of its nucleus. Most of an atom is an empty space, and this explains why a high-speed electron may go through many atoms before colliding with any of the components of an atom. It is interesting to visualize the hydrogen atom in terms of balls. Suppose the hydrogen nucleus (a proton) were a ball 3 in. in diameter. The electron (assuming the electron density to be equal to proton density) would be a ball $\frac{1}{4}$ in. in diameter. The K shell would have a diameter of 1.5 miles. A normal hydrogen atom would be visualized as a 3-in. ball with a $\frac{1}{4}$-in. ball moving on a spherical shell $\frac{3}{4}$ of a mile away. Furthermore, if all the electrons in the atoms of the world could be removed and the nuclei packed together (a condition that exists in the white dwarf stars), the diameter of the earth would be reduced to about 0.1 mile.

The production of x rays makes use of three properties of the tungsten atoms in the target of the x-ray tube: the electric field of the nucleus; the binding energy of orbital electrons; and the need of the atom to exist in its lowest energy state.

Processes of X-Ray Generation

X rays are produced by **energy conversion** when fast-moving electrons from the filament of the x-ray tube interact with the tungsten anode (target). The kinetic energy (E) of the electron in passing across a voltage (V) is increased by

$$E = eV$$

where e is the electronic charge. Because the electric charge (e) of the electron does not change (e = 1.60×10^{-19} Coulombs), it is apparent that increasing the voltage (V) across the x-ray tube will increase the kinetic energy of the electron. Voltage is expressed as the peak kilovoltage (kVp) applied across the x-ray tube (100 kVp = 100,000 peak volts). We must clearly distinguish between **kVp and keV** (kiloelectron volts). The expression 100 kVp means that the maximum voltage across the tube causing acceleration of the electrons is 100,000 volts. The expression keV denotes the energy of any individual electron in the beam (100 keV = 100,000 electron volts). When the x-ray tube is operated at 100 kVp, few electrons acquire a kinetic energy of 100 keV because the applied voltage pulsates between some lower value and the maximum value (kVp) selected. It takes the electrons something like 10^{-10} sec to go from the cathode to the anode, separated by 1 in., when the applied voltage is 100 kilovolts (kV). Each electron will acquire a kinetic energy (eV), where V is the instantaneous voltage across the tube. In a single-phase, full-wave rectified circuit, the voltage varies from 0 to the maximum (kVp) value selected, at a rate of 120 times per second. This will be discussed in more detail in Chapter 3. For the present discussion, it is adequate to state that the voltage (V) providing the potential to accelerate the electrons is pulsating, so that the energy (eV) of electrons that encounter the target (anode of the x-ray tube) covers a broad range. In other words, **the high-speed electrons striking the target do not have the same energy.**

X rays are generated by two different processes when the high-speed electrons lose energy in the target of the x-ray tube. One involves reaction of the electrons with the nucleus of the tungsten atoms, producing x rays that are termed **general radiation,** or **bremsstrahlung.** The second involves collision between the high-speed electrons and the electrons in the shell of the target tungsten atoms, producing x rays that are called **characteristic radiation.** To repeat, when high-speed electrons lose energy in the target of an x-ray tube x rays are produced by two different processes: (1) general radiation (bremsstrahlung), and (2) characteristic radiation.

General Radiation (Bremsstrahlung)

When an electron passes near the nucleus of a tungsten atom, the positive charge of the nucleus acts on the negative charge of the electron. The electron is attracted toward the nucleus and is thus deflected from its original direction. The electron may lose energy and be slowed down when its direction changes. The kinetic energy lost by the electron is emitted directly in the form of a photon of radiation. The radiation produced by this process is called

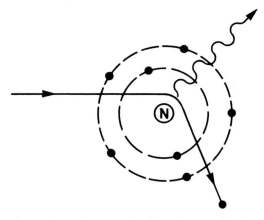

Figure 2–11 The production of general radiation (bremsstrahlung)

general radiation or bremsstrahlung (from the German for "braking radiation"). Figure 2–11 is a schematic representation of the production of bremsstrahlung.

Most electrons that strike the target give up their energy by interactions with a number of atoms. The electron gives up only part of its energy in the form of radiation each time it is "braked." Electrons penetrate through many atomic layers before giving up all their energy; therefore, not all x rays are produced on the surface of the target. Occasionally, the electron will collide head-on with a nucleus. In this type of collision all the energy of the electron appears as a single x-ray photon.

Usually an electron will undergo many reactions before coming to rest, and the energy it loses with each reaction is small. In addition, the electrons in the beam striking the target have widely different energies. These two factors cause a wide distribution in the energy of the radiation produced by this braking phenomenon. Most of the radiation will have little energy, and will appear as heat. Few x rays will appear, because over 99% of all reactions produce heat. The energy of the radiation is the amount of energy lost by the electrons. As discussed in Chapter 1, the energy of a photon of radiation is inversely related to its wavelength. The wavelength of x-ray photons produced when the electron is braked by the tungsten nuclei in the target is related to the energy (keV) of the electron. The energy of the electron is related to the potential difference (kVp) across the x-ray tube. Consider the case of a head-on collision between the electron and nucleus. All the energy of the electron is given to the resulting x-ray photon. The minimum wavelength (in Angstroms) of this x-ray photon can be calculated:

$$\lambda_{min} = \frac{12.4}{kVp}$$

For example, using 100-kVp x-ray potential, the maximum energy (eV) that an electron can acquire is 100 keV. An elec-

tron with this energy can produce an x-ray photon with a minimum wavelength of 0.124 Å:

$$\lambda_{min} = \frac{12.4}{100} = 0.124\ \text{Å}$$

Remember, 0.124 Å is the shortest wavelength (highest energy) x-ray photon that can be produced with an x-ray tube potential of 100 kVp. Another way to say this is that 100-keV electrons that strike a target can produce x-ray photons with 100 keV of energy (at most), but this is a rather rare event. Most of the x rays produced will have wavelengths longer than 0.124 Å. In fact, the wavelength of over 99% of the radiations will be so long that the radiation will produce only heat.

The energy of the emitted x-ray photon resulting from deceleration of electrons in the electric field of a nucleus depends on how close the electron passes to the nucleus, the energy of the electron, and the charge of the nucleus. Figure 2–12 is a graph of the distribution, or "continuous spectrum," of the wavelengths of x rays resulting from bombardment of the x-ray tube target by electrons. Notice that there will be a well-defined minimum wavelength (λ_{min}) of x rays produced; this λ_{min} will, of course, depend on the kVp used. The x-ray beam will also contain all wavelengths of x rays longer than the minimum wavelength. Filters (see Chap. 6) are used to remove the long wavelength low-energy x

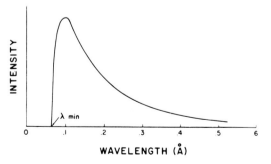

Figure 2–12 The continuous spectrum of x rays produced by bremsstrahlung

rays from the beam. Therefore, the highest energy x-ray photon leaving the x-ray tube depends on the kVp used; the lowest energy x-ray photon leaving the x-ray tube does not depend on kVp, but is determined by the filter used (or by the absorption of low-energy x rays by the glass envelope of the tube if no filter is used).

To review, **the wavelength of x rays in the continuous spectrum varies. The variation is produced by the different energies with which the electrons reach the target, and by the fact that most electrons give up their energy in stages.** The minimum wavelength x-ray photon is dictated by the x-ray tube voltage (kVp). The maximum wavelength (lowest energy) x rays escaping the tube will depend on the filtering action of the glass enclosure of the x-ray tube and on any added filtration.

Characteristic Radiation

Characteristic radiation results when the electrons bombarding the target eject electrons from the inner orbits of the target atoms. Removal of an electron from a tungsten atom causes the atom to have an excess positive charge, and the atom thus becomes a positive ion. In the process of returning to its normal state, the ionized atom of tungsten may get rid of excess energy in one of two ways. An additional electron (called an Auger electron) may be expelled by the atom and carry off the excess energy. The ejection of Auger electrons does not produce x rays, and so is not of much interest for this discussion. An alternative way to get rid of excess energy is for the atom to emit radiation that has wavelengths within the x-ray range. A tungsten atom with an inner shell vacancy is much more likely to produce an x ray than to expel an electron. X rays produced in this manner are called characteristic x rays because the wavelengths of the x rays produced are characteristic of the atom that has been ionized. For the purposes of illustration we will discuss ejection of an electron from the K shell of tungsten and then

apply the principles to electrons in other shells of the tungsten atom.

The binding energy of an electron in the K shell of tungsten is about 70 keV. Therefore, a cathode electron must have energy of more than 70 keV to eject the K shell electron from its orbit. A 60-kVp electron beam will not contain any electrons with enough energy to eject a K shell electron from tungsten. After an impinging electron uses 70 keV of its energy to eject the K shell electron, the remaining energy is shared between the initial electron and the ejected electron. Both these electrons leave the atom (Fig. 2–13). The ionized tungsten atom is unstable, and the K shell electron is rapidly replaced, usually with an electron from the L shell. The replacement electron may, however, come from other shells in the atom. The electron in the L shell has more energy than the K shell electron, as discussed earlier. In its transition from the L to the K shell, the electron must give up its excess energy. The energy lost by the L shell electron is radiated as a single x-ray photon. In tungsten, the energy of this x-ray photon is approximately 59 keV, which is the difference between the binding energy in the K shell (about 70 keV) and the L shell (about 11 keV). For tungsten, the energy of this x-ray photon will always be the same, regardless of the energy of the electron that ejected the K shell electron. Thus, the x-ray photon energy is a "characteristic" of the K shell of a tungsten atom. This process is illustrated in Figure 2–13.

When the L shell electron moves into the K shell, a vacancy is created. This vacancy may be filled from the M shell, and another x-ray photon will be produced. The energy of the L-characteristic radiation, however, will be much less than that of the K-characteristic radiation. In tungsten, L-characteristic x-ray photons have an energy of about 9 keV (L-shell binding energy is about 11 keV, and that of the M-shell about 2 keV). Characteristic radiations will also be generated from transitions involving the outer electron shells of tungsten. The en-

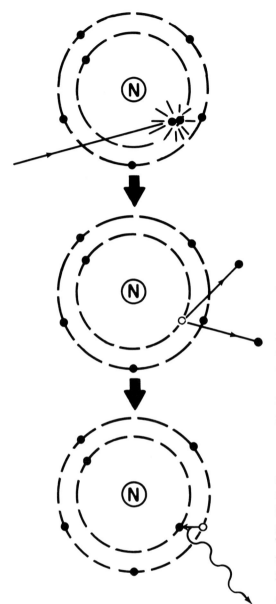

Figure 2–13 The production of characteristic radiation

than one binding energy for each inner shell in the tungsten atom except the K shell, and this causes the appearance of several different energies of characteristic radiation. In Figure 2–14 the α_1 (59.3 keV) and α_2 (57.9 keV) characteristic x rays arise from transition of L-shell electrons to the K shell. The β_1 (67.2 keV) results from an M-shell to K-shell transition, and the β_2 (69 keV) from an N-shell to K-shell transition. The dashed line in Figure 2–14 represents the low-energy x rays produced by bremsstrahlung that are removed from the x-ray beam by the glass enclosure of the x-ray tube and the added filtration.

What contribution does the characteristic radiation make to the total production of x rays by a standard x-ray tube? Below 70 kVp there is no K-shell characteristic radiation. Between 80 and 150 kVp characteristic radiation (K-shell characteristic) contributes about 10% (80 kVp) to 28% (150 kVp) of the useful x-ray beam. Above 150 kVp the contribution of characteristic radiation decreases, and it becomes negligible above 300 kVp.

Intensity of X-Ray Beams

The intensity of an x-ray beam is defined as the number of photons in the beam multiplied by the energy of each photon. The intensity is commonly measured in Roentgens per minute (R/min; see Chap. 27). The intensity of the x-ray beam varies with the kilovoltage, x-ray tube current, target material, and filtration.

Target Material

The target material used determines how much radiation (the quantity) will be produced by a given applied voltage (the next section will define the effect of this voltage on the radiation). **The higher the atomic number of the target atoms the greater will be the efficiency of the production of x rays.** For example, tungsten (Z = 74) would produce much more bremsstrahlung than tin (Z = 50) if both were used as the target of an x-ray tube

ergy of this radiation is small, and ionization in these outer shells produces mostly heat or x rays, which are absorbed by the glass walls of the x-ray tube.

Figure 2–14 diagrams the energy of the K-characteristic x rays of tungsten, superimposed on the continuous spectrum (bremsstrahlung). There is actually more

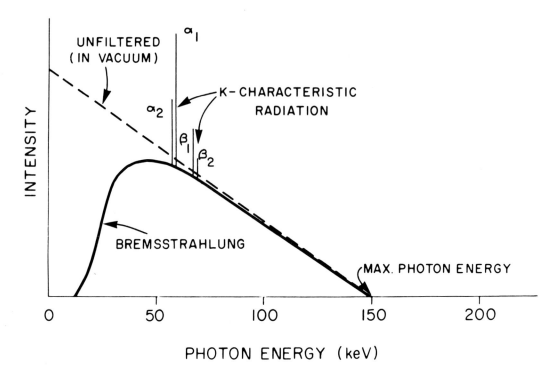

Figure 2–14 The spectrum of bremsstrahlung and K-characteristic radiation

and compared at identical tube potential (kVp) and current (mA). Earlier in this chapter we pointed out that tungsten is used as the target material because of its relatively high atomic number (74) and its high melting point (3370° C). Platinum, with a more favorable atomic number of 78, has a melting point of 1770° C, and stable gold (Z = 79) melts at 1063° C. Thus, **for the continuous spectrum, the atomic number of the target material partly determines the quantity of x rays produced.**

The relationship between atomic number and the production of characteristic radiation is quite different. **The atomic number of the target material determines the energy,** or quality, **of characteristic x rays produced.** For example, the K-shell characteristic x rays for tungsten (Z = 74) vary from 57 to 69 keV, those of tin (Z = 50) vary from 25 to 29 keV; and those of lead (Z = 82) have energies between 72 and 88 keV.

Molybdenum Target. With a high atomic number anode like tungsten, the x-ray beam consists almost entirely of bremsstrahlung radiation. The contribution from characteristic radiation varies somewhat with tube voltage, but it never makes up a large percentage of the total beam. With lower atomic number anodes, however, bremsstrahlung production is less efficient. Efficiency also diminishes as the tube voltage is decreased. The combination of a low atomic number anode and low tube voltage reduces the efficiency of bremsstrahlung production to the point at which characteristic radiation assumes a greater importance. Molybdenum anode tubes are designed to take advantage of this principle for breast radiography. Maximum tube voltages for mammography are approximately 40 kVp. At this voltage, the K-characteristic radiation of molybdenum forms an intense band between 17.9 and 19.5 keV, which is about optimum for mammography.

To summarize, the atomic number of the

target material determines the quantity (number) of bremsstrahlung produced and determines the quality (energy) of the characteristic radiation.

Voltage (kVp) Applied

We have reviewed how the energy of the photons emitted from the x-ray tube depends on the energy of the electrons in the electron stream that bombards the target of the x-ray tube. The energy of the electrons is, in turn, determined by the peak kilovoltage (kVp) used. Therefore, **the kVp determines the maximum energy** (quality) **of the x rays produced.** In addition, higher kVp techniques will also increase the quantity of x rays produced. The amount of radiation produced increases as the square of the kilovoltage:

Intensity is proportional to (kVp)²

The wavelength of the characteristic radiation produced by the target is not changed by the kVp used. Of course, the applied kilovoltage must be high enough to excite the characteristic radiation. For example, using a tungsten target, at least 70 kVp must be used to cause the K-characteristic x rays to appear.

X-Ray Tube Current

The number of x rays produced obviously depends on the number of electrons that strike the target of the x-ray tube. The number of electrons depends directly on the tube current (mA) used. The greater the mA the more electrons produced; consequently, more x rays will be produced. This principle was reviewed earlier in this chapter.

The effect of x-ray tube potential (kVp) and mA x-ray tube current on the wavelength (quality) and intensity of the x-ray beam is illustrated in Figure 2–15.

SUMMARY

X rays are produced by energy conversion when a fast-moving stream of electrons is suddenly decelerated in the target of an x-ray tube. An x-ray tube is a specially designed vacuum diode tube. The target of an x-ray tube is tungsten or an alloy of tungsten. Heat production in the x-ray

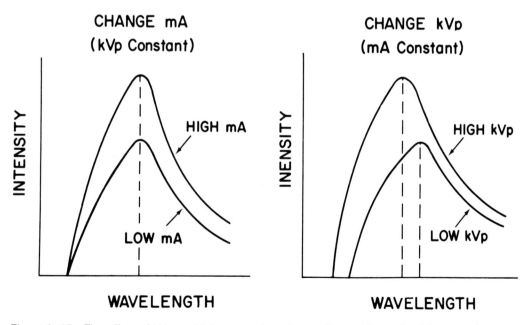

Figure 2–15 The effect of kVp and tube current on the quality and intensity of the x-ray beam

tube is minimized by using the line focus principle and a rotating anode.

X rays are generated by two different processes, resulting in (1) the production of a continuous spectrum of x rays (bremsstrahlung), and (2) characteristic x rays. The quantity (number) of the x rays generated is proportional to the atomic number of the target material (Z), the square of the kilovoltage [$(kVp)^2$], and the milliamperes of x-ray tube current (mA). The quality (energy) of the x rays generated depends almost entirely on the x-ray tube potential (kVp).

3

X-Ray Generators

An x-ray generator is the device that supplies electrical power to the x-ray tube. It is not an electrical generator in the strict sense of the word, because by definition a generator converts mechanical energy into electrical energy. An x-ray generator begins with a source of electrical energy (usually 120- or 220-volt, 60-Hertz alternating current) and then modifies this energy to meet the needs of the x-ray tube. The tube requires electrical energy for two purposes: to boil electrons from the filament; and to accelerate these electrons from the cathode to the anode. The x-ray generator has a circuit for each of these functions, and we will refer to them as the filament and high-voltage circuits. Also, the generator has a timer mechanism, a third circuit, which regulates the length of the x-ray exposure. These three circuits are all interrelated but, to simplify the discussion, we will describe them separately. We will not, however, discuss the overall design of the electric system but will leave the technical problems in the capable hands of the x-ray equipment manufacturer.

The mechanism of an x-ray generator is contained in two separate compartments: a control panel (box) and a transformer assembly. A representative control panel is shown in Figure 3–1. The panel contains a main switch to turn on the unit, three selector controls, two meters, and two exposure buttons. The controls allow the operator to select the appropriate kVp, mA, and exposure time for a particular radiographic examination. The meters measure the actual mA and kVp during the exposure. One exposure button (standby) readies the x-ray tube for exposure by heating the filament and rotating the anode, and the other button starts the exposure. The timing mechanism terminates the exposure.

The second component of the x-ray generator, the transformer assembly, is a grounded metal box filled with oil. It contains a low-voltage transformer for the filament circuit and a high-voltage transformer and a group of rectifiers for the high-voltage circuit. The potential differences in these circuits may be as high as 150,000 V, so the transformers and rectifiers are immersed in oil. The oil serves as an insulator and prevents sparking between the various components. By definition, **a transformer is a device that either increases or decreases the voltage in a cir-**

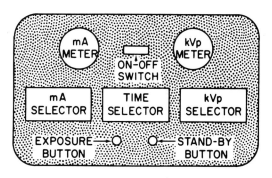
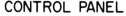
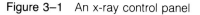

CONTROL PANEL

Figure 3–1   An x-ray control panel

33

cuit. **A rectifier changes alternating current into direct current.**

TRANSFORMERS

As mentioned earlier, the x-ray generator receives 120- or 220-volt, 60-Hertz (cycles per second) alternating current. Filament heating requires a potential difference of approximately 10 volts, while electron acceleration requires a potential difference that can be varied between 40,000 and 150,000 volts. Transformers are used to change the potential difference of the incoming electrical energy to the appropriate level.

Before we describe transformers, we must pause briefly to discuss the meaning of potential and potential difference. Potential is a relative term. For a discussion of electrical circuits, the earth (ground state) is considered to be at zero potential. A point in a circuit with an excess of electrons has a negative potential, while a point with a deficiency of electrons has a positive potential. Both potential and potential difference are measured in volts. If one point has a negative potential of 10 volts, and another point has a positive potential of 10 volts, the potential difference between them is 20 volts, and electrons will tend to flow toward the positive potential. Now suppose one point has a negative potential of 30 volts and another point a negative potential of 10 volts; the potential difference is still 20 volts. Electrons will flow toward the point with a negative potential of 10 volts. This flow of electrons represents a current, and is produced by a potential difference. A voltmeter is used to measure the potential difference between two points. The terms potential difference and voltage are synonyms, and will be used interchangeably.

A transformer consists of two wire coils wound around the opposite sides of an iron ring (Fig. 3–2A). The circuit containing the first coil is called the primary circuit, and that containing the second coil is called the secondary circuit. **When current flows**

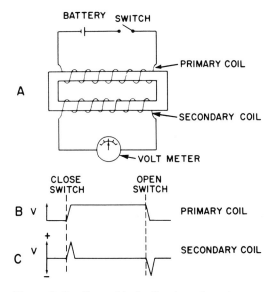

Figure 3–2 Current induction by a transformer

through the primary coil, it creates a magnetic field within the iron ring, and this magnetic field induces a current in the secondary coil. Current only flows through the secondary circuit when the magnetic field is changing (either increasing or decreasing), and no current flows while the magnetic field is in a steady state. We can demonstrate this principle with a simple experiment. In Figure 3–2A the primary circuit is connected to a battery and the secondary circuit to a voltmeter. When the switch in the primary circuit is closed, the battery drives current through the primary coil, which creates a magnetic field in the iron core. As the magnetic field increases, it induces a current through the secondary coil. Thus current builds up a potential difference between the two ends of the coil, and the voltmeter needle swings to one side. As soon as the magnetic field stabilizes, the potential across the secondary coil drops to zero and remains there until the switch in the primary coil is opened. When the switch is opened, the magnetic field decreases, and again this changing field induces a potential difference across the secondary coil. The polarity of the potential is reversed, and the voltmeter needle moves in the opposite direction. The voltage across the primary coil is shown in Figure 3–2B, and that across the secondary coil in Figure 3–2C. The important fact to remember is that a current only flows in the secondary circuit when the magnetic field is increasing or decreasing. No current flows while the magnetic field is stable. For this reason, steady direct current (like that from a battery) in the primary coil cannot be used to produce a continuous current through the secondary coil.

Alternating current is used for a transformer because it is produced by a potential difference (voltage) and changes continuously in magnitude and periodically in polarity (Fig. 3–3). Current flows in one direction while the voltage is positive and in the opposite direction while the voltage is negative. The most important characteristic of alternating current is that its voltage changes continuously, so it produces a continuously changing magnetic field. Therefore, an alternating current in the primary coil of a transformer produces an alternating current in the secondary coil.

Laws of Transformers

Two simple laws govern the behavior of a transformer.

1. **The voltage in the two circuits is proportional to the number of turns in the two coils.**

$$\frac{N_p}{N_s} = \frac{V_p}{V_s}$$

N_p = number of turns in primary coil
N_s = number of turns in secondary coil
V_p = voltage in primary circuit
V_s = voltage in secondary circuit.

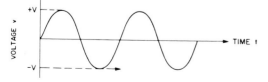

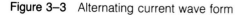

Figure 3–3 Alternating current wave form

For example, suppose the primary coil has 100 turns and the secondary coil has 30,000 turns. If the potential difference across the primary coil is 100 V, the potential difference across the secondary coil will be

$$\frac{100}{30,000} = \frac{100}{V_s}$$

and

$$V_s = 30,000 \text{ V}$$

A transformer with more turns in the secondary coil than in the primary coil increases the voltage of the secondary circuit and, appropriately, is called a step-up transformer. One with fewer turns in the secondary coil decreases the voltage and is called a step-down transformer.

2. The second law of transformers is simply a restatement of the law of the conservation of energy. A transformer cannot create energy. An increase in voltage must be accompanied by a correspondingly large decrease in current. **The product of the voltage and current in the two circuits must be equal.**

$$V_p I_p = V_s I_s$$

V_p = voltage in the primary coil
I_p = current in the primary coil
V_s = voltage in the secondary coil
I_s = current in the secondary coil.

In our previous example the voltage across the primary coil was 100 Volts and that across the secondary coil 30,000 Volts. If the current in the primary coil is 30 Amperes, then the current in the secondary coil will be

$$100 \times 30 = 30,000 \ I_s$$
$$I_s = 0.1 \text{ A (100 mA)}$$

The product of voltage and current is power. If the potential difference is in Volts and the current is in Amperes, then power will be in Watts:

$$W = V \times I$$

W = Watts
V = Volts
I = Amperes.

In the last example the power in the transformer is 3,000 Watts; it is the same on both the high-voltage (100 V × 30 A) and low-voltage (30,000 V × 0.1 A) sides of the transformer. The wire in the transformer must be large enough to carry the current without overheating. As a result, high-voltage transformers are both large and heavy, which also makes them very expensive.

In summary, a step-up transformer increases the voltage and decreases the current, while a step-down transformer decreases the voltage and increases the current. These laws assume 100% transformer efficiency, which cannot be achieved, but they are sufficiently accurate for our purposes.

Filament Circuit

The filament circuit regulates current flow through the filament of the x-ray tube. The circuit contains a variable resistor and a step-down transformer, as shown in Figure 3–4. The filament is a coiled tungsten wire. A potential difference of approximately 10 Volts produces a current of 3 to 5 Amperes through the filament. This current merely heats the filament, and does not represent the current across the x-ray tube. The potential difference of the incoming electrical supply (120 or 220 Volts) is considerably higher than the voltage required across the filament. The step-down transformer in the filament circuit has approximately ten time as many turns of wire in the primary coil as in the secondary coil, and it reduces the potential to the appropriate level of about 10 Volts.

The variable resistor in the primary circuit of the step-down transformer is the mA selector for the x-ray exposure (Fig. 3–4). It regulates the amount of current that flows through the x-ray filament. Decreasing the resistance increases the current flow and this increases the temperature of the filament. A hotter filament emits more electrons. Remember that the voltage across the x-ray tube is usually sufficient to accelerate all available electrons to the anode. Because these electrons represent the current (mA) through the tube, increasing the filament temperature actually increases the x-ray (cathode-anode) current.

High-Voltage Circuit

A simplified schematic of the high-voltage (cathode-anode) circuit is shown in Figure 3–5. The circuit has two transformers, an autotransformer and a step-up transformer. The autotransformer is actually the kVp selector and is located in the control panel. The voltage across the primary coil of the step-up transformer can be varied by changing the number of turns in the autotransformer. Only five selections are shown in Figure 3–5, but actually the kVp can be adjusted in steps from approximately 40 to 150 kVp.

The step-up transformer, which is sometimes called the high-voltage transformer, has many more turns in the secondary coil than in the primary coil, and it increases the voltage by a factor of approximately 600. The potential difference across the secondary coil may be as high as 150,000 Volts so the step-up transformer is immersed in oil in the transformer assembly for maximum insulation.

Two meters are incorporated into the high-voltage circuit, one to measure kVp and the other to measure mA. The meters themselves are located on the control panel, but their connections are in the high-voltage circuit as shown in Figure 3–5. They indicate the potential across the x-ray tube and the actual current flowing through the tube during an x-ray expo-

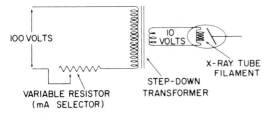

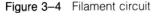

Figure 3–4 Filament circuit

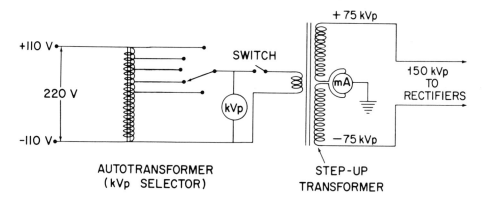

Figure 3–5 High-voltage (cathode-anode) circuit

sure. A voltmeter measures the difference in electrical potential (kVp) between two points. Electrons moving through the difference in potential constitute an electric current. In a closed circuit, the same number of electrons flows through all points. An ammeter merely counts the number of electrons flowing past a point per unit time, and it can be placed in the circuit wherever it is most convenient.

The ratio of the voltage across the primary and secondary coils in a transformer is proportional to the number of turns in the two coils. Some voltage is lost in the rectifier circuit, but with the appropriate calibrations the potential difference in the high-voltage side of the circuit (i.e., across the x-ray tube) can be measured indirectly on the low-voltage side of the transformer. Therefore, the kVp meter can be placed in the circuit between the autotransformer and step-up transformer, as shown in Figure 3–5. The voltage in this circuit is relatively small and the meter can be located on the control panel with a minimum of insulation, and without serious risk of electrical shock.

The connections for the mA meter must be in the secondary coil of the high-voltage transformer to record current flow accurately. Transformers are not 100% efficient, so the current through the primary coil is not an accurate representation of the current in the secondary coil. The mA

meter is in a circuit with a potential difference of up to 150 kVp and, to minimize the risk of an electric shock, the connections are made at the point at which the transformer is grounded, which is the center of the coil. With a voltage across the coil of 150 kVp, the potential on one side is + 75 kVp and on the other side − 75 kVp. The center of the coil is at zero potential and, if the meter is connected at this point, it may be placed on the control panel without risk of shock to the operator. Remember, even though the meter is remote from the x-ray tube, it measures the actual current flow across the tube, because the same number of electrons flows through all portions of a closed circuit.

The switch that opens and closes the high-voltage circuit is located between the autotransformer and high-voltage transformer (Fig. 3–5). This switch begins and terminates the x-ray exposure. It is operated by a timer mechanism, which we will discuss later in this chapter.

Rectification

Rectification is the process of changing alternating current into direct current, and the device that produces the change is called a rectifier. The circuits that we have described to this point are entirely capable of producing x rays. The current is still alternating, so the potential difference between the cathode and anode changes back and forth from positive to negative 60 times each second. When the cathode is negative with respect to the anode, electrons are propelled between the two, which of course produces x rays. During the next half of the electrical cycle the target of the x-ray tube is negative and the filament positive, so electrons would tend to flow away from the target. No electron cloud exists about the target, however, so no electrons are available to produce a current through the tube. By blocking current flow in the inverse half of the electrical cycle, the x-ray tube changes an alternating current into a direct current, so in effect it is a rectifier. Because only half of the electrical wave is used to produce x rays, the wave form is called **half-wave rectification.** Figure 3–6A shows the wave form of the incoming electrical supply, Figure 3–6B shows that of half-wave rectification, and Figure 3–6C shows that of full-wave rectification for comparison. Only the upper half of each electrical cycle is used to produce x rays. When the x-ray tube itself serves as a rectifier, the circuit is called self-rectified.

Self-rectification has two disadvantages. First, half of the available electrical cycle is not utilized to produce x rays, so exposure times need to be twice as long as they would if the whole cycle were utilized. Second, as repeated or prolonged exposures heat the

anode, it may become hot enough to emit electrons and to produce a current during the inverse half-cycle. The electrons in this current will bombard the filament and eventually destroy it. Therefore, to protect the x-ray tube and to improve the efficiency of x-ray production, special rectifiers are incorporated into the high-voltage circuit. Of course, the current must be rectified in the secondary circuit of the step-up transformer, because a transformer will not function with direct current in the primary circuit.

Rectifiers

A rectifier is a device that allows an electrical current to flow in one direction but does not allow current to flow in the other direction. Thus, if a voltage is applied across a rectifier with the negative potential at one end of the rectifier, the rectifier will allow current to flow, and almost no voltage is "dropped" across the rectifier, But, if the voltage is switched so that the positive potential is applied to that end of the rectifier, the rectifier blocks the flow of current and all the voltage is dropped across the rectifier.

Rectifiers are always incorporated into the x-ray circuit in series with the x-ray tube (Fig. 3–7). Exactly the same current flows through the x-ray tube and the rectifiers. When the applied voltage is as shown, the rectifiers have almost no resistance to the flow of electrons. (Electron flow

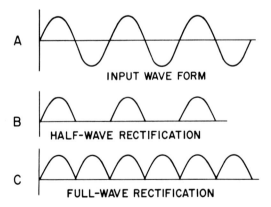

Figure 3–6 Electrical wave forms for full-wave and half-wave rectification

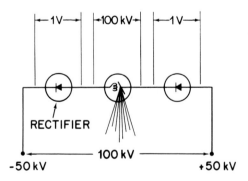

Figure 3–7 The circuit for half-wave rectification

is against the direction of the arrows in the diagram.) The x-ray tube filament produces relatively few electrons, and so the x-ray tube does impede the free flow of electrons. The result is that almost all the potential difference from the high-voltage transformer appears across the x-ray tube during the first half-cycle of the input alternating current wave form of Figure 3–6. When the voltage across the circuit is reversed (as on the other half-cycle of the input alternating current wave form), the rectifiers will block the flow of electrons through the x-ray tube.

Modern x-ray equipment uses solid-state silicon rectifiers. The advantage of these devices over earlier types of rectifiers are smaller size, lower cost, and increased life expectancy.

Half-Wave Rectification

We have already described one form of half-wave rectification, self-rectification by the x-ray tube. The same wave form is produced by two rectifiers connected in series with the x-ray tube, as shown in Figure 3–7. With the voltage shown in the illustration, electrons flow through the x-ray tube from the cathode to the anode. When the voltage reverses during the inverse half of the alternating cycle, the rectifier stops current flow. When rectifiers are used in this manner they produce half-wave rectification. The only advantage of the rectifiers is that they protect the x-ray tube from the full potential of the inverse cycle.

Full-Wave Rectification

Almost all modern x-ray generators employ full-wave rectification, which utilizes the full potential of the electrical supply. Figures 3–6C shows the wave form produced by full-wave rectification. Both halves of the alternating voltage are used to produce x rays, so the x-ray output per unit time is twice as large as it is with half-wave rectification.

Figure 3–8 is a schematic presentation of the high-voltage circuit for full-wave rec-

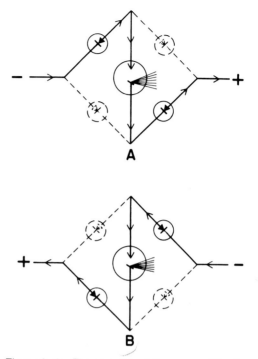

Figure 3–8   The circuit for full-wave rectification

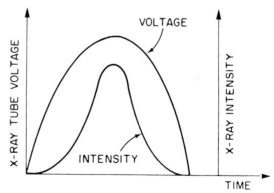

Figure 3–9   X-ray intensity superimposed on the electrical voltage

tification. The voltage across the circuit is supplied by the step-up transformer. Electrons flow along the solid lines and in the direction of the arrows. The rectifiers prevent flow along the dotted lines. The polarity is in one direction in (Fig. 3–8A) and in the opposite direction in (Fig. 3–8B). In both cases, current flows from the cathode to the anode of the x-ray tube. Thus, the current through the x-ray tube is a pulsating direct current (unidirectional), even though the input current is alternating. The voltage across the tube, however, still fluctuates from zero to its maximum level, and x rays are generated in 120 short bursts each second. Figure 3–9 shows the intensity of the x-ray beam superimposed on the electrical voltage of the x-ray tube during one half-cycle. As you can see, most of the x rays are generated during the central high-voltage portion of the cycle.

The principal disadvantage of pulsed radiation is that a considerable portion of the exposure time is lost while the voltage is in the valley between two pulses. The time spent bombarding the target with low-energy electrons does little except to produce heat in the target and to produce low energy x-rays, which are absorbed in the patient and raise patient dose. This disadvantage is not shared by three-phase generators, which we will discuss next.

TYPES OF GENERATORS

Three-Phase Generators

Three-phase generators produce an almost constant potential difference across the x-ray tube, and recently they have become more popular for both angiography and routine radiography.

Commercial electric power is usually produced and delivered by three-phase alternating current generators. It is easier to understand three-phase current if we think of each phase in terms of degrees rather than in terms of time. Figure 3–10 shows all three phases separately and superimposed on one another (*bottom*). Phase two lags 120° behind phase one, and phase three 120° behind phase two. Thus, a three-phase generator produces an almost constant voltage, because there are no deep valleys between pulses.

Three-phase generators are extremely complex, and we will not attempt to outline their circuits. Two wave forms can be produced by three-phase generators, depend-

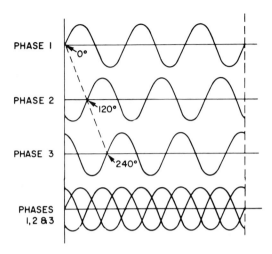

Figure 3–10   Three-phase alternating current wave forms

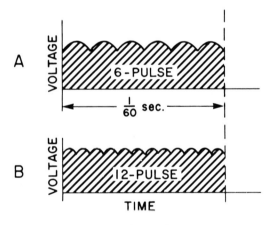

Figure 3–11   Wave forms from three-phase generators

ing on the manner in which the circuits are connected (Fig. 3–11). In Figure 3–11*A* the wave form has 6 pulses per cycle (1/60 sec), and in Figure 3–11*B* it has 12 pulses per cycle. As you can see, the voltage is more nearly constant with the 12-pulse generator.

The "ripple factor" is the variation in the voltage across the x-ray tube expressed as a percentage of the maximum value. The theoretic ripple factor for a 6-pulse generator is 13%, while for a 12-pulse generator the ripple factor is only 3%. In actual practice, the ripple is somewhat larger, but compared to the 100% ripple factor of a single-phase system, three-phase generators produce a nearly constant potential. This nearly constant potential gives three-phase generators a major advantage over single-phase generators that produce a pulsating direct current potential. Three-phase generators produce x rays efficiently throughout the exposure, and the average x-ray energy is somewhat higher because no time is spent bombarding the x-ray tube target with low-energy electrons.

A second major advantage of three-phase generators is a much higher tube rating for extremely short x-ray exposures. This is because near maximum loading is applied to the tube throughout the exposure, so the electron beam is spread across a sizable area of the rotating anode. Three-phase generators are now being built to deliver a tube current of up to 2000 mA. They make it possible to produce radiographs with extremely short exposure times and high repetition rates, so they are excellent for angiography.

Battery-Powered Generators

Some portable x-ray machines employ a series of batteries to generate the high voltage and filament currents. These units are designed to operate in areas in which the electrical supply is inadequate for conventional generators. Figure 3–12 shows a schematic outline of a battery-powered unit. Each cell in the battery pack supplies a potential difference of approximately 1.5 volts, about the same as a standard flashlight battery, so thousands of cells are required to produce the high voltages used in diagnostic radiology.

The controls on a battery generator are similar to those of a conventional generator. The kV selector in the high-voltage circuit regulates the potential difference across the x-ray tube by adding or subtracting batteries from the series. Note that the high-voltage selector is a kV, and not a kVp selector, because the batteries supply a constant potential. The filament current (milliampere selector) is adjusted by a variable resistor in the filament circuit. An ammeter (A) on the low-voltage side of the x-ray tube (near ground potential) measures the current in the circuit. A timing device simply breaks a connection (S) on the grounded side of the circuit, so no high-voltage timer is required. The batteries must be recharged periodically, but they carry enough energy to be used for numerous radiographic exposures.

Capacitor Discharge Generators

Another type of generator, a capacitor discharge unit, is now being used in clinical radiology. A capacitor is an electrical device for storing charge, or electrons. It consists of two metal plates separated by a space. The space is filled with a dielectric material but, for our purposes, we can picture the space as being filled with air. When a number of electrons is forced onto one plate of the capacitor, for instance from a storage battery, a like number is forced off the other plate. No current flows across the capacitor. In a capacitor discharge generator,

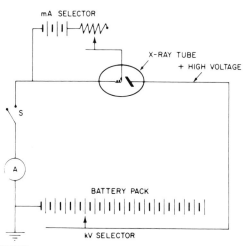

Figure 3–12 Circuit for a battery-powered generator

the capacitors are discharged through an x-ray tube.

The capacitors are charged to a high voltage by a step-up transformer-rectifier circuit such as the one shown in Figure 3–13. This circuit is exactly the same as the one shown earlier in our discussion of rectification, except that the x-ray tube has been replaced with a capacitor. The rectifiers change the alternating current from the transformer to a direct current through the capacitor limb of the circuit. A relatively small transformer-rectifier assembly can be used in the charging circuit because the charge on the capacitor builds up gradually over a period of time. In a conventional x-ray generator, the transformer and rectifiers must build up to full power (voltage times current) in a few milli-

seconds (thousandths of a second) and then maintain this power throughout the exposure. A capacitor discharge circuit may take several minutes to reach full charge, and then discharge in a relatively short time.

The voltage across the x-ray tube is maximum the instant the exposure begins. At this time the full charge of the capacitors is available, and a large current flows across the x-ray tube. As the current flows, the charge on the capacitors decreases and the voltage drops. Both capacitor discharge and single-phase generators produce a pulsed voltage, and consequently more relatively low-energy radiation than either battery-powered or three-phase generators, both of which produce a constant, or nearly constant, voltage.

TIMING X-RAY EXPOSURES

The length of an x-ray exposure is regulated by an exposure timer. The timer controls are located in the x-ray control panel, but the timer itself may be located in either the control panel or in the transformer assembly, depending on the design of the generator. The timer controls include a timer selector and two exposure buttons. Pushing the first button causes the filament to heat and the anode to rotate in preparation for an exposure. Pushing the second button activates the timer and closes a switch in the high-voltage circuit to begin the exposure. The timer automatically opens the switch and terminates the exposure at the preselected time. Timer switches are always located in the high-voltage circuit—that is, in the circuit supplying current between the cathode and anode of the x-ray tube. The filament circuit cannot be used to regulate exposure times. The filament heats and cools gradually, so its response time is relatively long. The high-voltage circuit has an almost instantaneous response time, so it is more practical to regulate the length of the exposure in the high-voltage circuit.

X-ray exposure timers and switches have

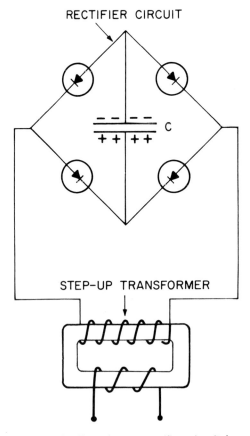

Figure 3–13 Transformer-rectifier circuit for a capacitor discharge generator

separate but interdependent functions. Timers are thinkers, and switches are workers. A timer tells a switch to close or open a circuit, and the switch responds to the best of its ability. A switch is not always capable of following the timer's instructions, however, and the actual exposure time may be considerably different than the anticipated time. For optimal results at the lowest possible cost, both the timer and switches should be designed for the same level of performance. Three factors must be considered in the design of a timer mechanism: (1) the minimum exposure time; (2) the current load of the circuit; and (3) the recycle time (the amount of time between exposures).

Early x-ray tubes had a low heat storage capacity, so they had to be operated with small tube currents (low mA). Exposure times were long, and a relatively simple timing mechanism was entirely adequate. With larger tubes came a need for faster, more accurate timers and switches. When series filming and cinefluorography were developed, use of the timer was confronted with a new problem, that of recycling to make ready for the next exposure. Each stage in the development of x-ray tubes and generators has demanded a more sophisticated timing system, and the circuitry of the newer timers is extremely complex.

Switches

An x-ray switch functions like the switch on a reading lamp; it turns the current in the x-ray tube on or off. When an electric current is started or stopped abruptly in an inductive (transformer) circuit, a sudden surge of current results. These abnormally high currents may damage the electrical components in the circuit. They also produce an unpredictably large x-ray output, which results in radiographs that are not uniform from one exposure to the next. This problem is not difficult to solve with a single-phase generator. The circuit can be opened and closed when the alternating current is at zero voltage. At this time there is no potential difference, and no current, so of course there is no inductive surge.

The problem of inductance is much more difficult to solve in a three-phase system. When one phase is at zero, the other two phases are at 87% of their maximum level. One approach to the problem is to "sequence switch," to switch each of the three phases individually as their voltages pass through zero. This does not work well with shorter exposure times, and usually three-phase generators are used to produce short exposures. Manufacturers have overcome the problem of inductive surges in three-phase circuits by a variety of complex means, mostly employing capacitors to store the surge. With newer timers and switches, it is possible to obtain exposure times as short as 0.001 second (1 millisecond).

Mechanical Switches

The simplest x-ray switches are mechanical contactors. They are usually opened and closed by solenoids (electromagnets) that are activated by the exposure timer. They are always connected into the low-voltage (primary) side of the high-voltage circuit, and perform satisfactorily with small currents and relatively long exposure times. The size of the contactor must be proportional to the amount of current it will carry. Large contactors have considerable inertia and require powerful electromagnets. They are noisy and tend to arc with large voltages. The maximum accuracy of mechanical contactors is one half-cycle of a full-wave rectified circuit (1/120 sec). They have a relatively slow recycle time, which limits them to two or three exposures per second.

Mechanical contactors may be used singly or in pairs. When they are used in pairs, one contactor closes the x-ray circuit and starts the exposure, and the second contactor opens the circuit and terminates the exposure.

Electronic Switches (Thyratrons)

The most important advance in the evolution of x-ray switches was the development of the thyratron tube. **A thyratron is a gas-filled triode that functions as an electronic switch.** The tube is filled with a small amount of inert gas (argon, neon, or mercury vapor). Thyratrons have three electrodes: an anode, a cathode, and a grid (Fig. 3–14). A heating element boils electrons from the cathode (thermionic emissions), and these electrons eventually form the current through the tube. Electron emission is similar to that of an x-ray tube, except that the cathode is heated indirectly. The electron cloud around the cathode is repelled by the third electrode, a grid, with a small negtive potential (− 3 volts) relative to the cathode. The grid behaves like a fine wire screen. Its negative potential creates an electrostatic field that blocks the flow of electrons, but it does not physically impede their flow. Even though the grid has a relatively small negative potential, it is able to hold back the electron stream because of its close proximity to the cathode. While the grid is sufficiently negative no current flows through the tube.

To start a current flowing through a thyratron tube, the grid voltage must be reduced (made less negative) below a critical level. This permits a few electrons to escape the grid's electrostatic field. These electrons are accelerated toward the anode and, as they move through the tube, they ionize gas molecules to form ion pairs, electrons (negative ions) and atoms with an electron deficiency (positive ions). These ions in turn ionize other atoms and create an avalanche effect. The positive ions migrate back to the grid and further diminish its negative potential. The grid loses control of the electron cloud as soon as ionization begins. If an outside force increases the grid's negative potential, it merely attracts more positive ions, which increases the efficiency and current flow through the tube. The only way that the current can be stopped is by removing the potential difference between the anode and cathode. Thus, a thyratron is like a trigger that can start, but cannot stop, a current flow.

Thyratrons are controlled by electronic timers. Because they are strictly one-way switches, they are always used in combination with either another thyratron or a mechanical switch. Frequently, the current from a thyratron is used to operate an electromagnet, in which case the current from an electronic switch (thyratron) operates a mechanical switch. Thyratrons are capable of conducting a large current with only a negligible drop in voltage. They have two obvious advantages over mechanical timers: (1) an almost instantaneous response time, because they have no inertia; and (2) an almost instantaneous recycling time. For this reason, they are capable of utilizing only a portion of an x-ray pulse, the intense central portion, so they can produce a nearly square wave form and exposure times as short as 1 millisecond.

In recent years, solid-state thyratrons have almost completely replaced gas-filled tubes. They are called either silicon-controlled switches or silicon-controlled rectifiers. Their characteristics are identical to those of gas-filled thyratrons, but they are smaller and do not require a heater. Even more recently high-voltage thyratrons have

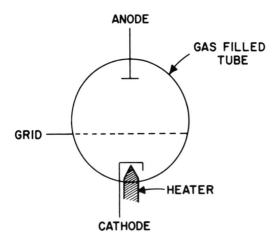

Figure 3–14   Thyratron tube

been developed, and they are occasionally incorporated into the secondary circuit of the high-voltage transformer with good results.

Grid-Controlled X-Ray Tubes

A grid-controlled x-ray tube is a triode tube (see Chap. 2). The focusing cup functions as the grid, and behaves like a switch much like the grid in the thyratron tube just discussed. The grid has a relatively small negative potential but it is close to the cathode, so it exerts a strong influence on the electron cloud. Grid-controlled tubes have the same advantages as thyratron switches but, in general, they cannot control as large a current flow. For this reason they are seldom used for routine radiography but they are used for cineradiography.

Exposure Timers

X-ray exposure timers have developed through several stages, beginning with simple mechanical timers and ending with highly sophisticated automatic electronic timers. All of the various stages are still in use, and we will discuss them in the order of their appearance.

Mechanical Timers

The simplest exposure timer is a mechanical device that functions much like a spring-driven clock. The timer is set by turning a dial to the appropriate time. Turning the dial winds a spring and opens a mechanical contactor to prepare for the exposure. When the timer button is pushed, the exposure begins and the spring drives the dial back to its starting position terminating the exposure. A mechanical timer activates a solenoid (electromagnet) in the x-ray circuit, and the solenoid opens and closes a single mechanical switch.

Mechanical timers are usually used in low-power dental and portable radiographic units. They are only accurate to approximately 0.25 seconds, so they cannot

be used to regulate the short exposures of high-power equipment.

Synchronous Timers

A synchronous timer is driven by a small synchronous motor. The speed of the motor is controlled by the frequency of the alternating current supplied by the electric power company, so it is fairly accurate. The motor drives a cam that activates an electromagnet to open and close a single contactor switch. Synchronous timers are accurate to 0.1 sec. They have a fairly long recycling time and cannot be used for rapid serial exposures.

Electronic Timers

As the power of x-ray generators increased, exposure times became too short to control with synchronous timers. Something better was needed, and the electronic timer was developed to meet this need. Electronic timers are far superior to any other timer, and they are incorporated into almost all modern x-ray generators.

All electronic timers operate on the same general principle. **The length of the x-ray exposure is determined by the time required to charge a capacitor** to a predetermined level. Electronic timers have two essential components, a variable resistor and a capacitor. The capacitor is always connected to the grid of a thyratron-type switch. Because all electron timers have a resistor and a capacitor, they are frequently called **resistance-capacitor (RC) circuits.** Figure 3–15 shows the basic RC circuit. The switch (S) is closed between exposures. This short-circuits the capacitor so that it does not accumulate a charge. At the beginning of an exposure, the switch is opened. At the same time that the timer

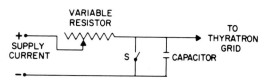

Figure 3–15 Electronic timer circuit

switch is opened, another switch closes the main x-ray circuit and begins the exposure. In the RC circuit, electrons migrate toward the lower plate and away from the upper plate of the capacitor. Electrons flowing away from the upper plate are impeded by the resistor and, the greater the resistance, the slower their flow. The upper plate is connected to the grid (third electrode) of a thyratron. While the thyratron grid remains negative it can contain the electron cloud about the cathode, and no current flows through the thyratron tube. As a positive charge accumulates on the upper plate of the capacitor, it lowers the negative potential of the thyratron grid. Eventually the grid reaches its critical level and, suddenly, a current flows through the thyratron. This current opens a switch in the x-ray circuit and terminates the exposure.

The amount of time required to reach the critical voltage of the thyratron depends on the resistance in the capacitor circuit. When we select an x-ray exposure time, we change the resistance in the capacitor circuit. Increasing the resistance increases the exposure time, and decreasing the resistance shortens the exposure time.

The basic resistor-capacitor circuit and thyratron tube produce an accurately timed electric current. This current can be used in various ways. It may be used to activate an electromagnet and thus open a mechanical contactor to terminate the x-ray exposure (impulse timer). When used in this manner, a second mechanical switch is employed to close the circuit at the beginning of the x-ray exposure.

Electronic timers may also be used entirely with electronic (usually silicon-controlled) switches, in which case they have a shorter activation time and an almost instantaneous recycling time. They are capable of delivering an x-ray pulse as short as 1 millisecond with an activation time (the time delay between the command to make an exposure and the beginning of execution) of 1 millisecond. They can control more than 60 exposures per second. Elec-tronic timers can be incorporated into either the primary or secondary circuit of the high-voltage transformer.

Phototimers

All the exposure timers that we have discussed to this point are subject to human error. The operator selects the exposure time that he believes will produce a film of the desired density. He can measure the patient's thickness, but he must estimate the density of the tissues that will be included in the radiographic field. If his estimate is incorrect, the resultant radiograph will be improperly exposed. Phototimers have been developed to eliminate human error. They measure the amount of radiation transmitted through the patient and terminate the exposure when the transmitted radiation reaches a predetermined level. Several types of radiation detectors could be used in phototimers, but only two are in common usage—photomultiplier tubes and ionization chambers. We will describe them separately.

Photomultiplier Tubes. Figure 3–16 shows the essential components of a photomultiplier tube-timer circuit. The tube is radiopaque, so it must be positioned beneath the film to prevent its image from appearing on the radiograph. The timing circuit consists of a photomultiplier tube,

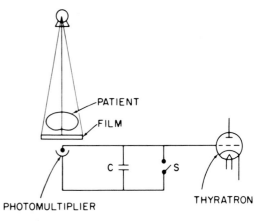

Figure 3–16 Photomultiplier timing circuit

capacitor (C), switch (S), and thyratron. After x rays pass through both the patient and film they strike the photomultiplier tube, which produces a small electric current. This current is used to charge the capacitor in the phototimer in a manner similar to that decribed for electronic timers. In fact, the only difference between a phototimer and an electronic timer is in the resistor. A phototimer does not require a resistor. The patient serves this function. In an electronic timer, the amount of resistance determines the time required to charge the capacitor. In a phototimer, the density of the patient determines the capacitor charge time. With a thick anatomic part, only a small amount of radiation is transmitted through the patient. a comparably small amount of current flows from the photomultiplier tube, the capacitor charges slowly, and the radiographic exposure is prolonged. The anode of the photomultiplier tube is connected to the grid of a thyratron tube, which serves as the switch for a phototimer.

Figure 3–17 is a schematic diagram of a photomultiplier tube. It consists of a small fluorescent screen, a photocathode, several intermediate electrodes (called dynodes) and an anode. The photocathode is coated with a photoemissive surface. When it is struck by light, it emits electrons in numbers proportional to the intensity of the light. The intermediate electrodes are coated with a material that emits secondary electrons when struck by another electron. The photocathode is at a more negative potential than any of the dynodes, and the potential difference between the electrodes diminishes in steps down to the anode.

Only three dynodes are shown in Figure 3–17, but there may be as many as ten. When x rays strike the fluoroscopic screen, the screen emits light. The light strikes the photocathode, and it in turn emits electrons. These electrons are accelerated toward the next electrode, and they acquire additional energy along the way. When they strike the electrode they emit a specific number of secondary electrons, and the process is repeated over and over down to the anode. At each step the number of electrons increases by a specific amount. It is important to realize that this is not an avalanche effect. **The output current is proportional to the amount of radiation striking the fluorescent screen.** The electrical signal is amplified as it passes through the photomultiplier tube, and this signal supplies the current to charge the capacitor.

Ionization Chambers. The ionization chambers for phototimers are designed to be as radiolucent as possible so that they can be positioned in front of the x-ray film (Fig. 3–18). The chamber casts its image on a film, but the image is so faint that it is lost in the stronger superimposed images of anatomic parts. This radiolucency gives ionization chambers a definite advantage

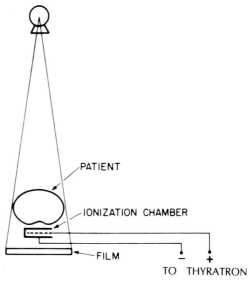

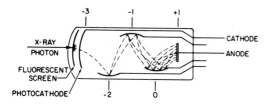

Figure 3–17 Photomultiplier tube

Figure 3–18 Ionization chamber timing circuit

over photomultiplier tubes, which must be placed behind the film because of their radiopacity. For example, an ionization chamber can be permanently mounted in the center of a fluoroscopic screen. In this position it is ideally positioned for spot film radiography (see Chap. 14), and yet does not interfere with routine fluoroscopy. A photomultiplier tube must be moved out of the radiographic field for fluoroscopy, and brought back for spot films. Even then its image obstructs the fluoroscopist's view of the spot film image. With the phototimer between the patient and the film, any type of cassette, regardless of the nature of its back, can be used to hold the film. Special cassettes with translucent backs must be used with photomultiplier tubes, because the detector measures the transmitted radiation. If a lead-back cassette is inadvertently used with a photomultiplier tube, the film will be overexposed.

Ionization chambers are filled with air, so they do not have to be enclosed in a glass envelope. The glass envelope around photomultiplier tubes is required to maintain a vacuum.

An ionization chamber consists of two electrodes, one a thin sheet of metal folded on itself to form two parallel plates, and the other a fine wire grid positioned equidistant between the plates (Fig. 3–18). Before the x-ray exposure the chamber is charged by applying a direct current voltage across the electrodes. As radiation passes through the chamber, air molecules are ionized. Each molecule produces an ion pair. The negative ions (electrons) move to the grid, which is the positive electrode, while the positive ions migrate to the negative plates. These moving electrons form an electric current. The current decreases the negative voltage on the grid of a thyratron tube; that is, it makes it more positive, and thus terminates the x-ray exposure.

Phototimer detectors (photomultiplier tubes and ionization chambers) are frequently used in pairs or triplets to sample several areas of the radiographic field. For example, paired detectors are used for PA chest films. The detectors are positioned on either side of the midline, hopefully in the upper lung fields. If the patient has a left upper lobe pneumonia, the detectors will average the readings from the two sides and expose the film accordingly. In this case the right lung will be a little overexposed, but not as much as it would have been with only a single detector positioned on the left side. For the lateral chest film the paired detectors are turned off and the exposure is regulated with a third detector placed near the center of the film.

The sensitivity of phototimers is adjusted empirically. Multiple radiographs are made on a test phantom until the desired density is achieved. The sensitivity of the phototimer is changed with a small variable resistor. Once adjusted, it should produce radiographs of uniform average density, regardless of the thickness of the patient. Phototimers usually have an automatic safety timer that controls the maximum exposure time. Safety timers are incorporated into the circuit to protect the x-ray tube, and they will terminate an exposure prematurely to prevent the anode from being overheated.

Testing X-Ray Timer Accuracy

With a pulsating x-ray beam, the accuracy of an x-ray exposure timer can be measured with the aid of a **spinning top** (Fig. 3–19A). It consists of a 3- to 4-in. metal disc attached to a stem and mounted on a base plate for support. The disc has a narrow slit (or hole) near its edge, and it must be free to rotate either on the stem or on the base plate. The disc may be made of lead, steel, brass, or any other rigid radiopaque material.

Spinning tops function best with pulsating radiation—that is, circuits with either half-wave or full-wave rectification. To test a timer, the spinning top is placed on an x-ray film (usually enclosed in a cassette). The top is manually rotated, and the film

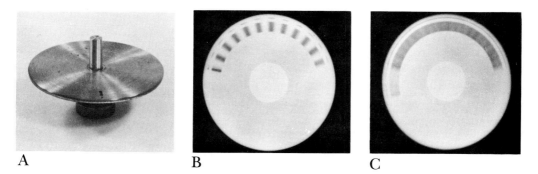

A   B   C

Figure 3–19   Spinning top (A); radiographs from a single-phase (B) and a three-phase (C) generator

is exposed by radiation that passes through the narrow slit. As the disc rotates, the x-ray pulses are recorded as a series of broad dashes (or dots). Each dash represents an exposure time of 1/120 sec with full-wave and 1/60 sec with half-wave rectification, so the number of dashes measures the length of the exposure. The speed of disc rotation is not important provided it is fast enough to separate the individual pulses on the radiograph, and not so fast that the disc makes a complete revolution during the exposure.

Figure 3–19B shows a test film made with the exposure timer set for 0.1 sec in a circuit with full-wave rectification. The 12 broad dashes on the film represent an exposure time of 12 × 1/120 sec, or 0.1 sec. Because both the anticipated and measured exposure times are the same, the timer is functioning properly.

Figure 3–19C shows a radiograph of a spinning top taken with a 12-pulse three-phase generator. The exposure is recorded as a broad continuous arc consisting of bands of varying density. These density variations represent ripple pulsations. The exposure timer was set for 1/30 sec, which is two cycles of alternating current. Because there are 12 pulses per cycle, 24 pulsations should be visible on the radiograph. The generator was not operating at full potential during the first portion of the exposure, however, so it is difficult to count the ripples. This points out another use for the

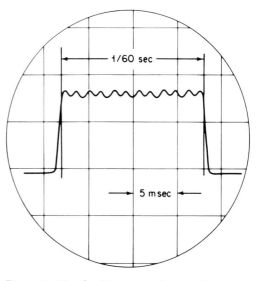

Figure 3–20   Oscilloscopic display of an x-ray exposure (12-pulse, three-phase generator)

spinning top: it provides a method of recording the intensity of an x-ray exposure at various instances in time.

A timer can also be evaluated with a photoconductor coupled to an oscilloscope. A photoconductor is a material that conducts a current when exposed to either light or to x rays. This current can be displayed on an oscilloscope in exactly the same way that electricity from the heart is displayed for an electrocardiogram. Figure 3–20 shows the x-ray output of a three-phase 12-pulse generator for an exposure set at 1/60 second. The exposure time can be calculated either by counting the pulses or by measuring the distances between the ascending and descending limbs of the exposure. Twelve pulses are shown on the oscilloscope, which is the correct number for a 1/60-sec exposure. The vertical lines on the oscilloscope are 5 milliseconds (msec) apart. A 1/60-sec exposure lasts 16.7 msec (1000 ÷ 60), so the ascending and descending limbs of the exposure should be 16.7 msec apart. The limbs are not perfectly vertical, so an exact measurement is impossible, but the timer is certainly functioning at an acceptable level of accuracy.

The height of the exposure on the oscilloscope is a measure of relative x-ray intensity. With careful calibration this height can be used as an exact measure of the x-ray exposure in Roentgens, but it is much easier to measure x-ray output with an ionization chamber or some similar device designed specifically for this purpose. In general, the height of the exposure on the oscilloscope is used only to compare the various parts of the exposure, which in this case is almost perfectly uniform except for ripple pulsations.

SUMMARY

An x-ray generator supplies electrical energy to the x-ray tube and regulates the length of the radiographic exposure. The x-ray tube requires two sources of energy, one to heat the filament and the other to accelerate electrons between the cathode and anode. The filament circuit contains a variable resistor, which is the current selector, and a step-down transformer. The cathode-anode circuit, called the high-voltage circuit, contains an autotransformer and a step-up transformer. The autotransformer is the kVp selector.

The incoming electrical supply to the x-ray generator has an alternating potential, which tends to move current from the anode to the cathode during half of each electric cycle. Rectifiers are electronic valves that transmit a current in only one direction. They are incorporated into the high-voltage circuit between the step-up transformer and the x-ray tube to prevent a reverse current. Half-wave rectification produces 60 x-ray pulses per second, while full-wave rectification produces 120 pulses.

Radiographic exposure timers open and close switches in the high-voltage circuit. These switches may be either mechanical (usually operated by an electromagnet) or electronic. Electronic switches, called thyratrons, have an almost instantaneous response and recycling time. Most modern x-ray generators have electronic timers. An electronic timer contains a variable resistor and a capacitor. The exposure time is determined by the amount of time required to charge the capacitor to a predetermined level. The variable resistor is the time selector. Phototimers are a special type of electronic timer in which the patient replaces the electrical resistor. The capacitor is charged by a current from a photomultiplier tube that measures the radiation transmitted through the patient. Another type of detector, an ionization chamber, can be used in place of the photomultiplier tube. Ionization chambers are radiolucent, so they can be permanently mounted in front of the x-ray film. Because of their radiolucency, they have replaced photomultiplier tubes in most installations.

4

Basic Interactions between X Rays and Matter

Atoms are bonded into molecules by electrons in the outermost shell. X-ray photons may interact either with orbital electrons or with the nucleus of atoms. In the diagnostic energy range, the interactions are always with orbital electrons. If these electrons happen to be the ones bonding atoms into molecules, the bonds may be disrupted and the molecular structure altered. The molecular bonding energies, however, are too small to influence the type and number of interactions. A group of oxygen atoms will stop the same number of x-ray photons, regardless of their physical state. It does not matter if the oxygen is free as a gas or is bound to hydrogen as water. The important factor is the atomic makeup of a tissue and not its molecular structure.

There are five basic ways that an x-ray photon can interact with matter. These are:

1. Coherent scattering
2. Photoelectric effect
3. Compton scattering
4. Pair production
5. Photodisintegration

As we discuss each of these interactions, you will see that at times x-ray photons are **absorbed,** while at other times they are merely **scattered.** When photons are absorbed, they are completely removed from the x-ray beam and cease to exist. When photons are scattered they are deflected into a random course, and no longer carry useful information. Because their direction is random, they cannot portray an image, and the only thing they produce on a film is blackness. In the language of the information transfer theorist, scatter radiation adds **noise** to the system. You can gain some insight into the effect of noise with a simple analogy. Imagine yourself listening to music on your car radio as you drive past an airport. As a plane approaches the music becomes more difficult to hear until finally, when the plane is directly overhead, it becomes completely inaudible. Even though the music is still there, you cannot hear it. Radiation noise does exactly the same sort of thing. It destroys image quality. We refer to the noise created by scatter radiation as film fog. When an x-ray film is badly fogged, the image may be completely obscured. It is still there, but we cannot see it. An understanding of the production of scatter radiation is of vital importance, so pay particular attention to it as we discuss the basic interactions between x rays and matter.

COHERENT SCATTERING

The name coherent scattering is given to those interactions in which radiation undergoes a change in direction without a change in wavelength. For this reason, the term "unmodified scattering" is sometimes used. There are two types of coherent scattering, Thomson scattering and Rayleigh scattering. In Thomson scattering a single electron is involved in the interaction. Rayleigh scattering results from a cooperative interaction with all the electrons of an atom. Both types of coherent scattering may be described in terms of a wave-particle interaction, and are therefore sometimes called classical scattering. Rayleigh scattering is shown in Figure 4–1. Low-energy radiation encounters the electrons of an atom and sets them into vibration at the frequency of the radiation. A vibrating electron, because it is a charged particle, emits radiation. The process may be envisioned as the absorption of radiation, vibration of the atom, and emission of radiation as the atom returns to its undisturbed state. This is the only type of interaction between x rays and matter that does not cause ionization. To produce an ion pair, a photon must transfer energy to the atom. No energy is transferred, and no ionization occurs with coherent scattering. Its only effect is to change the direction of the incident radiation. The percentage of radiation that undergoes coherent scattering is small compared to that of the other basic interactions; in general, it is less than 5%. Some coherent scattering occurs

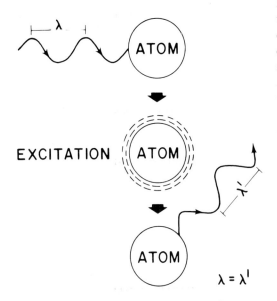

Figure 4–1   Coherent Rayleigh scattering

throughout the diagnostic energy range, but it never plays a major role. Even though it produces scattered radiation, which contributes to film fog, the total quantity is too small to be important in diagnostic radiology.

PHOTOELECTRIC EFFECT

Before beginning a discussion of the photoelectric effect, we are going to digress a moment to review a few points about atomic physics. Atomic structure is extremely complex, but we can greatly simplify it and still have a fairly good idea of how these interactions occur. The atom consists of a central nucleus and orbital electrons. The nucleus is important in our present discussion only as a means of keeping the electrons in the atom. The positively charged nucleus holds the negatively charged electrons in specific orbits, or shells. The innermost shell is called the K shell, and the more peripheral shells are named consecutively L, M, N, and so forth. These shells have a limited electron capacity. The K-shell can hold only two electrons. If more electrons are present in the atom they must move out to the L shell, which has a capacity of eight electrons. Each shell has a specific binding energy. The closer the shell is to the nucleus, the tighter the electrons in that shell are bound to the nucleus. The electrons in the outermost shell are loosely bound. They are essentially free and, appropriately, are called free electrons. The energy value of electronic shells is also determined by the atomic number of the atom. K-shell electrons are more tightly bound in elements with high atomic numbers than they are in elements with low atomic numbers. In fact, the differences are sizable. For example, the K-shell binding energy for lead is 88 keV, while the K-shell binding energy for calcium is only 4 keV. Electrons in the K shell are at a lower energy level than electrons in the L shell. If we consider the outermost electrons as free, than inner shell electrons are all in energy debt. Their energy debt is greatest when they are close to the nucleus in an element with a high atomic number.

The photoelectric effect is shown in Figure 4–2. We will quickly run through the whole interaction and then fill in some details later. An incident photon, with a little more energy than the binding energy of a K-shell electron, encounters one of these electrons and ejects it from its orbit. The photon disappears, giving up all its energy to the electron. Most of the photon's energy is needed to overcome the binding energy of the electron, and the excess gives the electron kinetic energy. The electron, which is now free of its energy debt, flies off into space as a photoelectron. It becomes a negative ion and is absorbed almost immediately, because charged particles have little penetrating power. The atom is left with an electron void on the K shell but only for an instant, because an electron immediately drops into the void

to fill the K shell. This electron usually comes from the adjacent L shell, occasionally from the M shell and, on rare occasions, from free electrons from the same, or another, atom. As an electron drops into the K shell it gives up energy in the form of an x-ray photon. The amount of energy is characteristic of each element, and the radiation produced by the movement of electrons within an atom is called characteristic radiation. When the K-shell void is filled by an outer shell electron from the same atom, the atom is left with a deficiency of one electron, and it remains a positive ion. If a free electron from another atom fills the void then the other atom becomes a positive ion, and the result is the same. The photoelectric effect always yields three end products: (1) characteristic radiation; (2) a negative ion (the photoelectron); and (3) a positive ion (an atom deficient one electron).

Probability of Occurrence

Three simple rules govern the probability of a photoelectric reaction.

1. The incident photon must have sufficient energy to overcome the binding energy of the electron. For example, the K-shell electrons of iodine have a binding energy of 33.2 keV. An x-ray photon with an energy of 33.0 keV absolutely cannot eject them from their shell. The photon may interact at the L or M shells but not at the K shell.

2. A photoelectric reaction is most likely to occur when the photon energy and electron binding energy are nearly the same, provided of course that the photon's energy is greater. A 34-keV photon is much more likely to react with a K-shell electron of iodine than a 100-keV photon. In fact, the probability of a photoelectric reaction drops precipitously as photon energy increases. It is inversely proportional to approximately the third power of energy, or, expressed in mathematical form:

$$\text{Photoelectric effect} \sim \frac{1}{(\text{energy})^3}$$

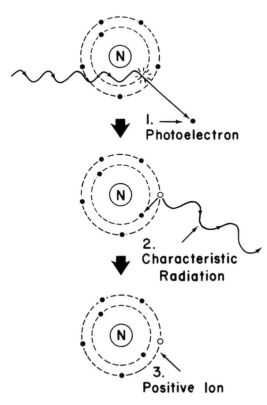

1. → Photoelectron

2. Characteristic Radiation

3. Positive Ion

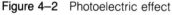

Figure 4–2   Photoelectric effect

3. **The tighter an electron is bound in its orbit, the more likely it is to be involved in a photoelectric reaction.** Electrons are more tightly bound in elements with high atomic numbers than in elements with low atomic numbers, as shown in Table 4–1. Most interactions occur at the K shell in elements with low atomic numbers, because the K shell contains the most tightly bound electrons. In elements with high atomic numbers, however, the energy of the incident photons is frequently insufficient to eject a K-shell electron, and many photoelectric reactions take place at the L and M shell levels. Because elements with high atomic numbers bind their electrons more tightly, they are more likely to undergo photoelectric reactions. The probability of the photoelectric effect increases sharply as the atomic number increases. In fact, it is roughly proportional to the third power of the atomic number:

Photoelectric effect ~ (atomic number)^3

In summary, photoelectric reactions are most likely to occur with low-energy photons and elements with high atomic numbers provided the photons have sufficient energy to overcome the forces binding the electrons in their shells. In fact, the photoelectric effect cannot take place with a "free" (not bound to an atom) electron. If you like, you may call this a "forbidden" interaction.

Characteristic Radiation

We first mentioned characteristic radiation when we discussed the production of x rays in Chapter 2. Characteristic radiation generated by the photoelectric effect is exactly the same. The only difference is in the modality used to eject the inner shell electron. In an x-ray tube a high-speed electron ejects the bound electron, while in a photoelectric interaction an x-ray photon does the trick. In both cases the atom is left with an excess of energy equal to the binding energy of the ejected electron. All physical systems seek the lowest possible energy state. For example, water always runs downhill. An atom with an electron deficiency in the K shell is in a higher energy state than an atom with an L-shell electron deficiency. The atom releases this excess energy in the form of photons. Usually an electron from an adjacent shell drops into an inner shell void, as shown for an iodine atom in Figure 4–3. The K-shell binding energy for iodine is 33.2 keV, while the L-shell binding energy is 4.9 keV, and more peripheral shells have even lower binding energies. When an electron from an L shell falls to the K shell, a 28.3-keV (33.2 − 4.9 = 28.3) photon is released. The void in the L shell is then filled with a photon from the M shell with the production of a 4.3-keV photon. This process is continued until the whole 33.2 keV of energy has been converted into photons. Of course, the lower energy photons are of no im-

Table 4–1. K-Shell Electron Binding Energies of Elements Important in Diagnostic Radiology

ATOMIC NUMBER	ATOM	K-SHELL BINDING ENERGY (keV)
6	Carbon	0.284
7	Nitrogen	0.400
8	Oxygen	0.532
13	Aluminum	1.56
20	Calcium	4.04
50	Tin	29.2
53	Iodine	33.2
56	Barium	37.4
74	Tungsten	69.5
82	Lead	88.0

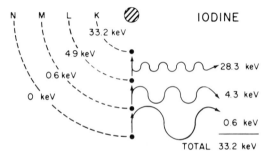

Figure 4–3 Characteristic radiation from iodine

portance in diagnostic radiology, because they are absorbed immediately. Occasionally an inner shell void is filled by an electron from distant peripheral shells, or even by free electrons. When a free electron moves into the K-shell void in iodine, a single photon of 33.2 keV is generated. This is the maximal energy characteristic radiation that iodine can produce.

The K-shell binding energies of some elements important in diagnostic radiology are shown in Table 4–1. Calcium, which has the highest atomic number of any element found in the body in significant quanity, emits a 4-keV maximal energy characteristic photon, which is little energy by x-ray standards. It is absorbed within a few millimeters of its site of origin. The contrast agents iodine and barium are the only elements encountered in diagnostic radiology that emit characteristic radiation energetic enough to leave the patient and fog an x-ray film.

Characteristic radiation is usually referred to as secondary radiation to differentiate it from scatter radiation, a distinction that hardly seems necessary because the end result is the same for both, a photon that is deflected from its original path.

Applications to Diagnostic Radiology

As diagnostic radiologists we can look at the photoelectric effect in two ways, one good and the other bad. Starting with the good, it produces radiographic images of excellent quality. The quality is good for two reasons: first, the photoelectric effect does not produce scatter radiation and second, it enhances natural tissue contrast. X-ray image contrast depends on some tissues absorbing more x rays than other tissues. Contrast is greatest when the difference in absorption between adjacent tissues is large. Because the number of reactions depends on the third power of the atomic number, the photoelectric effect magnifies the difference in tissues composed of different elements, such as bone and soft tissue. So, from the point of view of film qual-

ity, the photoelectric effect is desirable. From the point of view of patient exposure, though, it is undesirable. Patients receive more radiation from photoelectric reactions than from any other type of interaction. All the energy of the incident photon is absorbed by the patient in a photoelectric reaction. Only part of the incident photon's energy is absorbed in a Compton reaction, as you will see in the next section. Because one of our primary goals is to keep patient doses at a minimum, we must keep this point in mind at all times. The importance of the photoelectric effect can be minimized by using high-energy (kVp) techniques. In general, we should use radiation of the highest energy consistent with that of diagnostic quality x-ray films to minimize patient exposure.

In summary, the likelihood of a photoelectric interaction depends on two factors: the energy of the radiation and the atomic number of the absorber. The reaction is most common with low-energy photons and absorbers with high atomic numbers. Photons usually strike tightly bound K-shell electrons, and they must have more energy than the electron binding energy. Photoelectric reactions are desirable from the point of view of the film quality, because they give excellent contrast without generating signf。cant scatter radiation. Unfortunately, patient exposures are much higher than with any other type of interaction.

COMPTON SCATTERING

Almost all the scatter radiation that we encounter in diagnostic radiology comes from Compton scattering. Figure 4–4 diagrams this reaction. An incident photon with relatively high energy strikes a free outer shell electron, ejecting it from its orbit. The photon is deflected by the electron so that it travels in a new direction as scatter radiation. The photon always retains part of its original energy. The reaction produces an ion pair, a positive atom

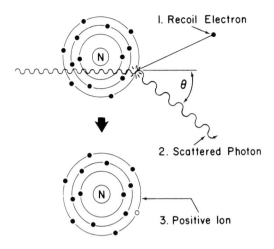

I. Recoil Electron

θ

2. Scattered Photon

3. Positive Ion

Figure 4–4   Compton scattering

and a negative electron, which is called a recoil electron.

The energy of the incident photon is distributed in two ways. Part of it goes to the recoil electron as kinetic energy, and the rest is retained by the deflected photon. Unlike a photoelectric reaction in which most of a photon's energy is expended freeing the photoelectron from its bond, in a Compton reaction no energy is needed for this purpose, because the recoil electron is already free. The incident photon always retains some of its original energy. Two factors determine the amount of energy the photon retains: its initial energy and its angle of deflection off the recoil electron. If you think of the Compton reaction as a collision between two billiard balls, the energy transfer is easier to understand. The cue ball is the incident photon, and the second ball is a free electron. When the cue ball strikes the second ball, they both deflect in a predictable manner. With a glancing blow the angle of deflection of the cue ball is small, and only a small quantity of energy is transferred to the second ball. The cue ball retains almost all its initial energy. With a more direct hit the cue ball deflects at a greater angle and loses more energy. Finally, with a direct hit, maximal energy is transferred to the second ball but, unlike the cue ball in billiards, a Compton

photon never gives up all its energy. The photon retains some energy and deflects back along its original path at an angle of 180°. Figure 4–5 shows the amount of energy a 75-keV photon retains as it is deflected through various angles. As you can see, more energy is lost with larger angles of deflection.

To make our comparison between a Compton reaction and billiard balls complete, we must make one last adjustment in the analogy. Billiard balls all have the same mass, but we want to compare them with photons whose energies vary. We can keep our analogy going by using cue balls of different masses. Thus, a lightweight cue ball simulates a low-energy photon, and a heavy cue ball simulates a high energy photon. Now, imagine both the lightweight and the heavy cue balls striking a second ball a glancing blow at an angle of 45°. The lightweight ball has little momentum, and it will deflect at a much greater angle than the heavy ball, which has more momentum. Photons also have momentum and, the higher the energy of the photons, the more difficult they are to deflect. With x-ray energies of 1 MeV (million electron volts), most scattered photons deflect in a forward direction. In the diagnostic energy range, however, the distribution is more symmetric. Figure 4–6 shows the pattern of distribution of scattered photons from a 100-keV x-ray beam. The distance from the point of the interaction is used to express

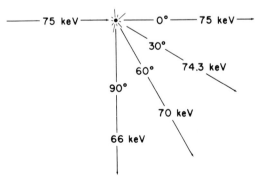

Figure 4–5   Energy of Compton-scattered photons

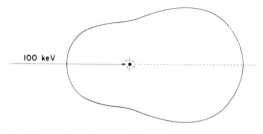

Figure 4–6 Distribution of Compton-scattered photons

Table 4–2. Energy of Compton-Scattered Photons for Various Angles of Deflection

ENERGY OF INCIDENT PHOTON (keV)	ENERGY OF SCATTERED PHOTONS (keV)			
	PHOTON DEFLECTION ANGLE			
	30°	60°	90°	180°
25	24.9	24.4	24	23
50	49.6	47.8	46	42
75	74.3	70	66	58
100	98.5	91	84	72
150	146	131	116	95

the percentage of scattered photons at various angles. Remember, this is a flat representation of events that are occurring in three dimensions. You can picture the three-dimensional distribution by rotating the pattern around its longitudinal axis. With lower energy radiation, fewer photons scatter forward and more scatter back at an angle of 180°. This distribution is fairly constant throughout the diagnostic energy range.

The classic formula for calculating the change in wavelength of a scattered photon is

$$\Delta\lambda = 0.024 \, (1 - \cos \theta)$$

$\Delta\lambda$ = change in wavelength (Å)
θ = angle of photon deflection

Most of us think in terms of kilovoltage and not wavelength. We can change wavelength from the above formula to kilovoltage with the following conversion factor:

$$kV = \frac{12.4}{\lambda}$$

λ = wavelength (Å)
kV = kilovoltage.

The amount of energy retained by scattered photons after a Compton reaction is shown in Table 4–2. In the diagnostic energy range up to 150 keV the photon retains most of its original energy, and very little is transferred to the recoil electron. At narrow angles of deflection, scattered photons retain almost all their original energy. This creates a serious problem in diagnostic radiology, because photons that are scattered at narrow angles have an ex-

cellent chance of reaching an x-ray film and producing fog. They are exceedingly difficult to remove from the x-ray beam. In fact, they cannot be removed by filters because they are too energetic, and they cannot be removed by grids because their angle of deflection is too small. Because we have no way of removing them from the useful beam, we must accept them and tolerate an image of diminished quality.

Scatter radiation from Compton reactions is also a major safety hazard. As you can see in Table 4–2, even after a photon has been deflected 90°, it still retains most of its original energy. This means that the scatter radiation that arises in the patient during a fluoroscopic examination is almost as energetic as the primary beam. It creates a real safety hazard for the fluoroscopist and other personnel who must be in exposure rooms.

Probability of Occurrence

The probability of a Compton reaction depends on the total number of electrons in an absorber, which in turn depends on its density and the number of electrons per gram. In Chapter 5 we will show that all elements contain approximately the same number of electrons per gram, regardless of their atomic number. Therefore, the number of Compton reactions is independent of the atomic number of the absorber. The likelihood of a reaction, however, does depend on the energy of the radiation and the density of the absorber. The number of reactions gradually diminishes as photon energy increases, so that a high-energy photon is more likely to pass through the body than a low-energy photon.

Because Compton reactions occur with free electrons, we must define this term a little more precisely. An electron can be considered free when its binding energy is a great deal less than the energy of the incident photon. With the photon energies used in diagnostic radiology (10 to 150 keV), only the outer shell electrons are free in the elements with high atomic numbers. For the elements with low atomic numbers, those found in soft tissues, all electrons can be considered free, because even those on the K shell are bound with an energy of less than 1 keV.

PAIR PRODUCTION AND PHOTODISINTEGRATION

The last two basic interactions, pair production and photodisintegration, do not occur in the diagnostic energy range. They have no importance in diagnostic radiology, and we will only discuss them briefly. In pair production, a high-energy photon interacts with the nucleus of an atom, the photon disappears, and its energy is converted into matter in the form of two particles. One is an ordinary electron and the other is a positron, a particle with the same mass as an electron but with a positive charge. Because the mass of one electron is equal to 0.51 MeV, and pair production produces two electrons, the interaction cannot take place with photon energies less than 1.02 MeV.

In photodisintegration, part of the nucleus of an atom is ejected by a high-energy photon. The ejected portion may be either a neutron, proton, alpha particle, or a cluster of particles. The photon must have sufficient energy to overcome nuclear binding energies of the order of 7 to 15 MeV.

Because pair production does not occur with photon energies less than 1.02 MeV, and photodisintegration does not occur with energies less than 7 MeV, neither of these interactions is of any importance in diagnostic radiology, where we rarely use energies above 150 keV.

RELATIVE FREQUENCY OF BASIC INTERACTIONS

Figure 4–7 shows the percentage of each type of interaction for water, compact bone, and sodium iodide, with photon energies ranging from 20 to 100 keV. The total number of reactions is always 100%. The contribution of each interaction is represented by an area in the illustration. Thus, if coherent scattering accounts for 5% of the interactions, Compton scattering for 20%, and the photoelectric effect for 75%, the total is 100%. Water is used to illustrate the behavior of tissues with low atomic numbers, such as air, fat, and muscle. The total number of reactions is less for air than for water, but the percentage of each type is approximately the same. Compact bone contains a large amount of calcium, and it represents elements with intermediate atomic numbers. Iodine and barium are the elements with the highest atomic numbers that we encounter in diagnostic radiology, and they are represented by sodium iodide.

As you can see in Figure 4–7, coherent scattering usually contributes around 5% to the total, and plays a minor role throughout the diagnostic energy range. In water, Compton scattering is the dominant interaction, except at very low photon energies (20 to 30 keV). The contrast agents, because of their high atomic numbers, are involved almost exclusively in photoelectric reactions. Bone is intermediate between water and the contrast agents. At low energies, photoelectric reactions are more common, while at high energies, Compton scattering is dominant.

SUMMARY

Only two interactions are important in diagnostic radiology, the photoelectric effect and Compton scattering. Coherent scattering is numerically unimportant, and

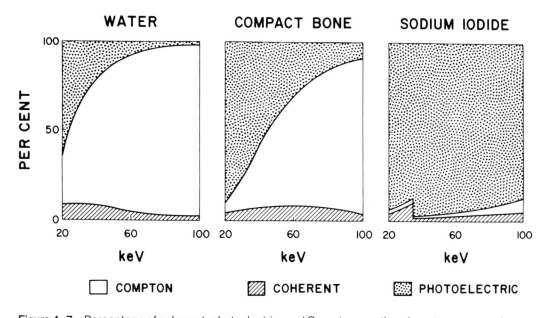

Figure 4–7   Percentage of coherent, photoelectric, and Compton reactions in water, compact bone, and sodium iodide

pair production and photodisintegration occur at energies above the useful energy range. The photoelectric effect is the predominant interaction with low-energy radiation and with high atomic number absorbers. It generates no significant scatter radiation and produces high contrast in the x-ray image but, unfortunately, exposes the patient to a great deal of radiation. At higher diagnostic energies, Compton scattering is the most common interaction between x rays and body tissues, and is responsible for almost all scatter radiation. Radiographic image contrast is less with Compton reactions than with the photoelectric effect.

5

Attenuation

Quantity and quality are two terms used to express the characteristics of an x-ray beam. Quantity refers to the number of photons in the beam, and quality refers to their energies. The intensity of a beam is the product of the number and energy of the photons, so it is dependent on both quantity and quality. A beam of 50-keV photons has a greater intensity than a beam made up of a comparable number of 20-keV photons. **Attenuation is the reduction in the intensity of an x-ray beam as it traverses matter by either the absorption or deflection of photons from the beam.** Because it is a measure of a change in x-ray intensity, attenuation depends on both the quantity and quality of the photons in a beam. For our purpose, it would be simpler to think of attenuation only in terms of quantity. Then a reduction in intensity would merely be a reduction in the number of photons in the beam. We can do this if we limit our discussion to the attenuation of monochromatic radiation. Later in the text, we will clarify why quality does not change with monochromatic radiation. To further simplify our discussion, we will disregard the attenuation of secondary radiation resulting from coherent or Compton scattering and the characteristic radiation of the photoelectric effect. Once a photon has undergone any of these reactions, it will be considered completely attenuated, that is, totally removed from the beam.

MONOCHROMATIC RADIATION

The attenuation of a beam of monochromatic radiation is shown schematically in Figure 5–1. A beam of 1000 photons is directed at a water phantom. The intensity of the beam is decreased to 800 photons by the first centimeter of water, which is an attenuation of 20%. The second centimeter of water decreases the intensity to 640 photons, which is 20% less than had passed through the first centimeter. With each succeeding centimeter of water, 20% of the remaining photons are removed from the beam.

The quality of monochromatic radiation does not change as it passes through an absorber. Remember, we are only discussing primary photons, the photons that, at most, have only one interaction. If we begin with a group of photons with an energy of 60 keV, then the transmitted photons will all have the same energy. Their numbers will be reduced, but their quality will not

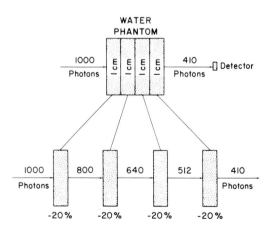

Figure 5–1 Attenuation of monochromatic radiation

60

be changed. So, when we talk about a change in the intensity of a monochromatic beam, we are really talking about a change in the number, or quantity, of photons in the beam. A 50% reduction in the number of photons is a 50% reduction in the intensity of the beam. The attenuation of polychromatic radiation is much more complicated, and we will not discuss it until the end of the chapter.

When the number of transmitted photons and absorber thickness are plotted on linear graph paper, a curved line results (Fig. 5–2A). The initial portion of the curve is steep, because more photons are removed from the beam by the first few centimeters of absorber. After the beam has passed through many centimeters of water, only a few photons remain. Although each centimeter continues to remove 20% of the photons, the total numbers are small, and the end of the curve is almost flat. The same numbers plot a straight line on semi-logarithmic graph paper (Fig. 5–2B). When the number of photons remaining in the beam decreases by the same percentage with each increment of absorber, as with monochromatic radiation, the attenuation is called exponential. Exponential functions plot a straight line on semilogarithmic graph paper.

ATTENUATION COEFFICIENTS

An attenuation coefficient is a measure of the quantity of radiation attenuated by a given thickness of an absorber. The name of the coefficient is determined by the units used to measure the thickness of the absorber. Four attenuation coefficients are described in classical texts on radiologic physics but only two are important in diagnostic radiology, the linear and mass attenuation coefficients.

Linear Attenuation Coefficient

The linear attenuation coefficient is the most important coefficient for diagnostic

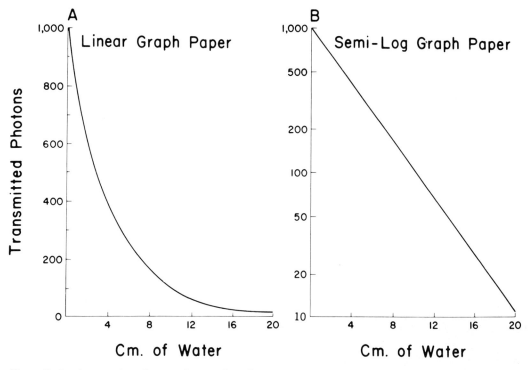

Figure 5–2 Attenuation of monochromatic radiation plotted on linear (A) and semilogarithmic graph paper (B).

radiology. It is a quantitative measurement of attenuation per centimeter of absorber, so it tells us how much attenuation we can expect from a certain thickness of tissue. Because we measure our patients in centimeters, it is a practical and useful attenuation coefficient. In the next section, after we have discussed the mass attenuation coefficient, you will understand why the linear coefficient is more useful. Its symbol is the Greek letter μ.

The unit of the linear attenuation coefficient is per centimeter, and thus the name **linear** attenuation coefficient, because a centimeter is a linear measurement. The expression per cm is the same as 1/cm, and is usually written cm^{-1}.

It is important to realize that **the linear attenuation coefficient (μ) is for monochromatic radiation,** and that it is specific both for the energy of the x-ray beam and for the type of absorber. Water, fat, bone, and air all have different linear attenuation coefficients, and the size of the coefficient changes as the energy of the x-ray beam changes. When the energy of the radiation is increased the number of x rays that are attenuated decreases, and so does the linear attenuation coefficient.

The mathematics involved in the derivation of the exponential equation for x-ray attenuation is beyond the scope of this book. The formula is

$$N = N_0 e^{-\mu x}$$

    N = number of transmitted photons
    N_0 = number of incident photons
    e = base of natural logarithm
    μ = linear attenuation coefficient
    x = absorber thickness (in centimeters).

This is a classic equation, and it has the same format as the equation for the decay of radionuclides. In fact, most people find it easier to think in terms of radionuclide decay, so we will digress for a moment. Radionuclides decay at an exponential rate. This rate is usually measured and defined in terms of half-life, which is the time that it takes a material to decay to one half

its original activity. For example, ^{131}I has a half-life ($T_{1/2}$) of 8.04 days. If we started with 100 units of activity, at the end of 8.04 days we would have 50 units, and at the end of another 8.04 days we would only have 25 units. The equation for this exponential decay is

$$N = N_0 e^{-\lambda t}$$

    N = activity of remaining radionuclide
    N_0 = activity of original radionuclide
    e = base of natural logarithm (2.718)
    λ = decay constant (seconds^{-1})
    t = time (seconds).

The decay constant (λ) can be easily related to half-life ($T_{1/2}$), which is a more familiar concept. After the elapsed time of one-half life ($T_{1/2}$), the quantity of remaining activity is $N_0/2$. The exponential decay equation can be rewritten as

$$\frac{N_0}{2} = N_0 e^{-\lambda T_{1/2}}$$

Dividing both sides by N_0, the equation becomes

$$\frac{1}{2} = e^{-\lambda T_{1/2}}$$

We would then go to a table of exponential values and find the value of the exponent $\lambda T_{1/2}$, which makes $e^{-\lambda T_{1/2}}$ equal to $\frac{1}{2}$ or, more simply, we could just look up the logarithm of $\frac{1}{2}$ in a table of natural logarithms. We would find this value to be -0.693. We can now rewrite the exponential decay equation:

$$\lambda \cdot T_{1/2} = 0.693 \text{ or } \lambda = \frac{0.693}{T_{1/2}}$$

The decay constant (λ) for any radionuclide can be calculated if we know its half-life. For example, the decay constant for ^{131}I ($T_{1/2} = 8.04$ days) is

$$\lambda = \frac{0.693}{8.04 \text{ days}} = 0.086/\text{day}$$

The attenuation of monochromatic radiation is exactly the same. All we need do is substitute thickness (cm of absorber) for time (seconds). The names are changed, but the concept remains the same. The decay constant (λ) becomes the linear attenuation coefficient (μ), and half-life ($T_{1/2}$) becomes the half-value layer (HVL). The product of the linear attenuation coefficient and half-value layer is equal to 0.693:

$$\mu \times HVL = 0.693, \text{ or } HVL = \frac{0.693}{\mu}$$

The half-value layer is the absorber thickness required to reduce the intensity of the original beam by one half. It is a common method for expressing the quality of an x-ray beam. A beam with a high half-value layer is a more penetrating beam than one with a low half-value layer.

If the values from the attenuation of the x-ray beam in Figure 5–1 are used in the exponential attenuation equation, the linear attenuation coefficient can be calculated as

$$N = N_0 e^{-\mu x}$$

where N is 800 photons transmitted, N_0 is 1000 initial photons, and x is 1 cm of water.

$$800 = 1000\, e^{-\mu(1)} = \frac{1000}{e^\mu}$$

$$e^\mu = \frac{1000}{800} = 1.25$$

$$\mu = 0.22/\text{cm}$$

The last step in the calculation requires a table of exponential values, or natural logarithms. After we have determined the linear attenuation coefficient, the half-value layer of the beam can be calculated as

$$HVL = \frac{0.693}{\mu} = \frac{0.693}{0.22} = 3.15 \text{ cm}$$

You can see from Figure 5–1 that the beam is reduced to one half its original intensity in the fourth 1-cm block of water, which confirms our calculations.

Calculating a linear attenuation coefficient is not of much practical value to a diagnostic radiologist, but the equation can be used for other purposes. There are tables available that list the linear attenuation coefficients for substances such as water, bone, sodium iodide, and most of the elements.[1] With the linear attenuation coefficient from these tables, we can calculate the percentage of transmitted photons for a whole variety of photon energies and for whatever thickness of tissue we may choose.

Mass Attenuation Coefficient

Another useful attenuation coefficient that is basic in the physics literature is the mass attenuation coefficient, which is used to quantitate the attenuation of materials independent of their physical state. For example, water, ice and water vapor, the three physical states of H_2O, all have the same mass attenuation coefficient. It is obtained by dividing the linear attenuation coefficient by the density (ρ), and has the symbol μ/ρ. The unit for the x-ray absorber is grams per square centimeter (g/cm^2), which contains a mass unit, and thus the name **mass** attenuation coefficient. Figure 5–3 illustrates the meaning of a gram per square centimeter by comparing aluminum and water. The density of water is 1 g/cm^3, so a square centimeter of water must be 1 cm thick to weigh 1 g. The density of aluminum is 2.7 g/cm^3, so a square centimeter of aluminum only has to be 0.37 cm thick to weigh 1 g. The arithmetic is simple. The thickness is merely the reciprocal of the density, or 1 divided by the density. A square centimeter of water 1 cm thick and a square centimeter of aluminum 0.37 cm thick both contain 1 g/cm^2.

The unit of the mass attenuation coefficient is per g/cm^2. It can be expressed in several ways: per g/cm^2 or $1/g/cm^2$ or cm^2/g; usually it is written cm^2/g.

A brief review should help to avoid confusion about units. When we talk about either the linear or mass attenuation coefficient, there are two separate units for each, one for the absorber and the other for the coefficient. The units for the absorber are cm for the linear attenuation coefficient and g/cm^2 for the mass attenuation coefficient. The units for the coef-

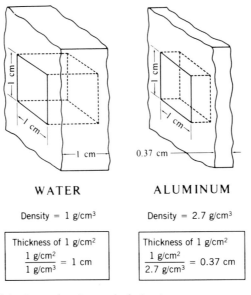

Figure 5–3 Thickness of 1 g/cm² of water and of aluminum

ficients themselves are cm⁻¹ for the linear and cm²/g for the mass attenuation coefficient. The unit of the coefficient is the reciprocal of the unit of the absorber.

A simple way to understand the relationship between the linear and mass attenuation coefficients is to compare the coefficients for water, ice, and water vapor (Fig. 5–4). The values in the illustration are for a 50-keV monochromatic beam. The linear attenuation coefficient for water is 0.214 cm⁻¹, and a 1-cm thickness of water absorbs 20% of the incidence beam. The same thickness of ice absorbs 18.5%, because ice is a little less dense than water. Water vapor has very little density, and a 1-cm thickness absorbs almost nothing. Density has a profound effect on x-ray attenuation at all energy levels.

The mass attenuation coefficient for water in Figure 5–4 is 0.214 cm²/g, which is the same as the linear attenuation coefficient. They must be the same, because the density of water is 1 g/cm³, and the mass attenuation coefficient is obtained by dividing the linear attenuation coefficient by the density (μ/ρ). The mass attenuation coefficient is the same for water, ice, and water vapor, which is logical because 1 g of all

three has exactly the same amount of mass. The thickness of 1 g/cm² of water is 1 cm, ice 1.09 cm, and water vapor 1670 cm. These thicknesses will all attenuate the same amount of x ray (i.e., 20%) because they all contain the same amount of mass. As you can see in Figure 5–4, the mass attenuation coefficient is independent of the density of the absorber. The coefficients for water, ice, and water vapor are all the same, but their densities vary considerably.

To say that a gram of water and a gram of water vapor both absorb the same amount of radiation is true, but the statement has no meaning to a diagnostic radiologist. In fact, it is misleading. We just do not deal with g/cm² of patient. We measure a patient's thickness in centimeters, and 1 cm of water absorbs a great deal more x ray than 1 cm of water vapor. When the effect of density is removed from the value of an attenuation coefficient, it is misleading in diagnostic radiology.

FACTORS AFFECTING ATTENUATION

Four factors determine the degree of attenuation of an x-ray beam as it passes

50 keV			
Linear Attenuation Coefficient (cm^{-1})	Mass Attenuation Coefficient (cm^2/gm)	Density (gm/cm^3)	Thickness of 1 gm/cm^2
0.214	0.214	1	WATER 1 cm
0.196	0.214	0.917	ICE 1.09 cm
0.000128	0.214	0.000598	WATER VAPOR 1670 cm

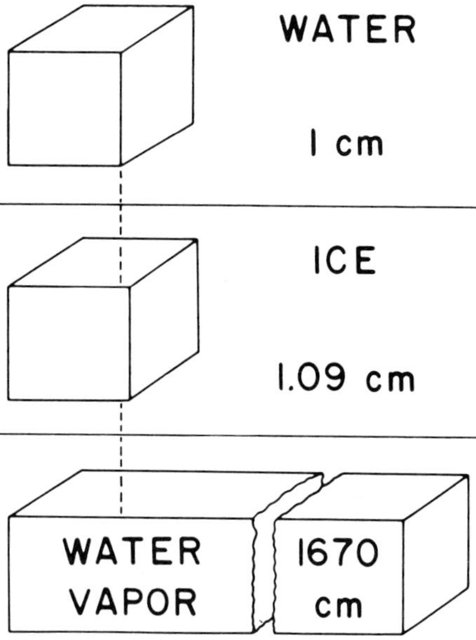

Figure 5–4   Comparison of linear and mass attenuation coefficients for water, ice, and water vapor

through matter. One involves the nature of the radiation, and three involve the composition of the matter:

RADIATION	MATTER
Energy	Density Atomic number Electrons per gram

Increasing the radiation energy increases the number of transmitted photons (and decreases attenuation), while increasing the density, atomic number, or electrons per gram of the absorber decreases the number of transmitted photons (and increases attenuation).

Relationships Between Density, Atomic Number, and Electrons per Gram

We will examine each of the four factors that affect attenuation separately, but first we must digress to review the relationships between density (ρ), atomic number (Z), and electrons per gram (e/g).

Density and Atomic Number

The relationship between density and atomic number is complex, and no simple rule covers all situations. In general, elements with high atomic numbers are denser than elements with low atomic numbers, but there are exceptions. Gold and lead provide a good example:

	ATOMIC NUMBER	DENSITY (g/cm^3)
Gold	79	19.3
Lead	82	11.0

There is no relationship between atomic number and density when different physical states of matter are considered. Water has an effective atomic number of 7.4 regardless of its state (ice, liquid, or vapor), but its density is different in each of these three forms.

Density and Electrons per Gram

Whenever a factor is expressed in the units per gram, the concept of volume is eliminated. Because density depends on volume (weight per unit volume), there is no relationship between density and electrons per gram. A gram of water has the same number of electrons, regardless of whether they are compressed together in a 1-cm cube as a liquid, or spread out over 1670 cm^3 as a vapor.

Atomic Number and Electrons per Gram

The number of electrons per gram is really a function of the number of neutrons in the atom. If the elements did not have neutrons, all materials would have 6.0×10^{23} e/g. Table 5–1 shows the relationships between atomic number and electrons per gram for various substances important in diagnostic radiology. Hydrogen, which has no neutrons, has 6.0×10^{23} e/g, which is twice as many as any other element. The elements found in soft tissue—carbon, nitrogen, and oxygen—all have 3.0×10^{23} e/g, and the higher atomic elements have even fewer e/g. In general, elements with low atomic numbers have more electrons per gram than those with high atomic numbers.

Effects of Energy and Atomic Number

Energy and atomic number, in combination, determine the percentage of each

Table 5–1. Electrons Per Gram for Several Elements Important in Diagnostic Radiology

ELEMENTS	ATOMIC NUMBER	NUMBER OF ELECTRONS PER GRAM
Hydrogen	1	6.00×10^{23}
Oxygen	8	3.01×10^{23}
Calcium	20	3.00×10^{23}
Copper	29	2.75×10^{23}
Iodine	53	2.51×10^{23}
Barium	56	2.45×10^{23}
Lead	82	2.38×10^{23}

Table 5–2. Percentage of Photoelectric Reactions

RADIATION ENERGY (keV)	WATER (Z = 7.4)	COMPACT BONE (Z = 13.8)	SODIUM IODIDE (Z = 49.8)
20	65%	89%	94%
60	7%	31%	95%
100	2%	9%	88%

type of basic interaction, so in this sense their effects on attenuation are inseparable. Table 5–2 shows the percentage of photoelectric reactions for various radiation energies in water, bone, and sodium iodide. You can easily calculate the percentage of Compton reactions by subtracting the percentage of photoelectric reactions from 100 (ignoring the small contribution from coherent scattering). As the radiation energy increases, the percentage of photoelectric reactions decreases for water and bone; as the atomic number increases, the percentage of photoelectric reactions increases. With extremely low-energy radiation (20 keV), photoelectric attenuation predominates, regardless of the atomic number of the absorber. As the radiation energy is increased, Compton scattering becomes more important until eventually it replaces the photoelectric effect as the predominant interaction. With high atomic number absorbers, such as sodium iodide, the photoelectric effect is the predominant interaction throughout the diagnostic energy range.

The linear attenuation coefficient is the sum of the contributions from coherent scattering, photoelectric reactions, and Compton scattering:

$$\mu = \mu_{coherent} + \mu_{PE} + \mu_{Compton}$$

For example, at 40 keV, the linear attenuation coefficient for water is 0.24 cm^{-1}. Of this total, 0.018 is from coherent scattering, 0.18 is from Compton scattering and the remaining 0.042 is from photoelectric attenuation. For water, the mass and linear attenuation coefficients are the same because the density of water is 1 g/cm^3. For other materials, however, the mass and linear attenuation coefficients are different, but the principle is exactly the same.

If we know the relative percentage of each type of interaction, we can predict the total amount of attenuation (or transmission). Attenuation is always greater when the photoelectric effect predominates. Perhaps the difference between photoelectric and Compton attenuation will be easier to understand with an analogy. Suppose we take a flat stone and slide it along the ground at a high speed. If we slide the stone over a rough surface, such as a concrete sidewalk, friction will stop it in a short distance. If we slide the stone over a frozen pond, friction is reduced, and the stone will travel a much greater distance. In this analogy, the x-ray beam is the moving stone and attenuation is the friction that stops the stone. Photoelectric attenuation is like the concrete sidewalk and Compton attenuation is like the frozen pond. The photoelectric effect attenuates a beam much more rapidly than Compton scattering.

Energy

In addition to its influence on the type of basic interaction, energy has its own effect on attenuation. Even when all the basic interactions are of one type, attenuation decreases as the radiation energy increases. Table 5–3 shows the percentage of photons transmitted through a 10-cm thick water phantom with various radiation energies. As you can see, the percentage of transmitted photons increases as the energy of the beam increases. With low-energy radiation (20 keV), most of the interactions are photoelectric, and few photons are transmitted. As the energy of the radiation increases photoelectric attenuation becomes less important, and completely ceases at 100 keV. Even when all attenuation is from Compton scattering, the percentage of transmitted photons continues to increase as the radiation energy increases. A larger percentage of photons is transmitted with a 150-keV than with a 100-keV beam.

As the energy of the radiation increases, photoelectric attenuation decreases sharply, while Compton attenuation decreases only slightly. In the low-energy range, a massive quantity of photoelectric attenuation is superimposed on a background of Compton attenuation. As the energy of the radiation increases, photoelectric attenuation diminishes until the background of Compton attenuation is all that is left. Once this happens, increasing the beam energy will cause only a slight decrease in attenuation (and slight increase in transmission).

As a general rule, the higher the energy of the radiation, the larger the percentage of transmitted photons, regardless of the type of basic interaction. The only exception to this rule occurs with high atomic number absorbers, which we will discuss next.

Atomic Number

Usually, as the radiation energy increases, x-ray transmission increases (and attenuation decreases) but, with high atomic number absorbers, transmission may actually decrease with increasing beam energy. This apparent paradox occurs because there is an abrupt change in the likelihood of a photoelectric reaction as the radiation energy reaches the binding energy of an inner shell electron. A photon cannot eject an electron unless it has more energy than the electron's binding energy. Thus, a lower energy photon is more likely

Table 5–3. Percent Transmission of Monochromatic Radiation Through 10 cm of Water

ENERGY (keV)	TRANSMISSION (%)
20	0.04
30	2.5
40	7.0
50	10.0
60	13.0
80	16.0
100	18.0
150	22.0

to be transmitted than a higher energy photon, provided one has slightly less and the other slightly more energy than the binding energy of the electron.

Table 5–4 shows the percentage transmission of monochromatic radiation through 1 mm of lead. A sudden change in transmission occurs at 88 keV, which is the binding energy of the K-shell electron. This is called the **K edge.** With a radiation energy just below the K edge, a fairly large percentage of the photons is transmitted (12%), while just above the K edge, transmission drops to nearly zero. Of course, the same thing is true for the low atomic number elements at the K edge, but the energies involved are usually less than 1 keV, far below those in the useful diagnostic energy range.

Figure 5–5 shows a plot of the mass attenuation coefficients of tin and lead over the range of energies used in diagnostic radiology. Remember, the higher the attenuation coefficient, the lower the number of transmitted photons. **Gram for gram, tin is a better absorber of x rays than lead between 29 and 88 keV.** This has a practical application. We are not usually concerned about attenuation per gram but, when we are carrying the gram on our back as a protective apron, our perspective changes. Because tin attenuates more radiation per unit weight than lead, it has recently come into use for this purpose. A lighter tin apron gives the same protection as a standard lead apron, or, if you have a

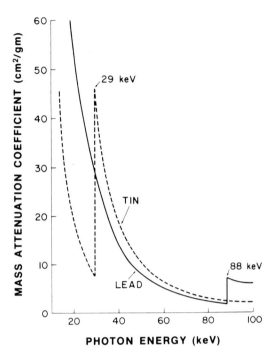

Figure 5–5 Comparison of the mass attenuation coefficients for tin and lead

strong back, you can use the same weight of tin for the apron and have more protection.

The commonly used contrast agents barium and iodine were originally selected because of their low toxicities. A better choice, however, could not have been made if they were selected for their physical properties. Both have ideal K-shell binding energies (iodine, 32 keV; barium, 34 keV). These binding energies are approximately the same as the mean energy of most diagnostic x-ray beams, so many interactions occur at the K-shell level. Attenuation is more intense than it would be for a higher atomic number element, such as lead. Most photons in a polychromatic beam are less energetic than the 88-keV K-shell binding energy of lead.

Table 5–5 shows the atomic numbers and K edges of most elements important in diagnostic radiology. When maximum x-ray absorption is desired, the K edge of an absorber should be closely matched to the

Table 5–4. Percent Transmission of Monochromatic Radiation Through 1 mm of Lead

ENERGY (keV)	TRANSMISSION (%)
50	0.016
60	0.40
80	6.8
88	12.0
—K edge for lead—	
88	0.026
100	0.14
150	0.96

Table 5–5. Atomic Numbers and K Edges of Elements Important in Diagnostic Radiology

ELEMENT	SYMBOL	ATOMIC NUMBER (Z)	K EDGE (keV)
Hydrogen	H	1	.013
Beryllium	Be	4	.11
Carbon	C	6	.28
Nitrogen	N	7	.40
Oxygen	O	8	.53
Sodium	Na	11	1.1
Aluminum	Al	13	1.6
Silicon	Si	14	1.8
Sulfur	S	16	2.5
Chlorine	Cl	17	2.8
Potassium	K	19	3.6
Calcium	Ca	20	4.0
Iron	Fe	26	7.1
Copper	Cu	29	9.0
Zinc	Zn	30	9.7
Germanium	Ge	32	11.1
Selenium	Se	34	12.7
Bromine	Br	35	13.5
Yttrium	Y	39	17.0
Molybdenum	Mo	42	20.0
Silver	Ag	47	25.5
Cadmium	Cd	48	26.7
Tin	Sn	50	29.1
Iodine	I	53	33.2
Cesium	Cs	55	36.0
Barium	Ba	56	37.4
Lanthanum	La	57	39.0
Gadolinium	Gd	64	50.2
Tantalum	Ta	73	67.5
Tungsten	W	74	69.5
Gold	Au	79	80.7
Lead	Pb	82	88.0

energy of the x-ray beam. For example, xeroradiography employs a selenium plate with a K edge of 12.7 keV as the x-ray absorber. This low K edge makes selenium an excellent absorber for the low-energy radiation (30 to 35 kVp) used for mammography. Selenium would be a poor choice, however, as an absorber for a high-energy beam, such as the 350 kVp used for chest radiography with a field emission unit. For high-energy radiation, tungsten, with a K edge of 59.5 keV, is a much better absorber. As we shall see later, the success of the rare earth intensifying screens and of the cesium iodide image intensifier is in large part related to excellent matching of their K edges to beam energies.

Effect of Density on Attenuation

Tissue density is one of the most important factors in x-ray attenuation, and a difference in tissue densities is one of the primary reasons why we see an x-ray image. Density determines the number of electrons present in a given thickness, so it determines the tissue's stopping power. The relationship between density and attenuation is linear. If the density of a material is doubled, attenuation doubles. This is easiest to understand in terms of a gas whose density can be changed by compression. If a quantity of gas in a closed container is doubled, the number of electrons doubles. The same thickness of material now has twice as much mass, and it will attenuate twice as many photons.

Effect of Electrons per Gram

The number of Compton reactions depends on the number of electrons in a given thickness. Absorbers with many electrons are more impervious to radiation than absorbers with few electrons. Unfortunately, the number of electrons is usually expressed in the unit e/g (a mass unit) rather than e/cm³ (a volume unit). In order for the number of electrons per gram to have meaning, we must know the density of the material. Density determines the number of electrons that will be present in a given thickness, and this is what determines x-ray attenuation as we think of it in clinical radiology. By multiplying electrons per gram and density, we get electrons per cubic centimeter:

$$\frac{e}{g} \times \frac{g}{cm^3} = \frac{e}{cm^3}$$

Now we are talking about a unit we can understand. A cubic centimeter represents a thickness of 1 cm, and this is the unit we use to measure a patient's thickness.

Table 5–6 summarizes the relationships

Table 5–6. Comparison of Physical Characteristics of Air, Fat, Water, and Bone

	EFFECTIVE ATOMIC NUMBER	DENSITY (g/cm³)	ELECTRONS PER GRAM	ELECTRONS PER CUBIC CENTIMETER
Air	7.64	0.00129	3.01×10^{23}	0.0039×10^{23}
Fat	5.92	0.91	3.48×10^{23}	3.27×10^{23}
Water	7.42	1.00	3.34×10^{23}	3.34×10^{23}
Bone	13.8	1.85	3.0×10^{23}	5.55×10^{23}

between density, e/g, and e/cm³ for air, fat, water, and bone.

When Compton reactions predominate, the number of e/cm³ becomes the most important factor in attenuation so, even though bone has fewer e/g than water, bone still attenuates more radiation, because it has more e/cm³.

The number of electrons per gram can be calculated by the equation:

$$N_0 = \frac{NZ}{A}$$

N_0 = number of electrons per gram
N = Avogadro's number (6.02×10^{23})
Z = atomic number
A = atomic weight.

When comparing one element with another, we can disregard Avogadro's number, because it is a constant and affects all elements equally. The relative number of electrons per gram then becomes the simple ratio

$$\frac{Z}{A} \text{ or } \frac{\text{number of electrons}}{\text{weight of the atom}}$$

The weight of the atom is the sum of the weights of the protons and neutrons. The number of electrons and protons is equal, so the only factor that varies independently is the number of neutrons, which add mass without affecting the number of electrons. As the atomic number increases, the number of neutrons increases faster than the number of electrons. Hydrogen has no neutrons, and it has twice as many electrons per gram as any other element. Oxygen has one neutron per electron, and half as many electrons per gram as hydrogen. Lead has more neutrons than electrons, so it has

even fewer electrons per gram than oxygen. In general, the high atomic number elements have about 20% fewer electrons per gram than the low atomic number elements. Table 5–1 shows the number of electrons per gram for various elements important in diagnostic radiology.

POLYCHROMATIC RADIATION

The attenuation of polychromatic radiation is more complex than the attenuation of monochromatic radiation. Polychromatic beams contain a whole spectrum of photons of various energies (see Fig. 2–14), with the most energetic being determined by the peak kilovoltage (kVp) used to generate the beam. **In general, the mean energy of polychromatic radiation is between one-third and one-half of its peak energy.** A 100-kVp beam has a mean energy of approximately 40 kV. This will vary somewhat depending on filtration.

As polychromatic radiation passes through an absorber, the transmitted photons undergo a change in both quantity and quality. The number of photons decreases because some are deflected and absorbed out of the beam, just as they are with monochromatic radiation. In contrast to monochromatic radiation, however, the quality of the beam also changes because the lower energy photons are more readily attenuated than the higher energy photons. As the low-energy photons are removed from the beam, the mean energy of the remaining photons increases.

The attenuation of polychromatic radiation is shown in Figure 5–6. The x-ray beam begins with 1000 photons having a mean energy of 40 kV. The first centimeter

kVp = 100

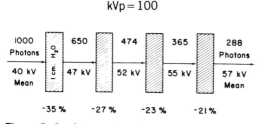

Figure 5–6   Attenuation of polychromatic radiation

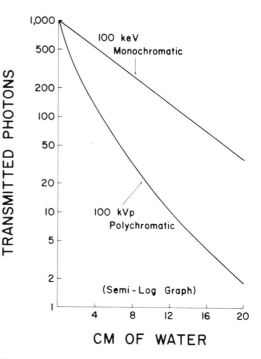

Figure 5–7   Comparison of the attenuation of polychromatic and monochromatic radiation

of absorber (water) reduces the number of photons by 35% and increases their mean energy to 47 kV. The second centimeter of water reduces the number of photons only 27%, because now the remaining photons are a little more energetic, and increases their mean energy to 52 kV. If the process is continued long enough, eventually the mean energy of the beam will approach its peak energy.

When the percentage of transmission of polychromatic radiation is plotted on semilogarithmic graph paper, it results in a curved line (Fig. 5–7). The initial slope of the curve is steep, because many low-energy photons are attenuated by the first few centimeters of water. Eventually, the slope of the curve becomes similar to the slope for a monochromatic beam as the mean energy of the polychromatic radiation approaches its peak energy.

APPLICATIONS TO DIAGNOSTIC RADIOLOGY

The photons in an x-ray beam enter a patient with a uniform distribution and emerge in a specific pattern of distribution. The transmitted photons carry the x-ray image, but their pattern also carries the memory of the attenuated photons. The transmitted and attenuated photons are equally important. If all photons were transmitted, the film would be uniformly black; if all photons were attenuated, the film would be uniformly white. In neither case would there be an x-ray image. Image formation depends on a differential attenuation between tissues. Some tissues attenuate more x rays than other tissues, and the size of this differential determines the amount of contrast in the x-ray image.

To examine differential attenuation we will consider a radiograph of a hand so we only have to discuss two tissue types, bone and soft tissue. Figure 5–8 shows the linear attenuation coefficients of compact bone and water. Water is used to represent the soft tissues. Remember, the higher the linear attenuation coefficient, the greater the attenuation. As you can see, x-ray attenuation is greater in bone than in water, so the bones show up as holes in the transmitted photon pattern. We see these holes as white areas on a film. With a 20-keV x-ray beam, water has a linear attenuation coefficient of 0.77 cm^{-1} and that of bone is 4.8 cm^{-1}. Bone has a greater linear attenuation coefficient by a factor of 6. With such a large differential, the x-ray image will display a great deal of contrast. At an x-ray beam energy of 100 keV, differential attenuation is not nearly as large. Bone still

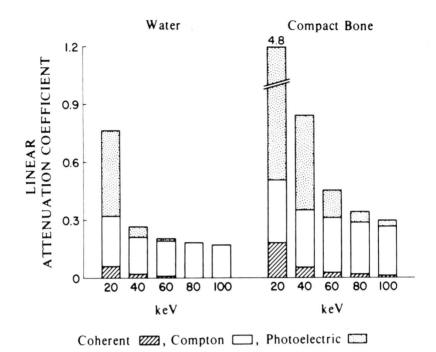

Coherent ▨, Compton ▭, Photoelectric ▢

Figure 5–8 Linear attenuation coefficients for water and compact bone

attenuates more x rays than water but now the difference is only by a factor of 0.6, so image contrast is considerably reduced.

Figure 5–8 illustrates another point. The total linear attenuation coefficient is actually made up of three separate coefficients, one for each of the basic interactions: coherent scattering, photoelectric effect, and Compton scattering. Each contributes its own component to the total linear attenuation coefficient. At low photon energies (20 keV) most of the difference in x-ray attenuation between bone and soft tisue results from a difference in the number of photoelectric reactions. More photoelectric reactions occur because bone contains calcium, which has a relatively high atomic number. At high photon energies (100 keV) the difference in x-ray attenuation between bone and soft tissues is almost entirely the result of the difference in the number of Compton reactions. Few photoelectric reactions occur in either bone or soft tissue at 100 keV. **When Compton reactions predominate, differential atten-uation is entirely dependent on differences in density.** The reason is that denser materials have more electrons available to undergo reactions.

Figure 5–9 shows the Compton linear attenuation coefficients for water, bone, and sodium iodide. The number of Compton reactions decreases only slightly with increasing x-ray energies. As the energy of an x-ray beam is increased from 20 to 100 keV, the Compton linear attenuation coefficient for bone decreases about 20% (while the photoelectric linear attenuation coefficient decreases more than 99%).

The shaded portion of Figure 5–9 shows the Compton mass attenuation coefficient. Remember, the mass attenuation coefficient indicates the amount of attenuation per gram, and it is not dependent on density. As you can see, a gram of water attenuates more x rays than a gram of either bone or sodium iodide by Compton reactions because water has more electrons per gram (it contains two atoms of hydrogen). Sodium iodide has even fewer electrons

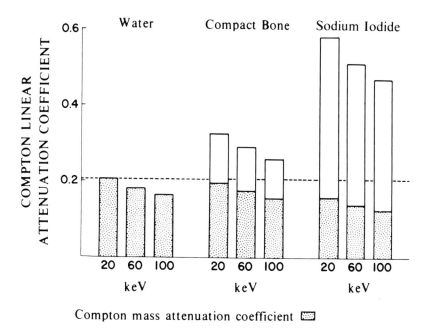

Compton mass attenuation coefficient ▨

Figure 5–9 Compton linear and mass attenuation coefficients for water, compact bone, and sodium iodide

per gram than bone because of the high atomic number of iodine, so a gram of sodium iodide attenuates fewer photons by Compton reactions than either a gram of water or bone. Nevertheless, even when Compton scattering is the only type of basic interaction, there is still a difference in x-ray attenuation between water, bone, and sodium iodide in favor of the higher atomic number absorber, but the difference is entirely dependent on density.

Fat and water are always difficult to differentiate radiographically. The effective atomic number of water (7.4) is slightly greater than that of fat (5.9), so they can be differentiated by photoelectric attenuation using low-energy techniques. With higher energy radiation, when Compton attenuation predominates, differentiation between fat and water depends on density and on the number of electrons per gram. Water has a greater density, but fewer electrons per gram. The net results, the number of electrons per cubic centimeter, are nearly the same for both water and fat (Table 5–6). Water has approximately 2%

more e/cm², which is too small a difference to demonstrate with only Compton reactions. A significant difference in attenuation between fat and water can only be demonstrated effectively using low-energy techniques.

SCATTER RADIATION

Our discussion of attenuation has only dealt with primary radiation, which either passes through the patient unchanged or is completely removed from the useful beam. The primary radiation carries the x-ray image. Now enters the villain, scatter radiation. It has nothing worthwhile to offer. Scatter radiation detracts from film quality and contributes no useful information.

How important is scatter radiation? How much of the density of an x-ray film is from scatter radiation? Several factors determine its importance. In most of our routine work it is important, frequently making up from 50 to 90% of the total number of photons emerging from the patient. The reason for the large number of scattered photons will be more apparent if we consider the fate of a diagnostic x-ray beam. With thick parts, such as the abdomen, only 1% of the photons in the initial beam reach the film. The rest are attenuated, the majority by Compton scattering. Fortunately, most of them do not reach the film. Nevertheless, those that reach the film make a major, and undesirable, contribution to total film blackening.

It would be more accurate to refer to all undesirable radiation as secondary radiation, which includes photons and electrons that might contribute to film fog. In actual practice, however, none of the electrons (photoelectric or recoil) have enough energy to reach the film, and the only characteristic radiation with sufficient energy to cause a problem occurs during contrast examinations with barium and iodine. The only secondary radiation of any significance comes from Compton scattering, and it has become common practice to refer to all undesirable radiation as scatter radiation, which is fairly accurate.

Factors Affecting Scatter Radiation

Three factors determine the quantity of scatter radiation. These are:
1. kilovoltage (kVp)
2. part thickness
3. field size.

Scatter radiation is maximum with high-kVp techniques, large fields, and thick parts and, unfortunately, is what we usually deal with in diagnostic radiology. We rarely have any control over part thickness and frequently must use large fields. The only variable we can control is kVp, but even here we have less control than we would like because patient doses increase sharply with low-kVp techniques.

Field size is the most important factor in the production of scatter radiation. A small x-ray field (usually called a narrow beam) irradiates only a small volume of tissue, so it generates only a small number of scattered photons. Most of them miss the film because they have a large angle of escape.

Figure 5–10 shows the angle of escape for a scattered photon originating at point P. As you can see, the escape angle is much larger than the narrow angle encompassed by the primary beam. Thus, the quantity of scatter radiation from a narrow beam is small to begin with, and most of it never reaches the plane of the film. For this reason, narrow beam attenuation is the method used to measure the attenuation of primary radiation, and the terms **narrow beam** and **primary** radiation are used synonymously.

As the x-ray field is enlarged, the quantity of scatter radiation increases rapidly at first, and then gradually tapers off until finally it reaches a plateau, or saturation point. A further increase in field size does not change the quantity of scatter radiation that reaches the film. The total number of scattered photons in the field increases, but the number that reaches any particular point on the film remains constant. For example, consider the central point of a circular field 4 cm in diameter. Scattered photons originating from the periphery of the field can easily penetrate 2 cm of tissue to reach the field's center. If the field is increased to a 30-cm circle, however, most scatter photons do not have sufficient range to penetrate the 15 cm of tissue between the field's margin and center. So, even though more scattered photons are generated in large fields, they do not increase the quantity reaching any particular area. The saturation point for scatter radiation occurs with a field approximately 30×30 cm, only a 12-in. square, which is not a large field for diagnostic radiology.

The quantity of scatter radiation reaches a saturation point with increasing **part thickness,** just as it does with increasing field size. The total number of scattered photons keeps increasing as the part becomes thicker, but photons originating in the upper layers of the patient do not have sufficient energy to reach the film. Unfortunately we have little control over part thickness and, except for the occasional use

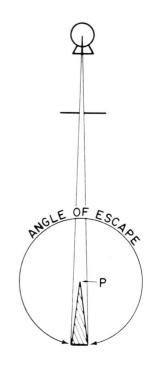

Figure 5–10   Angle of escape for scattered photons

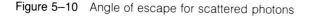

of a compressed band, we must accept the patient as he is.

The effect of **kilovoltage** (kVp) on the production of scatter radiation is probably not as important as part thickness, and certainly is not as important as field size. In the low-energy range (20 to 30 keV), in which the photoelectric effect predominates, extremely little scatter radiation is produced. As the radiation energy increases, the percentage of Compton reactions increases, and so does the production of scatter radiation. After Compton scattering becomes the predominant interaction, scatter radiation production tends to plateau, just as it does with increasing field size and part thickness. The energy of the point at which the plateau occurs depends on the atomic number of the tissue, but the plateau is not as well defined as it is with field size and part thickness. Even after Compton reactions predominate, the quantity of scatter radiation continues to increase with increasing beam energy because more photons scatter in the forward direction, and their greater energy allows them to penetrate greater thicknesses of tissue to reach the film.

Because we have so little control over the production of scatter radiation, we must find ways of keeping it from x-ray film after it has been generated. The most important of these is the x-ray grid, which we will discuss in Chapter 8.

SUMMARY

Attenuation is the reduction in the intensity of an x-ray beam as it traverses matter either by the absorption or deflection of photons from the beam. The attenuation of monochromatic radiation is exponential; that is, each layer of absorber attenuates the same percentage of the photons remaining in the beam. The attenuation of polychromatic radiation is not exponential. A large percentage of the low-energy photons are attenuated by the first few centimeters of absorber, so the quality (mean energy) of the remaining photons increases as the beam passes through an absorber.

The amount of attenuation depends on the energy of the radiation and three characteristics of the tissue: atomic number, density, and electrons per gram. Increasing the radiation energy increases the number of transmitted photons, while increasing the atomic number, density, or electrons per gram decreases transmission. Energy and atomic number together determine the relative percentage of photoelectric and Compton reactions. With low-energy radiation, and with high atomic number absorbers, a large amount of photoelectric attenuation is superimposed on a small background of Compton attenuation. As the energy of the radiation is increased, photoelectric attenuation diminishes, until the background of Compton attenuation is all that remains.

Density is one of the most important factors affecting attenuation, and radiographic image contrast is largely dependent on differences in tissue density. The high contrast between air and soft tissues occurs entirely because of density differences. The number of electrons per gram plays a lesser role. Generally, as the atomic number increases, the number of electrons per gram decreases, but the decrease is more than compensated by an even greater increase in density. Thus, high atomic number elements attenuate more radiation, even though they have fewer electrons per gram.

The amount of scatter radiation reaching an x-ray film increases with increasing field size, part thickness, and kilovoltage.

REFERENCE

1. Hubbell, J.H.: Photon Cross Sections, Attenuation Coefficients, and Energy Absorption Coefficients from 10 keV to 100 GeV. Washington, DC, U.S. Government Printing Office, National Bureau of Standards, Handbook 29, August 1969.

6

Filters

Filtration is the process of increasing the mean energy of polychromatic radiation by passing it through an absorber. Diagnostic x-ray beams are composed of photons that have a whole spectrum of energies; that is, they are polychromatic. Their mean energy is from one third to one half of their peak energy, so many photons fall in the lower energy range. As polychromatic radiation passes through a patient, most of the lower energy photons are absorbed in the first few centimeters of tissue, and only the higher energy photons penetrate through the patient to form the radiographic image. Because the patient's radiation dose is dependent on the number of absorbed photons, the first few centimeters of tissue receive much more radiation than the rest of the patient. This tissue can be protected by absorbing the lower energy photons from the beam before they reach the patient by interposing a filter material between the patient and the x-ray tube. Filters are usually sheets of metal, and their only function in diagnostic radiology is to reduce the patient's radiation dose.

In a radiologic examination the x-ray beam is filtered by absorbers at three different levels. Beginning at the x-ray source, these are as follows:

1. The x-ray tube and its housing (**inherent filtration**)
2. Sheets of metal placed in the path of the beam (**added filtration**)
3. The patient.

INHERENT FILTRATION

Filtration resulting from the absorption of x rays as they pass through the x-ray tube and its housing is called **inherent filtration.** The materials responsible for inherent filtration are the glass envelope enclosing the anode and cathode, the insulating oil surrounding the tube, and the window in the tube housing. Inherent filtration is measured in **aluminum equivalents,** which is the thickness of aluminum that would produce the same degree of attenuation as the thickness of the material in question. Table 6–1 shows the inherent filtration of a typical diagnostic x-ray tube. It usually varies between 0.5 and 1.0 mm aluminum equivalent, and the glass envelope is responsible for most of it.

In a few special circumstances, unfiltered radiation is desirable. Because filtration increases the mean energy of an x-ray beam, it decreases tissue contrast. The decrease is insignificant in the higher energy range but, with lower energy radiation, under 30 kVp, this loss of contrast may be detrimental to image quality. Beryllium window

Table 6–1. Inherent Filtration for a Typical Diagnostic X-Ray Tube

ABSORBER	THICKNESS (mm)	ALUMINUM EQUIVALENT (mm)
Glass envelope	1.40	0.78
Insulating oil	2.36	0.07
Bakelite window	1.02	0.05
Total		0.90

(From Trout, E.D.: The life history of an x-ray beam. Radiol. Technol., *35*:161, 1963.)

tubes are designed to produce an essentially unfiltered beam. The exit portal of the glass envelope is replaced with beryllium (atomic number 4), which is more transparent to low-energy radiation than glass. The radiation from these tubes has a minimum of inherent filtration, and it is excellent for soft tissue radiography, particularly mammography.

ADDED FILTRATION

Added filtration results from absorbers placed in the path of the x-ray beam. Ideally, a filter material should absorb all low-energy photons and transmit all high-energy photons. Unfortunately, no such material exists. A material can be selected, however, to absorb principally low-energy radiation by utilizing the proclivity of photoelectric attenuation for low-energy photons. Attenuation is most intense when the photoelectric effect is the predominant interaction and diminishes when Compton reactions predominate. The energy of the radiation filtered from the beam can be regulated by selecting a material with an appropriate atomic number. Aluminum and copper are the materials usually selected for diagnostic radiology. Aluminum, with an atomic number of 13, is an excellent filter material for low-energy radiation and a good general purpose filter. Copper, with an atomic number of 29, is a better filter for high-energy radiation. It is inconvenient to change filters between examinations, however, and there is a risk of forgetting to make the change. For practicality, most radiologists prefer to use a single filter material, usually aluminum.

Copper is never used by itself as the only filter material. It is always used in combination with aluminum as a **compound filter.** A compound filter consists of two or more layers of different metals. The layers are arranged so that the higher atomic number element, copper, faces the x-ray tube, and the lower atomic number element, aluminum, faces the patient. Most filtration occurs in the copper, and the pur-

pose of the aluminum is to absorb the characteristic radiation from copper. Photoelectric attenuation in copper produces characteristic radiation with an energy of about 8 keV, which is energetic enough to reach the patient and significantly increase skin doses. The aluminum layer absorbs this characteristic radiation. Its own characteristic radiation has so little energy (1.5 keV) that it is absorbed in the air gap between the patient and filter.

Compound filters of elements with atomic numbers even higher than that of copper have been developed for use in diagnostic radiology. These filters generally have photoelectric absorption K edges at energies of 30 to 50 keV, and can be used to alter radically the shape of the x-ray spectrum that reaches the patient. K edge filters are not yet in widespread clinical use, so we will not discuss them further here.

Filter Thickness

After selecting a filter material, usually aluminum, the next step is to determine the appropriate thickness for the filter. The percentages of x-ray attenuation with 1, 2, 3, and 10 mm of aluminum for photons of various energies are shown in Table 6–2. Two millimeters of aluminum absorb virtually all photons with energies less than 20 keV, so most of the advantages of filtration are achieved by this thickness. A filter of more than 3 mm thick aluminum offers no advantage; in fact, excess filtra-

Table 6–2. Percent Attenuation of Monochromatic Radiation by Various Thicknesses of Aluminum Filtration

PHOTON ENERGY (keV)	PHOTONS ATTENUATED (%)			
	1 mm	2 mm	3 mm	10 mm
10	100	100	100	100
20	58	82	92	100
30	24	42	56	93
40	12	23	32	73
50	8	16	22	57
60	6	12	18	48
80	5	10	14	39
100	4	8	12	35

tion has definite disadvantages. In Table 6–2, the column on the right shows the percentage of photons attenuated by 10 mm of aluminum, clearly excessive filtration. The effect is an overall attenuation of the beam, primarily by the absorption of high-energy photons, because all the low-energy photons have already been absorbed by thinner aluminum filters. The quality of the beam is not significantly altered, but its intensity is greatly diminished. This lengthens the time required to make an exposure, which increases the likelihood of the patient's moving during the examination.

The National Council on Radiation Protection and Measurements has recommended the following total filtration for diagnostic radiology.[1] The figures include both inherent and added filtration:

OPERATING kVp	TOTAL FILTRATION
Below 50 kVp	0.5 mm aluminum
50 to 70 kVp	1.5 mm aluminum
Above 70 kVp	2.5 mm aluminum

The effect of aluminum filtration on a 90-kVp polychromatic x-ray beam is shown graphically in Figure 6–1. The unfiltered beam is composed of a spectrum of photons, many of which have energies in the 10 to 20-keV range. The highest point in the curve occurs at 25 keV. Filtration reduces the total number of photons in the x-ray beam (area under the curve) but, more importantly, it selectively removes a large number of low-energy photons. The intensity on the low-energy side of the curve (*left*) is reduced considerably more than the intensity on the high-energy side of the curve (*right*), and the highest point in the curve is shifted from 25 to 35 keV. The overall effect is an increase in the mean energy of the x-ray beam.

Copper filters are always at least 0.25 mm thick, and they are backed with a 1.0-mm layer of aluminum. Thinner copper filters are not practical, because minor variations in thickness are difficult to eliminate, and produce a serious lack of uniformity in the transmitted radiation.

Effect of Filters on Patient Exposure

Trout and coworkers demonstrated the degree of patient protection afforded by filters with a series of tests, one of which is summarized in Table 6–3.[2] In this particular experiment, they made multiple radiographs of an 18-cm thick pelvic phantom using a 60-kVp x-ray beam. The initial radiograph was made without a filter and was then repeated with increasing thicknesses of aluminum filtration. Exposure times were adjusted to produce films of equal density, and the radiation dose to the skin over the pelvis was measured for each exposure. As you can see in Table 6–3, the decrease in patient exposure was remark-

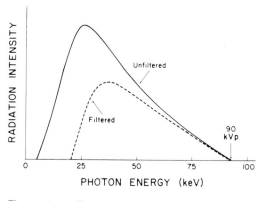

Figure 6–1 Energy and intensity of unfiltered and filtered polychromatic radiation

Table 6–3. Exposure Dose to the Skin for Comparable Density Radiographs of a Pelvic Phantom (18 cm Thick) With Various Thicknesses of Aluminum Filtration

ALUMINUM FILTRATION (mm)	60-kVp BEAM	
	EXPOSURE DOSE TO SKIN (mR)	DECREASE IN EXPOSURE DOSE (%)
None	2380	
0.5	1850	22
1.0	1270	47
3.0	465	80

(From Trout, E.D., Kelley, J.P., and Cathey, G.A.: The use of filters to control radiation exposure to the patient in diagnostic roentgenology. Am. J. Roentgenol., 67:942, 1952.)

able, up to 80% with 3 mm of aluminum filtration. These percentages are for a specific examination, but they should give you some insight into the degree of protection you can expect from adequate filtration.

Effect on Exposure Factors

The major disadvantage of filtration is a reduction in the intensity of the x-ray beam. Filters absorb some photons at all energy levels, and we must compensate for the loss of higher energy photons by increasing exposure factors, usually by increasing time. The percentage that the exposure time must be increased depends on the initial energy of the x-ray beam, as shown in Table 6–4. The table is based on one of the experiments of Trout and coworkers, in which they measured the percentage of increase in exposure time required to produce films of equal density with various thicknesses of aluminum filtration.[2] With low-energy radiation, represented by 60 kVp in Table 6–4, exposure time had to be increased up to 50% with 3 mm of aluminum but, with high-energy radiation, represented by 130 kVp in the

table, added filtration did not necessitate any increase in the exposure time. Even when it is necessary to increase exposure time because of filtration, the patient receives less radiation than he would from an unfiltered beam. The x-ray tube puts out more photons during longer exposures, but the filter absorbs many of them, and the total number reaching the patient actually decreases.

Wedge Filters

Wedge filters are occasionally used in diagnostic radiology to obtain films of more uniform density when the part being examined diminishes greatly in thickness from one side of the field to the other. The filter is shaped like a wedge. The relationship between the filter and patient is shown in Figure 6–2. When one side of the patient is considerably thicker than the other, the wedge compensates for the difference. Less radiation is absorbed by the thinner part of the filter, so more is available to penetrate the thicker part of the patient. Wedge filters have been used extensively in x-ray therapy, but their value has never been exploited in diagnostic radiology. They are occasionally used for lateral views of the pregnant abdomen in an attempt to obtain films of uniform density.

SUMMARY

Filters are sheets of metal placed in the path of the x-ray beam near the x-ray tube housing to absorb low-energy radiation before it reaches the patient. Their only function is to protect the patient from useless radiation, and they perform their function remarkably well, frequently reducing skin exposures by as much as 80%. Aluminum is usually selected as the filter material for diagnostic radiology. Most high-energy photons are transmitted through aluminum, while low-energy photons are absorbed by photoelectric interactions. The photoelectric effect selectively absorbs low-energy photons because of its dependence on energy and atomic number. The Na-

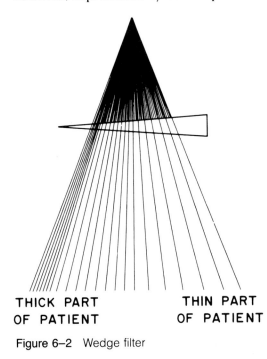

THICK PART OF PATIENT   **THIN PART OF PATIENT**

Figure 6–2   Wedge filter

Table 6–4. Exposure Times for Comparable Density Radiographs of a Pelvic Phantom (18 cm Thick) for Low- and High-Energy Radiation With Various Thicknesses of Aluminum Filtration

ALUMINUM FILTRATION (mm)	60 kVp · 100 mA		130 kVp · 100 mA	
	EXPOSURE TIME (seconds)	INCREASE IN EXPOSURE TIME (%)	EXPOSURE TIME (seconds)	INCREASE IN EXPOSURE TIME (%)
None	1.41		0.12	
0.5	1.61	14	0.12	0
1.0	1.64	17	0.12	0
3.0	2.14	52	0.12	0

(From Trout, E.D., Kelley, J.P., and Cathey, G.A.: The use of filters to control radiation exposure to the patient in diagnostic roentgenology. Am. J. Roentgenol., 67:942, 1952.)

tional Council on Radiation Protection and Measurement has recommended an equivalent of 2.5 mm of aluminum permanent filtration for diagnostic x-ray beams of energies greater than 70 kVp. Some higher energy useful photons are absorbed by filtration, and exposure factors must be increased to compensate for this loss. When filters are used in examinations employing lower energy radiation, exposure time may have to be increased up to 50%; with higher energy radiation, however, no ad-

justment in exposure factors is usually required. Filters are simple and inexpensive. Nowhere else in all of radiology do we gain so much for so little money.

REFERENCES

1. National Council on Radiation Protection and Measurements: Medical X-Ray and Gamma-Ray Protection for Energies up to 10 MeV. Washington, DC, U.S. Government Printing Office, Report No. 33, 1968.
2. Trout, E.D., Kelley, J.P., and Cathey, G.A.: The use of filters to control radiation exposure to the patient in diagnostic roentgenology. Am. J. Roentgen., 67, 942, 1952.

7

X-Ray Beam Restrictors

An x-ray beam restrictor is a device that is attached to the opening in the x-ray tube housing to regulate the size and shape of an x-ray beam. Beam restrictors can be classified into three categories:

1. aperture diaphragms
2. cones and cyclinders
3. collimators.

APERTURE DIAPHRAGMS

The simplest type of x-ray beam restrictor is an aperture diaphragm. It consists of a sheet of lead with a hole in the center, and the size and shape of the hole determine the size and shape of the x-ray beam. Its principal advantage is its simplicity. Lead is soft, so the aperture can be easily altered to any desired size or shape. The principal disadvantage of an aperture diaphragm is that it produces a fairly large penumbra at the periphery of the x-ray beam (Fig. 7–1A). The center of the x-ray field is exposed by the entire focal spot, but the periphery of the field (P in the illustration) "sees" only a portion of the focal spot; this partially exposed area is called the **penumbra.** The width of the penumbra can be reduced by positioning the aperture diaphragm as far away from the x-ray target as possible. This is usually accomplished by attaching the diaphragm to the end of a cone.

CONES AND CYLINDERS

The second type of x-ray beam restrictor comes in two basic shapes, conical and cylindric. The flared shape of a cone would seem to be the ideal geometric configuration for an x-ray beam restrictor but the flare of the cone is usually greater than the flare of the x-ray beam, in which case the base plate that attaches the device to the tube housing is the only part that restricts the x-ray beam (Fig. 7–1B). When used in this way, it is little more than an aperture diaphragm. Beam restriction with a cylinder takes place at the far end of the barrel, so there is less penumbra (Fig. 7–1C). Cylinders may be equipped with extensions to increase their length to give even better beam restriction. A major disadvantage of aperture diaphragms, cones, and cylinders is the severe limitation they place on the number of available field sizes. Even a large assortment cannot approach the infinite variety of field sizes needed in diagnostic radiology, and changing them is inconvenient.

COLLIMATORS

The collimator is the best all around x-ray beam restrictor. It has two advantages over the other types: (1) it provides an infinite variety of rectangular x-ray fields; (2) a light beam shows the center and exact configuration of the x-ray field. Two sets of shutters (S_1 and S_2) control the beam dimensions. They move together as a unit so that the second shutter aligns with the first to "clean up" its penumbra (Fig. 7–2). The shutters function as two adjustable aperture diaphragms. Each shutter consists of four or more lead plates (Fig. 7–3). These plates move in independent pairs.

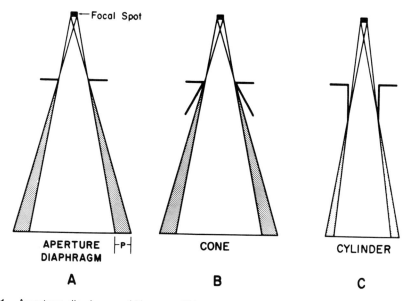

Figure 7–1   Aperture diaphragm (A), cone (B), and cylinder (C)

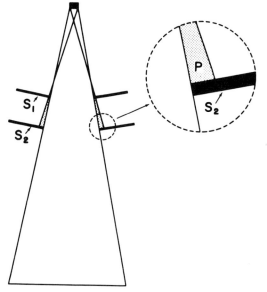

COLLIMATOR

Figure 7–2   Alignment of collimator shutters

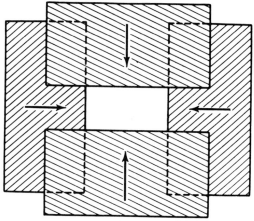

Figure 7–3   Collimator shutters (top view)

One pair can be adjusted without moving the other, which permits an infinite variety of square or rectangular fields. When the shutters are closed, they meet at the center of the x-ray field.

The x-ray field is illuminated by a light beam from a light bulb in the collimator. The light beam is deflected by a mirror mounted in the path of the x-ray beam at an angle of 45° (Fig. 7–4). The target of the x-ray tube and light bulb should be exactly the same distance from the center of the mirror. As the light beam passes through the second shutter opening, it is collimated to coincide with the x-ray beam. The distance from the mirror in the collimator to the target of the x-ray tube is critical. The collimator must be mounted so

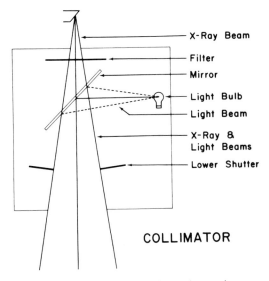

Figure 7–4   Alignment of light and x-ray beams

pose is to protect the patient from needless radiation.

Testing X-Ray Beam and Light Beam Alignment

The alignment of the x-ray beam and light beam should be checked periodically, because the mirror tends to get out of adjustment from daily use. The only equipment needed to test alignment includes four L-shaped wires (pieces of paper clips work nicely), a 14- to 17-in. x-ray film in a cassette, and a small lead letter "R." Place the film on the top of the x-ray table, open the collimator shutter to a convenient size (10 × 10 in.), carefully position the L-shaped wires at the corner of the light field, and place the "R" in the lower right corner. Then make an x-ray exposure (40 in., 3.3 mAs, 40 kVp) to mark the position of the x-ray field on the film. Without touching the film or wires, enlarge the field size to 12 × 12 in. and expose the film for the second time (same exposure factors).

Figure 7–5 shows a test film taken with a collimator whose mirror is out of adjustment. The dark center shows the position of the x-ray beam, and the wires indicate the position of the light beam. The second exposure (with an enlarged field) is made to ensure visibility of all the wires. The wire

that the x-ray target and light bulb are exactly the same distance from the center of the mirror. If the collimator is mounted too far from the x-ray target, the x-ray source will be further from the second shutter than the light source, and the x-ray beam will be smaller than the light beam.

A collimator can also identify the center of the x-ray field. This is accomplished by painting a cross line on a thin sheet of Plexiglas mounted on the end of the collimator. The light beam that illuminates the radiographic field also shows its center.

Collimators have a back-up system for identifying field size in case the light bulb should burn out. The x-ray field size for various target-film distances is indicated by a calibrated scale on the front of the collimator.

A federal regulation requires automatic collimators on all new x-ray installations. Automatic collimators are the same as other collimators except that their shutters are motor-driven by electronic sensors in the film holder. These sensors measure the film cassette and relay its size back to the collimator motor. The motor then positions the shutters to match the size of the x-ray field and cassette exactly. Their sole pur-

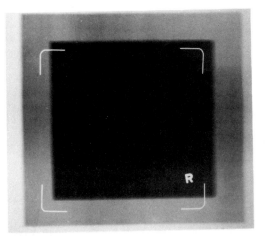

Figure 7–5   Test film of light and x-ray beam alignment

in the left lower corner of the illustration would not have been visible on the film without the second exposure.

To adjust a misaligned mirror, return the processed x-ray film to its original position on the x-ray table. The "R" in the lower right corner assists in orienting the film properly. Position the light beam to the images of the wires, as you did earlier for the film exposure, and adjust the mirror in the collimator until the light beam coincides exactly with the x-ray field (dark area on the film). Then repeat the test to make sure that the mirror adjustment has correctly aligned the light and x-ray beams.

FUNCTIONS OF RESTRICTORS

Collimators and other x-ray beam restrictors have two basic functions: to protect the patient and to decrease scatter radiation.

Although patient protection is the principal reason for using collimators today, it is interesting to note that the old-time radiologists restricted x-ray beams before they knew anything about the harmful effects of low doses of radiation. They used small fields because they obtained better films with small fields. Because they had no grids, their only means of controlling scatter radiation was to limit field size, so they collimated their x-ray beams and obtained excellent films.

Patient Protection

The mechanism by which collimators protect the patient is obvious; that is, the smaller the x-ray field, the smaller the volume of the patient that is irradiated. If a 20- × 20-cm field is collimated to 10 × 10 cm, the area of the patient that is irradiated decreases from 400 to 100 cm², a fourfold decrease in area and a corresponding decrease in volume. A decrease in field size is especially significant, because area is a square function. Trimming only a few centimeters off the edge of the field significantly decreases the exposed volume of the patient.

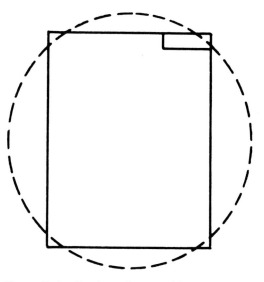

Figure 7–6 Overlap of a round field on a rectangular film

The ideal shape for a radiographic field for maximal patient protection has never been established. Initially, all x-ray beam restrictors were round (cones) and now they are usually square or rectangular (collimators). It was argued that x-ray films are rectangular. Round fields expose portions of the patient that are not even included on the film, as shown in Figure 7–6, so x-ray beam restrictors were made square. But the ideal field shapes should be dictated by the shape of the part being examined, and not by the shape of either the film or collimator. Some parts are better examined with round fields, such as gallbladders and paranasal sinuses. Certainly a circular field that is completely encompassed by the film is the most suitable shape when a round part is being examined.

Problems frequently arise, especially on board examinations, regarding beam restrictor sizes. These problems can be solved by setting up proportions between the comparable sides of similar triangles (Fig. 7–7). For example, if an aperture diaphragm (A) is 25 cm from the x-ray target, and the target film distance (B) is 100 cm, what size aperture (a) should be used to produce a 15-cm x-ray field (b) for a gallbladder ex-

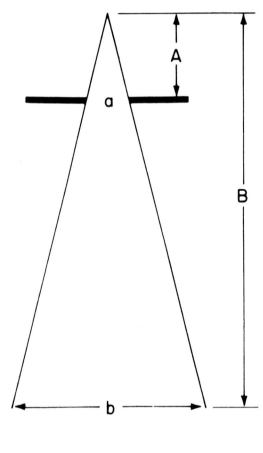

$$\frac{a}{b} = \frac{A}{B}$$

Figure 7–7 The sizes of the aperture and x-ray field are proportional to the target-aperture and target-film distances

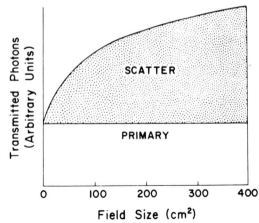

Figure 7–8 Transmitted radiation for various sizes of x-ray fields

amination? Using proportional triangles, the aperture hole should be

$$\frac{a}{15} = \frac{25}{100}, \text{ or } a = 15 \times \frac{25}{100} = 3.75 \text{ cm}$$

Decreased Scatter Radiation with Collimators

The quantity of scatter radiation reaching an x-ray film depends on field size; that is, the larger the field, the more scatter radiation. Figure 7–8 shows the general shape of the curves obtained when the number of transmitted primary and scat-

tered photons are plotted against field size. The exact contribution from scatter depends on the thickness of the part being examined and on the energy (kVp) of the x-ray beam. The amount of primary radiation at the plane of the film is independent of field size. The number of transmitted primary photons, per unit area, is the same for a 1- × 1-cm field and a 30- × 30-cm field, so the number of the primary photons in Figure 7–8 plots a straight line.

The number of scattered photons reaching the x-ray film depends on field size. Small x-ray fields generate little scatter radiation. As the field size is enlarged, the amount of scatter radiation increases rapidly at first, and then tapers off with larger fields. After the x-ray field reaches a size of about 30 × 30 cm, the total quantity of scatter radiation is near its maximum. Because collimators are only successful in decreasing scatter radiation with small fields, we should restrict the size of our x-ray beams as much as possible.

A final fact to remember about collimators is that they affect exposure factors. Small fields produce little scatter radiation, so the total quantity of blackening of the x-ray film decreases as the field size decreases. To keep film density constant, as you decrease the size of the x-ray field you must increase the exposure factors.

SUMMARY

There are three types of x-ray beam restrictors: aperture diaphragms, cones (cylinders), and collimators. Their basic function is to regulate the size and shape of the x-ray beam. Closely collimated beams have two advantages over larger beams. First, a smaller area of the patient is exposed and, because area is a square function, a decrease of one half in x-ray beam diameter effects a fourfold decrease in patient exposure. Second, well-collimated beams generate less scatter radiation and thus improve film quality. By decreasing the amount of scatter radiation, collimators also affect exposure factors. As the x-ray field size is decreased, the exposure factors must be increased to maintain a constant film density.

Collimators are the best general-purpose beam restrictors. They offer two advantages over the other types: the x-ray field is illuminated, which permits accurate localization on the patient; and the x-ray field can be adjusted to an infinite variety of rectangular shapes and sizes.

8

Grids

The radiographic grid consists of a series of lead foil strips separated by x-ray transparent spacers. It was invented by Dr. Gustave Bucky in 1913, and it is still the most effective way of removing scatter radiation from large radiographic fields. Figure 8–1 shows how a grid functions. Primary radiation is oriented in the same axis as the lead strips and passes between them to reach the film unaffected by the grid. Scatter radiation arises from many points within the patient and is multidirectional, so most of it is absorbed by the lead strips and only a small amount passes between them.

The interspaces of grids are filled either with aluminum or some organic compound. The main purpose of the interspace material is to support the thin lead foil strips. Aluminum interspace grids can probably be manufactured more precisely, and they are structurally stronger than grids with organic interspacers. Patient exposures are higher with aluminum because it absorbs more primary radiation. It also absorbs more secondary radiation, however, so contrast improvement is probably better. At the present time both materials are used, and there is no clear-cut differentiation as to which is better.

TERMINOLOGY

Grid ratio is defined as the ratio between the height of the lead strips and the distance between them. Figure 8–2 is a cross-sectional scale drawing of a grid with a ratio of 8:1. The lead strips are approximately 0.05 mm thick, so that they may appropriately be considered lead foil. The interspaces are much thicker than the lead strips. Grid ratios are usually expressed as two numbers, such as 10:1, with the first number the actual ratio and the second number always 1. The grid ratio is a parameter widely used to express a grid's ability to remove scatter radiation. Ratios usually range from 4:1 to 16:1. Generally, the higher the ratio, the better the grid functions. Grid ratios are indicated on the top of grids by manufacturers.

Grid pattern refers to the orientation of the lead strips in their longitudinal axis. It

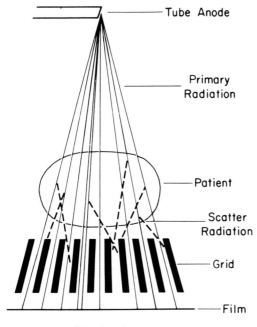

Figure 8–1 Grid function

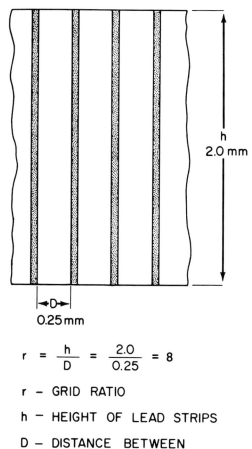

$$r = \frac{h}{D} = \frac{2.0}{0.25} = 8$$

r – GRID RATIO

h – HEIGHT OF LEAD STRIPS

D – DISTANCE BETWEEN
LEAD STRIPS

Figure 8–2 Cross section of a grid

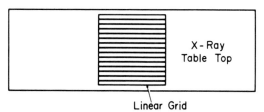

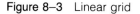

Figure 8–3 Linear grid

is the pattern of the grid that we see from a top view. The two basic grid patterns are linear and crossed.

In a **linear grid** the lead strips are parallel to each other in their longitudinal axis (Fig. 8–3). Most x-ray tables are equipped with linear grids. Their major advantage is

that they allow us to angle the x-ray tube along the length of the grid without loss of primary radiation from grid "cutoff."

A **crossed grid** is made up of two superimposed linear grids that have the same focusing distance (Fig. 8–4). The grid ratio of crossed grids is equal to the sum of the ratios of the two linear grids. A crossed grid made up of two 5:1 linear grids has a ratio of 10:1, and functions about the same as a linear grid with a 10:1 ratio. Crossed grids cannot be used with oblique techniques requiring angulation of the x-ray tube, and this is their biggest disadvantage.

A **focused grid** is a grid made up of lead strips that are angled slightly so that they focus in space (Fig. 8–5). A focused grid may be either linear or crossed, because the focusing refers to the cross-sectional plane of the lead strips. Most grids are focused. Linear focused grids converge at a line in space called the **convergent line.** Crossed grids converge at a point in space called the **convergent point.** The **focal distance** is the perpendicular distance between the grid and the convergent line or point. In practice, grids have a focusing range that indicates the distance within which the grid can be used without a significant loss of

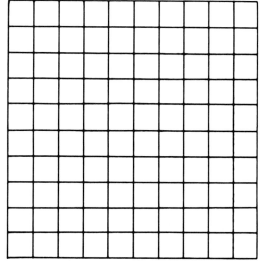

Figure 8–4 Crossed grid

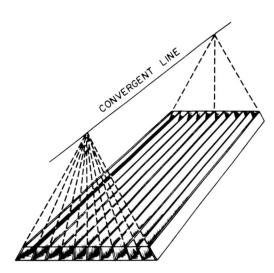

Figure 8–5 Focused linear grid

primary radiation. The **focusing range** is fairly wide for a low-ratio grid and narrow for a high-ratio grid. A 5:1 grid focused at 40 in. has a focusing range of approximately 28 to 72 in., while a 16:1 grid focused at 40 in. has a range of only 38 to 42 in. Focal ranges are indicated on the top of grids by manufacturers.

A **parallel grid** is one in which the lead strips are parallel when viewed in cross section. They are focused at infinity, so they do not have a convergent line. These grids can only be used effectively with either very small x-ray fields or long target-grid distances. They are frequently used in fluoroscopic spot film devices, but otherwise have little use in modern radiology.

Lines per inch is the number of lead strips per inch of grid. It can be calculated by adding the thickness of the lead strips and interspaces and dividing this sum into 1. Because the thickness of the lead strips and interspaces is usually expressed in millimeters, the answer must be multiplied by 25.4, which is the number of mm/in. The final equation is

$$\text{Lines/in.} = \frac{25.4}{D + d}$$

D = thickness of interspaces
d = thickness of lead strips
    (both in millimeters).

A grid (grid-front) cassette is a special x-ray cassette, usually used for portable radiography, with a grid built into the front of the cassette. Most grid cassettes are focused and have a fairly low grid ratio (4:1 to 8:1).

EVALUATION OF GRID PERFORMANCE

Grids are used to improve contrast by absorbing secondary radiation before it reaches the film. The "ideal grid" would absorb all secondary radiation and no primary radiation. It would give maximum film contrast without an unnecessary increase in patient exposure. The ideal grid does not exist, however, and the design of all grids is a compromise. The price of better film contrast is increased patient exposure. We must always compromise one for the other. Grids with high ratios give maximum contrast, but the improved contrast is not always worth the increased patient exposure. In every clinical situation we must weigh these two factors. To help in grid selection and design, several tests have been devised to evaluate grid performance. These tests also help us understand the way a grid functions. We will discuss three methods of evaluating performance:

1. primary transmission (Tp)
2. Bucky factor (B)
3. contrast improvement factor (K).

Primary Transmission

Primary transmission is a measurement of the percentage of primary radiation transmitted through a grid. Ideally, a grid should transmit 100% of the primary radiation, because it carries the radiographic image. The equipment for measuring primary transmission is shown in Figure 8–6. The x-ray beam is collimated to a narrow pencil of radiation, and the phantom is placed a great distance from the grid. With this arrangement, no scatter radiation reaches the grid. A small amount is pro-

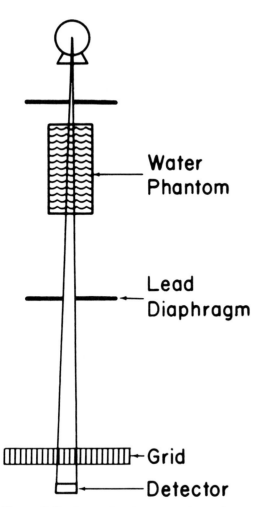

Figure 8–6 Apparatus for measuring primary transmission (Tp)

sion, which is multiplied by 100 to give the percentage of transmission:

$$T_p = \frac{I_p}{I'_p} \times 100$$

T_p = primary transmission (%)
I_p = intensity with grid
I'_p = intensity without grid.

Table 8–1 shows the primary transmission for eight different grids. There is a significant loss of primary radiation with grids. For the eight grids tested, the primary transmission varied between 57 and 72.5%, and was generally lower for cross grids.

The primary transmission as measured experimentally is less than would be anticipated. If the geometric relationship between the lead strips and the x-ray target is accurate, so that there is no grid cutoff, and if no primary radiation is absorbed in the interspaces, then the percentage of the grid's surface area that is made up of interspaces will be the percentage of anticipated primary transmission. This merely determines the percentage of the grid surface area that is not lead, and is as close as we will ever come to an ideal grid. The equation for calculating the anticipated primary transmission is

$$\text{Calc. Tp} = \frac{D}{D + d} \times 100$$

Tp = anticipated primary transmission (%)
d = thickness of lead strips
D = thickness of interspaces.

The measured primary transmission is always less than the calculated primary transmission.

The example in Figure 8–7 will help to demonstrate the magnitude of this difference. The dimensions are for grid number 8, shown in boldface in Table 8–1, which is a 15:1 grid with an experimentally determined primary transmission at 64%. Its lead strips are 60 μ thick and its interspaces are 390 μ wide. The calculated primary transmission is 87%, which is 23% more than the measured primary transmission. The difference is largely the result of ab-

duced in the phantom, but it diffuses out of the beam in the large air-gap between the phantom and the grid.

Two measurements must be made to determine the percentage of primary transmission. The first measurement is made with the grid in place to determine the intensity of the radiation transmitted through the grid, and the second measurement is made after removal of the grid to determine the intensity of the radiation directed at the grid. A simple ratio of the intensity with the grid to the intensity without the grid gives the fractional transmis-

Table 8–1. Primary Transmission (Tp)

GRID NO.	GRID RATIO	LEAD STRIP THICKNESS, d (μ)	INTERSPACE THICKNESS, D (μ)	PRIMARY TRANSMISSIONS (μ)
1	3.4	50	320	67.5
2	2 × 3.1*	50	350	57
3	11	30	220	69
4	7	60	290	72.5
5	6	80	370	72.5
6	9	50	380	67
7	2 × 7*	50	370	72.5
8	**15**	**60**	**390**	**64**

(Modified from Hondius Boldingh.[1])
*Crossed grids

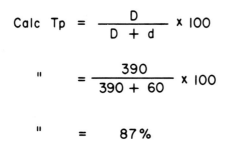
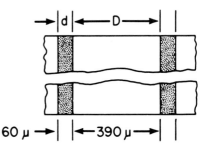

$$\text{Calc } Tp = \frac{D}{D + d} \times 100$$

$$" = \frac{390}{390 + 60} \times 100$$

$$" = 87\%$$

Figure 8–7 Anticipated primary transmission

sorption by the interspace material. Also, there is probably some loss in primary radiation because of manufacturing imperfections in the focusing of the lead strips.

Bucky Factor

The Bucky factor is the ratio of the incident radiation falling on the grid to the transmitted radiation passing through the grid. It is a practical determination, because it indicates how much we must increase exposure factors when we change from a nongrid to a grid technique. It also tells us how much the patient's exposure dose is increased by the use of a grid. The Bucky factor is similar to primary transmission except for one difference. Primary transmission indicates only the amount of primary radiation absorbed by a grid, while the Bucky factor indicates the absorption of both primary and secondary radiation. It is determined with a large x-ray field and a thick phantom (Fig. 8–8). The transmitted radiation is measured with the grid in place, and the incident radiation is meas-

ured after the grid has been removed. The equation for calculating the Bucky factor (B) is

$$B = \frac{\text{incident radiation}}{\text{transmitted radiation}}$$

The Bucky factor is a measure of the total quantity of radiation absorbed from an x-ray beam by a grid so, in part, it is a measure of the grid's ability to absorb scatter radiation. Table 8–2 shows the Bucky factors for several different grids with two different energies of radiation. Generally, high-ratio grids absorb more scatter radiation and have larger Bucky factors than low-ratio grids. The size of the Bucky factor also depends on the energy of the x-ray beam. High-energy beams generate more scatter radiation and place a greater demand on a grid's performance than low-energy radiation. The Bucky factor for the 16:1 grid in Table 8–2 increases from 4.5 to 6 as the radiation energy increases from 70 to 120 kVp. More scatter radiation is generated by the 120-kVp beam, and the

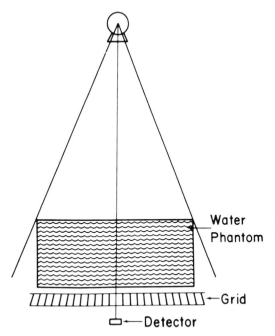

Figure 8–8 Apparatus for measuring the Bucky factor

Table 8–2. Bucky Factor (B)

GRID RATIO	70 kVp	120 kVp
No grid	1	1
5:1	3	3
8:1	3.5	4
12:1	4	5
16:1	4.5	6

16:1 grid successfully absorbs it. The 5:1 grid in Table 8–2, however, is not as efficient. Its Bucky factor is the same for both 70- and 120-kVp radiation. Low-ratio grids do not absorb scatter radiation from high-energy beams as well as high-ratio grids.

Although a high Bucky factor is desirable from the point of view of film quality, it is undesirable in two other respects. **The higher the Bucky factor, the greater the exposure factors and radiation dosage to the patient.** If the Bucky factor for a particular grid-energy combination is 5, then exposure factors and patient exposure both increase 5 times over what they would be for the same examination without a grid.

Contrast Improvement Factor

The contrast improvement factor (K) is the ratio of the contrast with a grid to the contrast without a grid:

$$K = \frac{\text{contrast with a grid}}{\text{contrast without a grid}}$$

This is the ultimate test of grid performance because it is a measure of a grid's ability to improve contrast, which is its primary function.

Unfortunately, the contrast improvement factor is dependent on kVp, field size, and phantom thickness. This is understandable, because these three factors determine the amount of scatter radiation. The larger the quantity of scatter radiation, the poorer the contrast, and the lower the contrast improvement factor. To permit comparison of different grids, the contrast improvement factor is usually determined at 100 kVp with a large field and a phantom 20 cm thick, as recommended by the International Commission on Radiologic Units and Measurements.[3] Table 8–3 shows the contrast improvement factor for eight different grids. It is more closely related to the lead content of the grid than any other factor. Generally, the higher the grid ratio, the higher the contrast improvement factor, but grid ratio is not as reliable an indicator as lead content.

Although the contrast improvement factor of a particular grid is dependent on kVp, field size, and part thickness, the relative quality of two grids appears to be in-

Table 8–3. Contrast Improvement Factor (K)

GRID NO.	GRID RATIO	LEAD CONTENT (mg/cm²)	CONTRAST IMPROVEMENT FACTOR (K)
1	3.4	170	1.95
2	2 × 3.1*	310	1.95
3	11	340	2.1
4	7	390	2.1
5	9	460	2.35
6	15	460	2.6
7	2 × 7*	680	2.95
8	15	900	2.95

(Modified from Hondius Boldingh.[1])
*Crossed grids.

dependent of these factors. A grid that has a high contrast improvement factor at 100 kVp will have a high factor at 50 or 130 kVp. In comparing two grids, the one that performs better with low-energy radiation will also perform better with high-energy radiation.

LEAD CONTENT

The lead content of a grid is expressed in g/cm². An easy way to understand what this means is to imagine cutting a grid up into 1-cm squares and then weighing one square. Its weight in grams is the lead content of the grid (ignoring the interspace material). The amount of lead in a grid is a good indicator of its ability to improve contrast, provided the grid is well designed. Poor design would be a solid sheet of lead.

There is a definite relationship between the grid ratio, lead content, and number of lines per inch (Fig. 8–9). If the grid ratio remains constant and the number of lines per inch is increased, the lead content must decrease. The only ways to increase the number of lines per inch is by decreasing the thickness of either the lead strips or interspaces. If the lead strips are made thinner, as in Figure 8–9B, compared to Figure 8–9A, the number of lines per inch increases without affecting grid ratio, because the thickness of lead strips is not considered in determining grid ratio. When the lead strips are made thinner, however, there is only a small increase in the number of lines per inch at a cost of a large decrease in lead content. If the number of lines per inch is increased by decreasing the width of the interspaces, as in Figure 8–9C, then the lead strips must be made shorter to keep the grid ratio constant and, again, the lead content of the grid decreases. This puts a limitation on the number of lines per inch a grid may have and still be effective. If a 10:1 grid could be constructed

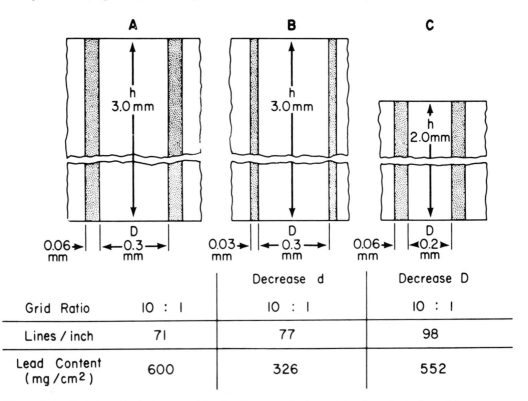

	A	Decrease d B	Decrease D C
Grid Ratio	10 : 1	10 : 1	10 : 1
Lines / inch	71	77	98
Lead Content (mg/cm²)	600	326	552

Figure 8–9 Relationship between grid ratio, lines per inch, and lead content of a grid

with 1000 lines per inch, it would be only 0.2 mm thick, and it would have too little lead to be of any real value.

In practice, when grids are constructed with many lines per inch, both the thickness and height of the lead strips are decreased. These grids are thinner, and improve contrast less than grids of comparable ratios with fewer lines per inch. A 133-line 10:1 grid improves contrast about the same as an 80-line 8:1 grid.

GRID CUTOFF

The primary disadvantage of grids is that they increase the amount of radiation that the patient receives. Another disadvantage is that they require careful centering of the x-ray tube because of the danger of grid cutoff. Grid cutoff is the loss of primary radiation that occurs when the images of the lead strips are projected wider than they would be with ordinary magnification (Fig. 8–10). It is the result of a poor geometric relationship between the primary beam and the lead foil strips of the grid. Cutoff is complete and no primary radiation reaches the film when the projected images of the lead strips are thicker

than the width of the interspaces. The resultant radiograph will be light in the area in which the cutoff occurs. With linear grids there may be uniform lightening of the whole film, one edge of the film, or both edges of the film, depending on how the cutoff is produced. The amount of cutoff is always greatest with high-ratio grids and short grid-focus distances. There are four situations that produce grid cutoff:

1. focused grids used upside down;
2. lateral decentering (grid angulation);
3. focus-grid distance decentering; and
4. combined lateral and focus-grid distance decentering.

Upside Down Focused Grid

All focused grids have a tube side, which is the side of focus of the lead strips. When a focused grid is used upside down, there is severe peripheral cutoff with a dark band of exposure in the center of the film and no exposure at the film's periphery. Figure 8–11A illustrates how cutoff occurs, and Figure 8–11B shows the resultant radiograph. The higher the grid ratio, the narrower the exposed area. When a crossed grid is used upside down, only a small square in the center of the film is exposed.

Lateral Decentering

Lateral decentering results from the x-ray tube being positioned lateral to the convergent line but at the correct focal distance (Fig. 8–12A). All the lead strips cut off the same amount of primary radiation, so there is **a uniform loss of radiation over the entire surface of the grid, producing a uniformly light radiograph.** This is probably the most common kind of grid cutoff, but it cannot be recognized by inspection of the film. All we see is a light film that is usually attributed to incorrect exposure factors. Figure 8–12B shows a series of film strips that were all taken with the same exposure factors, but with increasing amounts of lateral decentering. The x-ray tube was centered at the convergent line

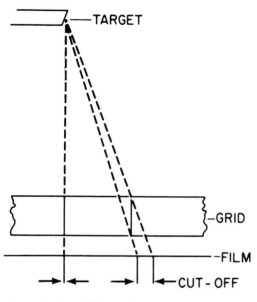

Figure 8–10 Grid cutoff

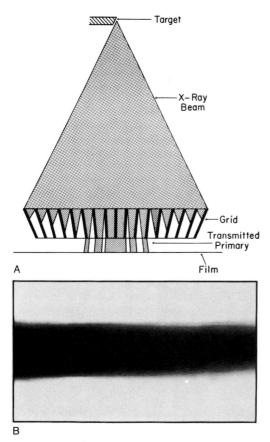

Figure 8–11 Cutoff from an upside down focused grid (A) and radiograph resulting from an upside down focused grid (B)

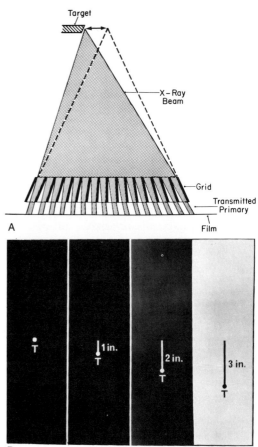

Figure 8–12 Cutoff from lateral decentering, (A) and series of radiographs resulting from increasing amounts of lateral decentering (B)

for the film strip on the left, and then laterally decentered 1, 2, and 3 in. for the next three strips. The films become progressively lighter as the amount of lateral decentering increases, but the exposure is still uniform. The center and both edges of the film are equally exposed, and it's impossible to recognize the cutoff from inspection of the film.

Three factors affect the magnitude of cutoff from lateral decentering: grid ratio, focal distance, and the amount of decentering. The equation for calculating the loss of primary radiation with lateral decentering is

$$L = \frac{rb}{f_0} \times 100$$

L = loss of primary radiation (%)
r = grid ratio
b = lateral decentering distance (inches)
f_0 = focal distance of grid (inches).

The amount of cutoff increases as the grid ratio and decentering distance increase, and cutoff decreases as the focal distance increases (Tables 8–4 and 8–5). The loss of primary radiation for any given amount of lateral decentering can be minimized with low-ratio grids and a long focal distance. With a 5:1 grid focused at 72

Table 8–4. Loss of Primary Radiation from Lateral Decentering for Grids Focused at 40 Inches

GRID RATIO	LOSS OF PRIMARY RADIATION (%)					
	LATERAL DECENTERING (in.)					
	1	2	3	4	5	6
5:1	13	25	38	50	63	75
6:1	15	30	45	60	75	90
8:1	20	40	60	80	100	
10:1	25	50	75	100		
12:1	30	60	90	100		
16:1	40	80	100			

Table 8–5. Loss of Primary Radiation from Lateral Decentering for Grids Focused at 72 Inches

GRID RATIO	LOSS OF PRIMARY RADIATION (%)					
	LATERAL DECENTERING (in.)					
	1	2	3	4	5	6
5:1	7	14	21	28	35	42
6:1	8	17	25	33	42	50
8:1	11	22	33	45	56	67
10:1	14	28	42	56	70	83
12:1	17	33	50	67	83	100
16:1	22	45	67	90	100	

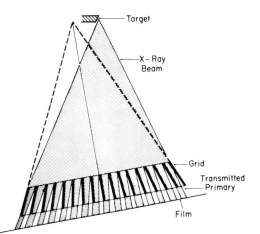

Figure 8–13 Cutoff from an off-level grid

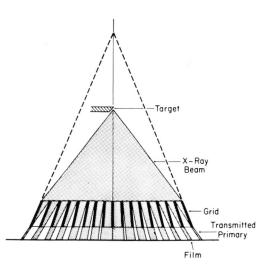

Figure 8–14 Cutoff from near focus-grid distance decentering

inches, there is a 14% loss of primary radiation with 2 inches of lateral decentering. If the grid ratio is increased to 16:1, the loss of primary radiation increases to 45%, and if the focal distance is then decreased to 40 inches, the loss of primary radiation goes up to 80%. When exact centering is not possible, as in portable radiography, low-ratio grids and long focal distances should be used whenever possible. It takes 8 inches of lateral decentering for 100% cutoff of primary radiation with a 5:1 grid focused at 72 inches, while it takes only 2.5 inches of lateral decentering for complete cutoff with a 16:1 grid focused at 40 inches.

Off-Level Grids

When a linear grid is tilted, as it frequently is in portable radiography, there is a uniform loss of primary radiation across the entire surface of the grid (Fig. 8–13). The effect on the film is the same as the effect of lateral decentering.

Focus-Grid Distance Decentering

In focus-grid distance decentering, the target of the x-ray tube is correctly centered to the grid, but it is positioned above or below the convergent line. If the target is above the convergent line, it is called **far** focus-grid distance decentering; if the target is below the convergent line, it is called **near** focus-grid distance decentering. The results are the same, but they differ in magnitude. The cutoff is greater with near than with far focus-grid distance decentering. Figures 8–14 and 8–15 show the cutoff be-

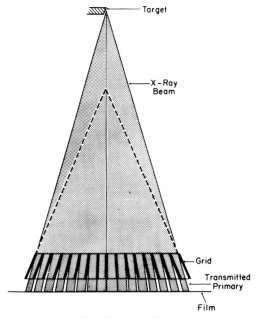

Figure 8–15   Cutoff from far focus-grid distance decentering

coming progressively greater with increasing distance from the film center. The central portion of the film is not affected, but the periphery is light. Because the fractional loss of radiation is not uniform, it must be calculated for a point, which actually represents two parallel lines running the length of the grid on either side of the center line. The loss of primary radiation is directly proportional to the grid ratio and distance from the center line.

The equations for calculating the loss of primary radiation for near and far focus-grid distance decentering are as follows:

Near Focus-Grid Distance Decentering	Far Focus-Grid Distance Decentering

$$L = rc\left(\frac{1}{f_1} - \frac{1}{f_0}\right) \times 100 \qquad L = rc\left(\frac{1}{f_0} - \frac{1}{f_2}\right) \times 100$$

  L = loss of primary radiation
        at point c (%)
  r = grid ratio
  f_0 = grid focusing distance
  f_1 = target-grid distance (below
        convergent line; inches),
  f_2 = the target-grid distance (above
        convergent line; inches)
  c = distance from center of grid (inches).

Table 8–6 shows the extent of cutoff at various distances from the center of grids focusing at 40 inches with a 10-inch focus-grid distance decentering error. The left half of the table indicates near (30 inches) and the right half far (50 inches) focus-grid distance decentering. The loss of primary radiation increases as the grid ratio increases and as the distance from the center of the grid increases; the loss is greater with near than with far focus-grid distance decentering. At the margin of a 14-inch wide film (7 inches from grid center), the loss of primary radiation is 35% for a 6:1 grid and 94% for a 16:1 grid with near focus-grid distance decentering. With far focus-grid distance decentering, the loss at the film margin decreases to 21% for a 6:1 grid and 64% for a 16:1 grid.

Parallel grids are focused at infinity so, of course, they are always used with near focus-grid distance decentering (Fig. 8–16). They usually have a low grid ratio to minimize cutoff. The only time there is no significant cutoff is with long target-grid distances or small fields. A film taken with a parallel grid has a dark center and light edges because of near focus-grid distance decentering.

Combined Lateral and Focus-Grid Distance Decentering

The most commonly recognized kind of grid cutoff is from combined lateral and focus-grid distance decentering. It is probably not as common as lateral decentering alone, but lateral decentering cannot be recognized as such on the resultant radiograph. Combined decentering is easy to recognize. It causes an uneven exposure, resulting in a film that is light on one side and dark on the other side. There are two kinds of combined decentering, depending on whether the tube target is above or below the convergent line. The amount of cutoff is directly proportional to the grid ratio and decentering distance, and inversely proportional to the focal distance of the grid. With high-ratio grids and large

Table 8–6. Loss of Primary Radiation from Near and Far Focus-Grid Distance Decentering for a Grid Focused at 40 Inches

	LOSS OF PRIMARY RADIATION (%)							
	TARGET AT 30 in.				TARGET AT 50 in.			
GRID RATIO	DISTANCE FROM GRID CENTER (in.)				DISTANCE FROM GRID CENTER (in.)			
	1	3	5	7	1	3	5	7
6:1	5	15	25	35	3	9	15	21
8:1	7	20	33	47	4	12	20	28
10:1	8	25	42	58	5	15	25	35
12:1	10	30	50	70	6	18	30	42
16:1	13	40	66	94	8	32	48	64

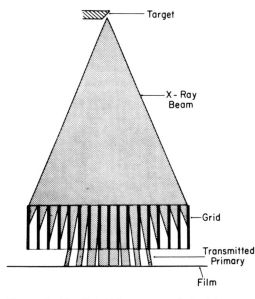

Figure 8–16 Cutoff from a parallel grid

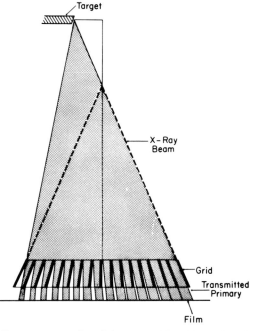

Figure 8–17 Cutoff from combined lateral and far focus-grid distance decentering

decentering errors, there is a large loss of primary radiation. With long focus-grid distances, there is less loss of primary radiation.

Combined lateral and focus-grid distance decentering above the convergent line is illustrated in Figure 8–17. The projected images of the lead strips directly below the tube target are broader than those on the opposite side, and the film is light on the near side. Cutoff is greatest on the side directly under the x-ray tube. Combined lateral and focus-grid distance decentering below the convergent line is illustrated in Figure 8–18. The projected images of the lead strips are broader on

the side opposite the tube target than on the same side, and the film is light on the far side. Cutoff is least on the side under the x-ray tube. With equal decentering errors the amount of cutoff is greater with combined decentering below the convergent line than with combined decentering above the convergent line.

MOVING GRIDS

The moving grid was invented by Dr. Hollis E. Potter in 1920 and, for many years, a moving grid was called a Potter-

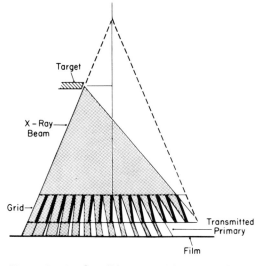

Figure 8–18 Cutoff from combined lateral and near focus-grid distance decentering

too slowly, you will see either the grid lines themselves or random density variations in the film that are just as distracting as the lines. Second, the transverse motion of the grid should be synchronous with the pulses of the x-ray generator. When this happens, the shadow of each lead strip is superimposed on the shadow of its neighbor. Each pulse produces a faint image of the lead strip on the film. Between pulses, the grid moves one interspace distance so that the next lead strip is over the position of the preceding strip and, with a new pulse, the two images are superimposed. Thus, even though the grid moves, the grid lines will be distinct.

Moving grids have several disadvantages. They are costly, subject to failure, may vibrate the x-ray table, and put a limit on the minimum exposure time because they move slowly. An even more serious disadvantage is that they increase the patient's radiation dose. There are two reasons for this, the first of which is lateral decentering. Because the grid moves 1 to 3 cm during the exposure, the tube is not centered directly over the center of the grid during most of the exposure. This lateral decentering may result in a loss of as much as 20% of the primary radiation with a high-ratio grid and a short focusing distance.

The second cause of increased patient exposure is more difficult to understand. The photons are spread out uniformly on the film by a moving grid. With the identical number of photons per unit area, a film is 15% darker with a stationary grid because the photons are concentrated be-

Bucky grid. In recent years the name has been shortened to Bucky grid, which is unfortunate, because the name of the inventor is omitted. Grids are moved to blur out the shadows cast by the lead strips. Most moving grids are reciprocating, which means they continuously move 1 to 3 cm back and forth throughout the exposure. They start moving when the x-ray tube anode begins to rotate. Older grids move only in one direction and must be cocked for each exposure. They also have timers that are set for a little longer than the exposure time to avoid grid lines. These single-stroke grids are inconvenient, and are seldom used in modern equipment.

Moving grids are advantageous because they eliminate grid lines from the film. Many years ago this was important, because the lead strips were thick and unevenly spaced. With improved manufacturing methods, however, grids have improved so that grid lines are not nearly as distracting, and many radiologists now prefer stationary grids.

If you are using a moving grid and want to avoid grid lines, you must take two precautions. First, the grid must move fast enough to blur its lead strips. If it moves

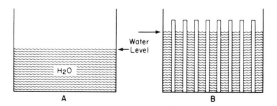

Figure 8–19 Analogy between water level and film density for moving and stationary grids

tween the lead strips. Figure 8–19 attempts to illustrate how this happens. The total quantity of density (blackness) on the film is represented by the water level in Figure 8–19A. This is the amount of density that is spread out uniformly over the film by a moving grid. In Figure 8–19B a grid is immersed in the water to represent the grid lines on a film. Now all the water is concentrated between the grid lines, and the water level rises just as the amount of blackness on the film rises. The total quantity of density on the film is the same with both moving and stationary grids, but with stationary grids the film is made up of many narrow voids (grid lines) containing no density, interspersed with black lines containing all the density.

GRID SELECTION

There is no simple rule to guide the clinician in choosing a grid for any particular situation. A compromise is always involved. The price of increased "cleanup" with high-ratio grids is that patient exposure is considerably increased and that x-ray tube

centering becomes more critical. You must weigh the value of a better-quality radiograph against your moral obligation to keep the patient's exposure at a minimum. There is little to be gained using high ratio grids in the low kVp range. Usually, **8:1 grids will give adequate results below 90 kVp. Above 90 kVp, 12:1 grids are preferred.** Crossed grids are only used when there is a great deal of scatter radiation, such as in biplane cerebral angiography.

The efficiency of scatter radiation absorption by various grids is shown in Figure 8–20, which plots the fractional transmission of scatter radiation against grid ratio. There is little decrease in transmitted scatter beyond an 8:1 ratio grid, and almost no change between 12:1 and 16:1. For this reason 12:1 grids are preferable to 16:1 grids for routine radiography. The improvement in film quality in going from a 12:1 to a 16:1 grid is not worth the greater patient exposure.

AIR GAP TECHNIQUES

The x-ray grid is the most important means of reducing scatter radiation with large radiographic fields but, under certain circumstances, an alternate method, an air gap, produces comparable results with less patient exposure. The basic principle of the air gap technique is quite simple. Scatter radiation arising in the patient from Compton reactions disperses in all directions, so the patient acts like a large light bulb (Fig. 8–21A). In the illustration, scattered photons are shown radiating out from a point source, but the point actually represents a tiny block of tissue. Each ray represents a separate scattering event, and numerous scatterings within the small block produce the array shown. The closer the patient is to the film, the greater the concentration of scatter per unit area. With an air gap, the concentration decreases because more scattered photons miss the film. The name "air filtration" has been applied to air gap techniques, but this is a misnomer. **Scatter radiation decreases not from**

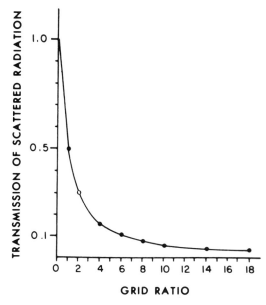

Figure 8–20 Fractional transmission of scatter radiation through grids (Courtesy of Sven Ledin and the Elema Shoenander Company)

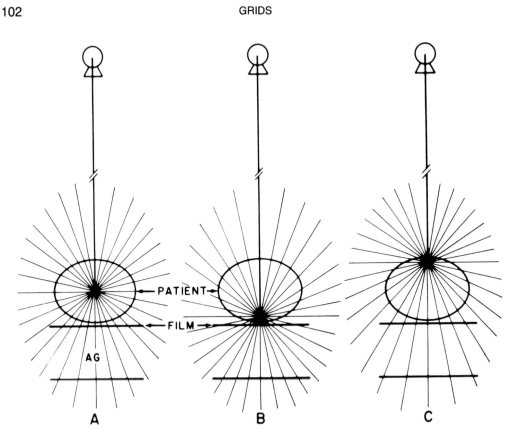

Figure 8–21 Air gap techniques

filtration but from scattered photons missing the film. Negligible quantities of radiation are absorbed in the gap, and the beam is not appreciably hardened, so the name air filtration should be discarded.

There is no strong bias for forward scattering in the diagnostic energy range, so the distribution of Compton scattering is nearly random. A photon is almost as likely to scatter at 90° as at 45°, or 180°. With increasing energy, more photons scatter in the forward direction, but the increase is negligible in the diagnostic range. When the energy of the incident photon is increased from 10 to 140 keV, a much greater change than is likely in clinical radiology, the most probable angle of scatter only changes from 53° to 45°.[4] With a strong forward bias, as in megavoltage therapy, air gaps are ineffective as a means of controlling scatter radiation.

Figure 8–21B and C compares the dis-

tribution of scattered radiation arising from superficial tissue blocks on opposite sides of the patient. More radiation reaches the film from scattering near the exit surface (Fig. 8–21B), because the film intercepts a larger angle of the scattered "beam." The angle of interception is smaller for scattering occurring on the input side of the patient (Fig. 8–21C), because a natural "gap" separates the film from the scattering site. The difference in the contribution from the two sides is even greater than the illustration implies. Many scattered photons from the input surface (Fig. 8–21C) are absorbed during their long journey through the patient, whereas those originating near the exit surface (Fig. 8–21B) have only a short escape distance. As a result of these two factors, a greater angle of capture and less tissue attenuation, most of the scattered photons reaching the film arise in the immediately adjacent superficial tissue layers, an ideal arrangement for an air gap technique. Your can see from the illustration that the air gap is most effective in removing scatter radiation when the scatter originates close to the film (Fig. 8–21*B*).

Optimum Gap Width

Air gap techniques are used in two clinical situations, magnification radiography and chest radiography. With magnification techniques the object-film distance is optimized for the screen-focal spot combination and the air gap reduces the scatter radiation to acceptable levels as an incidental bonus. In chest radiography the air gap is used instead of a grid and techniques are designed around the air gap. For example, image sharpness deteriorates as the gap widens, so the focal-film distance is usually lengthened from 6 to 10 feet to restore sharpness. Air gaps and grids have the same function, to remove as much scatter radiation and as little primary radiation as possible. As a measure of performance, gap width is analogous to grid ratio. A large air gap, like a higher ratio grid, removes a larger percentage of scatter radiation.

Figure 8–22 shows the ratio of scatter to primary radiation with air gap widths from ⅝ to 15 inches for three different absorber thicknesses. A ratio of 5 means that 5 scattered photons reach the film for each primary photon. At the ideal ratio of zero, all the transmitted photons are primary. As the gap increases, the ratio of secondary to primary radiation decreases, but the change is gradual without an abrupt transition point. The optimum gap width is a matter of judgment. The following four guidelines should be used to select a gap width:

1. The thicker the part, the more advantageous a larger gap. Figure 8–22 shows that a change from a 1- to a 15-inch width produces a more marked decrease in scatter radiation for a 22-cm phantom than for a 10-cm phantom.

2. The first inch of air gap improves

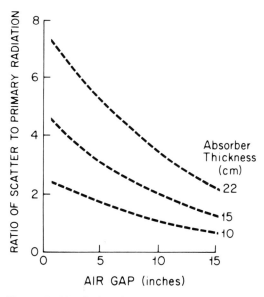

Figure 8–22 Ratio of scatter to primary radiation for various air gaps and absorber thicknesses

Table 8–7. Comparative Contrast Improvement Factors for Grid and Air Gap Techniques (100 kVp, 30- × 30-cm Field)

ABSORBER THICKNESS (cm OF WATER)	CONTRAST IMPROVEMENT FACTOR			
	AIR GAP		GRID	
	5 in.	10 in.	7:1	15:1
10	1.39	1.81	1.50	1.85
20	1.37	2.21	2.10	2.85

(Data from Gould and Hale.[4])

contrast more than any subsequent inch. The increase from a 1- to a 2-in. gap improves contrast more than an increase from a 14- to a 15-in. gap.

3. Image sharpness deteriorates with increasing gap width unless the focal-film distance is increased to compensate for the greater magnification. An increase in focal-film distance from 6 to 10 feet is customary in chest radiography to compensate for this loss of sharpness. A further increase in focal-film distance is usually not physically possible because of space limitations, or technically feasible at an acceptable exposure time because of the heat tolerance of the x-ray tube. Remember, a 50% increase in distance doubles the exposure factors.

4. If the gap is widened by moving the patient away from the film with a fixed focal-film distance, the patient is closer to the x-ray tube and his exposure increases. The increase can be corrected by a comparable increase in the focal-film distance, but this may not be a possible alternative for the reasons stated above.

Table 8–7 shows that a 5-inch air gap approaches the performance of a light (7:1) grid for thin patients. A 10-inch gap is the same as a heavy (15:1) grid for thin patients, but not as good for thicker patients. The final decision on air gap width is usually made empirically. Changing widths from patient to patient is inconvenient. Experience has shown that a 10-inch gap and a 10-foot focal-film distance with an energy from 110 to 150 kVp produces satisfactory results.

Exposure Factors with Air Gaps

Figure 8–23 compares a 6-foot focal-film distance (FFD) with a grid to a 10-foot focal film distance with a 10-inch air gap. The exposure factor, patient exposure, and transmitted primary radiation are all assigned a value of one for the grid technique, which is used as the standard for comparison. In this example, the primary transmission of the grid is 65%, and the experimental design was chosen to produce films of equal density (same total number of photons) and contrast (same ratio of primary to secondary photons). The x-ray tube exposure must be increased for the air gap technique because of the larger focal-film distance. Applying the inverse square law (constant KVp), exposures would have to be increased 2.8 times ($120^2 \div 72^2 = 2.8$) but the actual increase is somewhat less, because only 65% of the primary photons are transmitted through the grid. The increase is 1.8 times ($2.8 \times 0.65 = 1.8$), a substantial difference that taxes the heat capacity of the x-ray tube.

Patient exposures are usually less with air gaps than grids, because grids absorb primary photons. With the grid technique shown in Figure 8–23, 1.54 primary photons must pass through the patient for each one reaching the film ($1.0 \div 0.65 = 1.54$); the difference (35%) is absorbed in the grid. Only 1.19 primary photons need pass through the patient with the air gap technique to produce a comparable concentration per unit area of film; the difference ($1.19 - 1.0 = 0.19$ or 19%) is lost as a consequence of the inverse square law. The air gap loses less primary radiation, so the patient's exposure is less. If the patient exposure is unity with the grid, it will be 0.77 with the air gap ($1.19 \div 1.54 = 0.77$), a significant but not dramatic savings.

Magnification with Air Gaps

Two factors determine the amount of magnification, the object-film distance and the focal-film distance. Magnification is greatest with a short focal-film distance and a long object-film distance. As a general rule, image sharpness deteriorates with magnification. The objective with an air gap technique is to preserve image sharp-

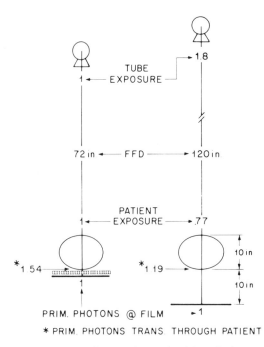

Figure 8–23 Comparison of grid and air gap techniques for chest radiography

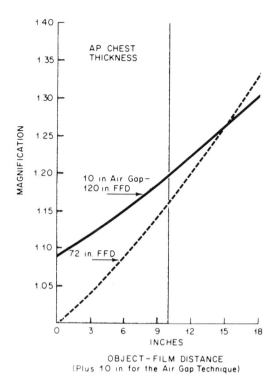

Figure 8–24 Magnification with 72-inch (no air gap) and 120-inch (air gap) focal-film distances (FFD)

ness by lengthening the focal-film distance until magnification returns to pre-air gap levels. Some deterioration is inevitable, however, for parts close to the film. Figure 8–24 shows that the objective is not accomplished with a 120-inch focal-film distance, at least not for a 10-inch air gap and a reasonably sized (10-inch thick) patient. Magnification is less with the 72-inch focal-film distance for all object-film distances up to 15 inches. The longer focal-film distance produces a more uniform magnification from the front to the back of the patient, a desirable characteristic. This uniformity is preserved with lesser air gaps. With a 5-inch gap, the curve would maintain its slope but would slide down the magnification scale to cross the 72-inch curve at a shorter object-film distance. Experienced chest radiographers do not feel that image sharpness deteriorates noticeably with air gap techniques.

SUMMARY

Radiographic grids consist of lead foil strips separated by x-ray transparent spacers. They are used to absorb scatter radiation and to improve radiographic image contrast. The grid ratio is defined as the ratio of the height of the lead strips to the distance between them, and it is the simplest way of characterizing a grid. Grids come in two patterns, linear and crossed. Crossed grids consist of two superimposed linear grids; their great disadvantage is that they cannot be used with oblique techniques. Most grids are focused to a line in space called a convergent line, but they can be used over a variable range of distances called the focal range.

Three tests have been devised to evaluate grid performance. (1) Primary transmission is a measurement of the percentage of primary radiation transmitted through a grid (usually between 60 and 70%). (2) The Bucky factor is a measurement of the total radiation (primary and scatter) absorbed by a grid. It indicates how much exposure factors must be increased because of grids, and also reveals how much more radiation the patient receives. Bucky factors range from 3 to 7, depending on the grid ratio. (3) The contrast improvement factor is a measurement of a grid's ability to improve contrast, and it is the best test of grid performance. Generally, high-ratio grids with a high lead content have the highest contrast improvement factors.

The grid ratio, lead content, and number of lines per inch are all interrelated. A grid with many lines per inch (over 100) is generally thinner and has a lower lead content than a grid of comparable ratio with fewer lines per inch.

Grid cutoff is the loss of primary radiation that occurs when the images of the lead strips are produced wider than they would be with ordinary magnification. The amount of cutoff with a particular decentering error is greatest with high-ratio grids that have a short focusing distance. Lateral decentering is the most common error, and it causes a uniform loss of primary radiation, so it is impossible to recognize on the film. With focus-grid distance decentering, the film is light on both sides, while with combined lateral and focus-grid distance decentering, the film is light only on one side.

Moving grids eliminate the image of the lead strips from the film, and this is their chief advantage. Generally, exposure factors are a little greater with moving grids than with stationary grids because of a lateral decentering error during a portion of the exposure, and because the exposure is spread out over the entire surface of the film. With properly positioned stationary grids there is no decentering error, and the exposure is concentrated between the lead strips.

Grid selection involves a compromise between film quality and patient exposure. High-ratio grids produce films with better contrast at a cost of increased patient exposure. Generally, low-ratio grids are adequate for low-energy radiation; 8:1 grids should be used with energies less than 90 kVp, and 12:1 grids for higher energy radiation.

Air gaps are an alternative method of eliminating scatter radiation with large radiographic fields. The intensity of scatter radiation is maximum at the patient's surface and diminishes rapidly at increasing distance from the surface. If the film is placed at a distance, the scatter simply misses the film. Focal-film distances are increased with air gap techniques in an attempt to maintain image sharpness and, as a consequence, x-ray exposure factors are greater with the air gaps than grids. Patient exposures are generally less with air gaps, however, because the grid absorbs some primary radiation.

REFERENCES

1. Hondius Boldingh, W.: Grids to reduce scattered x-ray in medical radiography. Eindhoven, Netherlands, Philips Research Laboratories, 1964, No. 1, Philips Research Reports Supplement.
2. Characteristics and Applications of X-Ray Grids, rev. ed. Liebel Flarsheim Company, 1968.
3. International Commission on Radiologic Units and Measurements: Methods of Evaluating Radiologic Equipment and Materials. Washington, DC, U.S. Government Printing Office, National Bureau of Standards, Handbook 89, August, 1963.
4. Gould, R.G., and Hale, J.: Control of scattered radiation by air gap techniques: Applications to chest radiography. Am. J. Roentgenol., *122*:109, 1974.

9

Intensifying and Fluoroscopic Screens

The x-ray photons making up the radiographic image cannot be seen by the human eye. This information is converted into a visual image by one of two methods. A photographic emulsion can be exposed to the x rays directly. More commonly, the energy of the x rays is converted into radiation in the visible light spectrum, and this light may be used to expose x-ray film (radiography or photofluorography), or the light may be viewed directly (fluoroscopy). The sensitivity of film to direct x-ray exposure is low. Direct exposure of film would require prohibitively large patient x-ray doses for most examinations. Therefore, almost all radiographic film examinations require that the radiographic image be converted into light at some stage by a luminescent screen.

FLUORESCENCE

Luminescence refers to the emission of light by a substance. It can be caused by varying kinds of stimuli (e.g., light, chemical reactions, or ionizing radiation). The term **fluorescence** is applied to that form of luminescence produced when light is emitted instantaneously (within 10^{-8} sec of the stimulation). If the emission of light is delayed beyond 10^{-8} sec, the term **phosphorescence** is used.

Fluorescence, as used in radiology, is **the ability of crystals of certain inorganic salts** (called phosphors) **to emit light when excited by x rays.** For many years the crystals, or phosphors, of importance in radiology were **calcium tungstate** (the phosphor in intensifying screens) and zinc cadmium sulfide (the phosphor in fluorescent and photofluorographic screens). Recent advances in technology have resulted in the introduction of a number of new phosphors, such as cesium iodide in image intensifer tubes and several new intensifying screen phosphors, including barium fluorochloride, barium strontium sulfate, yttrium, and the rare earths gadolinium and lanthanum.

Theories concerning the mechanism of luminescence are discussed in several textbooks of x-ray physics and will not be repeated here. The process is basically one in which a relatively small number of high-energy photons (x rays) is changed into a larger number of photons with much lower energy (light). At energies used in diagnostic radiology, almost all x-ray absorption in the screen is caused by the photoelectric effect in the high atomic number elements of the phosphor.

INTENSIFYING SCREENS

Intensifying screens are used because they **decrease the x-ray dose** (less mAs) to the patient, yet still afford a properly exposed x-ray film. Also, the reduction in exposure allows use of short exposure times, which becomes important when it is necessary to minimize patient motion.

107

The x-ray film used with intensifying screens has photosensitive emulsion on both sides. The film is sandwiched between two intensifying screens in a cassette, so that the emulsion on each side is exposed to the light from its contiguous screen. Remember, the screen functions to absorb the energy (and information) in the x-ray beam that has penetrated the patient, and to convert this energy into a light pattern that has (as nearly as possible) the same information as the original x-ray beam. The light, then, forms a latent image on x-ray film. The transfer of information from x-ray beam to screen light to film results in some loss of information. In this and subsequent chapters we will discuss some factors involved in the degradation of information and describe what can be done to keep this to a minimum.

Construction

An intensifying screen has four layers:

1. a base, or support, made of plastic or cardboard;
2. a reflecting layer (TiO_2);
3. a phosphor layer; and
4. a plastic protective coat.

The total thickness of a typical intensifying screen is about 15 or 16 mils (1 mil = 0.001 inch = 0.0254 mm).

Base

The screen support, or base, may be made of high-grade cardboard or of a polyester plastic. The base of Du Pont intensifying screens is a polyester plastic (Mylar*) that is 10 mils thick (10 mils = 254 μ). Kodak X-Omatic and Lanex screens have a similar (Estar†) base 7 mils thick.

Reflecting Coat

The light produced by the interaction of x-ray photons and phosphor crystals is emitted in all directions. Much of the light is emitted from the screen in the direction of the film. Many light photons, however, are also directed toward the back of the screen (i.e., toward the base layer) and would be lost as far as photographic activity is concerned. The reflecting layer acts to reflect light back toward the front of the screen. The reflecting coat is made of a white substance, such as titanium dioxide (TiO_2), and is spread over the base in a thin layer, about 1 mil thick. Some screens do not have a reflecting layer (e.g., Kodak X-Omatic fine and regular).

Phosphor Layer

The phosphor layer, containing phosphor crystals, is applied over the reflecting coat or base. The crystals are suspended in a plastic (polymer) containing a substance to keep the plastic flexible. We will discuss the phosphor in more detail later. The thickness of the phosphor layer is about 4 mils for par speed screens. The thickness of the phosphor layer is increased 1 or 2 mils in high-speed screens, and is decreased slightly in detail screens.

Protective Layer

The protective layer applied over the phosphor is made of a plastic, largely composed of a cellulose compound that is mixed with other polymers. It forms a layer about 0.7 to 0.8 mils thick. This layer serves three functions: it helps to prevent static electricity; it gives physical protection to the delicate phosphor layer; and it provides a surface that can be cleaned without damaging the phosphor layer.

Figure 9–1 shows a cross section of a typ-

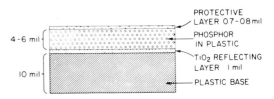

Figure 9–1 Par speed x-ray intensifying screen (cross section)

---

*Mylar is a trademark of E. I. du Pont de Nemours and Company, Inc.
†Estar is a trademark of Eastman Kodak Company.

ical par speed intensifying screen with a plastic base. Unlike the highly mechanized operation of x-ray film production, screens are largely a product of hand labor.

Phosphor

The original phosphor used in x-ray intensifying screens was **crystalline calcium tungstate** ($CaWO_4$). New (since about 1973) screen phosphor technology is being developed to increase screen speed over that available with calcium tungstate, and has resulted in the introduction of a bewildering variety of screens and corresponding films. Let us first consider calcium tungstate and then review some of the new phosphors.

Natural calcium tungstate (scheelite) is no longer used because synthetic calcium tungstate of better quality is produced by fusing sodium tungstate and calcium chloride under carefully controlled conditions. The first commercial calcium tungstate screens were made in England and Germany in 1896; they were first made in the United States in 1912. The calcium tungstate crystal must be absolutely free of any contaminant if it is to fluoresce properly. **It produces light primarily in the blue region of the visible spectrum,** with a wavelength range of 3500 to 5800 Å (1 Angstrom = 0.0001 μ = 0.00000001 cm) and a peak wavelength of about 4300 Å (430 nm), which is seen by the eye as a violet color. Although the eye is not sensitive to light of this wavelength, x-ray film emulsion exhibits maximum sensitivity to light from calcium tungstate screens. Figure 9–2 diagrams the spectrum of calcium tungstate fluorescence, the response of the eye to light of different wavelengths, and the sensitivity of x-ray film. Film sensitivity is seen to be high throughout most of the range of light emitted by the screen, a fact that ensures maximum photographic effect. Note that the film does not exhibit photosensitivity to red light, so red light can be used in the darkroom without producing any photographic effect on the film.

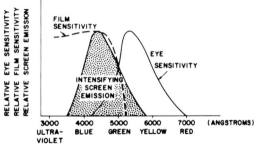

Figure 9–2 The spectral emission of a calcium tungstate x-ray intensifying screen compared to the spectral sensitivity of x-ray film and of the eye

Intensifying Action of Screens

An intensifying screen is used because it can convert a few absorbed x-ray photons into many light photons. The **efficiency with which the phosphor converts x rays to light is termed the intrinsic efficiency of the phosphor;** this is more accurately defined as the ratio of the light energy liberated by the crystal to the x-ray energy absorbed. The intrinsic efficiency of calcium tungstate is about 5%. If the energy of the absorbed x-ray photon, the wavelength of the emitted light, and the intrinsic efficiency of the phosphor are known, the number of light photons generated is easily calculated. For example, assume a 50-keV x-ray photon (50,000 electron volts) is absorbed in a calcium tungstate screen that emits most of its light at a wavelength of 4300 Å. The energy in electron volts (eV) of this light photon is calculated by

$$\lambda \text{ (wavelength)} = \frac{12.4}{keV}$$

$$4300 = \frac{12.4}{keV}$$

$$keV = \frac{12.4}{4300} \cong 0.003$$

$$eV = 3$$

The energy of a 4300 Å (430 nm) blue light photon is about 3 eV. At 100% intrinsic efficiency, a 50,000 eV x-ray photon would produce about 17,000 light photons of 3 eV energy:

$$\frac{50,000}{3} \cong 17,000$$

Because the intrinsic efficiency of calcium tungstate is only 5%, the actual number of light photons emitted by this phosphor is about 850 (17,000 × 0.05 = 850). One reason some new intensifying screen phosphors are faster than calcium tungstate is that the new phosphor has a higher intrinsic efficiency (up to 20%).

The ability of light emitted by the phosphor to escape from the screen and expose the film is termed the screen efficiency. For typical screens about half the generated light reaches the film; the rest is absorbed in the screen and is wasted. In the previous example, only half the 850 light photons generated would be able to escape from the screen and expose the film.

To examine the manner in which the screen amplifies the photographic effect of x rays, let us consider the case of a film-screen combination compared to a film alone, each irradiated by one thousand 50-keV x-ray photons. Of the 1000 photons, a high-speed calcium tungstate screen will absorb 40% (we will discuss this aspect in more detail later), or 400. Each of the 400 x-ray photons will produce 850 light photons, for a total of 340,000 light photons. Half of these light photons (170,000) will escape the screen and expose the film.

Let us assume that 100 light photons are needed to form one latent image center. The screen-film system in our example has caused the formation of 1700 latent image centers. (We will discuss the concept of the latent image in Chapter 10.) At this point, let us simply define a latent image center as the end product of the photographic effect of light or x rays on the film emulsion. It is possible to measure the magnitude of the photographic effect of an exposure by counting the number of latent image centers formed as a result of that exposure. In the case of x rays exposing film directly,

only about 5% of the x-ray photons are absorbed by the film, so our example will cause 50 x-ray photons to react with the film emulsion. It is usually considered that one latent image center is formed for each x-ray photon absorbed by a film emulsion. The result of the same 1000 x-ray photons acting directly on film is to produce only 50 latent image centers, versus 1700 latent image centers resulting from the use of intensifying screens. In our example, the ratio of the photographic effect of screen versus nonscreen, or direct, exposure is 34:1. If kVp remains constant, direct film exposure will require 34 times as many mAs as a film-screen exposure.

A review of the example of the intensifying effect of screens is presented in Table 9–1. Stated another way, patient exposure is decreased greatly when intensifying screens are used. A measure of this decrease in exposure is termed the intensification factor of the screen. **The intensification factor of a screen is the ratio of the x-ray exposure needed to produce the same density on a film with and without the screen** (intensification factor is commonly determined at a film density of 1.0).

$$\text{Intensification factor} = \frac{\text{exposure required when screens are not used}}{\text{exposure required with screens}}$$

The intensification factor of $CaWO_4$ screens will increase with kVp of the x-ray beam (Fig. 9–3). The K-absorption edges of silver and bromine in the film are 26 keV and 13 keV, respectively, while the K-absorption edge of tungsten is 69.5 keV. Photoelectric absorption of low-kVp x rays will be relatively greater in film because of the low-keV K-absorption edge of silver and bromine. High-kVp x rays will be more abundantly absorbed by the photoelectric process in calcium tungstate screens. For this same reason, a heavily filtered x-ray beam will increase the screen intensification factor by removing the low-energy components of the beam. Thus, $CaWO_4$ in-

Table 9–1. Comparison of the Photographic Effect of 1000 X-Ray Photons Used With and Without Intensifying Screens

	X-RAY PHOTONS ABSORBED BY SCREEN	X-RAY PHOTONS ABSORBED BY FILM	LIGHT PHOTONS GENERATED	LIGHT PHOTONS REACHING FILM	LATENT IMAGE CENTERS FORMED
Intensifying screen	400		340,000	170,000	1700
Direct exposure		50			50

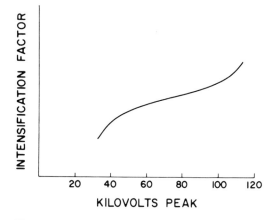

Figure 9–3 Variation of the intensification factor with kVp

tensifying screens are relatively faster in radiography of a thick body part, such as the lumbar spine, than when an extremity is examined. That is, only higher energy x rays can penetrate the thick part and reach the screen.

There will actually be a small number (3 or 4%) of x-ray photons directly absorbed by the film when a screen-film combination is exposed. This direct action of x rays would create so few latent image centers compared to those caused by the fluorescence of the screen that it may be ignored as having no detectable influence on total film response to the exposure.

Speed of Calcium Tungstate Intensifying Screens

Several factors determine how "fast" or "slow" a calcium tungstate screen will be. These include **thickness of the phosphor layer, size of the phosphor crystals,** presence or absence of **light-absorbing dye** in the phosphor layer, and **efficiency of fluorescence** of the crystal. Of course, the faster screen will allow a lower x-ray exposure to the patient, but a price for this speed must be paid. **The speed of a calcium tungstate screen and its ability to record detail are in reciprocal relationship;** that is, high speed means less detail. These screens are classified as fast, medium (par speed), and slow (detail), with intensification factors in the range of 100, 50, and 25, respectively.

A thicker phosphor layer will result in a faster screen because the thick layer will absorb more x-ray photons than a thin layer. Thick screens will be faster but will cause a decrease in the clarity of the image recorded on the film. This decrease in image clarity is primarily caused by **diffusion of light** in the phosphor layer. If a thick phosphor layer is employed, an x-ray photon may be absorbed in the phosphor at some distance from the film. **The light photons generated by this absorbed x-ray photon are emitted in all directions.** Not all the light will reach the film, but that which does will expose an area of the film that is much larger than the size of the calcium tungstate crystal that emitted the light (Fig. 9–4). In addition, some light scattering takes place in the screen, and further increases the area of illumination. The resultant light diffusion obviously causes images to have less sharp borders. Consider Figure 9–5. If an x-ray beam is directed onto a film-screen combination that has a thick lead block covering half the film, one would expect half the film to be exposed and half to be entirely unexposed, with the line between the two areas being

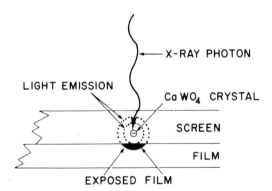

Figure 9–4   Screen unsharpness is caused by light diffusion in the intensifying screen

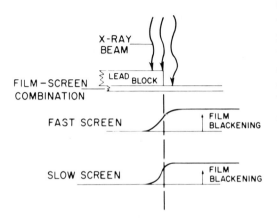

Figure 9–5   Unsharp image borders produced by light diffusion in intensifying screens

very sharp. If the x-ray beam were to expose film alone (without screens), the line between exposed and unexposed areas would be very sharp. If the film is sandwiched between intensifying screens, however, the border is less sharp because some light will diffuse into the area under the edge of the lead block and cause exposure of film in an area that actually receives no x-ray exposure. This light, which diffused under the edge of the lead block, is not available to expose the portion of the film that is not covered by the block. The final result is the production of a more gradual change in density, which is unlike the ideal abrupt transition from black to unexposed (clear) film. (Attempts to measure the magnitude of this problem of light diffusion

and scattering will lead us to consideration of the concepts of line spread function and modulation transfer function in Chapter 13.)

A thin screen causes less light diffusion than a thick one because light photons are produced closer to the film. Another way to decrease light diffusion is to incorporate a substance that absorbs light in the screen. The substance is commonly a yellow dye, but the question of which color is most effective has not been resolved. The light photons that emerge from the crystal immediately adjacent to the film will obviously travel the shortest distance before leaving the phosphor layer. Scattered photons must travel longer distances in the phosphor layer, and thus they have a better chance of being absorbed by the dye. The dye will decrease the speed of the screen because it decreases the amount of light emitted. Light absorbing dyes are included in screens designed to produce greater detail.

Resolving Power

The maximum number of line pairs per millimeter that can be resolved by the screen-film system is called the **resolving power.** A **line pair** means a line and a space. For example, two lines (or two line pairs) per mm means that there are two lines and two spaces per mm. Each line is $\frac{1}{4}$ mm wide, and each space is $\frac{1}{4}$ mm wide, thus making each line pair $\frac{1}{2}$ mm wide. (A more detailed discussion of resolving power is presented in Chapter 13.) X-ray film is able to record up to 100 line pairs per mm, but the slowest screens can record only a little over 10.

Temperature Effect

X-ray screens fluoresce more brilliantly at low temperature. At extremes of temperature this may have clinical significance. At 95° F an increase in exposure of about 25% may be necessary to produce the same film density as a similar radiograph done at 70° F.

Screen-Film Contact

The cassette in which the intensifying screens are mounted provides a light-tight container for the film. It also serves to hold the film in tight contact with the screens over its entire surface. With good film-screen contact a dot of light produced in the screen will be recorded as a comparable dot on the film. If contact is poor, this dot of light will diffuse before it reaches the film, so that its radiographic image is unsharp.

There is a simple method for testing film-screen contact. A piece of wire screen is placed on the cassette, and a radiograph of the wire screen is made. The sharpness of the image of the wire in all regions of the film is compared, and any areas of poor film-screen contact become obvious because the image of the wire appears fuzzy. The wire screen should be made of iron, brass, or copper (aluminum and plastic screens fail to absorb enough x rays), and should have a heavier wire than that used in ordinary window screen. It is best to mount the test wire screen between two pieces of plastic, composition board, or cardboard. Poor film-screen contact will occur quickly if the cassette is handled roughly, but eventually any cassette will wear out with routine use.

Cleaning

Intensifying screens must be kept clean. Any foreign material on the screen, such as paper or blood, will block light photons and produce an area of underexposure on the film corresponding to the size and shape of the soiled area. Cleaning will eliminate the "high spots" on a screen; these high points are the major source of excessive wear. The cause of screen failure is mechanical attrition. Under normal conditions of use, x-ray photons will not damage screens. Screens are best cleaned with a solution containing an antistatic compound and a detergent; the solution should be applied gently (never rub vigorously) with a soft lint-free cloth. The cassette should never be closed after cleaning until it is absolutely dry.

NEW PHOSPHOR TECHNOLOGY

It is usually agreed that the maximum useful speed of calcium tungstate screens has been achieved. New screen phosphors have permitted greater speed, but this changing technology is complex and perplexing.

Increasing Screen Speed

We must first consider how intensifying screen speed can be increased. There are three possible ways. The phosphor layer can be made thicker to absorb more of the x-ray beam. The phosphor may have a higher conversion efficiency of x rays to light. The phosphor may be able to absorb the x-ray beam more effectively. To review, there are three possible ways to increase screen speed:

1. thicker phosphor layer
2. higher conversion efficiency phosphor
3. higher absorption phosphor.

Before entering this long discussion of new phosphor technology, please review Table 9–2, which catalogs the noncalcium tungstate screens available from Du Pont and Kodak, listing phosphor composition and color of light emitted by the phosphor.

Thicker Phosphor Layer

Thick phosphor layers absorb more of the x-ray beam than thin layers. This is the major way in which the speed of calcium tungstate screens is increased. A pair of Du Pont Par Speed $CaWO_4$ screens absorbs about 20% of the x-ray beam. A pair of Du Pont Hi Plus screens absorbs about 40% of the x-ray beam (and is twice as fast as par speed). The Hi Plus screens are not twice as thick as par screens, though, they are about 2.3 times as thick as the par screens. Why is this? If 100 x-ray photons struck a pair of par screens, 80 photons would be transmitted through the screens (20 are ab-

Table 9–2. Non-Calcium Tungstate Intensifying Screens Manufactured by Du Pont and Kodak

MANUFACTURER	NAME	PHOSPHOR	SPECTRAL EMISSION
Du Pont	Cronex Quanta II	Barium fluorochloride:europium activated (BaFCl:Eu)	Blue
	Cronex Quanta III	Lanthanum oxybromide:thulium activated (LaOBr:Tm)	Blue
	Cronex Quanta V	Lanthanum oxybromide:thulium activated *plus* gadolinium oxysulfide:terbium activated (LaOBr:Tm *plus* Gd_2O_2S:Tb)	Blue and green
Kodak	X-Omatic Fine	Barium lead sulfate, yellow dye ($BaPbSO_4$)	Blue
	X-Omatic Regular	Barium strontium sulfate:europium activated, neutral dye ($BaSrSO_4$:Eu)	Blue
	Lanex Fine	Gadolinium oxysulfide:terbium activated, neutral dye (Gd_2O_2S:Tb)	Green
	Lanex Medium	Gadolinium oxysulfide:terbium activated, yellow dye (Gd_2O_2S:Tb)	Green
	Lanex Regular	Gadolinium oxysulfide:terbium activated (Gd_2O_2S:Tb)	Green

sorbed). A second set of par screens placed in the path of the 80 transmitted photons would absorb 20%, or 16 photons, allowing 64 to pass through. Thus, a double thickness of par speed screens does not absorb 40% of the x-ray beam. It is possible to continue to increase the speed of $CaWO_4$ screens by increasing screen thickness, but unsharpness caused by light diffusion in the thick phosphor layer becomes unacceptable. Thus, **calcium tungstate screens may be considered a compromise between speed** (needing thick screens) **and sharpness** (needing thin screens). Because of the emphasis being given new screen phosphors, it is not difficult to overlook the fact that currently available $CaWO_4$ screens offer a wide range of speeds. For example, Table 9–3 lists the Du Pont family of Cronex* $CaWO_4$ intensifying screens, which cover a range of 16 in speed. (We will consider the term "speed class" in detail in Chapter 11.)

Conversion Efficiency

In 1972, reports describing rare earth oxysulfide phosphors for use in intensify-

Table 9–3. Speed Class of Various $CaWO_4$ Screens with Cronex 4 Film

CALCIUM TUNGSTATE SCREEN (Du Pont CRONEX)	SPEED CLASS
Detail	25
Fast detail	50
Par speed	100
Hi Plus	250
Lightning Plus	400

ing screens were published.[9] This work was supported by a contract from the Atomic Energy Commission to the Lockheed Corporation, and this class of phosphors is sometimes referred to as the Lockheed rare earth phosphors. Rare earth intensifying screens have been commercially available since about 1973.

Chemists divide the periodic table of the elements into four basic groups: alkaline earths, rare earths, transition elements, and nonmetals. The term "rare earth" developed because these elements are difficult and expensive to separate from the earth and each other, not because the elements are scarce. The rare earth group consists of elements of atomic numbers 57 (lanthanum) through 71 (lutetium), and includes thulium (atomic number 69), ter-

---

*Cronex is a trademark of E. I. du Pont de Nemours and Company, Inc.

bium (atomic number 65), gadolinium (atomic number 64), and europium (atomic number 63). Because lanthanum is the first element, the rare earth group is also known as the lanthanide series. Lanthanum (La) and gadolinium (Gd) are used in the rare earth phosphors. A related phosphor, yttrium (Y), with atomic number 39, is not a rare earth but has some properties similar to those of the rare earths.

The rare earth phosphors are produced as crystalline powders of **terbium-activated gadolinium oxysulfide** (Gd_2O_2S:Tb) and **thulium-activated lanthanum oxybromide** (LaOBr:Th). Unlike $CaWO_4$, the rare earth phosphors do not fluoresce properly in the pure state. Maximum rare earth light production occurs when approximately 0.3% of the atoms are terbium (another rare earth) replaces gadolinium.

The x ray to light conversion efficiency of rare earth phosphors is significantly greater than that of $CaWO_4$. It is generally correct to state that the x ray to light conversion efficiency of $CaWO_4$ is about 5%, while that of the rare earth phosphors is about 20%. Stated another way, one absorbed x-ray photon in a $CaWO_4$ intensifying screen will produce about 1000 light photons, and the same photon absorbed in a rare earth screen will produce about 4000 light photons. The conversion efficiency of yttrium oxysulfide screens is about the same as that of gadolinium. In the literature, actual conversion efficiency figures quoted are $CaWO_4$ 5%, LaOBr:Th 18%, Gd_2O_2S:Tb 18%, and Y_2O_2S:Tb 18%. The Du Pont Quanta II screen has a phosphor of barium fluorochloride:europium activated (BaFCl:Eu), which also owes part of its increased speed to a more efficient conversion of x-ray energy to light.

Higher Absorption

The fraction of the x-ray beam absorbed by a pair of par speed $CaWO_4$ screens is about 20%, high-speed $CaWO_4$ screens about 40%, and rare earth screens about 60%. The increased absorption in the faster $CaWO_4$ screens occurs because a thicker screen is used; the increased absorption in rare earth screens is a result of improvement in the absorption characteristics of the phosphor.

At diagnostic x-ray energies, absorption is almost entirely caused by the **photoelectric effect** in the high atomic number elements of the phosphor. As discussed in Chapter 4, a photoelectric reaction is most likely to occur in elements with high atomic numbers, and when the x-ray photon energy and the binding energy of the ejected K-shell electron are almost the same.

A phosphor with a higher atomic number would have higher absorption. Because the atomic numbers of tungsten (74) and lead (82) are almost at the end of the periodic table the potential for this type of improvement is limited. It is interesting to note that the improvement in the input phosphor of image intensifier tubes involved a change from zinc sulfide (atomic numbers 30 and 16) to cesium iodide (atomic numbers 55 and 53). Actually, each of the phosphors used in the new fast intensifying screens has an atomic number lower than that of tungsten. Table 9–4 lists some of the elements found in intensifying screens, together with their atomic number (Z) and K-shell binding energy.

Figure 9–6 diagrams the approximate x-ray absorption curve of a calcium tungstate screen. Notice that the screen is less absorbing as radiation energy increases until the 70 keV K-edge of tungsten is reached.

In Figure 9–7 the approximate absorption curve of Gd_2O_2S:Tb is added to the $CaWO_4$ curve. Up to 50 keV, both phos-

Table 9–4. Atomic Number and K-Shell Binding Energy of Some Screen Phosphors

ELEMENT	ATOMIC NUMBER (Z)	K-SHELL BINDING ENERGY (keV)
Yttrium (Y)	39	17.05
Barium (Ba)	56	37.4
Lanthanum (La)	57	38.9
Gadolinium (Gd)	64	50.2
Tungsten (W; wolfram)	74	69.5

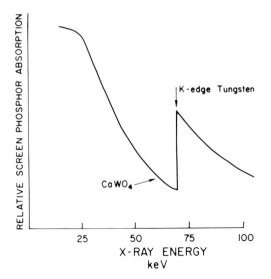

Figure 9–6 Approximate x-ray absorption as a function of x-ray photon energy in a calcium tungstate intensifying screen

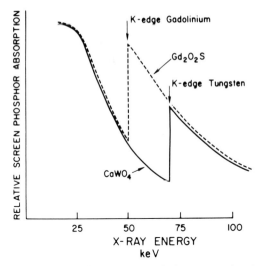

Figure 9–7 Comparison of the approximate x-ray absorption as a function of x-ray photon energy in $CaWO_4$ and Gd_2O_2S

phors absorb about the same. But, at the 50.2-keV K-edge of Gd, the rare earth screen develops a four- or fivefold advantage over $CaWO_4$, which persists until the 70-keV K edge of W is reached. It is apparent that Gd, which has a lower atomic number than W, enjoys an absorption advantage over W in the x-ray energy range of 50 to 70 keV because of the differences

in photoelectric absorption related to the K-shell electron binding energies of these two elements. In diagnostic radiology, however, a large percentage of x rays in the beam will have an energy less than 50 keV, making the advantage of gadolinium much less. This is why lanthanum is added to the phosphor of some rare earth screens (such as the Du Pont Cronex Quanta V). Lanthanum, with its K edge at 39 keV, effectively "closes the window" between 39 and 50 keV.

In Figure 9–8 the approximate x-ray absorption curves of LaOBr, Gd_2O_2S, and $CaWO_4$ are compared. By combining the two rare earth phosphors, the rare earth screen has a significant absorption advantage over $CaWO_4$ in the 39- to 70-keV range.

Figure 9–9 shows the approximate absorption of yttrium oxysulfide (Y_2O_2S:Tb is the phosphor in the GAF Rarex B Midspeed screens) compared to that of $CaWO_4$. Notice that $CaWO_4$ and Y_2O_2S match from 17 to 70 keV. Although these two phosphors absorb about the same x-ray energy, the Y_2O_2S screen produces more light photons because of its higher x ray to light conversion efficiency (18 versus 5%). The

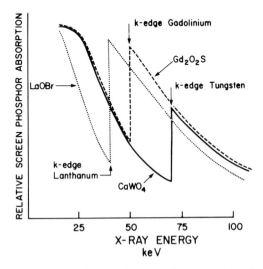

Figure 9–8 Comparison of the approximate x-ray absorption curves of $CaWO_4$, LaOBr, and Gd_2O_2S

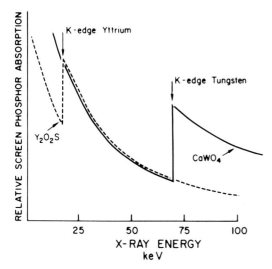

Figure 9–9 Comparison of the approximate x-ray absorption curves of $CaWO_4$ and Y_2O_2S.

absorption of BaFCl is almost the same as that of LaOBr, showing an absorption advantage over $CaWO_4$ from 38 keV (K edge of Ba) to 70 keV (K edge of W).

Let us summarize this section. The K edges of Ba, La, and Gd correspond closely to the maximum intensity of x rays in the primary beam, causing much of the energy in the primary beam to decrease in the region of increased absorption for these phosphors. This is the principal reason that these phosphors have higher absorption of x rays used in diagnostic radiology as compared with $CaWO_4$, even though the atomic number of tungsten (74) is higher than that of barium (56), lanthanum (57), or gadolinium (64). The absorption for yttrium (39) is the same as that of tungsten from 17 to 70 keV, but yttrium is "faster" because of a higher conversion efficiency.

Perhaps you have noticed that there has been a change in the phosphor composition of the Kodak Lanex family of screens. At the time our second edition was published, Lanex screens contained terbium-activated gadolinium oxysulfide ($Gd_2O_2S:Tb$) and terbium-activated lanthanum oxysulfide ($La_2O_2S:Tb$). The phosphor used in currently manufactured

Kodak Lanex screens contains only $Gd_2O_2S:Tb$. The reason for this change had to do with difficulty in obtaining pure supplies of lanthanum. You will recall that the rare earths are difficult and expensive to separate from the earth and from each other.

Emission Spectrum

This section will deal with the wavelength (color) of light emitted by the various phosphors, an important consideration because **the light output of the screen and the maximum sensitivity of the film used must be matched.**

The spectrum of light emitted by some of the new screen phosphors is quite different from that of $CaWO_4$, which produces a continuous spectrum of light in the blue region with a peak wavelength of about 4300 Å (430 nm) shown in Figure 9–2. Some phosphors other than calcium tungstate also produce light in the blue-violet range. Table 9–5 lists some of these phosphors. Natural silver halide films are maximally sensitive to light of this wavelength. Figure 9–10 shows in graphic form the approximate spectral emission of the screen phosphors listed in Table 9–5, compared to the sensitivity of natural silver halide film (such as Du Pont Cronex films and Kodak X-Omatic films). Keep in mind that the speed of these screens covers a wide range.

We must now consider the light emission of the rare earth phosphor $Gd_2O_2S:Tb$. The spectral emission of this earth phosphor is produced by the terbium ion. The terbium emission is not a continuous spectrum (as is $CaWO_4$) but is concentrated in narrow lines with a very strong peak at 544 nm, which is in the green light part of the spectrum. There are less intense emission peaks in the blue, blue-green, yellow, and red areas. Because standard x-ray silver halide film will not absorb (i.e., is not sensitive to) light in the green area, a special film must be used with these screens. Such films are Kodak Ortho G and Du Pont Cro-

Table 9–5. Spectral Emission of Several Screen Phosphors

PHOSPHOR	SPECTRAL EMISSION, PEAK WAVELENGTH (nm)	EXAMPLE
Tungsten	430	Du Pont Cronex family
Barium lead sulfate	360	Kodak X-Omatic Fine
		Du Pont Hi Speed
Barium strontium sulfate	380	Kodak X-Omatic Regular
Barium fluorochloride	390	Du Pont Quanta II

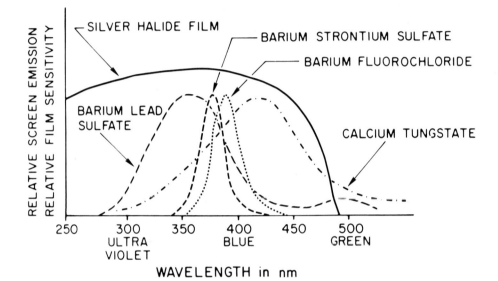

Figure 9–10 Approximate spectral emission of several different intensifying screen phosphors compared to the natural sensitivity of silver halide

nex 8. (This subject will be explored in more detail in Chapter 11.) Figure 9–11 is a graph of the spectral emission of the Kodak Lanex regular screen (which contains Gd_2O_2S:Tb in its phosphor) and the sensitivity of Kodak Ortho G film. Because the sensitivity of natural silver halide film stops at about 500 nm, use of this film with some rare earth screens would result in loss of much of the speed of these screens because the film would be insensitive to much of the light produced.

The spectral emission of yttrium oxysulfide screens is similar to that of the rare earth screens in that it shows line emission, but a large fraction of the emission from a Y_2O_2S:Tb screen falls within the sensitivity range of natural silver halide films. The principal emission of the terbium at 544

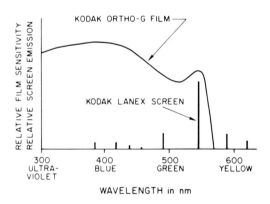

Figure 9–11 Approximate spectral emission of the Kodak Lanex Regular screen (rare earth) compared to the sensitivity of Kodak Ortho G film. (This is similar to charts supplied through the courtesy of the Eastman Kodak Company)

nm, though, is still present. Yttrium oxysulfide screens may be used with natural silver halide films, but will exhibit even more speed when used with green sensitive films.

A more recently introduced intensifying screen, the Du Pont Cronex Quanta V, contains two phosphors, terbium-activated gadolinium oxysulfide ($Gd_2O_2S:Tb$) and thulium-activated lanthanum oxybromide (LaOBr:Tm). It is interesting to note that the color of light emitted by a rare earth phosphor depends on the activator used; terbium (Tb) produces green light and thulium (Tm) blue. For example, $Gd_2O_2S:Tb$ is a green-emitting intensifying screen phosphor, and LaOBr:Tm is a blue-emitting intensifying screen phosphor. The spectral emission of LaOBr:Tm is illustrated in Figure 9–12. The Du Pont Quanta V intensifying screen is interesting in that it contains both a blue (LaOBr:Tm) and a green ($Gd_2O_2S:Tb$) emitting phosphor. This "double" spectral emission allows a wider choice of suitable films, because both blue- and green-sensitive films are matched to the spectral emission of the screens.

An example of a rare earth screen with a blue-emitting phosphor is the Du Pont Cronex Quanta III, which has LaOBr:Tm at its phosphor (see Fig. 9–12). Recent advances in separating rare earths have made suitably pure supplies of lanthanum available for use in intensifying screens.

Table 9–6 is an attempt to compare roughly the relative speed (speed class) of the newer screens we have been discussing. (The term "speed class" will be discussed in more detail in Chapter 11.) It is common to express the speed of an intensifying screen relative to that of a par speed calcium tungstate screen (specifically, the Du Pont Cronex Par Speed screen). In our speed class scheme the speed of the par speed $CaWO_4$ screen is assigned a value of 100. Remember that a film that matches the spectral emission of the screen must be used. In Table 9–6 Du Pont Cronex 4 and Kodak XRP are films sensitive to blue light. Green light-sensitive films are represented by Du Pont Cronex 8 and Kodak Ortho G films. When comparing the relative speed of various intensifying screens, the films that were used must be specified. (In Chapter 11 the characteristics of these films will be presented in more detail, and in Chapter 13 we will examine potential problems associated with very fast screens.)

Response to Kilovoltage

In the past we compared the speeds of other screens to that of $CaWO_4$ as if the $CaWO_4$ screen had a constant response to kilovoltage. The response of $CaWO_4$ to kVp is not flat, but drops down at low kVp. This is illustrated in Figure 9–13, which shows the kVp response of $CaWO_4$, LaOBr:Tm, and a combined $Gd_2O_2S:Tb$ and LaOBr:Tm phosphor. Figure 9–13 shows that the speed of the rare earth screens varies much more with kVp than does the $CaWO_4$ screen. Note that the rare earth screens show maximum speed at about 80 kVp, with less speed at both low and high kilovoltages. The need for exposure technique adjustment because of screen speed variation with kVp is not great, and is usually of little importance

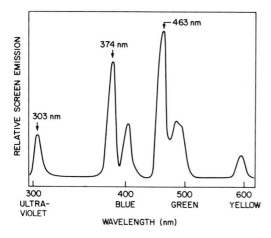

Figure 9–12 Approximate spectral emission of LaOBr:Tm. (Data courtesy of E.I. du Pont de Nemours & Company, Inc.)

Table 9–6. Speed Class of Various Intensifying Screens

MANUFACTURER	NAME	PHOSPHOR	SPECTRAL EMISSION	FILM	SPEED CLASS
Du Pont	Cronex Par Speed	CaWO$_4$	Blue	Cronex 4	100
	Cronex Hi Plus	CaWO$_4$	Blue	Cronex 4	250
	Cronex Quanta II	BaFCl:Eu	Blue	Cronex 4	500
	Cronex Quanta III	LaOBr:Tm	Blue	Cronex 4	800
	Cronex Quanta V	LaOBr:Tm and	Blue	Cronex 4	320
		Gd$_2$O$_2$S:Tb	Green	Cronex 8	400
Kodak	X-Omatic Fine	BaPbSO$_4$, yellow dye	Blue	XRP	32
	X-Omatic Regular	BaSrSO$_4$:Eu, neutral dye	Blue	XRP	200
	Lanex Fine	Gd$_2$O$_2$S:Tb, neutral dye	Green	Ortho G	100
	Lanex Medium	Gd$_2$O$_2$S:Tb, yellow dye	Green	Ortho G	250
	Lanex Regular	Gd$_2$O$_2$S:Tb	Green	Ortho G	400

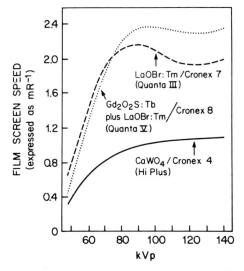

Figure 9–13 Response to kVp of a Du Pont CaWO$_4$ (Hi Plus), LaOBr:Tm (Quanta III), and dual phosphor Gd$_2$O$_2$S:Tb plus LaOBr:Tm (Quanta V) screen. (Data courtesy of E.I. du Pont de Nemours & Company, Inc.)

speed is often expressed as the reciprocal of the exposure in milliroentgens required to produce a net film density of 1.0. This explains the numbers used to express film-screen speed. The speed of a film-screen system depends on the speed of the screen and on the speed of the film. The films used to determine the curves in Figure 9–13 were a medium-speed and half-speed blue-sensitive film (Cronex 4 and Cronex 7) and a medium-speed green-sensitive film (Cronex 8). We will repeat Figure 9–13 in Chapter 11; don't worry if these areas are not entirely clear now.

Phototimers

Some phototimers being used today will not work well with rare earth screens. Many of these phototimers have a response time of about 30 milliseconds (i.e., it takes 30 milliseconds for the phototimer to measure the radiation and terminate the exposure). With fast screens a response time of 3 milliseconds is recommended.[3] In addition, the phototimer must be able to recognize differences in screen speed caused by variation in kVp. If a photomultiplier-type phototimer is used, the fluorescent screen (photocathode) used in the photomultiplier tube will probably have to be the same

unless kilovoltage lower than 70 kVp is used. It is generally advisable to establish constant kVp (with variable mAs) exposure technique charts when using noncalcium tungstate screens.

Figure 9–13 introduces two areas we will not explain until Chapter 11. Film-screen

phosphor as that used in the intensifying screen. It is also probable that ionization chamber-type phototimers can be made to work satisfactorily. Use of phototimers with very fast screens will usually require special consideration, and one should plan for appropriate changes in advance.

Screen Asymmetry

Some intensifying screens, such as the Du Pont Cronex Quanta II, have a thinner phosphor layer on the front screen than on the back screen. (Kodak Lanex screens no longer use screen asymmetry; both front and back screens are the same.) With this very fast screen a significant fraction of the incident x-ray beam is absorbed by the front screen. Thus, a thicker back screen is required if it is to absorb the same number of photons as the front screen (i.e., fewer x rays arrive at the back screen, so it must absorb a larger percentage of its part of the beam). Asymmetry also helps to produce equality in sharpness of the image produced by the front and back screens. Because of the differential absorption of x rays in the thickness of the screen phosphor, more x rays are absorbed (and light produced) in that portion of the screen closest to the source of the x rays. This means that x rays absorbed by the front screen are more likely to cause light production near the base (and reflecting coat) of the screen, and this light produced deep in the phosphor will undergo significant diffusion before reaching the film. X-ray absorption in the back screen, for the same reason, will be greater nearer the film (or screen protective coat) and will produce light near the outer surface of the screen that will not undergo much diffusion before reaching the film. For very fast screens, sharpness of the rear screen would be better than that of the front screen for screens of equal thickness.

To review, some companies make asymmetric front and back screens to cause equal amounts of light production by each screen and equal sharpness of the image produced by each screen.

Quantum Mottle

Quantum mottle, commonly called "noise," results from statistical fluctuation in the number of x-ray photons absorbed by the intensifying screens to form the light image recorded on film. With the fast screens and films now available, it is possible to use a film-screen system so fast (i.e., the screen does not have to absorb many x rays) that noise makes the resulting image unsatisfactory. (This subject will be reviewed in painful detail in Chapter 13.) At this time, we only wish to emphasize that any discussion of fast screens demands careful evaluation of system noise. One pays a price for speed.

FLUOROSCOPIC SCREENS

The major difference between fluoroscopic and intensifying screens is related to the wavelength of the fluorescent light. The light from the fluoroscopic screen must have a wavelength corresponding to the maximum sensitivity of the eye, which is from 500 to 600 nm. From 1914 to 1933 cadmium tungstate was the phosphor used. In 1933 the Patterson type B fluoroscopic screen was introduced in the United States. This screen was made of zinc cadmium sulfide, silver activated. Unlike calcium tungstate, which fluoresces in the pure state, crystals of zinc cadmium sulfide will luminesce effectively only if they contain a small amount of a metallic impurity, called an activator. The activator used is silver, and a change in its concentration of as little as one part per million may change the color of light produced. Zinc sulfide has a natural blue fluorescence, but the addition of activators and cadmium can vary this color through the entire visible color range to red. Both zinc sulfide and zinc cadmium sulfide are efficient in converting the energy of x rays into light, with a fluorescence efficiency of about 10 to 15%. The phosphor now used in fluoroscopic screens is silver-activated zinc cadmium sulfide that is synthesized to fluoresce in the yellow-green range, with a peak at about 530 nm. The screen is similar in physical construction to intensifying screens, but the phosphor layer is thicker, averaging 7 to 8 mils. Phosphor particle size may vary from 25 to 40 μ. The resolving power of fluoroscopic screens is no more than 3 line pairs/mm.

When a fluoroscopic screen is viewed directly, the examiner must be protected from any x rays transmitted through the screen. This protection is afforded by lead glass, which is glass containing a large proportion of lead (about 60% by weight). This glass is transparent to visible light but effectively absorbs x rays. The protection afforded by this glass is expressed as its lead equivalent. By lead equivalent is meant the thickness of lead that will produce the same degree of attenuation of the x-ray beam as the lead glass in question.

The edges of fluoroscopic screens are sealed so as to be watertight, so these screens require little care as compared to intensifying screens.

The input screens used in some x-ray image intensifiers contain zinc cadmium sulfide as the phosphor, and are similar to fluoroscopic screens. The input screen phosphor in the new generation of image intensifiers is composed of cesium iodide. The output screen of all image intensifiers is zinc cadmium sulfide.

PHOTOFLUOROGRAPHY

Photofluorography is frequently called mass miniature radiography. This is the method usually employed in projects such as mass chest x rays for tuberculosis control. In this technique the image of a fluorescent screen is recorded on film by means of a camera. The film used is of small size. Some units use cut film 4 inches by 4 inches in size. More commonly, roll film is used; the film is usually 70 mm wide but may be 90 or 100 mm.

Two types of fluorescent screens are used. The phosphor may be silver-acti-vated zinc sulfide, which emits a blue light (440 nm), or zinc cadmium sulfide (the same as a fluoroscopic screen). Particle size and phosphor thickness are about the same as those employed in fluoroscopic screens, and resolving power ranges between 2 and 5 line pairs per mm. The film emulsion used with zinc sulfide screens must be blue sensitive, and that for zinc cadmium sulfide yellow-green sensitive.

SUMMARY

Intensifying screens are used in diagnostic radiology because they reduce x-ray dose to the patient. Also, the lower exposures required (less mAs) allow the shorter exposure times needed to reduce motion unsharpness. Until about 1971, calcium tungstate was the phosphor used in most screens. New technology has resulted in very fast rare earth and other phosphors. There are three ways in which screens can be made "faster":

1. thicker phosphor layer
2. higher conversion efficiency phosphor
3. higher absorption phosphor.

$CaWO_4$ screen speed is determined largely by the thickness of the phosphor layer. The newer fast phosphors exhibit a higher conversion efficiency. Higher absorption of x rays in the diagnostic range is a function of the matching of the K-absorption edge of the screen phosphor to the energy spectrum in the x-ray beam. The spectral emission of some phosphors requires that an appropriately sensitized film be used, or much of the light will be wasted. Intensifying screens are usually used in pairs, with a double-emulsion x-ray film sandwiched between the two screens in a light-tight cassette. System noise becomes important when the fastest film-screen systems are used.

A fluoroscopic screen converts the x-ray image into light to be viewed by the eye, and must fluoresce with a yellow-green light to which the eye is most sensitive. The phosphor used is silver-activated zinc cadmium sulfide. The input screen for the new generation of x-ray image intensifiers is cesium iodide.

REFERENCES

1. Alves, R.V., and Buchanan, R.A.: Properties of Y_2O_2S:Tb x-ray intensifying screens. Presented at the IEEE meeting in Miami, December, 1972.
2. Balter, S., and Laughlin, J.S.: A photographic method for the evaluation of the conversion efficiency of fluoroscopic screens. Radiology, 86:145, 1966.
3. Bates, L.M.: Properties of radiographic films and intensifying screens which influence the efficacy of a film-screen combination. Contained in the syllabus of the joint BRH-ACR Conference: First Image Receptor Conference: Film/Screen Combinations, Arlington, Virginia, November 13–15, 1975. Washington, DC, U.S. Government Printing Office, HEW Publ. No. (FDA) 77-8003, 1975, p. 123.
4. Buchanan, R.A., Finkelstein, S.I., and Wickersheim, K.A.: X-ray exposure reduction using rare-earth oxysulfide intensifying screens. Radiology, 105:85, 1972.
5. Castle, J.W.: Sensitivity of radiographic screens to scattered radiation and its relationship to image contrast. Radiology, 122:805, 1977.
6. Coltman, J.W., Ebbighausen, E.G., and Alter, W.: Physical properties of calcium tungstate x-ray screens. J. Appl. Physics, 18:530, 1947.
7. Holland, R.S.: Image analysis. Contained in the syllabus of the AAPM 1975 Summer School, The Expanding Role of the Diagnostic Radiologic Physicist, Rice University, Houston, July 27–August 1, 1975, p. 103.
8. Lawrence, D.J.: Kodak X-Omatic and Lanex screens and Kodak films for medical radiography. Rochester, N.Y., Radiography Markets Division, Eastman Kodak Company File No. 5.03, June 1976.
9. Ludwig, G.W., and Prener, J.S.: Evaluation of Gd_2O_2S:Tb as a phosphor for the input screen of x-ray image intensifier. IEEE Trans. Biomed. Eng., 19:3, 1972.
10. Meredith, W.J., and Massey, J.B.: Fundamental Physics of Radiology. Baltimore, Williams & Wilkins, 1968.
11. Morgan, R.H.: Characteristics of x-ray films and screens. Radiology, 49:90, 1947.
12. Patterson, C.V.S.: Roentgenography: Fluoroscopic and intensifying screens. In Medical Physics. Vol. 2. Edited by O. Glasser. Chicago, Year Book Medical Publishers, 1950.
13. Patterson, C.V.S.: Roentgenography: Fluoroscopic and intensifying screens. In Medical Physics. Vol. 3. Edited by O. Glasser. Chicago, Year Book Medical Publishers, 1960.
14. Patterson X-Ray Screens: Sales Manual for Du Pont Patterson X-Ray Screen Dealers. Wilmington, Photo Products Department, E.I. du Pont de Nemours and Company, Inc., 1952.
15. Properzio, W.S., and Trout, E.D.: The deterioration of x-ray fluoroscopic screens. Radiology, 91:439, 1968.
16. Roth, B.: X-ray intensifying screens. Contained in the syllabus of the AAPM 1975 Summer School, The Expanding Role of the Diagnostic Radiologic Physicist, Rice University, Houston, July 27–August 1, 1975, p. 120.
17. Stevels, A.L.N.: New phosphors for x-ray screens. Medicamundi 20:12, 1975.
18. Ter-Pogossian, M.: The efficiency of radiographic intensifying screens. In Technological Needs for Reduction of Patient Dosage from Diagnostic Radiology. Edited by M.L. Janower. Springfield, IL, Charles C Thomas, 1963.
19. Thompson, T.T., Radford, E.L., and Kirby, C.C.: A look at rare-earth and high-speed intensifying screens. Appl. Radiol., 6:71, 1977.

10

Physical Characteristics of X-Ray Film and Film Processing

When an x-ray beam reaches the patient, it contains no useful medical information. After the beam passes through and interacts with the tissues in the part examined, it contains all the information that can be revealed by that particular radiographic examination. This is represented by variation in the number of x-ray photons in different areas of the emergent beam. We are unable to make direct use of the information in this form, however, and must transfer it to a medium suitable for viewing by the eye. The method of transfer might involve a magnetic tape or disc, a fluoroscopic screen, or xerography. The most important material used to "decode" the information carried by the attenuated x-ray beam is photographic film. The film may be exposed by the direct action of x rays. More commonly, the energy of the x-ray beam is converted into light by intensifying screens, and this light is used to expose the film.

It is unfortunate that the transfer of information from the x-ray beam to the screen-film combination always results in a loss of information. In reviewing x-ray film, we must examine both the film and those factors that influence the amount of information lost in the transfer process.

FILM

X-ray film is photographic film consisting of a photographically active, or radia-

tion-sensitive, emulsion that is usually coated on both sides of a transparent sheet of plastic, called the base. Firm attachment between the emulsion layer and the film base is achieved by use of a thin layer of adhesive. The delicate emulsion is protected from mechanical damage by layers known as the supercoating (Fig. 10–1).

Film Base

The only function of the film base is to provide a support for the fragile photographic emulsion. Three characteristics of the base must be considered. First, it must not produce a visible pattern or absorb too much light when the radiograph is viewed. Second, the flexibility, thickness, and strength of the base must allow for ease of processing (developing) and produce a radiograph that "feels right" when handled (a film too "floppy" to "snap" under the hangers of a viewbox gets a cool reception). Third, the base must have **dimensional stability;** that is, the shape and size of the base must not change during the developing

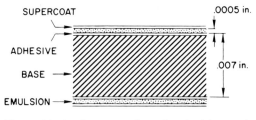

Figure 10–1 Cross section of a double emulsion x-ray film

process or during the stored life of the film. Figure 10–2 illustrates a radiograph in which the base has slowly diminished in size over a period of 22 years. Notice how shrinking of the base has thrown the unshrinking emulsion into folds, producing a wrinkled appearance.

Original x-ray "plates" consisted of a glass plate with the emulsion coated on one side. It is no longer possible to make a "flat plate of the abdomen," because x-ray plates are not available. The onset of World War I cut off the supply of photographic glass from Belgium and, additionally, created a demand for a less fragile x-ray film for use by the Army. Cellulose nitrate, previously used as a base for photographic film, was adapted for use in x-ray film in 1914. Cellulose nitrate is quite flammable, however, and several fires were caused by improper handling and storage of the film. Because of this fire hazard a new "safety base" film was urgently sought and, in 1924, a "safety" film with a cellulose triacetate base was developed. This acetate-base safety film (cellulose acetate will burn if held directly in a flame) is still widely used. In 1960 the first medical radiographic film using a polyester base was introduced. **Polyester** as a film base offers the advantage of improved dimensional stability, even when stored under conditions of varying humidity, and it is much stronger than acetate.

What is polyester? It is similar to Dacron* polyester fiber used in clothing. The raw materials, dimethyl terephthalate (DMT) and ethylene glycol, are brought together under conditions of low pressure and high temperature to form a molten polymer that is then literally stretched into sheets of appropriate size and thickness to form film base. Cronex* film is an example of a polyester-base film, and the characteristics of polyester may be appreciated by examining a piece of "cleared" Cronex film.

Triacetate and polyester bases are clear and colorless. In 1933 the first commercialized blue tint was added to x-ray film in an effort to produce a film that was "easier" to look at, causing less eyestrain. Present x-ray film is tinted blue. The blue dye may be added to the film base or to the emulsion.

Triacetate base is about 0.008 inch (8 mils) thick, and polyester base is 7 mils thick. The slightly thinner polyester base has handling properties approximately equal to those of the thicker acetate.

Photographic emulsion would not adhere to the finished base if applied directly. Therefore, a thin layer of adhesive substance is applied to the base to ensure perfect union between base and emulsion.

Emulsion

The two most important ingredients of a photographic emulsion are **gelatin** and **silver halide**. The exact composition of the various emulsions is a closely guarded industrial secret. Most x-ray film is made for use with intensifying screens, and has

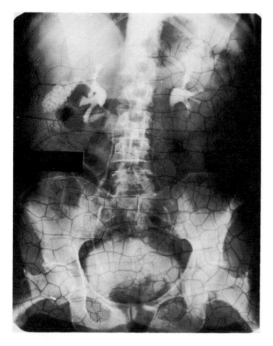

Figure 10–2 Wrinkled emulsion resulting from shrinking of the film base

*Dacron and Cronex are trademarks of E.I. du Pont de Nemours and Company, Inc.

emulsion coated on both sides of the base. Emulsion thickness varies with film type, but is usually no thicker than 0.5 mil. A thicker emulsion would not be useful because of the inability of light to penetrate to the deeper layers.

Gelatin

Photographic gelatin for x-ray film is made from bone, mostly cattle bone from India and Argentina. (Useless information: India and Argentina do not have better cows, but they have a lot of them. They also have inexpensive labor to process the bones.) Gelatin satisfies several exacting requirements better than any other suspension medium. It keeps the silver halide grains well dispersed and prevents the clumping of grains. Processing (developing and fixing) solutions can penetrate gelatin rapidly without destroying its strength or permanence, and gelatin is available in a reasonably large quantity and uniform quality.

Silver Halide

Silver halide is the light-sensitive material in the emulsion. The halide in medical x-ray film is about 90 to 99% silver bromide and about 1 to 10% silver iodide (the presence of AgI produces an emulsion of much higher sensitivity than a pure AgBr emulsion). The silver iodobromide crystals are precipitated and emulsified in the gelatin under exacting conditions of concentration and temperature, as well as the sequence and the rate at which these chemicals are added. The method of precipitation determines crystal size, structural perfection, and concentration of iodine. In general, the precipitation reaction involves the addition of silver nitrate to a soluble halide to form the slightly soluble silver halide:

$$AgNO_3 + KBr \rightarrow AgBr + KNO_3$$

The silver halide in a photographic emulsion is in the form of small **crystals** suspended in the gelatin. The crystal is formed from ions of silver (Ag^+), ions of

bromine (Br^-), and ions of iodine (I^-) arranged in a cubic lattice (Fig. 10–3). These grains, or crystals, in a medical x-ray film emulsion are small but still relatively large compared to fine-grain photographic emulsions. Crystal size might average 1.0 to 1.5 microns (1 micron = 0.001 millimeter) in diameter with about 6.3×10^9 grains per cubic centimeter of emulsion, and each grain contains an average of 1,000,000 to 10,000,000 silver ions.

The silver iodobromide grain is not a perfect crystal because a perfect crystal has almost no photographic sensitivity. There are several types of crystal defects. A point defect consists of a silver ion that has moved out of its normal position in the crystal lattice; these interstitial silver ions may move in the crystal (Fig. 10–4). A dislocation is a line imperfection in the crystal,

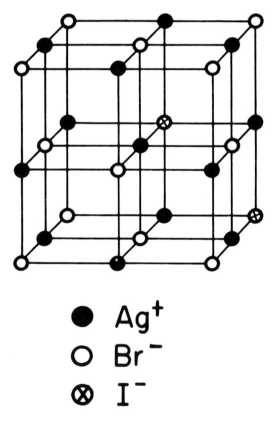

● Ag^+

○ Br^-

⊗ I^-

Figure 10–3 The silver iodobromide crystal lattice

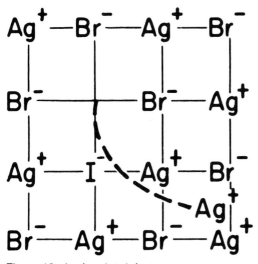

Figure 10–4 A point defect

and may be thought of as a brick wall that contains one row in which the bricks are not the same size as all the other bricks, thus causing a strain in the wall structure. This may be the way in which the iodine ion strains the crystal.

Chemical sensitization of a crystal takes several forms. It is commonly produced by adding a sulfur-containing compound, such as allylthiourea, to the emulsion, which reacts with silver halide to form silver sulfide. The silver sulfide is usually located on the surface of the crystal and is referred to as the **sensitivity speck.** It is the sensitivity speck that traps electrons to begin formation of the latent image centers.

Latent Image

Metallic silver is black. It is silver that produces the dark areas seen on a developed radiograph. We must explain how exposure of the sensitized silver iodobromide grains in the film emulsion to light (from x-ray intensifying screens), or to the direct action of x rays, initiates the formation of atomic silver to form a pattern. The energy absorbed from a light photon gives an electron in the bromine ion enough energy to escape. The electron can move in the crystal for relatively large distances as long as

it does not encounter a region of impurity or fault in the crystal.

$$Br^- + light\ photon \rightarrow Br + electron$$

A site of crystal imperfection, such as a dislocation defect, or an AgS sensitivity speck, may act as an electron trap where the electron is captured and temporarily fixed. The electron gives the sensitivity speck a negative charge, and this attracts the mobile interstitial Ag^+ ions in the crystal. At the speck, the silver ion is neutralized by the electron to form a single silver atom:

$$Ag^+ + electron \rightarrow Ag$$

This single atom of silver then acts as an electron trap for a second electron. The negative charge causes a second silver ion to migrate to the trap to form a two-atom silver nucleus. Growth of silver atoms at the site of the original sensitivity speck continues by repeated trapping of electrons, followed by their neutralization with interstitial silver ions. The negative bromine ions that have lost electrons are converted into neutral bromine atoms, which leave the crystal and are taken up by the gelatin of the emulsion. Figure 10–5 diagrams the development of a two-atom latent image according to the Gurney-Mott hypothesis.[6]

A single silver halide crystal may have one or many of these centers in which atomic silver atoms are concentrated. The presence of atomic silver is a direct result of the response of the grain to light exposure, but no visible change has occurred in the grain. These small clumps of silver can, however, be seen with electron microscopy. These clumps of silver atoms are termed **latent image centers,** and are the sites at which the developing process will cause visible amounts of metallic silver to be deposited. The difference between an emulsion grain that will react with the developing solution and thus become a visible silver deposit and a grain that will not be "developed" is the presence of one or more latent image centers in the exposed grain. At least two atoms of silver must be present

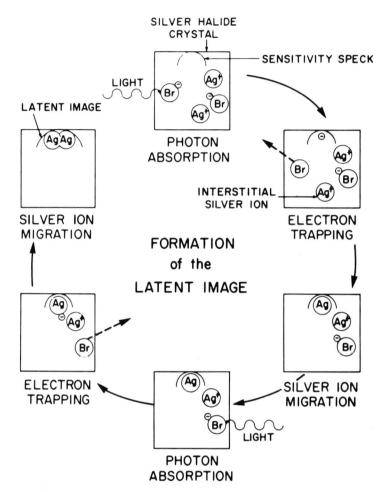

Figure 10–5   Formation of the latent image

at a latent image center to make a grain developable (i.e., to become a visible deposit of silver). In practical terms the minimum number to produce developability is probably between three and six. The more silver atoms that exist at a latent image center, the greater the probability that the grain will be developed. Some centers will contain several hundred silver atoms. Under the usual conditions, the absorption of one quantum of light by a silver halide grain will produce one atom of silver and one of bromine.

Direct X-Ray Exposure

The photographic effect of direct absorption of x rays by the emulsion is not caused by electromagnetic radiation itself but by electrons emitted when the x-ray photon interacts with the silver halide in the emulsion. These electrons come from photoelectric absorption or Compton scattering, and have rather long ranges in the emulsion. In fact, an electron produced in this way may react with many grains in an emulsion. The manner in which the energy of the electrons is imparted to the photographic emulsion is complex and will not be considered in detail. The final result is freeing of electrons from the bromide ion, producing bromine atoms and an electron that can move to a trapping site and begin the process of latent image formation. The energy of one absorbed x-ray photon can produce thousands of silver atoms at latent image sites in one or several grains. Even this large number of silver atoms is low, considering the energy of the absorbed photon. Most of the energy of the absorbed photon is lost in processes that do not produce any photographic effect (such as losses to gelatin). Only 3 to 10% of the photon energy is used to produce photolytic silver. The photographic effect of direct x-ray exposure on an emulsion can be increased by a factor of almost 100 by proper chemical sensitization of the emulsion.

The sensitivity of film to direct x-ray exposure varies markedly (by a factor of 20 to 50) with the energy (kVp) of the x-ray beam. This x-ray spectral sensitivity is most important when considering use of film to measure x-ray exposure dose (i.e., film badge monitoring). Above 50 kVp, the efficiency with which absorbed x-ray photons are utilized to produce a photographic effect decreases significantly with increasing photon energy. At about 50 kVp the average keV of the x rays produced will be close to the K-shell binding energy of silver (25.5 keV) and bromine (13.5 keV). This will cause the film to exhibit maximum photoelectric absorption of 50-kVp x rays. Figure 10–6 shows, in a rough graphic form, the way in which the x-ray sensitivity of film varies with kVp.

The sensitivity also varies greatly with the way in which the film is developed. The amount of blackening (density) on the developed film may be used as an indication of how much x-ray exposure (i.e., how many milliroentgens) the film has received. Because the sensitivity of the film varies greatly with the energy (kVp) of the x rays, however, blackening of a piece of film does not give an accurate estimation of the exposure to which the film has been subjected. For example, a film subjected to an exposure of 50 mR at an x-ray energy of 50 kVp will, after development, exhibit a much higher density (amount of blackening) than an identical film subjected to an exposure of 50 mR by 200-kVp x rays. The

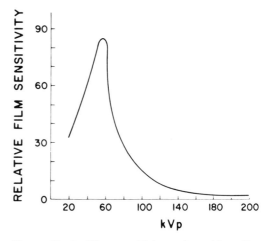

Figure 10–6 Film sensitivity varies with radiation quality

problem of variation of film sensitivity with radiation energy is partially solved by placing various metal filters in front of the film in an attempt to control the energy (kVp) of the x rays that reach different areas of the film. The accuracy of film badge monitoring of x-ray exposure is about ±20%. Film badge monitoring of personnel exposure offers several advantages over other methods, such as ionization chambers. The film badge provides a permanent record, and is small in size and weight, rugged, and inexpensive.

Supercoating

Covering the emulsion is a thin layer, commonly gelatin, that serves to protect the emulsion from mechanical damage. In special types of film this supercoat, or anti-abrasive coating, may contain substances that make the film surface smooth and slick. This is a desirable quality in film that must be transported through a cut film rapid film changer.

FILM PROCESSING
Development

Development is a chemical process that amplifies the latent image by a factor of millions (about 100,000,000) to form a visible silver pattern. The basic reaction is reduction (addition of an electron) of the silver ion, which changes it into black metallic silver:

$$Ag^+ + electron \rightarrow Ag$$

The developer is the reducing agent. Development is generally an all-or-none phenomenon, because an entire grain is developed (reduced) once the process begins. The process is usually initiated at the site of a latent image speck (commonly on the surface of the grain). It is believed that the action of the silver atoms in the latent image is to accelerate (catalyze) the reduction of the silver ions in the grain by the developing chemicals. The silver in a grain that does not contain a latent image can be reduced by the developer, but at a much slower rate. Thus, **time is a fundamental factor in the developing process.** Development should be discontinued when the differential between exposed developed grains and unexposed undeveloped grains is at a maximum.

Modern developing solutions contain two developing agents, hydroquinone and phenidone. Two agents are used because of the phenomenon of **synergism,** or superadditivity. The mixture results in a development rate greater than the sum of the developing rate of each developing agent. The reasons for development synergism are complex and not fully understood, so we will not explore the details.

The chemistry of developing is not our chief interest, but the formulas for the basic reactions help in gaining a good understanding of the process. As shown in Figure 10–7, the developing agent reduces silver ions to metallic silver, causing oxidation and inactivation of the developing agent and the liberation of hydrogen ions. Note that the reaction must proceed in an alkaline solution. When hydroquinone is oxidized to quinone, two electrons are liberated to combine with the two silver ions to form metallic silver (Fig. 10–7A). The reaction of phenidone is similar (Fig. 10–7B).

The silver thus formed is deposited at the latent image site, gradually enlarging this initially microscopic black spot into a single visible black speck of silver in the emulsion.

In addition to **developing agents,** the developing solution contains (1) an **alkali** to adjust the pH, (2) a **preservative** (sodium sulfite), and (3) **restrainers,** or antifoggants. The **alkali** adjusts the hydrogen ion concentration (pH), which greatly affects the developing power of the developing agents, especially hydroquinone. In addition, the alkali serves as a buffer to control the hydrogen ions liberated during the development reaction. Most radiographic developers function at a pH range of 10 to 11.5. Typical alkalies include sodium hydroxide, sodium carbonate, and borates (sodium metaborate and sodium tetraborate).

Sodium sulfite is added for two reasons. The oxidation products of the developing agents decompose in alkaline solution and form colored materials that can stain the emulsion. These products react rapidly with sodium sulfite to form a colorless soluble substance. In addition, sodium sulfite acts as a preservative. In alkaline solution the developing agent will react with oxygen from the air. The sulfite acts as a preservative by decreasing the rate of oxidation, especially that of hydroquinone.

Fog is the **development of unexposed silver halide grains** that do not contain a latent image. In a complex manner, dilute concentrations of soluble bromide (potassium bromide) decrease the rate of fog formation. To a lesser degree the bromide also decreases the rate of development of the latent image. The development reaction in a 90-sec x-ray processor must be completed in about 20 sec. This rapid rate of development requires that the temperature of the developing solution be quite high, usually between 90 and 95° F. This rapid, high-temperature rate of developing requires that modern x-ray developers contain additional antifoggants to permit rapid development of exposed grains but minimize

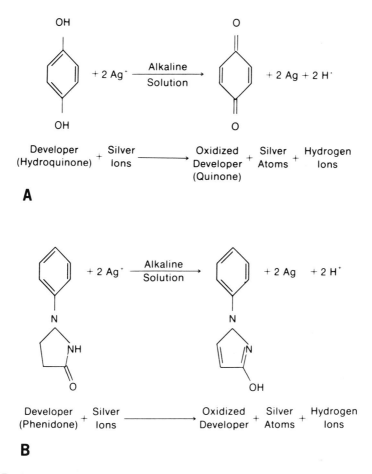

Figure 10–7 Basic chemical reactions involved in the development process. Hydroquinone (*A*) or phenidone (*B*) may be used as the developer

fog development. The most significant difference in commercial x-ray developing solutions is in the antifoggants present.

Developer formulas also contain other ingredients designed to influence swelling of the x-ray film emulsion, development rate, and physical properties. All developers contain the same basic functional components: developer (reducing agent), alkali, preservatives, and bromide. Differences in antifoggants and other ingredients are often proprietary, so we cannot give specific examples.

The bromide ions released by the reduction of silver ions to silver atoms pass into the developing solution. It is mainly this increase in bromide concentration that limits the life of developing solutions.

Replenishment

We have seen that, during use, developing solutions consume developing agents and preservatives, but acquire hydrogen ions and bromide ions. Replenishing solutions used to maintain the activity of the developer must be free of bromide, contain alkaline agents and buffers and, to a lesser extent, restore depleted preservative and developing agents.

Three developer problems may occur: underreplenishment, overreplenishment, and normally replenished but oxidized developer. In underreplenished developing solutions, bromide ions released from the processed films build up, hydroquinone is oxidized but insufficiently replaced, and the pH is decreased. Overreplenishment reduces bromide concentration and raises the pH. One cause of overreplenishment is processing an unusually high percentage of smaller films, such as 105-mm roll film. Normally replenished but oxidized developer causes the hydroquinone concentration to be low, the bromide level to be normal, and the pH to be high. The developer is oxidized when solutions sit in a processor that receives little or intermittent use. This situation has become relatively common as larger radiology departments acquire more and dispersed processors, resulting in a lower volume per unit, or when isolated CT and ultrasound areas have their own processors with relatively low volumes of films. For this reason Du Pont has recently marketed its HSD (High Stability) developer for use in low-volume units. Table 10–1 reviews the effects of aerial oxidation, overdevelopment, and underdevelopment.

The consequence of an abnormal composition of developer ingredients is to produce developed films with a sharp decrease in toe gradient (see Chap. 13; Fig. 13–5 shows the sensitometric effect caused by a significant change in developer concentration).

Fixing

Only part of the silver halide in the emulsion is reduced to silver during developing. The remaining silver halide impairs both the immediate usefulness and permanence of the developed radiograph. Therefore it must be removed, but the fixing solution must remove silver halide without damaging the image formed by metallic silver.

The solubility of silver halide (we will use silver bromide as an example) in a water solution is controlled by the concentration of silver and halide ions. Silver bromide is only slightly soluble in water. The product of the silver and bromide ions in solution is always constant for any given temperature, and may be expressed by the equation

Silver ion × bromide ion = constant

If the concentration of silver ions could be reduced, the concentration of bromide ions would have to increase, which means that more silver bromide would have to dissolve from the emulsion. Thus, the solubility of silver halide would increase. The function of the fixing agent is to form water-soluble complexes in which silver ions are tightly bound. The soluble complex thus formed effectively removes silver ion from solution.

Two agents form satisfactory stable complexes with silver ions, cyanides and thiosulfates. Cyanides are poisonous and are not generally used. **Thiosulfate** in the form of the sodium or ammonium salt is the common fixing agent, or "hypo." Why is it called hypo? In earlier chemical nomenclature, the compound we call sodium thiosulfate ($Na_2S_2O_3$) was given the name hyposulfite of soda, and "hypo" it remains to photographers. At least three silver thiosulfate complexes are formed in the fixing solution; their identities need not concern us. A typical reaction might be

Silver bromide + sodium thiosulfate →

silver thiosulfate complex + sodium bromide

Table 10–1. Changes in Developer Composition Caused by Wrong Replenishment or Aerial Oxidation

ERROR	HYDROQUINONE CONCENTRATION	BROMIDE CONCENTRATION	pH
Underreplenishment	Decreased	Increased	Low
Overreplenishment	Increased	Decreased	High
Aerial oxidation	Decreased	Normal	High

The ammonium thiosulfate salt is more active, and is used in fixer supplied in the form of a liquid concentrate.

In addition to thiosulfate, the fixing solution contains a substance to harden the gelatin. Hardening results in a decrease in the swelling of gelatin, making it tougher and more resistant to abrasion. The hardener is usually a chromium or aluminum compound. The fixing bath also contains an acid, stabilizers, and a buffer to maintain the acidic pH level.

An incompletely fixed film is easily recognized because it has a "milky" or cloudy appearance. This is a result of the dispersion of transmitted light by the very small silver iodobromide crystals that have not been dissolved from the emulsion.

Washing

After developing and fixing, the film must be well washed with water. Washing serves primarily to remove the fixing-bath chemicals. Everyone has seen an x-ray film that has turned brown with age. This is the result of incomplete washing. Retained hypo will react with the silver image to form brown silver sulfide, just as silverware acquires a brown tarnish when exposed to the hydrogen sulfide produced by cooking gas. The general reaction is

Hypo + silver → Silver sulfide (brown)

+ Sodium sulfite

SUMMARY

X-ray film is a photographic film coated with emulsion on both sides of the film base. The light-sensitive material in the emulsion is a silver iodobromide crystal. X-ray film is only slightly sensitive to direct x-ray exposure. Impurities in the silver halide crystal structure increase the light sensitivity of the film emulsion. Light, or x-ray, exposure causes the grains in the emulsion to develop an invisible latent image. The developing process magnifies the latent image to produce a visible pattern of black metallic silver.

The sensitivity of x-ray film to direct x-ray exposure varies with the kVp of the x-ray beam.

REFERENCES

1. Baines, H., and Bomback, E.S.: The Science of Photography. 2nd Ed. London, Fountain Press, 1967.
2. Fuchs, A.W.: Evolution of roentgen film. Am. J. Roentgenol., 75:30, 1956.
3. James, T.H., and Higgins, G.C.: Fundamentals of Photographic Theory. 2nd Ed. New York, Morgan and Morgan, 1968.
4. Martin, F.C., and Fuchs, A.W.: The historical evolution of roentgen-ray plates and films. Am. J. Roentgenol., 26:540, 1931.
5. Mees, C.E.K., and James, T.H.: The Theory of the Photographic Process. 3rd Ed. New York, Macmillan, 1969.
6. Neblette, C.B.: Photography, Its Materials and Processes. 6th Ed. New York, Van Nostrand, 1962.
7. Wayrynen, R.E., Holland, R.S., and Trinkle, R.J.: Chemical Manufacturing Considerations and Constraints in Manufacturing Film, Chemicals and Processing. Proceedings of the Second Image Receptor Conference: Radiographic Film Processing, Washington, DC, March 31–April 2, 1977, pp. 89–96. Washington, DC, U.S. Government Printing Office, 1977, Stock No. 017-015-00134-2.

11

Photographic Characteristics of X-Ray Film

The diagnostic accuracy of a radiographic film examination depends, in part, on the visibility of diagnostically important information on the film. Understanding the relationship between the exposure a film receives and the way the film responds to the exposure is essential to intelligent selection of proper exposure factors and type of film to provide maximum information content of the radiograph.

What is meant by the term "exposure" of an x-ray film or film-screen combination? Exposure is proportional to the product of the milliamperes of x-ray tube current and the exposure time. Thus, an exposure of 100 milliamperes for 1 second is expressed as 100 milliampere-seconds, usually written 100 mAs. An exposure of 100 mAs could also be produced by using 50-mA tube current for 2 seconds, 200 mA for 0.5 second, 500 mA for 0.2 second, and so forth. In this chapter, film exposure is assumed to mean exposure of the x-ray film by light from x-ray intensifying screens, unless otherwise stated.

Exposure (mAs) of the x-ray film produces film blackening, or density. The quality of the x-ray beam (kVp) has more effect on image contrast. Two general but not completely accurate statements should be kept in mind:

1. mAs controls film density.
2. kVp controls image contrast.

This chapter will discuss the response of the x-ray film to exposure.

PHOTOGRAPHIC DENSITY

When the x-ray beam passes through body tissues, variable fractions of the beam will be absorbed, depending on the composition and thickness of the tissues and on the quality (kVp) of the beam. The magnitude of this variation in beam intensity is the mechanism by which the x-ray beam acquires the information transmitted to the film. This pattern of varying x-ray intensity has been called the x-ray image. Webster's Collegiate Dictionary defines an image as "a mental representation of anything not actually present to the senses." This definition is particularly applicable to the idea of the x-ray image. The x-ray image actually exists in space, but it cannot be seen or otherwise detected by the natural senses. The x-ray image is the pattern of information that the x-ray beam acquires as it passes through and interacts with the patient; that is, the beam is attenuated by the patient. The x-ray image is present in the space between the patient and the x-ray film (or x-ray intensifying screen). The information content of the x-ray image must be transformed into a visible image on the x-ray film with as little loss of information as possible. We have seen how the energy of the x-ray beam may be used to produce a visible pattern of black metallic silver on the x-ray film, with the degree of film blackening being directly related to the intensity of radiation reaching the film or intensifying screen. The measurement of film blackness is called photographic density; usually, only the word **density** is used. Density is expressed as a number that is actually a **logarithm,** using the common base 10. Photographic density is defined by

$$D = \log \frac{I_0}{I_t}$$

D = density
I_0 = light incident on a film
I_t = light transmitted by the film

Refer to Figure 11–1. If ten arrows (photons) of light strike the back of the film, and only one photon passes through the film, then $I_0 = 10$ and $I_t = 1$:

$$\text{Density} = \log \frac{10}{1} = \log 10 = 1$$

Note that $\frac{I_0}{I_t}$ measures the **opacity** of the film (the ability of film to stop light). The reciprocal of density, $\frac{I_t}{I_0}$, measures the fraction of light transmitted by the film, and is called **transmittance.** Useful densities in diagnostic radiology range from about 0.3 (50% of light transmitted) to about 2 (1%

of light transmitted). A density of 2 means that $\log \frac{I_0}{I_t} = 2$. Because the log of 100 = 2, $\frac{I_0}{I_t} = 100$. Thus, for every 100 light photons incident on the film, only 1 photon, or 1%, will be transmitted. Table 11–1 lists some common values for opacity $\left(\frac{I_0}{I_t}\right)$, density $\left(\log \frac{I_0}{I_t}\right)$, and percentage of light transmission. Note that an increase in film density of 0.3 decreases transmitted light to 50% of its previous value. For example, an increase in density from 0.6 to 0.9 decreases the amount of transmitted light from 25 to 12.5%. This emphasizes the fact that the number used to signify a certain density has no units, but is a logarithm. The number 0.3 is the logarithm of 2. Thus, an increase in density of 0.3 $\left(\log \frac{I_0}{I_t}\right)$ means an increase in opacity $\left(\frac{I_0}{I_t}\right)$ of 2; opacity is doubled by a density increase of 0.3.

Higher density means a blacker film (less light transmission). In routine x-ray work, a density of 2 (1% of light transmitted) is black when viewed on a standard viewbox, and a density of 0.25 to 0.3 (50% of light transmitted) is very light.

If an unexposed x-ray film is processed, it will demonstrate a density of about 0.12. This density consists of base density and

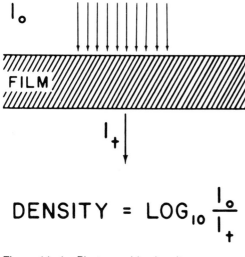

Figure 11–1   Photographic density

Table 11–1. Percentage of Light Transmitted by X-Ray Films of Various Densities

OPACITY $\left(\frac{I_0}{I_t}\right)$	DENSITY $\left(\log \frac{I_0}{I_t}\right)$	LIGHT TRANSMITTED (%)
1	0	100
2	0.3	50
4	0.6	25
8	0.9	12.5
10	1.0	10
30	1.5	3.2
100	2	1
1,000	3	0.1
10,000	4	0.01

fog. The plastic material used to make the film base absorbs a small amount of light. Also, the blue dye used to color some film base adds slightly to base density. Total base density will average about 0.07. A few of the silver halide grains in an x-ray film emulsion develop without exposure. These unexposed but developed grains comprise the density known as fog. Fog density of a fresh x-ray film averages about 0.05. We will refer to the subject of base and fog density several times in this chapter and in Chapter 13.

Why is density expressed as a logarithm? There are three primary reasons. First, logarithms conveniently express large differences in numbers on a small scale. For example, the difference in the light transmission represented by going from a density of 1 (10% of light transmitted) to a density of 2 (1% of light transmitted) is a factor of 10.

Second, the physiologic response of the eye to differences in light intensities is logarithmic (Fig. 11–2). Assume that a film having regions of density that equal 0.3, 0.6, and 0.9 is transilluminated by a light source of 1000 photons. The number of light photons transmitted will be 500, 250, and 125, respectively. The difference in transmitted light photons between density 0.3 and density 0.6 is 250 (500 to 250), but between density 0.6 and density 0.9 it is

only 125 photons (250 to 125). The eye will interpret density 0.3 as being exactly as much brighter than density 0.6, as density 0.6 is brighter than density 0.9. The eye has "seen" the equal differences in density rather than the unequal differences in the number of light photons transmitted.

The third reason for expressing density as a logarithm deals with the addition or superimposition of densities. If films are superimposed, the resulting density is equal to the sum of the density of each film. Consider two films, one of density 2 and one of density 1, which are superimposed and put in the path of a light source with an intensity of 1000 units (Fig. 11–3). The film of density 1 absorbs 90% of the light (100 units are transmitted) and the film of density 2 absorbs 99% of these 100 units, to allow final transmission of 1 unit of light. We started with 1000 units ($I_0 = 1000$) and ended with 1 unit of light ($I_t = 1$), so we may calculate density:

$$D = \log \frac{I_0}{I_t} = \log \frac{1000}{1} = 3$$

The effect of superimposing films with a density of 2 and 1 is the same as using a single film of density 3. Almost all the film

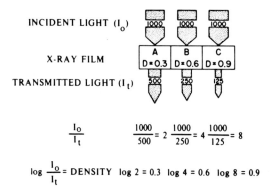

Figure 11–2 The reduction in intensity caused by three films having densities of 0.3, 0.6, and 0.9

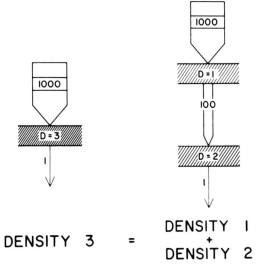

Figure 11–3 The density of superimposed films is the sum of the density of the individual films

used in radiology has two emulsions, one on each side of the base. The total density exhibited by the radiograph is the sum of the density of each emulsion.

CHARACTERISTIC CURVE

It is necessary to understand the relationship between the exposure a film receives and the density produced by the exposure. The relationship between exposure and density is plotted as a curve, known as the characteristic curve or H and D curve (named after F. Hurter and V.C. Driffield, who first published such a curve in England in 1890). The concept of the characteristic curve of an x-ray film exposed by light from x-ray intensifying screens is illustrated in Figure 11–4. Film density is plotted on the vertical axis and film exposure on the horizontal axis. The shape and location of this curve on the graph are important and will, we hope, take on some meaning as this chapter progresses.

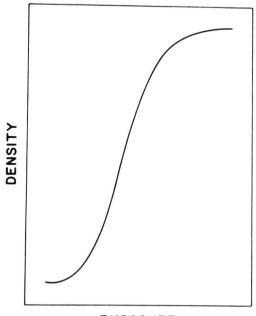

Figure 11–4 Typical characteristic curve of a screen-type x-ray film, exposed with x-ray intensifying screens

Characteristic curves are derived by giving a film a series of exposures, developing the film, and plotting the resulting density against the known exposure. The actual exposure the film received may be measured in the laboratory, but such measurements are not important to use and understand the characteristic curve. (Using medium-speed intensifying screens and 80-kVp x rays, a density of 1.0 on the x-ray film requires that about 3×10^4 x-ray photons hit each square mm of the screen.) By **film exposure** we refer to the product of the intensity of the exposure (milliamperes of x-ray tube current) and time of exposure (expressed in seconds). Exposure is expressed in terms of milliampere seconds, usually abbreviated mAs. One way to produce a characteristic curve is to expose different areas of a film with constant kilovoltage and milliamperage while varying the time of exposure (e.g., with constant kVp and mA, doubling the time of exposure will double the mAs). The exposure is recorded as the relative exposure.

The term **relative exposure** tends to create confusion. Actually, the radiologist and technologist think in terms of relative exposure when evaluating radiographs. For example, if a radiograph of the abdomen exposed with factors of 70 kVp and 75 mAs is judged to be underexposed, the correction might involve increasing the mAs to 150. In other words, the correction involves doubling the exposure. The actual exposure (such as the number of milliroentgens or the number of x-ray photons per square mm) is not known, and does not have to be. The relationship between the two exposures, however, is important. One function of the characteristic curve is to allow the amount of change necessary to correct an exposure error to be predicted. For example, if a film with the characteristic curve shown in Figure 11–5 is underexposed so that its average density is 0.35, the corresponding relative exposure is 4. If the exposure (mAs) is doubled (relative exposure is increased to 8), it can be pre-

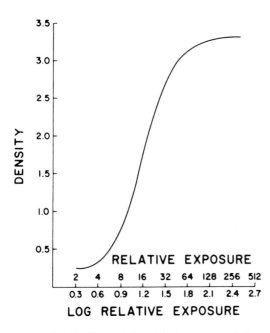

Figure 11–5 The relationship between relative exposure and the corresponding log relative exposure

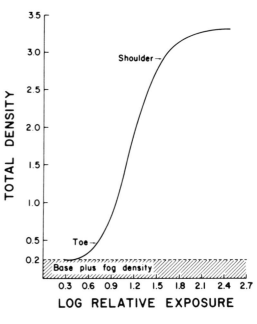

Figure 11–6 The regions of the characteristic curve

dicted that the average density will increase to about 0.8. The exposure is also recorded as the logarithm of the relative exposure, mainly for two reasons. First, use of a logarithmic scale allows a very wide range of exposures to be expressed in a compact graph. Second, use of log relative exposure makes analysis of the curve easier. Two exposures whose ratio is constant (e.g., one is twice the other) will always be separated by the same distance on the exposure scale, regardless of their absolute value. Refer to Figure 11–5, in which both the relative exposure and the log relative exposure are indicated, and note that **an increase in the log relative exposure of 0.3 always represents a doubling of the relative exposure.**

Analysis of the characteristic curve of a particular x-ray film provides information about the contrast, speed (sensitivity), and latitude of the film. Please refer to Figure 11–6. Even at 0 exposure the film density is not 0 but will usually be 0.2, or less. This density is made up of fog (development of unexposed grains of silver halide in the emulsion) and base densities (opacity of the film base), which have been previously discussed. Therefore, total density on an exposed and developed film will include base and fog densities. The minimum density caused by base and fog in a "fresh" film is about 0.12. To evaluate density produced by the exposure alone, base and fog densities must be subtracted from the total density. Second, note that at low density (toe) and high density (shoulder), the film shows little change in density despite a relatively large change in log relative exposure (Fig. 11–6). The important part of the characteristic curve is between the toe and shoulder, and in this region the curve is almost a straight line. In this "straight line" portion the density is approximately proportional to the log relative exposure. For example, if log relative exposure 1.1 produces a density of 1.0, and log relative exposure 1.3 produces a density of 2.0, we can predict that a density of about 1.5 will be produced by a log relative exposure of

1.2 (these figures correspond roughly to the characteristic curve of Figure 11–6).

Film Contrast

The information content of the invisible x-ray image is "decoded" by the x-ray film into a pattern of variations in optical density, known as radiographic contrast. Radiographic contrast is the density difference between image areas in the radiograph. There are many definitions of contrast, but we will use the simple definition that contrast is the difference in density existing between various regions on the film. Radiographic contrast depends on subject contrast and on film contrast. Subject contrast depends on the differential attenuation of the x-ray beam as it passes through the patient. The discussion of attenuation in Chapter 6 has already introduced the important aspects of subject contrast. Subject contrast was seen to be affected by the thickness, density, and atomic differences of the subject, the radiation energy (kVp), contrast material, and scatter radiation. The major theme of the remainder of this chapter will be film contrast.

The information content of the x-ray image is the pattern of varying intensity of the x-ray beam caused by differential attenuation of x rays by the subject. Few x rays reach the film through areas of bone or opaque contrast material, while many photons are transmitted through soft tissue, and the air around the patient stops almost no x-ray photons. The kVp must be selected with care so that the numbers of photons attenuated by bone and soft tissue are in the proper proportion to produce an x-ray image of high information content for the film intensifying screen to "decode." The correct kVp is tremendously important in producing proper subject contrast. This relationship (kVp and contrast) will be examined in detail in Chapter 13. Using the correct mAs causes the total number of x rays in each part of the attenuated x-ray beam to be sufficient to produce correct overall density in the processed film. Because exposure (mAs) determines the total number of x rays in the beam, mAs may be considered analogous to light in producing an ordinary photograph. Too little, or too much, mAs results in an underexposed or overexposed radiograph.

Subject contrast may be thought of as one factor that controls the log relative exposure which reaches the film. That is, film directly under a bone receives a low exposure, while a high exposure reaches the film under soft tissue areas of the subject. A consideration of film contrast must examine how the film responds to the difference in exposure produced by subject contrast. Film contrast depends on four factors:

1. characteristic curve of the film
2. film density
3. screen or direct x-ray exposure
4. film processing.

Shape of the Characteristic Curve

The shape of the characteristic curve tells us how much change in film density will occur as film exposure changes. The slope, or gradient, of the curve may be measured and expressed numerically. One such measurement is called **film gamma.** The gamma of a film is defined as the maximum slope of the characteristic curve, and is described by the formula

$$\text{Gamma} = \frac{D_2 - D_1}{\log E_2 - \log E_1}$$

where D_2 and D_1 are the densities on the steepest part of the curve resulting from log relative exposures E_2 and E_1. Figure 11–7 shows an example of how film gamma is calculated. The gamma of x-ray films exposed with intensifying screens ranges from 2.0 to 3.5.

In radiology the concept of film gamma is of little value because, as illustrated in Figure 11–7, the maximum slope (steepest) portion of the characteristic curve is usually

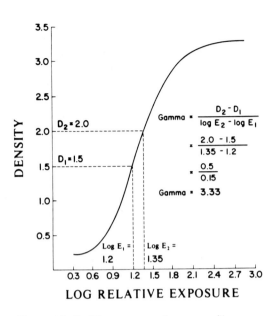

Figure 11–7   The gamma of an x-ray film

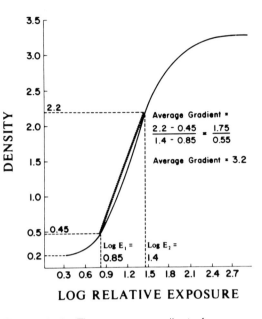

Figure 11–8   The average gradient of an x-ray film

very short. We are interested in the slope of the curve over the entire range of useful radiographic densities (0.25 to 2.0). The slope (gradient) of a straight line joining two points of specified density on the characteristic curve is called the **average gradient.** The average gradient is usually calculated between density 0.25 and 2.0 above base and fog for radiographic films. Such a calculation is shown in Figure 11–8, which is the same curve from which gamma was calculated in Figure 11–7. In calculating average gradient, D_1 is always 0.25 and D_2 is 2.0; therefore, $D_2 - D_1$ is always 1.75. In Figure 11–8, log E_2 and E_1 are 1.4 and 0.85, respectively.

If the average gradient of the film used is greater than 1, the film will exaggerate subject contrast and, the higher the average gradient, the greater this exaggeration will be. A film with average gradient of 1 will not change subject contrast; a film with an average gradient of less than 1 will decrease subject contrast. Because contrast is very important in radiology, x-ray films all have an average gradient of greater than 1. For example, consider a radiograph of the hand (exposed with a screen-film com-

bination) made with an x-ray beam of proper energy (kVp) to cause the bones to absorb four times as many photons as the soft tissue. This means that four times as many x-ray photons will reach the film under soft tissues as will reach the film under bone. The difference in log relative exposure, between bone and soft tissue reaching the film under the hand is 0.6 (log 4 = 0.6). If we assign a value of 1.5 as the log relative exposure in the soft tissue area (E_S), then the log relative exposure corresponding to the bones (E_B) is 0.9 (Fig. 11–9). These two exposures will produce film densities of 0.8 (bone density) and 2.8 (soft tissue density) on the hypothetical film's characteristic curve depicted in Figure 11–9. This is a density range of 2.0, corresponding to an overall brightness range of 100:1 when the film is transilluminated and viewed (100 is the antilog of 2.0). Thus, subject contrast resulting in an exposure range to the x-ray film of 4:1 has been exaggerated, or amplified, in the viewed radiograph into a brightness range (radiographic contrast) of 100:1.

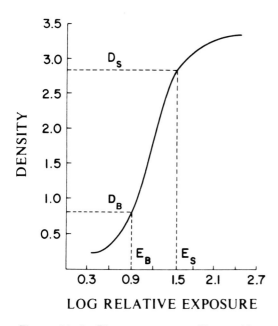

Figure 11–9 Film contrast amplifies subject contrast if the average gradient is greater than one

Film Density

The slope of the characteristic curve (i.e., film contrast) changes with density. This is especially true in the toe and shoulder regions (see Fig. 11–5). Let us emphasize that the ratio of the difference in log relative exposure is determined by the kVp selected (such as the 4:1 ratio between soft tissue and bone in the example of the hand). If the kVp remains constant, this ratio will remain constant for any one examination despite change in exposure time, milliamperes, or focus-film distance. All these last mentioned factors, however, will determine the actual value of the exposure, thereby determining the location of the exposure on the log relative exposure axis of the characteristic curve of the film.

Let us consider an x-ray study of the abdomen in which the kVp chosen results in one area transmitting about 1.6 times more radiation than another. This means a log relative exposure difference of 0.2 (log 1.6 = 0.2). We will assume that the film used

for this study has the characteristic curve depicted in Figure 11–10. If the factors of time, milliamperes, and focus-film distance (the inverse square law) are correct, the log relative exposures will produce film density falling along the steep portion of the characteristic curve. This will produce a density difference (radiographic contrast) of 0.6, or a difference in light transmission of 4:1 (antilog 0.6 = 4). If the exposure puts the developed densities on the toe of the curve, however, the film is underexposed (not enough mAs), and the density difference will fall to 0.13, or a difference in light transmission of 1.35:1 (antilog 0.13 = 1.35). Note that the exposure ratio has remained the same (i.e., log relative exposure difference of 0.2) because the kVp has not been changed. Similarly, overexposure, or too many mAs, will result in densities in the shoulder region of the characteristic curve of our hypothetic film-screen combination. As shown in Figure 11–10, this will result in a density difference (contrast)

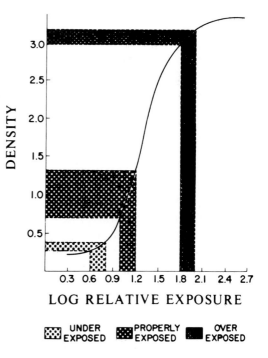

Figure 11–10 Incorrect exposures result in loss of contrast

of 0.2, corresponding to a difference in light transmission of 1.59:1 (antilog 0.2 = 1.59). Exposures producing density at the level of 3 (0.1% of light transmitted) also produce less visible contrast under ordinary viewing conditions, because the human eye has low sensitivity to contrast at low brightness levels. This is why a spotlight must be used to aid in viewing regions of high density.

Screen or Direct X-Ray Exposure

If a film designed for exposure by light from intensifying screens is exposed to x rays directly, its characteristic curve has a considerably different shape than the curve obtained from exposure with screens. Remember, considerably more exposure (mAs) is required if no screens are used, because the intensification factor of screens may range from about 15 to 50 or more. Films exposed with par speed intensifying screens will require an x-ray exposure of approximately 1 mR to produce a density of 1; this value will rise to 30 mR or more with direct x-ray exposure.

At the same density, contrast is always lower for a film exposed to x rays only than for the same film exposed by light from intensifying screens. The reason for this difference in contrast is not precisely known. It probably is related to the complex manner in which the film emulsion responds to the energy of absorbed x-ray photons.

In addition, intensifying screens are relatively more sensitive than film to higher energy x rays. The primary x-ray beam transmitted through the patient is of higher energy than the secondary, or scatter, radiation. Scatter radiation decreases contrast, as will be discussed in detail in Chapter 13. Because intensifying screens are relatively less sensitive to the lower energy of the scatter radiation, decrease in contrast will be minimized by screens. X-ray film, because it is more sensitive to lower kVp x rays, may record the scatter radiation better than the higher energy, in-

formation-containing primary beam. The variation in film sensitivity to x rays between 50 and 100 kVp is not very great, however, and can usually be ignored in clinical radiology.

Stated another way, the average gradient of a double-emulsion x-ray film will be greatest when the film is exposed with intensifying screens. Direct x-ray exposure will produce a lower average gradient. The photochemical reasons for this phenomenon are unknown.

Film Processing (Development)

Increasing the time and/or temperature of development will, up to a point, increase the average gradient of a film (film speed is also increased). If development time is only 40% of normal, the gradient will be reduced to about 60% of maximum. Fog will also be increased with increased development time or temperature, though, and fog decreases contrast. Therefore, it is important to adhere to the manufacturer's standards in processing film. Automatic film processing equipment has eliminated some problems associated with temperature of solutions and development time. To summarize, increasing the time or temperature of development will

1. increase average gradient (increase film contrast),
2. increase film speed (increase density for a given exposure),
3. increase fog (decrease film contrast).

Figure 11–11 shows the effect of development time (or temperature) on average gradient, film speed, and fog.

Speed

The speed of a film-screen system is defined as the reciprocal of the exposure in Roentgens required to produce a density of 1.0 above base plus fog density:

$$\text{Speed} = \frac{1}{\text{Roentgens}}$$

As an example we will consider the speed

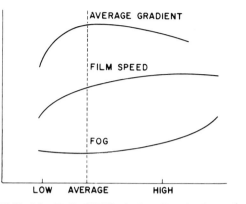

Figure 11–11 Development time influences average gradient, speed, and fog

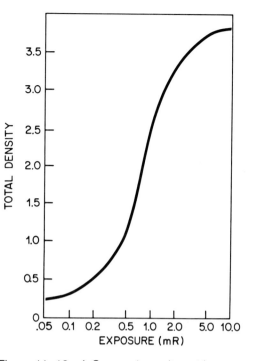

Figure 11–12 A Cronex 4 sensitometric curve (70-kVp exposure, Hi Plus screens) shows that 0.57 mR is used to reach a 1.0 net density. The system speed for 70 kVp is

$$\frac{1}{0.00057} = 1750 \text{ R}^{-1}$$

(Modified from the Cronex 4 medical x-ray film data sheet available from E.I. du Pont de Nemours Company, Inc. Modified with the help of Russell S. Holland, Ph.D.)

of a commonly used film-screen system, Du Pont Cronex 4 film combined with Du Pont Cronex Hi Plus (CaWO₄) screens. Analysis of the curve in Figure 11–12 shows that an exposure of 0.57 mR (0.00057 R) was required to produce a net density of 1.0 above base and fog. Therefore, the speed (S) of the film-screen system for this kVp is

$$S = \frac{1}{0.00057 \text{ R}} = 1750 \text{ R}^{-1}$$

The shape of the characteristic curve is controlled by film contrast; the film speed determines the location of the curve on the log exposure scale.

Figure 11–13 shows the curves of two films that are identical except that film B is 0.3 log relative exposure units to the right of film A. Both films will show identical film contrast, but film B will require twice (antilog 0.3 = 2) as much exposure (mAs) as film A. Because the gradient of a characteristic curve varies with density, the relative speed between two films will be found to vary with the density at which speed is measured. For example, if a low-contrast and a high-contrast film are compared for speed, as in Figure 11–14, the relative speed between the two films might actually reverse with change in density. In our example, speed calculated at a density

of 1.0 will show the low-contrast film (film B) to be the fastest (i.e., film B requires a lower log relative exposure to produce a density of 1.0 than film A). At a density of 1.5 both films have the same speed, and above density 1.5 the higher contrast film A is faster than film B. For medical x-ray films, relative film speed is usually compared at a density of 1.0 above base and fog.

Speed Class System

The measured speed of a film-screen system depends on a number of variables, such as the kVp, amount of scatter radiation, x-ray absorption by the cassette or

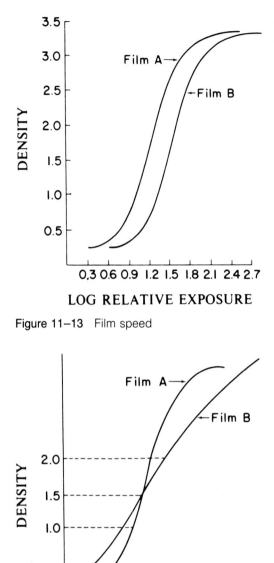

Figure 11–13 Film speed

Figure 11–14 Relative film speed varies with the density at which speed is measured

x-ray table top, and the way in which the film is processed. The American National Standards Institute (ANSI) has attempted to standardize the way in which speed (and contrast) of medical x-ray film-screen systems is measured.[1] This standard defines test objects that are used to simulate ra-

diography of the chest, the skull or pelvis, and the extremities. Various exposures are made at four kilovoltages, approximately 125, 80, 70, and 60 kVp. Film processing is strictly controlled. If all manufacturers followed such a rigid standard to determine speed, direct comparison of products would be easy and meaningful. As things exist now, however, published measurements of speed must be used as approximations only. For this reason, we suggest that the "speed class system" concept be used to assign relative speeds to various film-screen systems.

Refer to Table 11–2, which is the same as Table 9–6. Notice that film-screen speed is listed as speed class.* The numbers in the speed class system make up a sequence in which the logarithm of each number differs from the next number by 0.1 (i.e., this is a 0.1 log system). Table 11–3 lists the sequence from 100 to 1000 and gives the logarithm of each number. Note that the log of each number increases or decreases by 0.1 (this makes each number approximately 25% greater or less than its neighbor). Thus, the ratio between numbers in the sequence is a constant. Because log 2 = 0.3, addition of 0.3 to the log of a number multiplies the number by 2 (e.g., log 160 = 2.2, log 320 = 2.5, etc.). All of us who use a camera have used this 0.1 log system, usually without realizing it. Consider the speed of the film you use in your camera. Don't the numbers ASA 25, 32, 64, 125, 200, and 400 sound familiar? Table 11–3 does not list the sequence below 100, but simply divide by 10 to go on down (i.e., 100, 80, 64, 50, 40, 32, 25, 20, 16, and so forth).

Why propose this speed class system? First, it is a handy number sequence. It is easy to multiply or divide by 10, the numbers increase or decrease by an easily de-

---

*This idea was proposed to us by Robert Wayrynen, Ph.D.: Reid Kellogg, Ph.D.; and Russell Holland, Ph.D., of the photo products department of E.I. du Pont de Nemours & Company, Inc.

Table 11–2. Speed Class of Various Intensifying Screens

MANUFACTURER	NAME	PHOSPHOR	SPECTRAL EMISSION	FILM	SPEED CLASS
Du Pont	Cronex Par Speed	$CaWO_4$	Blue	Cronex 4	100
	Cronex Hi Plus	$CaWO_4$	Blue	Cronex 4	250
	Cronex Quanta II	BaFCl:Eu	Blue	Cronex 4	500
	Cronex Quanta III	LaOBr:Tm	Blue	Cronex 4	800
	Cronex Quanta V	LaOBr:Tm and	Blue	Cronex 4	320
		Gd_2O_2S:Tb	Green	Cronex 8	400
Kodak	X-Omatic Fine	$BaPbSO_4$, yellow dye	Blue	XRP	32
	X-Omatic Regular	$BaSrSO_4$:Eu, neutral dye	Blue	XRP	200
	Lanex Fine	Gd_2O_2S:Tb, neutral dye	Green	Ortho G	100
	Lanex Medium	Gd_2O_2S:Tb, yellow dye	Green	Ortho G	250
	Lanex Regular	Gd_2O_2S:Tb	Green	Ortho G	400

Table 11–3. Speed Class System of Numbers from 100 to 1000

Number	100	125	160	200	250	320	400	500	640	800	1000
Logarithm	2	2.1	2.2	2.3	2.4	2.5	2.6	2.7	2.8	2.9	3.0

fined ratio, and a change in log of 0.3 doubles or halves a number. The other reason is that the currently available measurements of film-screen system speed are not standardized. Published values are accurate for the conditions under which they were determined, but such conditions vary. Until rigid standards (such as the ANSI method[1]) are adopted by industry, assigning a particular film-screen system speed to one of the numbers in the 0.1 log system appears reasonable. There are more than 1000 film-screen combinations on the market today, so some "lumping" of an otherwise enormous variety of expressions of speed seems necessary. Some of you may have also noticed that the mAs stations of some x-ray generators now use an 0.1 log sequence of steps.

Latitude

Unlike average gradient and speed, film latitude is not expressed in numeric terms. Latitude refers to the range of log relative exposure (mAs) that will produce density within the accepted range for diagnostic

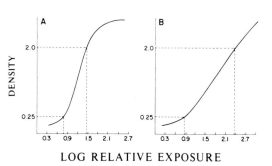

LOG RELATIVE EXPOSURE

Figure 11–15 Film B has greater latitude than film A

radiology (usually considered to be density 0.25 to 2.0). Let us consider two hypothetical films (Fig. 11–15), one a high-contrast film (film A) and one a lower contrast film (film B). If the density recorded on the film is to remain in the range of 0.25 to 2.0, film A will be limited to a log relative exposure range of 0.75 to 1.42, or a difference in log relative exposure of 0.67 corresponding to an actual ratio of 4.68 to 1 (antilog 0.67 = 4.68). Film B will remain in the designated density values over a range of log relative exposure from 0.85

to 2.35, or a difference in log exposure of 1.50 corresponding to an actual ratio of 31.6:1. Film B is said to have greater latitude than film A in that it will accept a wider range of exposures. Note that film B has greater latitude but less film contrast. Generally speaking, **the latitude of a film varies inversely with film contrast.** There are two practical aspects to this concept of film latitude. For the technologist exposing a film, the film with more latitude makes the exposure less critical; if he has picked the proper kVp for adequate penetration, he has more room for error in his choice of exposure (mAs). Generally, the radiologist is interested in high contrast, which means films of less latitude. But there may be situations in which a wide range of subject contrast (such as in the chest) must be recorded, and in such cases the film with the lower contrast but higher latitude may produce a radiograph in which many small changes in film exposures (i.e., subject contrast) can be recorded. Such lower contrast but higher latitude films are available to the radiologist. (We will discuss another aspect of exposure latitude as it pertains to kVp and subject contrast in Chapter 13.)

Double-Emulsion Film

Films used for routine radiography have photosensitive emulsion coated on both sides of the base support. There is a physical and photographic reason for this. The emulsion is applied to the base in liquid form. When the emulsion dries, it shrinks to about one tenth of its original volume. Most of the decrease in volume causes a decrease in thickness of the emulsion, but there is also a slight tendency to shrink in area. If emulsion were put on only one side of the base, shrinking of the emulsion would cause the film to curl toward the emulsion side. An identical emulsion on each side of the base prevents this curling. The photographic advantage of a double emulsion is important only when the film is exposed with intensifying screens. We may assume that each emulsion receives an

identical exposure from each screen, because any filtering action of the front screen that might act to decrease the intensity of x rays reaching the back screen is small.

Consider the case of a single-emulsion film in a cassette, which receives two exposures, log E_1 and E_2, and responds with densities D_1 and D_2. Film contrast for this exposure difference may be expressed as

$$\text{Contrast} = \frac{D_2 - D_1}{\log E_2 - \log E_1}$$

If this same exposure is now used to expose a double-emulsion film with light from intensifying screens, each emulsion will respond with densities D_1 and D_2. When two films are superimposed, the resulting density is the sum of the densities of each film. Therefore, when the double-emulsion film is viewed, the densities of each emulsion are added, and the resulting total density will now be $D_1 + D_1 = 2D_1$ and $D_2 + D_2 = 2D_2$. The exposures E_2 and E_1 have not changed, but we have allowed two emulsions to respond to the exposure. The contrast that the eye now sees is

$$\text{Contrast} = \frac{2D_2 - 2D_1}{\log E_2 - \log E_1} = \frac{2(D_2 - D_1)}{\log E_2 - \log E_1}$$

Because $\log E_2 - \log E_1$ is the same for each exposure, we may compare contrast without the $\log E_2 - \log E_1$ term:

$$\text{Single emulsion contrast} = D_2 - D_1$$

$$\text{Double emulsion contrast} = 2(D_2 - D_1)$$

The double-emulsion film has produced twice the contrast of a single-emulsion film. Obviously, the overall density of the double-emulsion film is increased, resulting in increased film speed. For a film being exposed to x rays directly, a similar effect could be produced by making a single-emulsion film with a thicker emulsion. Because light photons are easily absorbed by the emulsion, however, only the outer layer of the emulsion is affected by light from intensifying screens. This is one reason why x-ray film designed for exposure by light from two intensifying screens (in a cassette) has a thin emulsion on each side of the base, rather than a single thick emulsion.

EMULSION ABSORPTION

To expose an x-ray film with intensifying screens, it is necessary for the silver halide grains in the film to absorb the light emitted by the screen phosphor. The ability of the film grains to absorb light depends on the wavelength, or color, of the light. **Standard silver halide films absorb light in the ultraviolet, violet, and blue regions of the visible spectrum.** Used with calcium tungstate or barium lead sulfate screens, such films worked well because these phosphors emitted light that was absorbed by natural silver halide (Fig. 11–16). Note that natural silver halide film does not absorb in the green and yellow portions of the visible spectrum, where much of the light from some rare earth phosphors is emitted (see Fig. 11–18). You will recall that the peak wavelengths from some rare earth screens, such as Kodak Lanex screens, are produced by the terbium ion with about 60% of its energy at about 544 nm (green light). It is possible to extend the sensitivity of film to the green wavelengths by coating

the silver halide grains with a thin layer of dye that absorbs the green light and then transfers this absorbed energy to the grain. Such green-sensitive film is called **ortho** film. Similarly, the silver halide grain can be coated with a dye that absorbs red light, and this is called a **pan** film (panchromatic: sensitive to light of all colors). This is illustrated in Figure 11–17. When rare earth screens are used, an appropriate film should be used if one is to take advantage of all the light emitted by the screen. Such a combination is the Kodak Lanex screen and Ortho G film (Fig. 11–18).

Please look back at Figure 9–12, which shows the spectral emission of LaOBr:Tm (found in Du Pont Cronex Quanta III and Quanta V screens). Remember that this

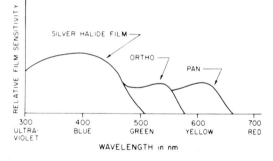

Figure 11–17 Relative spectral sensitivity of natural silver halide, ortho, and pan films

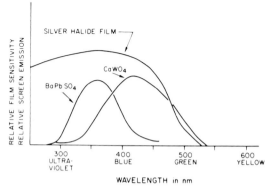

Figure 11–16 The spectral emission of barium lead sulfate and calcium tungstate intensifying screens compared to the spectral sensitivity of natural silver halide (not drawn to scale)

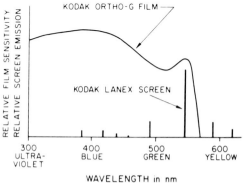

Figure 11–18 Spectral emission of Kodak Lanex Regular screens and the spectral sensitivity of Kodak Ortho G film (the bars and curve are approximations used for illustration only, and no attempt to achieve accuracy was made)

rare earth, activated by thulium, produces light to which natural silver halide film is sensitive. Compare the twin peaks of 374 nm and 463 nm in Figure 9–12 to the sensitivity of silver halide as shown in Figure 11–17. Some rare earth phosphor screens use green-sensitive film, some use blue-sensitive film, and some (e.g., Cronex Quanta V) may use either.

Darkroom Safelight

The use of ortho films requires that the correct darkroom safelight be used. For many years an amber safelight (such as the Kodak Type 6B filter) has been used with blue-sensitive films. The amber safelight emits light to which ortho film is sensitive, however, and will produce "safelight fog" if used with such film. With ortho films a safelight filter shifted more toward the red is required (this removes the green light to which ortho film is sensitive). Such a red safelight filter is the Kodak GBX-2 filter. Figure 11–19 illustrates the approximate sensitivity of regular silver halide film and ortho film as compared to the transmission of an amber (6B) and a red (GBX-2) safelight filter.

Crossover Exposure

Crossover exposure occurs when a double-emulsion x-ray film is exposed in a cassette containing two intensifying screens. Ideally, each film emulsion would receive

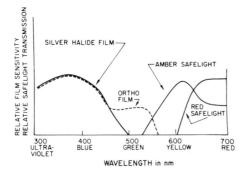

Figure 11–19 Spectral sensitivity of natural silver halide and ortho film compared to the transmission of an amber and a red safelight filter

light only from the screen in contact with the emulsion. Crossover is the exposure of a film emulsion to light emitted by the screen opposite the emulsion. The main cause of this crossover is incomplete absorption of light by the adjacent emulsion. This unabsorbed light passes through the film base to reach the opposite emulsion. The crossover light is spread because of diffusion, scattering, and reflection caused by the film base and interfaces between the emulsions and film base. Crossover exposure is a significant contributing factor to unsharpness in film-screen systems.

How important is this crossover light in terms of total film exposure? With green-sensitive films, up to 40% of the total exposure is attributed to print-through. Blue-sensitive emulsions (natural silver halide) are slightly more efficient light absorbers and, with blue light systems, crossover comprises less than one third of the total exposure (about 30 to 32% with $CaWO_4$ screens, and only 23% with $BaSrSO_4$ screens).

At present, there is only one x-ray film designed to reduce crossover exposure (3M XUD film). This film contains a light-absorbing layer coated on both sides of a film base, between the base and each emulsion. This anticrossover coating absorbs light attempting to diffuse through the base into the opposite emulsion. The coating is rendered invisible during film processing and is not visible on the radiograph. With XUD film, only about 13% of total film darkening is caused by crossover. System speed is decreased by 40% when the anticrossover film is used. The ideal way to decrease crossover without decreasing film speed would be to increase light absorption in the film emulsion, because this would improve image quality without reducing system speed.

It must be pointed out that the effect of crossover on the diagnostic usefulness of the radiographic image is unknown. When examining thin body parts (e.g., the hand), anticrossover film produces a superior image. When thicker body parts are examined, the increase in geometric unsharpness and scatter tend to deemphasize the difference in imaging properties of different film-screen systems.

Low-Dose Mammography

The photo products department of the E.I. du Pont de Nemours & Company has developed a film-screen system designed specifically to provide the diagnostic clarity needed for mammography; this is marketed as the Lo-Dose system. Perhaps a brief technical description of the Lo-Dose system will illustrate a practical application of some of the tedious details in the chapters dealing with films and screens. (Other manufacturers also market systems appropriate for mammography.)

The Lo-Dose system uses a single-emulsion x-ray film, a single high-definition calcium tungstate intensifying screen, and a flexible vacuum cassette. The mammography screen is made with a calcium tungstate phosphor because its x-ray absorption in the energy range used in mammography (15 to 30 keV) is at least as high as that of other phosphors. The single-screen phosphor layer is 0.1 mm (0.004 in.) thick and contains a yellow dye. Sharpness and resolution of the screen permit imaging calcifications as small as 0.1 mm, while x-ray absorption is high enough to allow minimum quantum noise (mottle) and maximum speed. The single emulsion x-ray film used with this screen eliminates parallax and crossover as causes of unsharpness. Using the screen in the rear position, so that x rays pass through the film first, allows a small but perceptible gain in sharpness compared with the reverse position. Speed of the film is about half that of standard medium-speed x-ray film; use of a faster film was found to cause a perceptible increase in quantum mottle. The use of a vacuum cassette ensures intimate film-screen contact, eliminating another potential cause of unsharpness. This system will record a log exposure scale of 1.4 (i.e., an

exposure range of 25:1), which is needed to visualize all breast tissue from the chest wall to the edge of the breast as well as abnormal soft tissue structures and calcifications. The density scale allows all detail in the breast image to be recorded at densities less than 3.0 to minimize the need for using high-intensity light to view the film. The exposure required with this system is about one seventh that required with direct x-ray exposure of high-speed industrial (single-emulsion) films.

The preceding describes the Du Pont Lo-Dose/1 system. In 1975 Du Pont introduced the Lo-Dose/2 intensifying screen. The Lo-Dose/2 is also a calcium tungstate screen but does not contain the yellow light-absorbing dye found in the Lo-Dose/1 screen, resulting in a faster intensifying screen that sacrifices some screen sharpness. (If a par speed calcium tungstate screen is assigned a relative speed of 1.0, the relative speed of a Lo-Dose/1 screen is 0.062, and that of a Lo-Dose/2 screen is 0.125). In addition, a film called MRF31 can be used rather than Lo-Dose film. MRF31 is a single-emulsion film coated on a blue-tinted base that is twice as fast as Lo-Dose film. The higher contrast film has less latitude, so a more limited exposure range can be recorded. This smaller exposure range became useful as a result of better use of compression devices, which make the breast tissue more uniform in thickness. Use of Lo-Dose/2 and MRF31 film can reduce patient exposure by a factor of 4 as compared to that of the original Lo-Dose system. But remember the compromise. Faster screens (by eliminating the dye) mean more unsharpness. Increasing film speed by 2 means that only half as many x-ray photons are used; this increases quantum noise by the square root of 2 (quantum mottle is a subject for Chapter 13).

In 1975 Kodak announced a film-screen combination for mammography called Min-R. This combination uses a single gadolinium oxysulfide intensifying screen and a single-emulsion orthochromatic film, and has a system speed comparable to that of the Lo-Dose/2. The Kodak Min-R screen is the same as the Lanex Fine screen. The Min-R screen may be used with Min-R film to obtain a slow speed system, or with Ortho M film to double the system speed (Ortho M film is twice as fast as Min-R film and has significantly higher contrast). Other film-screen systems for mammography have been announced by other manufacturers.

TRANSPARENCY VERSUS PRINT

Why is a radiograph viewed as a transparency rather than as a print, like an ordinary photograph? The density of a print is related to the amount of light reflected or absorbed by the paper. The density of the maximum black of most photographic printing papers is between 1.3 and 1.7. A few papers give density values as high as 2.0 (glossy-surfaced paper gives the highest maximum black). Obviously, such a limitation on maximum density would be intolerable in radiology, in which densities up to 2.0, and occasionally greater, are commonly encountered. This limitation is overcome by viewing the radiograph as a transparency, which permits use of density ranges up to a maximum of 3.0 or more for diagnostic radiology films and up to 6.0 for industrial x-ray use.

SUMMARY

The amount of blackening of an x-ray film is expressed by the term photographic density. The most useful range of density in diagnostic radiology is 0.25 to 2.0, although densities up to 3.0 are sometimes used.

Analysis of the characteristic curve of a film provides information about the contrast, speed, and latitude of the film. Film contrast amplifies subject contrast if the average gradient of the film is greater than 1. Film contrast will vary with the amount of exposure (density), the way the film is exposed (intensifying screens or direct action of x rays), and the way the film is developed.

Double-emulsion films produce greater contrast than single-emulsion films (assuming light is used to expose the film).

X-ray film is viewed as a transparency because of the greater range of density available.

The film must be able to absorb the wavelength of light emitted by the intensifying screen. Some of the newer intensifying screen phosphors must be used with an appropriately sensitized (i.e., ortho) x-ray film.

REFERENCES

1. American National Standards Institute: American National Standard Method for the Sensitometry of Medical X-Ray Screen-Film-Processing Systems. New York, American National Standards Institute, 1982. (Available as ANSI PH2.43-1982 from the American National Institute, 1430 Broadway, New York, NY 10018.)
2. Bates, L.M.: Some Physical Factors Affecting Radiographic Image Quality: Their Theoretical Basis and Measurement. Washington, DC, U.S. Government Printing Office, 1969, Public Health Service Pub. No. 999-RH-38.
3. Doi, K., Loo, L.N., Anderson, T.M., and Frank, P.H.: Effect of crossover exposure on radiographic image quality of screen-film systems. Radiology, *139*:707, 1981.
4. Lawrence, D.J.: Kodak X-Omatic and Lanex screens and Kodak films for medical radiography. Rochester, NY, Eastman Kodak Company, Radiography Markets Division, File No. 5.03, June 1976.
5. Meredith, W.J., and Massey, J.B.: Fundamental Physics of Radiology. Baltimore, Williams & Wilkins, 1968.
6. Ostrum, B.J., Becker, W., and Isard, H.J.: Low-dose mammography. Radiology, *109*:323, 1973.
7. Presentation Script: New Screen Technology. Prepared by Photo Products Department. Wilmington, Del., E.I. du Pont de Nemours & Company.
8. Rao, G.U.V., Fatouros, P.P., and James, A.E.: Physical characteristics of modern radiographic screen-film systems. Invest. Radiol., *13*:460, 1978.
9. Seeman, H.E.: Physical and Photographic Principles of Medical Radiography. New York, John Wiley and Sons, 1968.
10. Sensitometric Properties of X-Ray Films. Rochester, NY, Eastman Kodak Company, Radiography Markets Division.
11. Thompson, T.T.: Selecting medical x-ray film. Part 1. Appl. Radiol., *4*:47, 1974.
12. Thompson, T.T.: Selecting medical x-ray film. Part II. Appl. Radiol., *4*:51, 1974.
13. Wayrynen, R.E.: Radiographic film. Contained in

the syllabus of the 1975 AAPM Summer School: The Expanding Role of the Diagnostic Radiologic Physicist, Rice University, Houston, July 27–August 1, 1975, p. 112.

14. Wayrynen, R.E.: Fundamental aspects of mammographic receptors film process. *In* Reduced Dose Mammography. Edited by W.W. Logan and E.P. Muntz. New York, Masson Publishing USA, 1979, pp. 521–528.

15. Weiss, J.P., and Wayrynen, R.E.: Imaging system for low-dose mammography. J. Appl. Photogr. Eng., *2*:7, 1976.

12

Geometry of the Radiographic Image

We must briefly consider some geometric and trigonometric factors that influence the quality of the image of a radiograph. We will only consider examples of x rays originating at the x-ray tube and directed at the patient (or test object) and an x-ray film. We will assume that any object placed in the x-ray beam will absorb all the x-ray photons that hit the object. This is a very unlikely situation, but it makes examples easier to draw and understand. Because x rays travel in straight lines, the x-ray beam can be drawn as a straight line that hits the object or the film. The fact that x rays are emitted in all directions from the target of the x-ray tube has been previously discussed. In our examples we will assume the ideal situation, in which proper collimation has produced a beam that is perfectly cone-shaped, and the object is placed in the x-ray beam at a varying distance from the film. We will observe the beam from one side so its shape can be drawn as a triangle, with the focal spot of the x-ray tube as the apex (origin of x rays) and the object or the film as the base of the triangle (Fig. 12–1). In Figure 12–1, h represents the focal spot-object distance, and H is the focal spot-film distance. This type of diagram will allow us to consider two triangles, one with the object as its base and the other with the film as its base (Fig. 12–2). The two triangles have the same shape but are of different sizes, and are known as **similar**

triangles. The sides and altitudes of similar triangles are proportional. This means that, in Figure 12–2,

$$\frac{a}{A} = \frac{b}{B} = \frac{c}{C} = \frac{h}{H}$$

The altitude of a triangle is a perpendicular dropped from a vertex to the opposite side or to an extension of the opposite side.

By using simple line drawings to represent the conditions of our idealized x-ray object-film conditions, and by applying the rule of similar triangles, it is possible to develop an understanding of the basic

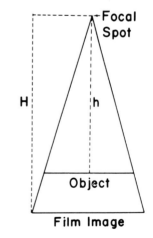

Figure 12–1 Schematic drawing of the relationship between an x-ray beam, the object being examined, and the image of the object on the film

152

principles of magnification, distortion, and penumbra.

MAGNIFICATION

When an object is placed in the x-ray beam, it will cast a "shadow" on the film that will show some degree of enlargement. Because it is assumed that the object absorbs all the x rays that hit it, the developed film will show a clear area corresponding to the shape of the object, surrounded by blackened (exposed) film. If the object is round and flat, shaped like a coin, its magnified image will be round but larger than the coin. The image has been magnified, and the amount of magnification (M) can be defined as

$$M = \frac{\text{size of the image}}{\text{size of the object}}$$

In the clinical situation the object may be

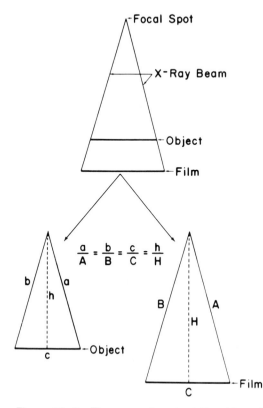

$$\frac{a}{A} = \frac{b}{B} = \frac{c}{C} = \frac{h}{H}$$

Figure 12–2 The proportional relationships of similar triangles

a structure or foreign body within the patient that is not available for measurement. It is usually possible to determine the distance of the source of x rays (focal spot of the x-ray tube) from the film, however, as well as the distance of the object from the film, and the image size can be measured directly. By determining the degree of magnification, the true size of the object can be calculated. Refer to Figure 12–1, which shows a simple line drawing of an object placed some distance from the x-ray film, causing its image to be magnified by the diverging x-ray beam. The altitude of the large triangle (H) represents the distance from the focal spot of the x-ray tube to the film, often termed **focus-film distance.** The altitude of the smaller triangle (h) represents the distance from the focal spot to the object, or the **focus-object distance.** Because the sides and altitudes of similar triangles are proportional,

$$\frac{h}{H} = \frac{\text{object size}}{\text{image size}}$$

Because focus-film distance, image size, and focus-object distance can be measured directly, object size is easy to calculate. Notice that calculating simple magnification problems does not require that any formulas be learned. Consider a simple example. Using a 40-inch focus-film distance, the image of an object that is known to be 8 inches from the film measures 10 cm in length. What is the true length of the object, and how much magnification is present? Using Figure 12–1, we see that H = 40, h = 32 (40 − 8 = 32), and image size = 10 cm. Setting up the proportion:

$$\frac{40}{32} = \frac{10 \text{ cm}}{\text{object size}}$$

Solving for object size:

$$\text{Object size} = \frac{(32)\,(10)}{40} = 8 \text{ cm}$$

$$M = \frac{\text{size of the image}}{\text{size of the object}} = \frac{10}{8} = 1.25$$

What if the object is not placed directly

beneath the focal spot, but is displaced to one side so that the more oblique x rays are used to form an image? If the object is flat, and remains parallel to the film, magnification will be exactly the same for the object whether central or oblique x rays are used. Consider Figure 12–3, in which the coin is not directly beneath the x-ray tube but is still parallel to the film. The altitude of the two triangles is exactly the same as it was when the object was directly under the focal spot (see Fig. 12–1), so the ratio of object to image size will be the same in each circumstance. In Figure 12–4 the three coins are parallel to, and the same distance above, the film. The image of each coin will be a circle, and all the circles will be the same size.

Under usual radiographic situations, magnification should be kept to a minimum. Two rules apply: (1) **Keep the object as close to the film as possible,** and (2) **Keep the focus-film distance as large as possible.**

Consider Figure 12–1 again. Because magnification is determined by the ratio of

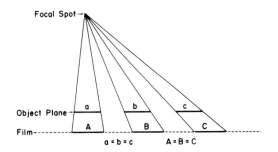

Figure 12–4 The magnification of three coins (a, b, c) all parallel to the film and the same distance above the film produces three round images (A, B, C) of equal size

the altitude of the two triangles, we may write

$$M = \frac{H}{h}$$

If H:h = 1.0, there is no magnification. The closer the object is to the film, the closer the magnitude of altitude h will approach the value of altitude H. An increase in focus-film distance (increasing H while leaving object-film distance unchanged) will also bring the ratio H:h closer to 1. To illustrate, assume an object is 6 inches from the film. What will be the magnification if the focus-film distance is (1) 40 inches, and (2) 72 inches? At 40 inches focus-film distance:

$$M = \frac{H}{h} = \frac{40}{34} = 1.18$$

At 72 inches focus-film distance:

$$M = \frac{H}{h} = \frac{72}{66} = 1.09$$

To review, magnification depends on two factors: **object-film distance** and **focus-film distance.**

DISTORTION

Distortion results from unequal magnification of different parts of the same object. Consider Figure 12–5, in which one coin (*dashed line*) is parallel to the film and the other coin (*solid line,* AB) is tilted with respect to the plane of the film. The tilted

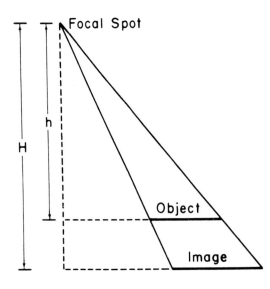

Figure 12–3 Magnification of an object by oblique rays

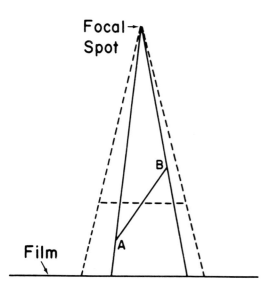

Figure 12–5 Distortion of an object (line AB) that is not parallel to the film

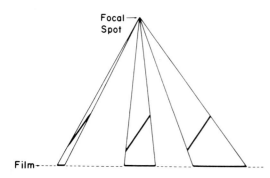

Figure 12–6 Distortion of the shape and size of the image of a tilted object depends on the position of the object in the x-ray beam

coin undergoes distortion because of unequal magnification (side A is closer to the film than side B). The shape of the image of the tilted coin will be an ellipse, and its exact size and shape will vary with the amount of tilting.

Distortion of the image of an object will be different in different parts of the x-ray beam. Figure 12–6 shows how distortion of the shape and size of three equally tilted coins will vary in different parts of the x-ray beam.

Distortion of thick objects occurs if they are not directly in the central part of the x-ray beam. Because different parts of thick objects are different distances from the x-ray film, each part will be magnified by a different amount. This will cause the shape of the image of most thick objects to be distorted. Only the part of a thick object that is parallel to the film will be undistorted. Figure 12–7 illustrates the relative size and shape of the image of three spheres (such as steel ball bearings) that are in different parts of the x-ray beam. The sphere that lies in the center of the beam will exhibit a round (undistorted) magnified image. The image of each of the two laterally placed spheres will be an ellipse because the x-ray beam "sees" a diameter of each of these spheres that is not parallel to the film. The x-ray beam "sees" a laterally placed spherical object in the same way it "sees" a round flat object (a coin) that is tilted with respect to the plane of the film. Notice the similarity between Figures 12–6 and 12–7.

Distortion of the relative position of the image of two objects may occur if the objects are at different distances from the film. For example, in Figure 12–8 two opaque objects, A and B, are present inside a circle. Object A is more medial than B, but A is farther from the film. The film image of object A will be lateral to the image of object B. This is because the distance between A and the midline (line a) has been magnified much more than has the distance between B and the central beam (line b). Distortion of position is minimal when the object is near the central part

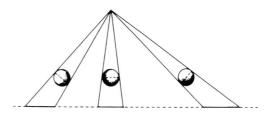

Figure 12–7 The size and shape of the image of a spherical object depends on the position of the object in relation to the central part of the x-ray beam

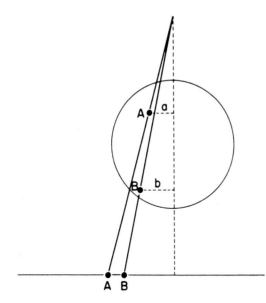

Figure 12–8   Distortion of position

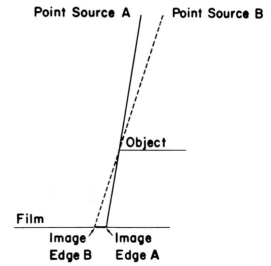

Figure 12–9   The focal spot acts as if it were composed of many point sources of x rays

of the x-ray beam, and the object is placed as close to the film as possible.

PENUMBRA

Penumbra (from the Latin *pene*, meaning almost, and *umbra*, meaning shadow), often termed **edge gradient,** is defined as the region of partial illumination that surrounds the umbra, or complete shadow. In the discussion of magnification and distortion, it was assumed that the source of x rays (focal spot) was a point source. Actually, the focal spot is not a point. It has finite dimensions, usually ranging from 0.3 to 2.0 mm square. The focal spot acts as if it were composed of many point sources of x rays, with each point source forming its own image of an object. The edges of each of these images will not be in exactly the same spot on the film. In Figure 12–9 the edge of an object, as formed by two x-ray sources (A and B), which represent the opposite ends of a focal spot, is shown. The x rays must travel in a straight line from each point source to the film. Image edges A and B are not in the same place, and an image formed in this way has a fuzzy, or unsharp, margin. This zone of unsharpness is called **geometric unsharpness, pen-**

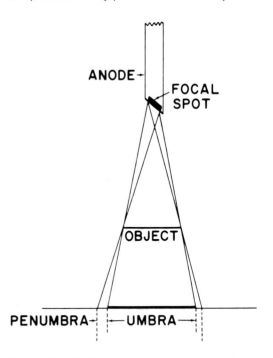

Figure 12–10   Penumbra (geometric unsharpness)

umbra, or **edge gradient,** and represents the area at which the margins caused by the many "point sources" of x rays in the focal spot overlap. Figure 12–10 shows how the zone of penumbra is formed from an angled rotating anode; focal spot size has been exaggerated. The region of complete image is called the **umbra.** These terms are used in astronomy to describe a solar eclipse, in which the umbra is the area of complete shadow within which a spectator can see no portion of the sun's disc, and the penumbra is the zone of partial shadow between the umbra and the full light. Note that, as shown in Figure 12–10, the width of the penumbra is less on the anode side than on the cathode side of the x-ray tube. This effect can be used to achieve maximum sharpness by placing the object of greatest interest toward the anode side of the x-ray tube.

The width of blurring caused by pen-umbra can be calculated. Figure 12–11 shows the penumbra (P) caused by focal spot F (dimensions are exaggerated for illustration). Note that two similar triangles are again formed, with the apex of each triangle at the object (labeled point X), the base of the upper triangle being the width of the focal spot and the base of the lower triangle being the width of the penumbra.

Because the sides and altitudes (H and h) of similar triangles are proportional, a simple proportion can be established between focal spot size (F), penumbra (P), focus-object distance (H), and object-film distance (h):

$$\frac{P}{F} = \frac{h}{H}$$

Using a 2-mm focal spot and a focus-film distance of 40 inches, calculate the penumbra if the object is (1) 4 inches above the film and (2) 10 inches above the film. In case (1) focus-object distance (H) = 40 − 4 = 36 inches:

$$\frac{P}{2} = \frac{4}{36}$$

$$P = \frac{(4)\,(2)}{36}$$

$$P = 0.22 \text{ mm}$$

In case (2) H = 40 − 10 = 30 inches:

$$\frac{P}{2} = \frac{10}{30}$$

$$P = \frac{(2)\,(10)}{30}$$

$$P = 0.67 \text{ mm}$$

In case (2), if object-film distance remains 10 inches, but focus-film distance is increased to 72 inches, what will be the penumbra?

$$\frac{P}{2} = \frac{10}{62}$$

$$P = \frac{(2)\,(10)}{62}$$

$$P = 0.32 \text{ mm}$$

The importance of focal spot size may be appreciated by substituting a focal spot size of 1 mm in each of the preceding examples.

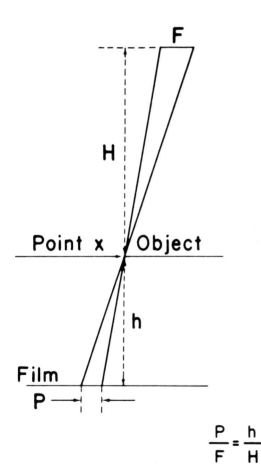

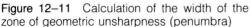

Figure 12–11 Calculation of the width of the zone of geometric unsharpness (penumbra)

The width of the penumbra will be half of that caused by a 2-mm focal spot. These situations illustrate the factors that will decrease penumbra:

1. Put the object as close to the film as possible (make h small).
2. Use as large a focus-object distance as possible (make H large).
3. Use as small a focal spot as possible.

Keeping the object as close to the film as possible, and using a long focus-film distance, also decreases magnification. The use of the magnification technique, which we will discuss in Chapter 20, causes an increase in geometric unsharpness.

MOTION UNSHARPNESS

This term is used to describe image unsharpness caused by motion of the examined object during the exposure. Object motion will produce the same type of image unsharpness as penumbra. Object motion may be minimized by immobilizing the patient or by using a short exposure time. Similar motion unsharpness will result if the focal spot moves during the exposure. X-ray tube motion is much less important than object motion, unless considerable magnification is present. (The relationship between motion and magnification will be discussed in more detail in Chapter 20.)

ABSORPTION UNSHARPNESS

Absorption unsharpness is caused by the way in which x rays are absorbed in the subject. This type of unsharpness arises from the gradual change in x-ray absorption across the boundary, or edge, of an object. To illustrate the meaning of absorption unsharpness, let us again assume that x rays originate from a point source (F). Figure 12–12 shows a truncated cone, cube, and sphere, which all have the same thickness and are assumed to be made of the same material. The cone will show little absorption unsharpness because its edges are parallel to the diverging beam, and its edge will be sharply defined on the film. It

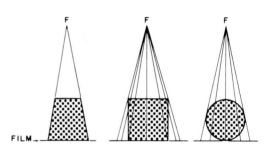

Figure 12–12   The origin of absorption unsharpness

is apparent in Figure 12–12 that the absorption of x rays by the cube will vary along the outer edge of its upper surface, with fewer x rays being absorbed along the sides, and more in the region of the lower corners. With the sphere, absorption unsharpness occurs across the entire image, with maximum x-ray absorption occurring only in the center.

Absorption unsharpness produces a poorly defined margin in the image of most solid objects because there is a gradual change in film density along the image edge. The cone shows high contrast (density difference) along its edge because there is a well-defined line on the film at which x-ray exposure changes from high (no absorption by the object) to low (high absorption by the object). In the case of the cube and the sphere, however, there is no abrupt change in the film exposure, only a gradual change, the magnitude of which depends on the shape of the object.

The effect of absorption unsharpness is particularly important when the accurate measurement of small round or oval structures is necessary, as in coronary angiography. Because absorption unsharpness is caused by the shape of the object being examined, it will occur no matter how exacting the conditions of generating and recording the radiographic image. Perhaps the term "subject unsharpness" would be more accurate.

INVERSE SQUARE LAW

X rays obey the physical laws of light. There is a well-known law of light propagation that states that the intensity of light falling on a flat surface from a point source is inversely proportional to the square of the distance from the point source. The principle is illustrated in Figure 12–13.

The number of x-ray photons emitted at the anode remains constant. At a distance of 1 foot, the diverging x-ray beam covers an area (A) represented by the square with each side of dimension x, or an area of $x \cdot x = x^2$. At 2 feet the diverging beam covers a square (B) in which each side is now twice as long as it was at 1 foot. The area covered by the beam at 2 feet is therefore $2x \cdot 2x = 4x^2$, which is four times the area at 1 foot. Because the intensity of the beam originating at the anode is constant, the intensity falling on square A must spread out over an area four times as large by the time it reaches square B. For example, assume that an x-ray tube has an output such that the intensity 1 foot from the tube is 144 units per square inch. At 2 feet, the 144 units are now divided between 4 square inches, or 36 units per square inch. Likewise, the intensity per square inch at 3 feet is

$$\frac{144}{3^2} = \frac{144}{9} = 16 \text{ units/in.}^2$$

and so forth. At 4 feet the intensity will be $(\frac{1}{4})^2$ or $\frac{1}{16}$ that at 1 foot.

A practical example will illustrate use of the inverse square law. Assume that an exposure of 100 mAs (100 mA for 1 sec) is needed for a film of the abdomen using a 40-inch focus-film distance. Employing portable equipment, the maximum focus-film distance that can be obtained at the bedside is 30 inches. What mAs must be used to maintain the same radiographic density as that obtained at a 40-inch distance (kVp remains constant)? Because the intensities (mAs) of the x-ray beam at 40 and 30 inches are proportional to the squares of these distances,

$$\frac{100 \text{ mAs}}{X \text{ mAs}} = \frac{40^2}{30^2} = \frac{1600}{900}$$

$$X = \frac{(100)(900)}{1600} = 56.25 \text{ mAs}$$

The distance from the x-ray tube to the film should be kept as large as practical to minimize the geometric unsharpness caused by penumbra. This greater distance will increase the exposure (mAs) needed to maintain proper film density. Older techniques called for a 36-inch focus-film distance but, with x-ray tubes capable of increased output, a 40-inch distance is now routine. The increased exposure required in going from 36 to 40 inches is

$$\frac{40^2}{36^2} = \frac{1600}{1296} = 1.23$$

or a 23% increase in mAs. As the output of x-ray tubes increases, techniques using up to 60-inch focus-film distance may become routine.

SUMMARY

Geometric factors that influence the quality of the radiographic image include magnification, distortion, penumbra, and motion. Absorption unsharpness produces a similar effect. Factors that will decrease unsharpness caused by

MAGNIFICATION
1. small object-film distance
2. large focal spot-film distance

PENUMBRA
1. small focal-spot size
2. small object-film distance
3. large focal spot-film distance

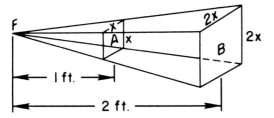

Figure 12–13 The inverse square law

MOTION

1. short exposure time
2. maximum possible limitation of actual object motion

To minimize distortion, the object of interest should be kept parallel to the film and near the central portion of the x-ray beam, and magnification should be minimized.

The intensity of the x-ray beam varies inversely as the square of the distance from the x-ray tube.

REFERENCES

1. Bookstein, J.J., and Steck, W.: Effective focal-spot size. Radiology, *98*:31, 1971.
2. Fuchs, A.W.: Principles of Radiographic Exposure and Processing. 2nd Ed. Springfield, IL, Charles C Thomas, 1958.
3. Meredith, W.J., and Ramsey, J.B.: Fundamental Physics of Radiology. Baltimore, Williams & Wilkins, 1968.
4. Method of focal spot image and measurements. Report of the International Commission on Radiological Units and Measurements. Radiology, *76*:125, 1961; and Am. J. Roentgenol., *85*:191, 1961.
5. Seeman, H.E.: Physical and Photographic Principles of Medical Radiography. New York, John Wiley and Sons, 1968.

13

The Radiographic Image

The basic tool of diagnostic radiology is the radiographic image. The radiologist must be thoroughly familiar with the factors that govern the information content of these images. R. E. Wayrynen* has suggested that the term **image clarity** be used to describe the visibility of diagnostically important detail in the radiograph.[21] Two basic factors determine the clarity of the radiographic image, contrast and image quality.

Image clarity
↙   ↘
Contrast   Image quality

A discussion of image clarity is difficult because there are so many subjective factors involved. Many problems concerning image visibility are the result of the physiologic and psychologic reactions of the observer rather than of the physical properties of the image. There is no well-defined relationship between the amount of information on a film and the accuracy of interpretation of the film. Many overlooked lesions are large and easy to see in retrospect. In this chapter the physical properties of contrast and image quality will be considered.

CONTRAST

The term **radiographic contrast** refers to the difference in density between areas in the radiograph. Differing degrees of grayness, or contrast, allow us to "see" the information contained in the x-ray image. Radiographic contrast depends on three factors:

1. subject contrast
2. film contrast
3. fog and scatter.

Subject Contrast

Subject contrast, sometimes called **radiation contrast,** is the difference in x-ray intensity transmitted through one part of the subject as compared to that transmitted through another part. In Figure 13–1, assume that a uniform beam of x rays strikes an object made up of a block of muscle (A) and a block of bone (B) of equal thickness. Few x rays are transmitted through the bone, but most go through the muscle. The attenuated x-ray beam now contains many x rays in the area beneath muscle and few

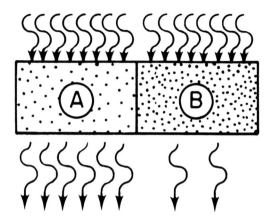

Figure 13–1 Equal thickness of muscle (A) and bone (B) do not equally attenuate an x-ray beam

*Technical Manager, X-ray Markets, E.I. du Pont de Nemours & Company.

beneath bone; this difference of intensity in the beam caused by the object is subject contrast.

Obviously, the effect of subject contrast on the x-ray beam cannot be seen directly. Because the x-ray beam exposes the film, however, anything that attenuates the x-ray beam will similarly affect the radiographic image on the film. As has been previously discussed, variations in the intensity of the x-ray beam caused by subject contrast are greatly amplified by the film. Subject contrast is the result of the attenuation of the x-ray beam by the patient, and attenuation has been discussed in detail in Chapter 5. A brief review will emphasize the pertinent points.

Subject contrast depends on

1. thickness difference
2. density difference
3. atomic number difference
4. radiation quality (kVp).

Thickness Difference

If an x-ray beam is directed at two different thicknesses of the same material, the number of x rays transmitted through the thin part will be greater than the number transmitted through the thick part. This is a relatively simple but important factor contributing to subject contrast. If I_S is the intensity of the x-ray beam (I) transmitted through the thin (small) segment, and I_L is the intensity transmitted through the thick (large) segment, subject contrast may be defined in the following way (Fig. 13–2):

$$\text{Subject contrast} = \frac{I_S}{I_L}$$

Another less obvious cause of difference in tissue thickness is the presence of a gas-filled cavity. Because gas attenuates almost no x rays, the presence of a pocket of gas in a soft tissue mass has the same effect on the x-ray beam as decreasing the thickness of the soft tissue mass. In ventriculography the brain ventricles are visible because they are filled with air. The x-ray beam then

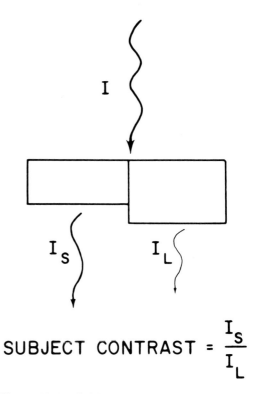

$$\text{SUBJECT CONTRAST} = \frac{I_S}{I_L}$$

Figure 13–2   Subject contrast

"sees" the cross section of brain containing a gas-filled ventricle as being "thinner" than that of the adjacent solid brain substance.

Density Difference

The difference in density between body tissues is one of the most important factors in causing subject contrast. The greater the density (i.e., mass per unit volume) of a tissue, the greater is its ability to attenuate x rays. Consider ice and water. Because ice floats in water, it is less dense than water. Water is about 9% more dense than ice. Equal thicknesses of ice and water will demonstrate subject contrast to an x-ray beam because the water attenuates 9% more of the beam than does the ice.

Atomic Number Difference

Subject contrast depends on the relative difference in attenuation of the x-ray beam by different tissues in the body. In diagnostic radiology, attenuation of the x-ray beam by the photoelectric effect makes the most important contribution to subject contrast. Photoelectric absorption is increased in substances with high atomic numbers, especially when low-kVp x rays are used. The effective atomic numbers of bone, muscle (water), and fat are

Bone	13.8
Muscle	7.4
Fat	5.9

Bone will attenuate many more x rays than muscle or fat, assuming equal thicknesses. Subject contrast between bone and muscle is high. Muscle and fat, with little difference in atomic number, show little difference in their ability to attenuate x rays by the photoelectric absorption process, and less difference by Compton reactions. Use of low-kVp (below 30) x rays produces the greatest possible difference in photoelectric x-ray absorption between muscle and fat. Soft-tissue radiography, such as mammography, requires the use of low-kVp x rays because the small differences in atomic number between breast tissues produce no subject contrast unless maximum photoelectric effect is used.

Contrast Media

The use of contrast materials with high atomic numbers (53 for iodine and 56 for barium) gives high subject contrast. Photoelectric absorption of x rays in barium and iodine will be proportionally much greater than that in bone and tissue because of the large differences in atomic number.

Radiation Quality

The ability of an x-ray photon to penetrate tissue depends on its energy; high-kVp x rays have greater energy. Selecting the proper kVp is one of the most important matters to consider in choosing the proper exposure technique. If the kVp is too low, almost all the x rays are attenuated in the patient and never reach the film.

The kilovoltage selected has a great effect on subject contrast. Low kVp will produce high subject contrast, provided the kVp is high enough to penetrate the part being examined adequately.

In general terms, the reason low kVp produces greater subject (or radiation) contrast than high kVp can be explained by a simple example. In Figure 13–2, subject contrast was defined as $\dfrac{I_S}{I_L}$. Assume that 100 x rays of low kVp (such as 50 kVp) strike the object (Fig. 13–3A). Most of these low-energy x rays are attenuated by the thick part, but quite a few can penetrate the thin part. Assume the numbers to be 25 (thick) and 40 (thin). By the definition of subject contrast,

$$\text{Subject contrast} = \frac{40}{25} = 1.60,$$

which states that the thin part transmits 60% more x rays than the thick part at 50 kVp. If the kVp is then increased to 80 (Fig. 13–3B), more x rays will get through both the thick and thin parts. Both I_S and I_L will increase, but I_S will increase more than I_L, so $\dfrac{I_S}{I_L}$ becomes smaller, and subject contrast is decreased. Figure 13–3B assumes values of $I_S = 80$ and $I_L = 60$, giving subject contrast of $\dfrac{80}{60} = 1.33$, or only 33% difference in transmitted radiation intensity.

As a general rule, low kVp gives high subject contrast. This is often called **short-scale contrast** because everything is black or white on the film, with fewer shades of gray in between. High kVp gives lower subject contrast, called **long-scale contrast,** because there is a long scale of shades of gray between the lightest and darkest portions of the image.

Exposure Latitude

A low-contrast film (shallow slope of the characteristic curve) has greater exposure

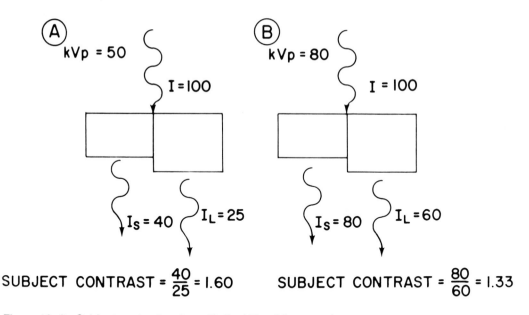

SUBJECT CONTRAST = $\frac{40}{25}$ = 1.60 SUBJECT CONTRAST = $\frac{80}{60}$ = 1.33

Figure 13–3 Subject contrast varies with the kVp of the x-ray beam

latitude. That is, a wider range of mAs settings will produce proper film density if the kVp is satisfactory. Similarly, kVp will also have an effect on exposure latitude. High-kVp techniques will allow a wider range of mAs settings (wide exposure latitude) but will result in relatively less contrast. **Low-kVp techniques produce high subject contrast** because there is a large variation in the intensity of the transmitted x-ray beam in different parts of the patient. The x-ray film must then "decode" a range of exposure from low to high. This wide range of exposure (log relative exposure) must fall within the steep portion of the characteristic curve (Fig. 13–4A). When a low kVp is used, the mAs must be carefully selected. Figure 13–4A shows that if the exposure (mAs) is only a little too low, the low-exposure areas (i.e., under bone) will produce exposures in the toe area of the curve. Likewise, excessive mAs will rapidly move high-density exposures onto the shoulder of the curve. Both these mistakes will decrease film contrast. High-kVp exposures produce less difference in intensity between areas of the attenuated x-ray beam; this is why **high kVp gives less subject contrast.** With a high-kVp technique, the film has to "decode" a smaller difference in log relative exposure between the low- and high-exposure areas.

Figure 13–4B diagrams how a high-kVp technique (using the same object and film-screen system) will "use up" a much shorter portion of the steep portion of the film's characteristic curve. Using high kVp, the technologist has considerable room for error in the choice of mAs, because the exposure range can move up or down on the curve and still fall within the steep portion of the curve.

To review, **kVp influences subject contrast** (exposure differences) **and exposure latitude; mAs controls film blackening** (density). Consider a specific example. A chest film (par speed film-screen combination, 6-feet distance, no grid, exposed with factors of 70 kVp and 6.6 mAs [400 mA, 1/60 sec]) would result in a radiograph with high contrast. The exposure of 6.6 mAs, however, is critical at 70 kVp. An error of ±50% would probably produce a radiograph with a great deal of its density on the toe or shoulder of the film curve, resulting in an unacceptable loss of con-

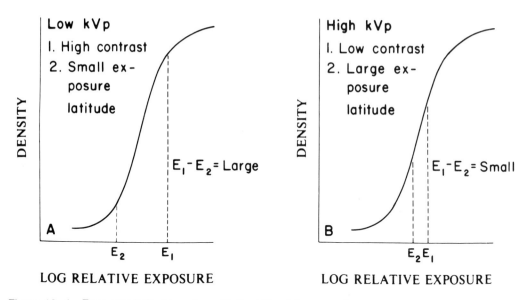

Figure 13–4 Exposure latitude varies with the kVp of the x-ray beam

trast. Another chest examination exposed at 100 kVp and about 3 mAs would result in a low-contrast radiograph, but changing the exposure (3 mAs) by a factor of ± 100% would probably not reduce radiographic contrast. Obviously, fewer mAs or more mAs produces a lighter (less density) or darker (more density) radiograph, but the density range still falls on the steep portion of the film curve. At 100 kVp the exposure can be varied considerably; this is termed **large exposure latitude.** At 70 kVp, the exposure must fall within a narrow range (i.e., there is small exposure latitude).

To make matters more complicated, kVp does have an effect on film blackening. This effect is approximately equal to the fourth power of the kVp. For example, if kVp is increased from 50 to 60 the change in film density (if mAs remains constant) will be about

$$\frac{60^4}{50^4} = 2.07$$

Because kVp has doubled film density, mAs would have to be cut in half. An old rule says: "If you add 10 kVp, cut mAs in half." This holds true around 50 to 60 kVp, but kVp change has less effect on film den-

sity at higher ranges. For example, at 85 kVp, an increase of 15 kVp is required to double the film blackening power of the beam.

Subject contrast thus is seen to vary with the makeup of the subject (thickness, density, atomic number), the use of contrast material, and the kVp of the x-ray beam.

Film Contrast

Film contrast has been discussed as a photographic property of x-ray film (see Chap. 11). **X-ray film will significantly amplify subject contrast** provided the exposure (mAs) is correct (keep away from the toe and shoulder of the characteristic curve). Under good viewing conditions, a density difference of about 0.04 (difference in light transmission of 10%) can be seen.

Fog and Scatter

The effect of fog and scatter is to reduce radiographic contrast.

Scattered radiation is produced mainly as a result of **Compton** scattering. The amount of scatter radiation increases with increasing part thickness, field size, and energy of the x-ray beam (higher kVp). Scatter is minimized by collimation of the x-ray beam (use as small a field size as possible) and the use of grids or air gaps. **Scatter radiation that reaches the x-ray film or film-screen combination produces unwanted density.**

Fog is strictly defined as those silver halide grains in the film emulsion that are developed even though they were not exposed by light or x rays. The amount of fog in an unexposed x-ray film can be demonstrated easily. Cut the unexposed film in half. Develop (fully process) one-half of the film and clear (fix, wash, and dry only) the other. The density difference between the two film halves represents the amount of fog present. **Fog produces unwanted film density, which lowers radiographic contrast.**

Another type of unwanted film density may result from accidental exposure of film to light or x rays. This is usually also called "fog" or "exposure fog" and, although the term is not absolutely correct, it has established itself by common usage. These two types of "fog" are different in origin, but both lower film contrast in the same manner.

True fog is increased by the following conditions:

1. Improper film storage (high temperature or humidity).
2. Contaminated or exhausted developer solution.
3. Excessive time or temperature of development.
4. Use of high-speed film (highly sensitized grains).

Fog, "exposure fog," and scatter add density to the film. By knowing the magnitude of this density and the characteristic curve of the film, it is possible to calculate the effect of the added density on radiographic contrast accurately. Figure 13–5 shows how fog and scatter change the slope of the characteristic curve of a film. Note that the slope of the curve is decreased (contrast is decreased) most at lower levels

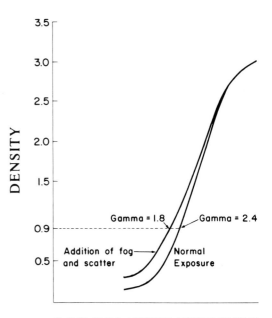

LOG RELATIVE EXPOSURE

Figure 13–5 Fog and scatter decrease radiographic contrast. (Courtesy of R. E. Wayrynen[21])

of density. These are the densities used most frequently in diagnostic radiology. In Figure 13–5 the gamma of the normal film, at a density of 0.9, is 2.4. When fog and scatter are added, the gamma drops to 1.8. At a density of 2.5, fog and scatter have no significant effect on the shape of the curve, but densities as high as 2.5 are seldom used in diagnostic radiology.

To repeat, fog and scatter are undesirable because they decrease radiographic contrast by decreasing film contrast.

IMAGE QUALITY

The second basic factor determining image clarity is image quality. The quality of the radiographic image may be defined as the ability of the film to record each point in the object as a point on the film. In radiology this point-for-point reproduction is never perfect, largely because of the diffusion of light by intensifying screens. There is no general agreement as to what should be included in a discussion of image quality. Our approach will involve almost no mathematics.

Image quality is influenced by

1. radiographic mottle
2. sharpness
3. resolution.

Radiographic Mottle

If an x-ray film is mounted between intensifying screens and exposed to a uniform x-ray beam to produce a density of about 1.0, the resulting film will not show uniform density but will have an irregular mottled appearance. This mottled appearance (caused by small density differences) is easily detected by the unaided eye, and may be seen, if looked for, in any area of "uniform" density in a radiograph exposed with screens (e.g., the area of a chest film not covered by the patient). This uneven texture, or mottle, seen on a film that "should" show perfectly uniform density is called **radiographic mottle.** Radiographic mottle has three components:

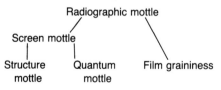

Only **quantum mottle** is of any importance in diagnostic radiology.

Film Graininess

Film graininess makes no contribution to the radiographic mottle observed in clinical radiology. Film graininess can be seen when the film is examined with a lens producing magnification of 5 to 10 ×. With this magnification, the image is seen to be made up of a nonhomogeneous arrangement of silver grains in gelatin. Because a radiograph is almost never viewed at an enlargement of 5 ×, film graininess is not seen.

Screen Mottle

Screen mottle has two components, **structure mottle** (unimportant) and **quan-**

tum mottle (important). Structure mottle is caused by defects in the intensifying screen, such as varying thickness or physical imperfections in the phosphor layer. Such screen irregularities can occur, but the quality control used in screen manufacturing is so good that structure mottle may be dismissed as making no contribution to radiographic mottle.

Quantum mottle is the only important cause of radiographic mottle. **Quantum** refers to a discrete unit of energy and, in this discussion, it may be considered as the energy carried by one x-ray photon. An x-ray beam may be thought of as containing a certain number of x-ray photons, or an equivalent number of quanta.

By showing a pattern of mottle, or nonuniform density, the x-ray film is telling us that it has "seen" a nonuniform pattern of light on the surface of the intensifying screen. The nonuniform pattern of light on the screen is caused by fluctuations in the number of photons (or quanta) per square millimeter in the beam that arrived at the screen. What this means is that a "uniform" beam of x rays is not uniform at all. Suppose a "uniform" x-ray beam could be frozen in space and cut into cross sections. If the number of x-ray photons per square millimeter were counted, it would be unlikely that any two square mm would contain exactly the same number of photons. The "uniform" beam is not uniform.

The actual number of x-ray photons per mm^2 obeys the law of probability, because the emission of x rays by the x-ray tube is a random event. The average number of photons per mm^2 can be calculated by adding the number in each mm^2 and dividing by the number of squares. It will then be found that the actual number in any square will almost never be the average value, but that all numbers will fall within a certain range (percent fluctuation) of the average. The law of probability says that the magnitude of this fluctuation is plus or minus the square root of the average number of photons per mm^2. (The square root of the average number of photons is usually referred to as the standard deviation.) For example, if an x-ray beam contains an average of 10,000 photons per mm^2, the number in any one square mm will fall in the range

$$10,000 \pm \sqrt{10,000} = 10,000 \pm 100$$

or any mm^2 may be expected to contain between 9,900 and 10,100 photons. In some of the squares (32%) the variation will be even greater than this.

The percent fluctuation in the actual number of photons per mm^2 becomes greater as the average number becomes smaller. If 100 photons are used, fluctuations will be $\pm \sqrt{100}$, or ± 10, giving a percent fluctuation of $\frac{10}{100}$, or 10%. Using 10,000 photons, fluctuation is ± 100, or a percent fluctuation of $\frac{100}{10,000}$ or 1%.

Quantum mottle is caused by the statistical fluctuation in the number of quanta per unit area absorbed by the intensifying screen. The fewer quanta (x-ray photons) used, the greater will be the quantum mottle (more statistical fluctuation). Intensifying screens are used because they decrease the x-ray exposure (number of photons) needed to expose the x-ray film. Quantum mottle is seen when intensifying screens are used. Quantum mottle will be greater with high-kVp x rays because they produce a higher screen intensification factor.

The concept of quantum mottle is illustrated in Figure 13–6. The model consists of the cardboard top of a hatbox, small cardboard figures in the shape of a circle, square, and triangle placed in the hatbox top, and 1000 pennies. The pennies represent x-ray quanta, and were dropped into the hatbox top in a completely random manner. Radiographs of the model were made after 10, 100, 500, and 1000 pennies had been dropped into the hatbox top. Notice that the radiograph of 10 pennies shows no information about the makeup of the model; 100 pennies show that the hatbox top is probably round; 500 pennies show three filling defects in the hatbox top, which is definitely round; and all 1000 pennies clearly define the shape of each filling defect. In other words, a lot of pennies (quanta) provided a lot of information about the model, fewer pennies provided less information, and too few pennies provided no useful information.

Quantum mottle is difficult to see unless a high-quality radiograph is produced. A film of high contrast and good quality will show visible quantum mottle. If film contrast and quality are poor, such as produced by poor film-screen contact, quantum mottle will not be visible. Thick intensifying screens may show less visible mottle on the film because of greater diffusion of light. A radiograph with poor visibility of image detail will also exhibit poor visibility of quantum mottle.

In summary, let us define radiographic mottle as the radiographic recording of the statistical fluctuations in a beam of x-ray photons.

Speed Versus Noise

Radiographic mottle is often called **noise.** Allow us to repeat an important but poorly understood fact: **noise (quantum mottle) results from statistical fluctuation in the number of x-ray photons used (absorbed) by the intensifying screens to form the image.** With currently available films and screens it is possible to obtain a film-screen system so fast that noise makes the resulting image unsatisfactory except for a few special applications such as pelvimetry. Two basic premises must be remembered:

1. High-contrast images are **SHARPNESS**-limited.
2. Low-contrast images are **NOISE**-limited.

Because low-contrast images comprise most diagnostically important information,

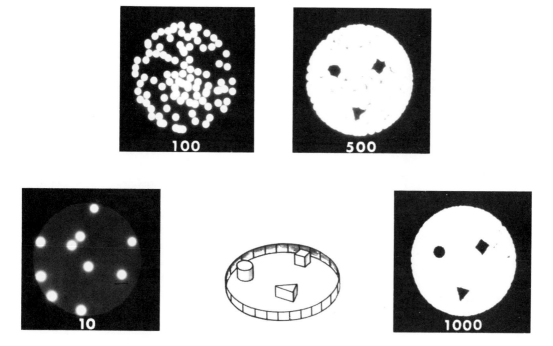

Figure 13–6 The "pennies-in-the-hatbox" model illustrating the concept of quantum mottle

noise may seriously compromise a radiograph.

The two ways to increase the speed of a film-screen radiographic system are obvious:

1. Use a faster screen.
2. Use a faster film.

The way the increase in speed affects system noise (quantum mottle) is not so obvious or easy to understand. Let us illustrate this difficulty by posing a question that experience has shown almost everyone answers incorrectly. Assume that two radiographs of an abdomen are made. Both exposures use the same medium-speed x-ray film. The first exposure is made using par speed calcium tungstate screens. The second exposure is made using high-speed calcium tungstate screens, which are exactly twice as fast (i.e., require only half the mAs) as the par speed screens. Now for the question. Which exposure (par speed or high-speed screens) will produce the radiograph with the most noise (quantum mottle)? If you answer "the high-speed sys-

tem," you are wrong, in company with most of your colleagues. The correct answer is that the noise is the same for both radiographs (the noise will be more difficult to see when the thick fast screen is used because of more light diffusion, which causes decreased visibility of image detail).

The rest of this section will attempt to explain this relationship between noise and system speed, a concept made important in film-screen radiography by the introduction of noncalcium tungstate high-speed intensifying screens and fast x-ray film.

Let us try to simplify the problem by stating that, with regard to noise, there are two ways to increase the speed (i.e., lower the x-ray dose to the patient) of a film-screen radiographic system:

1. Increase speed with no change in noise.
2. Increase speed and increase noise.

We need to examine each of these two methods in some detail.

1. **Increased speed with no change in noise can be done in two ways:**

Par

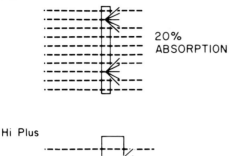

20% ABSORPTION

Hi Plus

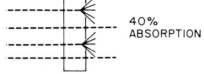

40% ABSORPTION

LESS PATIENT EXPOSURE
SAME NUMBER OF PHOTONS USED
SAME NOISE

Figure 13–7 Increasing speed by increasing the stopping power of the intensifying screen will not change noise

a. Increase phosphor layer thickness.
b. Use a phosphor with a higher absorption coefficient for x rays.

Both these methods will increase the stopping power of the intensifying screen. Refer to Figure 13–7, which diagrams a par speed and a Du Pont Hi Plus (twice the speed of par) calcium tungstate screen. If 10 x-ray photons arrive at the par speed screen, 2 photons are absorbed (assume 20% absorption). If a Hi Plus $CaWO_4$ screen is used, the screen will absorb 40% of the x-ray beam because it is thicker than a par speed screen. Thus, to cause the high-speed screen to absorb 2 photons, we need only cause 5 photons to arrive at the screen (the amount of light produced per absorbed photon is the same in each screen). Because only half as many photons are required, exposure to the patient is cut in half and we speak of the Hi Plus screen as being twice as "fast" because we were able to decrease patient exposure by half (i.e., we cut the mAs in half). The only factor determining noise, however, is **THE NUMBER OF PHOTONS USED BY THE SCREEN.**

Both the par and Hi Plus $CaWO_4$ screens have **USED** the same number of photons. The faster screen has a thicker phosphor layer, which absorbs a higher percentage of the x-ray beam. Stated another way, if the screen phosphor is the same, changes in screen speed will not result in any change in noise. This last statement has an exception. Addition of a light-absorbing dye to the screen phosphor layer will prevent some light from reaching the film. Because some light is lost, more photons must be absorbed by the screen to produce enough light to expose the film (i.e., use of dye in slow screens decreases noise).

The price that must be paid for increased speed in $CaWO_4$ screens is more **unsharpness** caused by light diffusion in the thicker phosphor layer. Thus, the choice of which $CaWO_4$ screen to use is a compromise between:

SHARPNESS vs. SPEED.

A phosphor with higher inherent absorption of x rays could give more speed without an increase in unsharpness (thicker screen not required) or noise (same x ray to light conversion efficiency as $CaWO_4$). The potential for this type of improvement is limited. Lead (atomic number 82) is the highest atomic number nonradioactive element. Tungsten (atomic number 74) is so close to lead that there is little room in the periodic table to discover phosphors with a higher atomic number. We have previously discussed how some of the new phosphors do gain some of their speed through higher inherent absorption of x rays by use of a favorably located K-absorption edge. Screen speed obtained in this manner is desirable because patient exposure is then decreased without any increase in noise or unsharpness.

2. **Increased speed with increased noise can be done in two ways:**
   a. Use a phosphor with a higher x ray-to-light conversion efficiency.
   b. Use a faster film.

Both these processes will have identical effects on the noise content of the finished radiograph. The system cannot distinguish between a phosphor having a higher conversion efficiency and the use of a faster film. In each case the faster system will provide an image produced by use (absorption) of fewer photons in the screen, with a corresponding increase in noise. This is illustrated in Figure 13–8, in which a par speed calcium tungstate screen (20% absorption of the x-ray beam) is compared to a rare earth screen (such as gadolinium oxysulfide), which also absorbs 20% of the x-ray beam but produces twice as much light per absorbed photon (in this example). Note that the rare earth screen, by absorbing only one x-ray photon, has produced as much light as the $CaWO_4$ screen produced by absorbing two x-ray photons. It is this difference in photons absorbed by the screen that causes a change in the quantum noise (mottle). Similarly, if one uses identical screens but a film that is twice as fast, the faster film will be properly exposed with half as much light, which the

screen produces by absorbing half as many photons.

The new fast screen phosphors are faster than calcium tungstate because they:

1. Absorb (use) a larger percentage of the x-ray beam (no change in quantum noise).
2. Have a higher x ray-to-light conversion efficiency (with an increase in quantum noise).

It is possible to use a film-screen combination in which system quantum mottle (noise) will produce a perceptible decrease in the visibility of low contrast images on the radiograph. In choosing one of the noncalcium tungstate very fast screens a compromise must thus be reached between:

SPEED vs. NOISE.

Another way to look at quantum noise is to examine a terribly complex function called the **Wiener spectrum.** This may be thought of as the modulation transfer function (MTF) of the noise of an image, and we will briefly examine this concept after the discussion of MTF later in this chapter.

We will summarize the concept of quantum noise in film-screen radiography in outline form:

1. Increase speed with no change in noise.
   a. Increase phosphor layer thickness.
   b. Use a phosphor with a higher absorption coefficient for x rays.
2. Increase speed with increased noise.
   a. Use a phosphor with a higher x ray-to-light conversion efficiency.
   b. Use a faster film.

Calcium Tungstate

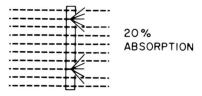

20% ABSORPTION

Rare Earth

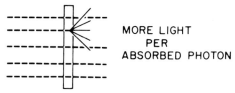

MORE LIGHT PER ABSORBED PHOTON

LESS PATIENT EXPOSURE
SMALLER NUMBER OF PHOTONS USED
MORE NOISE

Figure 13–8 Increasing speed by increasing the x ray-to-light conversion efficiency of the phosphor will increase noise

Sharpness

Sharpness is the ability of the x-ray film or film-screen system to define an edge. The inability of a film-screen system to record a sharp edge because of light diffusion in the intensifying screen has been previously discussed. Sharpness and contrast are closely related in the subjective response they produce. An unsharp edge can be easily seen if contrast is high, but a sharp edge may be poorly visible if contrast is low.

Most of the causes of unsharpness have been previously discussed. We will review them briefly.

Geometric Unsharpness

Penumbra is minimized by using a small focal spot and by keeping magnification as small as possible. If you understand why the term "edge gradient" (rather than penumbra) is now preferred, you really understand what geometric unsharpness means.

Motion Unsharpness

Subject motion can be minimized by using a short exposure time. Motion of the x-ray tube during the exposure will cause unsharpness, but it is not as important as motion of the object.

Absorption Unsharpness

Absorption unsharpness results because a patient is not made up of objects that have nice sharp edges. Absorption unsharpness is greatest for round or oval objects.

Screen Unsharpness

X-ray intensifying screens cause unsharp borders because of **light diffusion** in the screen phosphor layer. Good screen-film contact is essential.

Parallax Unsharpness

Parallax unsharpness is seen only with double-emulsion films. There is an image on each emulsion, and the images are separated by the width of the film base (0.007 or 0.008 inches). When viewed from an angle, these two image edges will not overlap exactly. Parallax makes a negligible contribution to image unsharpness.

Total Unsharpness

In a radiographic image, all types of unsharpness are present. The proper method of calculating the total unsharpness is not known, but it is known that simple addition does not give the correct result. For example, assume that total unsharpness is given by

$$U_T = \sqrt{U_g^2 + U_a^2 + U_m^2 + U_s^2}$$

where U_T = total unsharpness
U_g = geometric unsharpness
U_a = absorption unsharpness
U_m = motion unsharpness
U_s = screen unsharpness

This formula is probably incorrect, but will illustrate an important point. Assume an examination in which $U_g = 0.5$ mm, $U_a = 4$ mm, $U_m = 1$ mm, and $U_s = 0.6$ mm. What is total unsharpness?

$$U_T = \sqrt{(0.5)^2 + 4^2 + 1^1 + (0.6)^2} = 4.2 \text{ mm}$$

Note that total unsharpness of 4.2 mm is largely determined by the single largest cause of unsharpness, which is 4 mm of absorption unsharpness in this example. If any unsharpness is significantly larger than the others, the largest cause of unsharpness almost completely controls total unsharpness. In our example absorption unsharpness of 4 mm is the most important. Decreasing U_g (smaller focal spot), U_m (shorter exposure time), or U_s (detail screens) would not significantly improve image sharpness. Attempts to improve the image must be directed toward the factor most responsible for a poor image. Absorption unsharpness cannot be changed, but the unsharp image edge may be made more easily visible by increasing contrast. Therefore, by increasing contrast with a lower kVp technique, it is possible that actually increasing U_g (geometric unsharpness) and U_m (motion unsharpness) by using higher mAs (larger focal spot and longer exposure time) will produce a radiograph with better visibility of fine detail. The infinite variety of boundaries encountered in the patient compounds the problem of absorption unsharpness. No matter how good the geometric conditions, absorption unsharpness may make exact delineation of the borders of small objects (such as opacified blood vessels) all but impossible.

Resolution

Imagine a photograph of a pastoral scene in which a barn and a windmill are depicted against the background of a dark blue sky. If the top edge of the roof of the barn is sharply outlined against the sky, the photograph has good sharpness. The term **sharpness** is used to describe the subjective response of crisp, or abrupt, edges (the objective correlate of sharpness is termed acutance). If each vane of the windmill is easily counted, the photograph has good resolution, or resolving power. Sharpness is the ability of an imaging system to record sharply defined margins, or abrupt edges. **Resolving power is the ability to record separate images of small objects that are placed very close together.** An imaging system may have the ability to record sharp edges but be unable to resolve fine details. Another system may yield fuzzy unsharp edges but still be able to show much fine detail. Sharpness and resolving power are different, but they are related in the subjective response they produce.

Until recently, x-ray imaging systems were evaluated by their resolving power. For example, a par speed intensifying screen might be described as having a resolving power of 8 lines per mm. Several methods of determining resolving power are used. One method uses a resolving power target made up of a series of parallel wires or lead strips, placed so that the space between each lead strip is equal to the width of the strip (Fig. 13–9). In this system, a "line" actually means a line and a space, more appropriately termed a "line pair." For example, 4 lines per mm means that there are 4 lead strips or wires per mm, with each line $\frac{1}{8}$ mm wide and each space $\frac{1}{8}$ mm wide, so that each line pair is $\frac{1}{4}$ mm

Figure 13–9 A resolving power target consists of a series of lines and spaces

wide. A commonly used resolving power target is the Buckbee-Meers resolution plate, which consists of line pairs varying from 1.0 to 9.6 per mm in 18 steps.[1]

A film-screen system is evaluated by how many line pairs per mm can be clearly seen in the developed radiograph. Another testing device uses a slit of adjustable width between two blocks of lead. After each x-ray exposure, this apparatus is moved across the film or film-screen combination a distance equal to the width of the slit, producing in this way a series of lines and spaces on the developed film.[6] All these systems depend on an observer determining how many line pairs per mm he can see, and the number will vary among observers. It is argued that these measurements only evaluate the ability of the system to depict the image of a wire, or lead strip or slit, and do not necessarily pertain to the complex shapes and varying contrasts presented to a film-screen system (or fluoroscopic system) in clinical practice. Also, the resolving power only measures a limit. Knowing that a film-screen system will resolve 8 line pairs per mm tells us that it will not produce an image of 10 line pairs per mm, but says nothing about how good or bad a job it does at 2, 4, or 6 line pairs per mm.

The basic question to consider is this. When the information in the x-ray image is transferred to the x-ray film (usually with light from intensifying screens), how much information is lost? The answer is now being sought by evaluation of the line spread function and the modulation transfer function. The physics and mathematics involved in these determinations are highly complex. We hope to present the basic concepts in an understandable form without the use of any mathematics.

LINE SPREAD FUNCTION

The fact that light diffusion by intensifying screens causes blurred, or unsharp, image edges has been discussed. The line spread function provides a way to measure this effect.

The line spread function is determined as follows. A narrow slit is formed between two jaws made of metal highly opaque to x rays, such as platinum. The width of the slit is usually 10 microns, and the metal jaws are about 2 mm thick. X rays passing through this slit are so severely collimated that they may be considered as a "line source" x-ray beam. The slit apparatus is placed in intimate contact with a film-screen system, and an exposure is made. Only the x rays passing through the 10-micron slit reach the intensifying screens. A perfect imaging system would produce an image of a line 10 microns wide on the developed film. Because of light diffusion in the screens, however, the developed film will actually show density extending out for several hundred microns on each side. The photographic effect of the x-ray beam is spread over a total distance of 800 or more microns (0.8 mm).[11] This technique provides a way to express the line spread function (LSF) numerically. Figure 13–10 shows line spread function graphs in which the relative density is shown to decrease with distance away from the 10-micron line source of x rays. Measuring film density over such a small area requires the use of a microdensitometer, which reads the density of an extremely small area of the film.

Notice on the hypothetic curves of Figure 13–10 (based on the work of Rossmann and Lubberts[13]) that the tailing off of image density is much more marked when high-speed screens are used than when medium-speed screens are used to produce the same density in the center. The shape of the curves in Figure 13–10 allows us to predict accurately that image boundaries will be less faithfully recorded when the image resulting from the use of high-speed screens is compared to that resulting from the use of slower screens. The less light diffusion, the sharper, or more abrupt, will be image edges. Sharper image edges allow imaging of finer detail in the radiograph.

The line spread function can also be used to measure the influence of factors on the image other than that of intensifying screens. These factors include x-ray film, fluoroscopic screens, focal spots of x-ray tubes, x-ray image intensifiers, motion unsharpness, and scatter radiation.

The LSF of x-ray film exposed without screens (direct x-ray exposure) is difficult to measure. There is almost no diffusion of x rays and secondary electrons in the film, so the LSF is narrow. The grain size of an x-ray film may be as large as 2.0 microns. If an x-ray photon were to pass between two grains that were side by side, it might cause both grains to be developed, producing an image 4 μ wide. The image of a line source x-ray beam exposing a film directly will be slightly broadened because of slight radiation diffusion and the finite size of the developed silver halide grains. Image diffusion is so small, however, that the LSF of film exposed to x rays is difficult to measure.

Is the determination of the line spread function of a screen-film system of any practical value? Through a series of complex mathematical manipulations the modulation transfer function of the screen-film system can be calculated from the line spread function, and the modulation transfer providing a way to measure the image quality that can be produced.

MODULATION TRANSFER FUNCTION

We have discussed how the clarity of the x-ray image is influenced by **contrast, sharpness,** and **resolution.** Each of these terms may be defined separately, but their complex interrelationships that ultimately

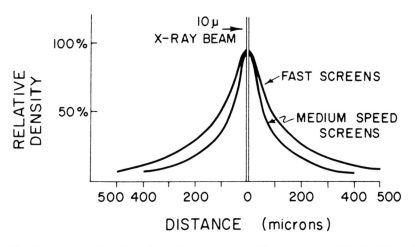

Figure 13–10 Line spread function of medium-speed and fast screens. (Modified from Rossman and Lubberts[13])

determine image clarity are much more difficult to evaluate. The modulation transfer function (MTF) is a concept that has been formulated to provide an objective measurement of the combined effects of sharpness and resolution. Let us consider that modulation means a change in the amplitude (or intensity, or amount) of an information-carrying signal. Imagine a can that contains an unknown amount of thick oil. The oil is measured by pouring it into a graduated beaker. Some of the oil will stick to the sides of the can and escape detection. The information signal seen is the oil in the beaker. The amount of information (oil) seen is less than the total amount of information in the can; the signal has been modulated (changed) because some information was lost in the transfer of oil from the can to the beaker. If careful laboratory measurements determine that the can holds 500 ml of oil, but only 400 ml is measured, the information-detecting system used will detect $\frac{400}{500}$, or 0.8, of the total information. Similarly, the MTF is an attempt to measure the amount of information transferred from the invisible x-ray image to the detecting system (x-ray film, television image, etc.). The MTF repre-sents a ratio between the information recorded and the total amount of information available, or

$$MTF = \frac{information\ recorded}{information\ available}$$

Because recorded information can never be greater than available information, the MTF can never be greater than 1.

The MTF of a screen-film system is usually calculated from the corresponding line spread function by a complex mathematical operation known as a Fourier transformation. In practice, a computer may do the calculations from information it receives from the microdensitometer used to measure the densities making up the line spread function. A complete discussion of the specialized physics and mathematics involved in developing an MTF curve is far beyond the scope of this text, and most radiologists (including the authors) lack the specialized background necessary to understand such a treatment of the subject. We are indebted to R. E. Wayrynen for developing the following discussion of what the modulation transfer means, expressed in simple examples.[21]

Consider a resolving power target (Fig. 13–11). A radiograph of the target should produce a film with "square wave" changes

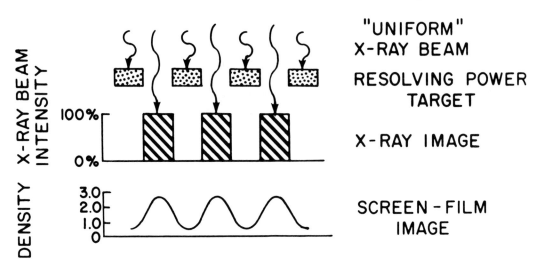

Figure 13–11 Information is lost when the x-ray image of a resolving power target is recorded by a screen-film combination

in density, completely black in the area corresponding to the spaces and completely unexposed in areas corresponding to the metal strips, with abrupt density changes (i.e., sharp margins). Using a screen-film combination, the blackest black will have a density of about 3.0, and unexposed film will have a density of about 0.2 (base and fog densities). Because of light scattering by the screens, the actual radiograph will not show square waves. The maximum density will be less than expected, "unexposed" areas of the film will react as if they had received exposure, and the transition from minimum to maximum density will be gradual, producing the sine wave density pattern expressed graphically in Figure 13–11. Light scattering causes density to be "shoveled off" the density peaks and "poured into" the valleys, causing a **decrease in image sharpness** (less abrupt image borders) and a **decrease in contrast** (density difference between the peaks and valleys).

Now consider a resolving power target in which the widths of the opaque metal strips and the spaces become progressively smaller. The more line pairs per unit length, the greater the amount of information presented to the screen-film sys-

tem. The amount of information is usually expressed as a certain number of line pairs per mm, or a certain number of cycles per mm, both being the same. Figure 13–12 is a diagram of what happens to the image of the resolving power target recorded by the screen-film combination as information content increases. The difference in density (contrast) on the developed film between areas of maximum exposure (under the spaces) and minimum exposure becomes less as information content increases. This is caused almost entirely by light scattering in the intensifying screens. Eventually, the screen-film system becomes unable to show any density difference between lines and spaces. This represents the limit of the resolving power of the system—that is, the ability to record lines and spaces.

When an x-ray beam is directed onto a resolving power target, most x rays that encounter a space pass through the space, while those that encounter a metal strip are absorbed. In the laboratory it is possible to measure the intensity of the x-ray beam under spaces (maximum exposure) and lead strips (minimum exposure). The intensity may be expressed in milliroentgens, and represents the exposure received by the screen-film combination. A character-

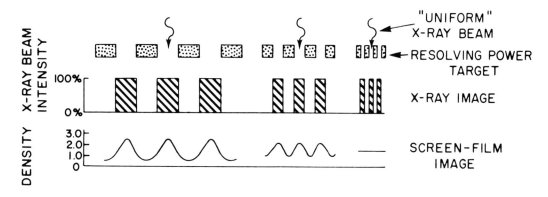

Figure 13–12 As the information content of a resolving power target increases, the ability of the screen-film system to record the x-ray image of the target decreases

istic curve may be prepared in which the logarithm of the actual exposure (rather than relative exposure) is used to prepare the density-log E curve. On such a curve (Fig. 13–13) the measured maximum (E_{max}) and minimum (E_{min}) exposures reaching the film are recorded. Then the exposed film is processed, and the developed maximum and minimum densities are carefully measured and plotted on the curve, shown as the obtained densities D'_{max} and D'_{min} in Figure 13–13. Note that the maximum and minimum densities actually produced by the exposure are not the same as the densities expected from the measured exposures. The observed maximum density is less than predicted, and the observed minimum density is more than predicted. This is another way of graphically representing the effect of light scattering by the intensifying screens. Expressed another way, the film has acted as if it received a lower maximum exposure and a higher minimum exposure, as shown by the dotted lines in Figure 13–13.

The amplitude of the exposure input ($E_{max} - E_{min}$) to the film is known from actual measurement. The amplitude of the exposure "equivalent" output ($E'_{max} - E'_{min}$) has been calculated by knowing the characteristic curve of the film and by measuring film density produced by the exposure. In addition, the width of the lines and

spaces of the resolving power target are obviously known. Therefore, we may now calculate the modulation transfer function (MTF) of the screen-film system at a known frequency (lines per mm) as follows (Fig. 13–13):

$$MTF = \frac{\text{exposure amplitude output}}{\text{exposure amplitude input}}$$

Using this rather laborious procedure, the MTF of a screen-film system could be calculated for 1, 2, 4, 6, 8, etc., line pairs per mm by using the appropriate resolving power target, measuring exposure input, and calculating the exposure "equivalent" output. A curve similar to that shown in Figure 13–14 would be developed, and this is the MTF curve of our hypothetical screen-film system. This curve tells us that, at 1 line pair per mm, the $\frac{\text{output}}{\text{input}}$ = about 0.8 (or 80%), which is good. At 4 line pairs per mm $\frac{\text{output}}{\text{input}}$ = about 0.3, and at 8 line pairs per mm it is about 0.1, or 10%. Remember, MTF curves are usually calculated from the line spread function, but the meaning of the MTF curve is easier to understand if it is discussed in terms of its derivation based on the use of resolving power targets.

How is an MTF curve useful? There are no "units" of MTF. It does not measure

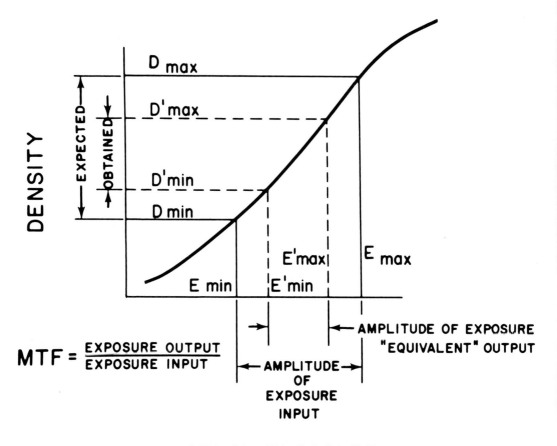

Figure 13–13   The modulation transfer function of a screen-film system may be calculated by using a resolving power target

contrast or sharpness or resolution. For the clinical radiologist, MTF curves may be useful as a more accurate way to compare the imaging qualities of competing systems, to help choose the system that best suits his needs. Consider intensifying screens again. We have discussed the fact that resolving power measures only a limit. Assume that Figure 13–14 is the MTF curve for a par speed intensifying screen. The 10% response on the MTF curve corresponds roughly to the resolving power of the imaging system. In Figure 13–14 the 10% response is about 8 line pairs per mm, so this screen would have a resolving power of 8 lines (or line pairs) per mm. But the curve also allows us to compare the relative im-

aging properties of the screen at frequencies lower than the resolving power.

Now consider Figure 13–15, in which hypothetic MTF curves for two x-ray intensifying screens are shown; the differences in the curves are exaggerated for the purposes of illustration. Screen A has a resolving power (10% MTF) of 6 lines per mm, while the resolving power of screen B is 14 line pairs per mm. From resolving power figures, screen B is apparently a much better screen. However, the MTF curves show that, at 4 lines per mm, screen A has a response of 80%, while screen B has fallen to 30%, and at 2 lines per mm the values are 90% and 50%, respectively. Under normal viewing conditions the eye

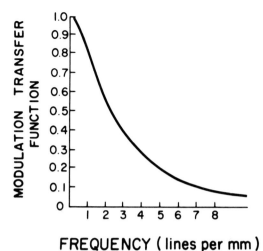

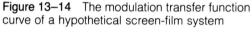

Figure 13–14 The modulation transfer function curve of a hypothetical screen-film system

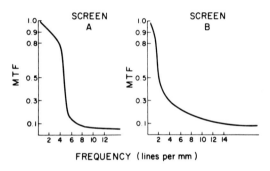

Figure 13–15 Hypothetical MTF curves of two x-ray intensifying screens

usually sees structures of a size corresponding to an information content between 2 and 4 line pairs per mm. For routine radiography, the information recorded by screen A will probably produce radiographs of greater diagnostic accuracy than those produced by screen B. On the other hand, an attempt to record very small structures would require the use of screen B. Obviously, the true difference in the characteristics and clinical applications of these screens can be appreciated only from a comparison of the respective MTF curves. Resolving power may be thought of as a single point on the MTF curves.

Modulation transfer function curves are being developed for all the imaging sys-

tems used in radiology, including screen-film systems, x-ray image amplifiers, cine and 70, 90, and 105-mm systems, and television viewing, including tape and disc image storage systems.

The MTF plays an important role in the evaluation of a complex imaging system. Consider, for example, a film-screen system that has a front screen, first film emulsion, film base, second film emulsion, and back screen. In optical terms this is called a cascaded system, or a series of cascaded imaging processes. In Chapter 20, dealing with magnification radiography, we will consider the film, the x-ray tube focal spot, the x-ray intensifying screens, and the motion of the object being radiographed as four components in a cascaded system. Each component of a cascaded system has its own imaging properties, and it is often possible to express these properties in terms of the MTF of the particular component. Once the MTFs of the components of a complex system are known, the total MTF of the entire system may be obtained by multiplying the MTFs of each of the components (this concept will be considered in some detail in Chapter 20).

As an example, if one knows that, at an object frequency of 2 line pairs per mm, the MTF of x-ray film is 1.0 (i.e., the film is perfect), the MTF of the intensifying screens is 0.7, and the MTF of the focal spot of the x-ray tube is 0.8, then total system MTF will be $1.0 \times 0.7 \times 0.8 = 0.56$. The MTF concept allows each component of an imaging system to be studied so that the optimum system may be designed. Unfortunately, in diagnostic radiology it is difficult to define the "optimum system" objectively because the elements in a radiograph that allow one to arrive at a correct diagnosis are not easily defined. It is not correct to assume that by measuring the MTF for different imaging systems radiologists can compare and decide which system to buy. The ultimate practical use of MTF measurements to both radiologists and industry is still being evaluated.

NOISE AND THE WIENER SPECTRUM

We previously introduced the concept of quantum mottle (or noise) caused by the fact that film-screen radiography is quantum-limited (i.e., the radiograph may be formed with a relatively small number of x-ray photons). This noise may be apparent visually, and it can also be measured in the laboratory. The radiologist generally considers a radiograph made with average speed film and par speed screens as being pretty good. Such radiographs require that about 50,000 x-ray photons per square millimeter be absorbed by the screen to produce an average density of 1.0. In photography this would not be considered a good image, because a typical aerial photography film will use about 20 times as many photons to form its image.

One way to describe noise objectively is by the Wiener spectrum, sometimes called the power spectrum of noise. The mechanics of measuring radiographic mottle (noise) present difficult problems. In one method the radiographic mottle is scanned by a microdensitometer, and the sampled density fluctuation is analyzed by a computer. Another method involves putting the "noisy" film into a type of microdensitometer in which it can be spun in a circle and illuminated from one side. The transmitted light is collected by a photomultiplier behind a scanning aperture. The fluctuation in transmitted light intensity caused by radiographic mottle is converted to a voltage fluctuation in the photomultiplier tube. Electronic analysis of this voltage fluctuation performs what amounts to a Fourier analysis, which can determine the frequency content in the noise pattern.

Let us consider for a moment what noise looks like on a microdensitometer scan. In previous discussions we assumed that such a scan across the image of a small object would produce a nice smooth scan of density change versus distance, as shown in Figure 13–11. This is not a true picture of the situation. In Figure 13–16 we show how a real microdensitometer scan across an image will appear. Assume that identical screens are used, but in Figure 13–16A a slow film (low noise) and in Figure 13–16B a fast film (high noise) is used. The small square aperture of the microdensitometer (e.g., 5 to 10 microns) will "see" the small irregular density variations that constitute radiographic mottle superimposed on the larger density change caused by the image of the object being radiographed. In fact, it is difficult to make accurate microdensitometer scans of noisy and unsharp images because of the presence of quantum mottle. Nice smooth microdensitometer scans of objects such as opacified blood vessels simply do not exist.

We must retreat for a moment and review the components of radiographic mottle. You will recall that there is both screen mottle (for practical purposes this is quantum mottle) and film graininess. Although the eye does not normally see film grain, the microdensitometer is able to "see" the nonhomogeneous arrangement of clumps of silver in the gelatin. Thus, a microdensitometer will detect noise of two types:

1. Quantum mottle (statistical fluctuation of x-ray quanta absorbed in the screen).
2. Film grain (noise caused by the inherent grain distribution in the film).

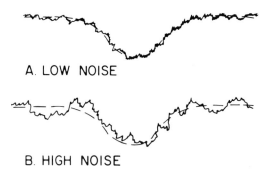

A. LOW NOISE

B. HIGH NOISE

Figure 13–16 Schematic depiction of a microdensitometer scan of the image of a blood vessel made with a low-noise (A) and a high-noise (B) imaging system

The Wiener spectrum is a measure of the total noise recorded by the film, **the sum of the grain noise and the quantum noise.** How does one distinguish film grain from screen mottle (quantum mottle)? This requires that two "flash" exposures of a film-screen system be made. The film in its cassette is simply placed under an x-ray tube and exposed at a reasonable kVp (one author uses 80 kVp) and low milliampere seconds to produce a density on the processed film of about 0.7. If the film and screen (or screens) are in intimate contact, the film will record quantum mottle resulting from the nonuniform absorption of x-ray quanta (and thus nonuniform production of light) in the screen, so the resulting noise will be made up of recorded quantum noise superimposed on the inherent film grain. To measure film grain alone a specially designed cassette is used. This cassette holds the screen (or screens) 13 or 14 mm away from the film, causing the individual light flashes (scintillations) from the screen to be blurred into a pattern of completely uniform illumination before the light reaches the film. In such a circumstance the film has been exposed with a truly uniform light source (i.e., quantum mottle has become undetectable in the light pattern by the time it reaches the film), so any noise in the processed film must originate from inherent film grain. In all these experiments we assume (virtually always correctly) that the screens used are free of any structural defects that could produce noise.

Schematic representation of the Wiener spectrum of a film-screen system will depict

1. total system noise (quantum plus grain noise),
2. film grain noise (grain noise), and
3. ability of the system to record the noise at increasing spatial frequency (recorded noise) (Fig. 13–17).

Note in Figure 13–17 that the lines depicting total (quantum plus grain) noise and grain noise are straight lines. This

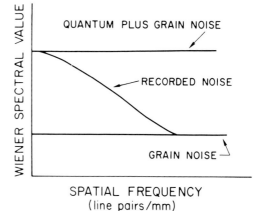

Figure 13–17 Schematic representation of the Wiener spectrum of a film-screen system

means that the amount of noise is the same at all spatial frequencies; this is termed white noise. Considering only noise, we may consider quantum mottle as the information input that we have asked the film-screen system to record. If the system were perfect, the amount of recorded quantum noise would be the same (white noise input) at all spatial frequencies. The MTF of the film-screen system limits the ability of the system to record information input, however, whether that information is the image of a skull, opacified blood vessel, or quantum mottle. The ability of the film-screen system to record noise decreases as the spatial frequency (line pairs per mm) increases, exactly as the ability of the system to record any image decreases with increasing spatial frequency. Depending on the MTF of the screen being used, a point is reached at which quantum noise is no longer imaged, and at this point only inherent film grain remains for the microdensitometer to detect (this might occur at about 6 to 10 line pairs per mm with typical screens). Let us not concern ourselves with a unit for measuring the Wiener spectrum, but be content to compare the position of a curve along the vertical axis to indicate more noise or less noise.

Some examples may make this topic easier to understand. Figure 13–18 shows the

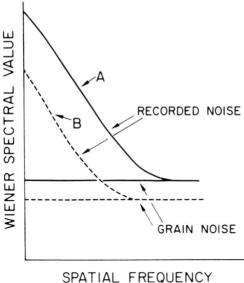

SPATIAL FREQUENCY
(line pairs/mm)

Figure 13–18 Schematic representation of the Wiener spectrum of a sharp screen combined with a fast film *(A)*, and a less sharp screen combined with a slower film *(B)*

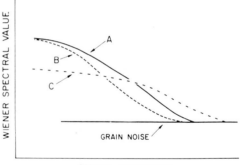

Figure 13–19 Schematic representation of the Wiener spectral curves of three different calcium tungstate intensifying screens used with the same film (see text)

Wiener spectrum of radiographic mottle for two film-screen systems. System A uses a sharp (thin) screen combined with a fast film. System B uses a less sharp (thicker) screen combined with a slower film. Note that the inherent film grain white noise is greater for the fast film (i.e., larger clumps of silver more unevenly distributed in the gelatin) than the slow film. System A has an increased Wiener spectral noise value because fewer x-ray quanta were absorbed (i.e., the fast film required less light). The point at which the total recorded noise curve merges with the film grain noise level indicates the relative MTF of each screen. The screen used in system A has the better MTF because it is able to record noise out to higher frequencies than system B. Without assigning any value units to the Wiener spectrum, a lot of information may still be derived from these two curves (i.e., compare total noise, film graininess, and system MTF).

Now consider Figure 13–19, which shows the Wiener spectral curves of three different screens used with the same film. Because systems A and B have the same total system noise at very low spatial frequency we can conclude that these two screens use the same number of x-ray quanta to expose the film. Likewise, because system A records nose at higher spatial frequencies, we know that screen A has a better MTF than screen B (probably because it is thinner). In fact, these two curves are similar to curves obtained with two par speed calcium tungstate screens made by different manufacturers.[20] Curve C represents a screen with significantly less total noise than that of the other two systems. This might be accomplished by using a less efficient screen phosphor (requiring absorption of more x-ray quanta to make an equal amount of light), or by using the same phosphor and including a light-absorbing dye in the phosphor layer. System C has a better MTF than that of the other systems because it records noise at a higher spatial frequency. This improved MTF might result from a thinner screen or from use of a dye in the screen to minimize light diffusion (acutance dye). This curve (C) is similar to a published Wiener spectral value curve of a detail calcium tungstate screen containing a yellow acutance dye to minimize light diffusion in the phosphor layer.[20]

As is true with MTF measurements, it is difficult to define the ultimate use of Wiener spectral curves in diagnostic radiology. It is clear that new developments in design regarding system optics, noise, and speed are offering the radiologist great flexibility in choice of an imaging system. Unfortunately, this greater flexibility creates a problem that requires greater understanding of the relation between system speed, noise, and detail visibility.

SUMMARY

Image clarity is defined as the visibility of diagnostically important detail in the radiographic image. Image clarity is determined by contrast and image quality. Radiographic contrast depends on three factors: subject contrast, film contrast, and scatter radiation plus fog. Image quality is a difficult subject to discuss because there is no good definition of what actually constitutes diagnostically important detail. Quantum mottle interferes with the smallest perceptible contrast, and is inversely proportional to the number of photons used to form an image. Sharpness is the ability of an imaging system to define a sharp edge. Resolving power is the ability of an imaging system to record separate images of small objects that are placed very close together. Use of the line spread function, modulation transfer function, and Wiener spectrum concepts help to develop a better understanding of the physical factors that control the information content of the radiographic image. We have attempted to introduce the fundamentals of the LSF, MTF, and Wiener spectrum in simple terms. The bibliography lists a number of excellent articles that explore these concepts in more detail.

REFERENCES

1. Bookstein, J.J., and Steck, W.: Effective focal spot size. Radiology, 98:31, 1971.
2. Cleare, H.M., Splettstosser, H.R., and Seeman, H.E.: An experimental study of the mottle produced by x-ray intensifying screens. Am. J. Roentgenol., 88:168, 1962.
3. Doi, K., and Rossman, K.: Measurement of optical and noise properties of screen-film systems in radiography. SPIE Medical X-Ray Photo-Optical Systems Evaluation, 56:45, 1975.
4. Gopala Rao, U.V., and Bates, L.M.: The modulation transfer function of x-ray focal spots. Phys. Med. Biol., 14:93, 1968.
5. Holm, T.: Some aspects of radiographic information. Radiology, 83:319, 1964.
6. Morgan, R.H.: The frequency response function. Am. J. Roentgenol., 88:175, 1962.
7. Morgan, R.H., Bates, L.M., Gopala Rao, U.V., and Marinaro, A.: The frequency response characteristics of x-ray films and screens. Am. J. Roentgenol., 92:426, 1964.
8. Roesch, W.C., Mellins, H.Z., and Gregg, E.C.: Improvements in the radiological image: A report from the Radiation Study Section of the National Institutes of Health. Radiology, 97:442, 1970.
9. Rossman, K.: Image-forming quality of radiographic screen-film systems: The line spread-function. Am. J. Roentgenol., 90:178, 1963.
10. Rossman, K.: Image quality. Contained in the syllabus of the proceedings of the AAPM 1971 Summer School. Physics of Diagnostic Radiology, Trinity University, San Antonio, July 12–17, 1971, pp. 220–281.
11. Rossman, K.: Image quality. Radiol. Clin. North Am., 7:419, 1969.
12. Rossman, K.: Point spread-function, line spread-function and modulation transfer function. Radiology, 93:257, 1969.
13. Rossman, K., and Lubberts, G.: Some characteristics of the line spread-function and modulation transfer function of medical radiographic films and screen-film systems. Radiology, 86:235, 1966.
14. Rossman, K., and Sanderson, G.: Validity of the modulation transfer function of radiographic screen-film systems measured by the slit method. Phys. Med. Biol., 13:259, 1968.
15. Seeman, H.E.: Factors which influence image quality and speed of film-screen combinations. In Technological Needs for Reduction of Patient Dosage from Diagnostic Radiology. Edited by M. L. Janower. Springfield, IL, Charles C Thomas, 1963.
16. Seeman, H.E.: Physical and Photographic Principles of Medical Radiography. New York, John Wiley and Sons, 1968.
17. Seeman, H.E.: Physical factors which determine roentgenographic contrast. Am. J. Roentgenol., 80:112, 1958.
18. Strum, R.E., and Morgan, R.H.: Screen intensification systems and their limitations. Am. J. Roentgenol., 62:617, 1949.
19. Wagner, R.F., and Denny, E.W.: A primer on physical parameters affecting radiographic image quality. Contained in the syllabus of the joint BRH-ACR conference, First Image Receptor Conference: Film/Screen Combinations, Arlington, VA, November 13–15, 1975, pp. 35–58.
20. Wagner, R.F., and Weaver, K.E.: Prospects for x-ray exposure reduction using rare earth intensifying screens. Radiology, 118:183, 1976.
21. Wayrynen, R.E.: Personal communication.

14

Fluoroscopy

X rays were discovered because of their ability to cause fluorescence, and the first x-ray image of a human part was observed fluoroscopically. Dr. Glasser, in his book, *Dr. W. C. Röntgen*, recounted:

> To test further the ability of lead to stop the rays, he selected a small lead piece, and in bringing it into position observed to his amazement, not only that the round dark shadow of the disc appeared on the screen, but that he actually could distinguish the outline of his thumb and finger, within which appeared darker shadows—the bones of his hand.[1]

During the years immediately following the discovery of x rays, film emulsions were of inferior quality and tube performance was unpredictable. Fluoroscopy was more reliable and probably more important than radiographic techniques. In the ensuing years, equipment improved and radiography moved to the forefront while fluoroscopy slipped to the subordinate role that it now maintains, that is, principally for the study and detection of moving parts, and secondarily to position a part optimally to obtain better radiographs.

Recently a large amount of accessory equipment has been developed to enhance and record the fluoroscopic image. These include x-ray image intensifiers, cine, television, and spot film cameras. Conventional fluoroscopy with x-ray intensifying screens has almost entirely disappeared. The image intensifiers that have replaced the screens will be discussed in Chapter 15. The basic fluoroscopic system (including the x-ray dose to the patient) is essentially the same, however, whether the image receptor is an image intensifier or an x-ray intensifying screen.

THE FLUOROSCOPE

A fluoroscope has two essential components, an x-ray tube and a fluoroscopic screen (or some other image receptor). All the other parts are designed either to protect the patient and operator from stray radiation or to facilitate the performance of an examination. The tube and screen are usually mounted at the opposite ends of a C arm to maintain their alignment (Fig. 14–1). The operator moves the fluoroscopic screen over the patient, and the x-ray tube follows the screen beneath the tabletop. The only motion between the two occurs along a slip joint in the C arm, which allows the screen to be raised and lowered to accommodate patients of various sizes.

A fluoroscopic x-ray tube is a standard rotating anode tube, the same as those used for radiography, but it is operated at a much lower tube current. Instead of the 100 to 1000 mA used in radiography, fluoroscopes are operated at currents ranging from 0.5 to 5.0 mA. The tube is equipped with shutters (an x-ray collimator) so that the operator can regulate the size and shape of the x-ray beam. The collimator is electrically driven. Controls for the collimator are located at the position from which the fluoroscopist moves the x-ray tube and intensifying screen. Permanent filtration equivalent to 2.5 mm of aluminum is recommended for fluoroscopy. A protective barrier (lead glass for intensifying screens, lead for image intensifiers) is used to intercept radiation that passes through the image receptor. Electrical interlocks prevent the x-ray tube from operating unless this protective barrier for operator protection is in place to intercept the beam entirely.

One of the principal reasons for employing fluoroscopy is to position a part optimally so as to isolate its image from obscuring shadows. Most fluoroscopes are equipped with a spot film device to record this image. To expose a spot film, the operator adjusts the field size and moves a film from a lead-shielded storage compartment into the fluoroscopic field. Usually a small motor drives the film cassette into position in a slot between the fluoroscopic screen and the grid, as shown in Figure 14–1. The fluoroscopic x-ray tube current automatically increases from approximately 3.0 mA to conventional radiographic levels (100 to 1000 mA) for the exposure. Most fluoroscopes are equipped with grids to absorb scatter radiation. Some units have specially designed shutters that automatically adjust the x-ray beam to the exact size selected for a spot film.

A large variety of fluoroscopic tables have been designed to meet the needs of particular examinations. Two important safety factors are common to all of them. The first protects the patient—the x-ray tube target should be at least 18 inches below the tabletop. Exposure rates are measured at the tabletop, and they are excessively large if the tube is closer than 18 inches. Remember that the inverse square law is in effect during fluoroscopy, so the input side of the patient receives more radiation per unit area than the output side (disregarding the difference resulting from attenuation). The input dosage is unnecessarily large with short tube-tabletop distances. The tabletop exposure rate should not exceed 10 Roentgens per minute, and with well-designed equipment it should be considerably lower. The second safety factor applies only to tables that have a Bucky grid mechanism. Cassettes are slid into a tray beneath the grid through an opening in the side of the table. Most tables have a hinged lead strip that fills this opening when the grid is parked at either end of the table. If the opening is not shielded, scatter radiation originating from the undersurface of the tabletop has an unimpeded route to the fluoroscopist. Lead

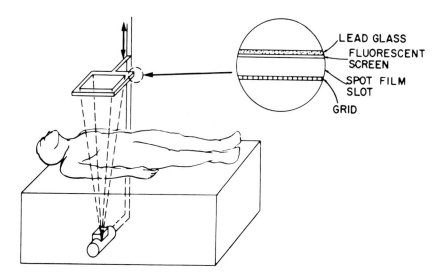

LEAD GLASS
FLUORESCENT SCREEN
SPOT FILM SLOT
GRID

Figure 14–1 Fluoroscope

rubber drapes hung from the image receptor are another common type of barrier used when a sterile field is not needed. The lead drapes intercept x rays scattered from within the patient.

Another feature included in most systems, and required by law in many states, is a 5-minute safety timer. It measures the accumulated fluoroscopic time during an examination and sounds an alarm or turns off the unit after 5 minutes. It is only a safety timer if it is coupled with good judgment on the part of the fluoroscopist, because it can be reset with little effort.

CONVENTIONAL SCREENS

Screen Illumination

In 1941, at a meeting of the Radiologic Society of North America in Chicago, Dr. W. Edward Chamberlain startled his audience when he announced that the light reflected from the piece of paper he was holding in his hand was 30,000 times brighter than the illumination of a fluoroscopic screen.[3] Radiologists had always known that the fluoroscopic screen was poorly illuminated, but no one before Chamberlain had ever bothered to measure it. How can we see anything with so little light? The answer is found in the eye's amazing ability to adapt to low levels of illumination.

Radiographs of average density are illuminated by an x-ray viewbox to a brightness that is three to four orders of magnitude brighter than the fluoroscopic screen. The fluoroscopic image is too poor to salvage by simply increasing exposure factors. Patient exposures of thousands of Roentgens per minute would be needed to bring the brightness of the fluoroscopic screen to ideal levels, clearly an intolerable situation. When conventional fluoroscopic screens were used, very low levels of illumination had to be accepted. Fluoroscopists had to use night vision for fluoroscopy.

Visual Physiology

Before progressing further with a discussion of fluoroscopy, we will digress for a brief review of visual physiology, especially as it relates to night vision.

The retina contains two different types of light receptors, rods and cones. Cones function most efficiently in bright light, while rods function best with low levels of illumination. Daylight (cone) vision is called photopic vision, and night (rod) vision is called scotopic vision. The differences between day and night vision are so great that humans can be considered to have two almost totally separate vision systems.

Photopic Vision

The cones are concentrated very densely in the fovea at the center of the retina, and are sparsely scattered over the rest of the retina. The dense concentration of cones gives high visual acuity for direct vision, and the sparse population in the remainder of the retina contributes to daylight peripheral vision. The cones are almost completely blind to low levels of illumination.

Scotopic Vision

There are no rods in the fovea, so scotopic vision is entirely peripheral vision. Also, the density of rods (and the interconnecting network of nerves) is less over the remainder of the retina than the density of cones in the fovea. The result is that scotopic (rod) vision is less acute than photopic (cone) vision. In addition, rods are most sensitive to changing levels of illumination. Night vision is best when the scene is changing (by moving the fluoroscopic unit) or when the eye scans over the scene. Rods can be extremely sensitive, however, to low levels of illumination. The human visual system can function at illumination levels more than a billion times larger than the lowest levels detectable. Of course, a transition from cone vision to rod vision is necessary. Rods are most sensitive to blue-green light, and daylight levels of these wavelengths of light greatly reduce the sensitivity of rods to low (night) illumination levels. Fluoroscopists had to "dark adapt" by wearing red goggles to filter out blue-green wavelengths for periods of over half an hour to allow the rods to recover peak sensitivity before fluoroscopy.

Integration Time

The integration time of the eye is the time over which it can store information. An x-ray film can integrate over a long period of time; the eye cannot. The integration time of the eye is only 0.2 second.[5] This short time is a serious disadvantage during fluoroscopy, a disadvantage that is not shared by radiographic techniques. For example, if a radiographic image is too light, it can be darkened by lengthening the exposure time. If necessary, the exposure time can be increased to several seconds, and the film will gradually accumulate enough radiation to reach an optimum density. The eye cannot build a picture in this way. It can only integrate for 0.2 second and then it must begin over on a whole new picture. If the fluoroscopic image is not bright enough to be of good quality, it cannot be improved by prolonged observation. Nothing is gained by gazing at a fluoroscopic image for an extended period of time.

STATISTICAL QUALITY OF FLUOROSCOPIC IMAGE

When we talk about fluoroscopic image quality, we must consider two different aspects of quality: the statistical quality of the image itself and the quality of the image that is actually perceived. A statistically superb image is of no value if the eye cannot capture it. In conventional fluoroscopy image quality is severely limited by the poor visual acuity of scotopic vision.

The fluoroscopic image exists at three different levels: (1) as an x-ray image; (2) as a light image on the fluoroscopic screen; and (3) as a light image on the retina of the eye. We will examine statistical quality (i.e., the number of photons making up the image) at each of these levels.

Compared to a standard roentgenogram, fluoroscopy begins with an inferior x-ray image. A simple way to demonstrate its inferiority is by comparing fluoroscopic and spot film exposure factors. No correction is needed for distance, grids, or other variables because they are the same for both systems. The following exposure factors were used in our department for abdominal fluoroscopy of a fairly large patient:

	SPOT FILM	FLUOROSCOPY
kVp	85	85
mA	150	3
Time (sec)	0.4	0.2*
mAs	60	0.6
Ratio	**100**	**1**

A fluoroscopic time (*) of 0.2 seconds, the integration time of the eye, is used for the comparison. The number of mAs (product of milliamperes and seconds) is proportional to the total number of photons involved in the two techniques. The ratio is 100 to 1; i.e., the x-ray image contains 100 times as many photons as the fluoroscopic image. Even if 150 mA are used for fluoroscopy, image quality is still inferior, because the spot film can integrate over a longer period of time.

One last point about the comparison between fluoroscopy and spot films is worth mentioning, even though it is not related to our present discussion. With the factors given above, each spot film results in a 60-mAs exposure to the patient, which is equivalent to 20 seconds of fluoroscopic time. With very large patients and long exposure times, one spot film may be equal to more than a minute of fluoroscopic time. We do not mean to condemn spot films, but merely to point out their cost in exposure to both the patient and fluoroscopist.

Sturm and Morgan have measured the number of photons in each link of the flu-

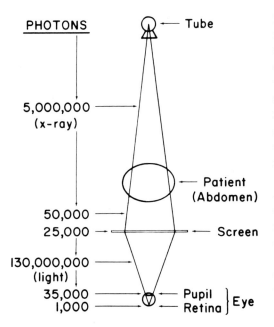

PHOTONS

Tube

5,000,000
(x-ray)

Patient
(Abdomen)

50,000
25,000 →

Screen

130,000,000
(light)

35,000
1,000

Pupil
Retina } Eye

Figure 14–2 The number of x-ray and light photons per square millimeter of fluoroscopic screen per second. (Adapted from the measurements of Sturm, R.E., and Morgan, R.H.: Screen intensification systems and their limitations. Am. J. Roentgenol., 62:613, 1949)

oroscopic chain; their results are summarized in Figure 14–2.[6] The numbers are for abdominal fluoroscopy, and of course they will vary depending on the thickness and density of the patient. Their reference point was 1 square millimeter of fluoroscopic screen, that is, the number of x-ray photons directed at, and the number of light photons emitted from, 1 mm² of screen. The x-ray tube delivers 5,000,000 photons per second, and 99% of them are absorbed in the patient. Half of the remaining 50,000 photons pass through the screen, and contribute nothing to image formation. Approximately 25,000 photons are absorbed by the screen.

Each x-ray photon produces many light photons, so the 25,000 x-ray photons are swelled to 130,000,000 light photons, quite enough to produce a good image if the eye could capture them. The eye is the weakest link in the chain. It defines the lowest level of photon flux. From a viewing distance of

20 cm, only one photon out of approximately 100,000 is absorbed by the retina, and the rest are lost. From each millimeter of screen only about 1000 photons reach the retina each second. Two factors are responsible for this tremendous loss. The first and most important is the narrow angle subtended by the eye from a viewing distance of 20 cm. Each millimeter of the fluoroscopic screen is like a tiny light bulb. It sends out light photons in all directions, and they obey the inverse square law. The only ones that enter the eye are those falling on an area 20 cm away that is the size of the pupil (50 mm²). The second reason for the loss of photons is absorption in the conducting system of the eye (cornea, lens, vitreous, and aqueous) and incomplete absorption by the retina. The eye does not transmit all the photons that enter the pupil, and the retina does not absorb all the photons it receives. Perhaps these are defense measures to protect the retina from the damaging effects of bright light.

In summary, photons are lost from the x-ray beam by attenuation in the patient and by transmission through the fluoroscopic screen. Their numbers are greatly increased in the conversion from x-ray to light photons, but unfortunately most of these never reach the retina. They are lost either by diffusion according to the inverse square law or within the eye itself. Only about 1000 photons are absorbed by the retina each second. By the standards of the eye, a second is a long time. It can only integrate for 0.2 second, so its image is made up of the photons that it can gather in 0.2 second, which in this example represents only 200 photons.

Statistical fluctuations in the number of photons in the x-ray beam are more important in fluoroscopy than they are in radiography because the total numbers are smaller in fluoroscopy. The production of x rays is a random process. The x-ray beam is not perfectly uniform in two adjacent areas, nor is it identical in the same area from one instant to the next. The same is true of light photons from the fluoroscopic screen. The number of photons fluctuates according to the law of statistics (i.e., the square root of the total number generated). We can examine the importance of statistical fluctuations by comparing two x-ray (or light) beams. Let us suppose that the first beam has 100 photons and the second, being more intense, has 10,000 photons. Their square roots are

Beam 1	Beam 2
$\sqrt{100} = 10$	$\sqrt{10,000} = 100$

It appears that the statistical fluctuations are greater in the more intense beam, but in actual fact the opposite is true. The percentage fluctuation is what is important, and not the absolute numbers. We can compare percentages by dividing the square root by the total intensity and multiplying by 100:

Beam 1	Beam 2
$\frac{10}{100} \times 100 = 10\%$	$\frac{100}{10,000} \times 100 = 1\%$

As you can see, the less intense beam fluctuates considerably more than the more intense beam.

The number of light photons absorbed on the retina of the eye will also show statistical fluctuations. In the example above, with 200 photons per square millimeter of fluoroscopic screen, the statistical fluctuation is the square root of 200, or $\pm$ 14. At one instant 214 photons may make up an image, and the next instant only 186. Variations of this magnitude can completely obscure an image, especially if the inherent contrast is low.

SUMMARY

A fluoroscope has only two essential components, an x-ray tube and a fluorescent screen, and they are usually mounted on a C arm to maintain their alignment.

The following safety features are recommended: 2.5 mm aluminum equivalent of permanent filtration, shutters to regulate field size, lead glass to absorb radiation transmitted through the screen, and an 18-inch minimum distance between the x-ray target and the tabletop. The exposure dose at the tabletop should not exceed 10 Roentgens per minute.

The illumination of a fluoroscopic screen is only 0.0001 as bright as that used to view average density radiographs. The screen illumination is such that the fluoroscopic image can only be seen with night (scotopic) vision, with its associated diminished visual acuity and the inconvenience of dark adaptation. The statistical quality of the fluoroscopic image is poor to begin with, because it is composed of a relatively small number of photons, and its quality is further reduced by the eye's inability to gather the light photons that are available. The whole problem is compounded by scotopic vision, a physiologically inferior viewing system. The result is an image that is too poor to be salvaged by increasing exposure factors, and the only way to improve its quality significantly is by a system of light amplification, the image intensifier, which we will discuss in the next chapter.

REFERENCES

1. Glasser, O.: Dr. W. C. Röntgen. Springfield, IL, Charles C Thomas, 1945.
2. Medical X-Ray and Gamma-Ray Protection for Energies up to 10 MeV. Washington, DC, National Council on Radiation Protection and Measurements, 1968, Report No. 33.
3. Chamberlain, W.E.: Fluoroscopes and fluoroscopy. Radiology, *38*:383, 1942.
4. Last, R.J.: Eugene Wolff's Anatomy of the Eye and Orbit. 6th Ed. Philadelphia, W.B. Saunders, 1968.
5. Davson, H.: The Physiology of the Eye. Boston, Little, Brown and Company, 1963.
6. Sturm, R.E., and Morgan, R.H.: Screen intensification systems and their limitations. Am. J. Roentgenol., *62*:613, 1949.

15

X-Ray Image Intensifiers

Conventional fluoroscopy has two serious limitations: a statistically inferior image and too little light for photopic (daylight) vision. Radiologists have always been aware of these limitations, but there was nothing they could do to improve the situation. They had to wait for a major technologic breakthrough, which occurred in the early 1950s, after a wait of more than 50 years. This breakthrough came with the development of the x-ray image intensifier, which has revolutionized fluoroscopy. Its image is bright enough for scotopic vision and small enough to be conveniently coupled to cine, television, or spot film cameras.

IMAGE INTENSIFIER DESIGN

The components of an x-ray image intensifier are shown in Figure 15–1. The tube itself is an evacuated glass envelope, a vacuum tube, which contains four basic elements:

1. input phosphor and photocathode
2. electrostatic focusing lens
3. accelerating anode
4. output phosphor.

After an x-ray beam passes through the patient, it enters the image intensifier tube. The input fluorescent screen absorbs x-ray photons and converts their energy into light photons. The light photons strike the photocathode, causing it to emit photoelectrons. These electrons are immediately drawn away from the photocathode by the high potential difference between it and the accelerating anode. As the electrons

flow from the cathode toward the anode, they are focused by an electrostatic lens, which guides them to the output fluorescent screen without distorting their geometric configuration. The electrons strike the output screen, which emits the light photons that carry the fluoroscopic image to the eye of the observer. In the intensifier tube, the image is carried first by x-ray photons, then by light photons, next by electrons, and finally by light photons.

Input Phosphor and Photocathode

First-generation image intensifiers had silver-activated zinc-cadmium sulfide crystals (ZnS-CdS:Ag) in the **input fluorescent screen.** Second-generation intensifiers

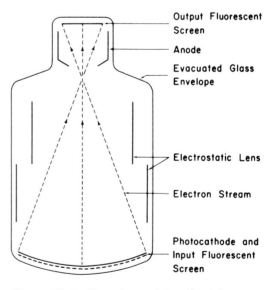

Figure 15–1   X-ray image intensifier tube

Output Fluorescent Screen

Anode

Evacuated Glass Envelope

Electrostatic Lens

Electron Stream

Photocathode and Input Fluorescent Screen

have cesium iodide (CsI) input screens. We will compare the relative merits of the two later in the chapter. The screen must be in intimate contact with the photocathode so that the system does not lose resolution. Figure 15–2A shows the arrangement of the input screen and photocathode. They are separated by a thin transparent layer, which prevents the fluorescent screen from reacting chemically with the photocathode. Remember that these layers are thin, only a small fraction of a millimeter, and little information is lost as the image is transferred from the screen to the photocathode.

The **photocathode** is a photoemissive metal (usually a combination of antimony and cesium compounds). When light from the fluorescent screen strikes the photocathode, it emits photoelectrons in numbers proportional to the brightness of the screen.

In addition to functioning as a photoemissive surface, the photocathode also serves as the cathode of the image tube. It is usually kept at ground potential.

Electrostatic Focusing Lens

This is made up of a series of positively charged electrodes that are usually plated onto the inside surface of the glass envelope. These electrodes focus the electron beam as it flows from the photocathode toward the output phosphor. Electron focusing inverts the image. Each point on the input phosphor is focused to a specific point on the opposite side of the output phosphor. For undistorted focusing, all photoelectrons must travel the same distance. The distance between corresponding points in the image on two phosphors is equalized by curving the input phosphor. The image on the output phosphor is reduced in size, which is one of the principal reasons why it is brighter, a point to which we will return later.

Accelerating Anode

This is located in the neck of the image tube (see Fig. 15–1). Its function is to draw

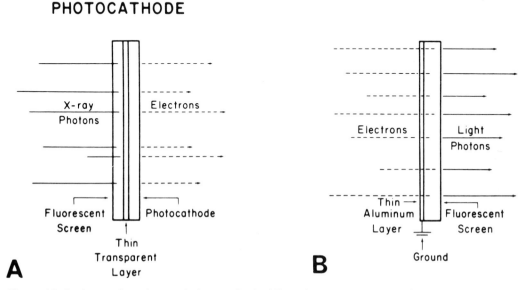

INPUT PHOSPHOR and PHOTOCATHODE

OUTPUT PHOSPHOR

Figure 15–2 Input phosphor and photocathode (*A*) and output phosphor of an image intensifier (*B*)

electrons from the photocathode and accelerate them toward the output screen. The anode has a positive potential of 25,000 volts (25 kV), so it accelerates electrons to a tremendous velocity.

Output Phosphor

The **output fluorescent screen** of all image intensifiers is silver-activated zinc-cadmium sulfide, the same material used in first-generation input phosphors, but the crystal size and layer thickness are reduced to maintain resolution in the minified image. Because the electrons are greatly accelerated, they emit more light photons from the output screen than were originally present at the input screen. The number of light photons is increased approximately 50-fold. The fluoroscopist observes this brighter image through a viewing system, usually a series of mirrors or a television camera.

A thin layer of aluminum is plated onto the fluorescent screen (Fig. 15–2*B*) to prevent light from moving retrograde through the tube and activating the photocathode. The aluminum layer is very thin, and high-energy photoelectrons easily pass through it en route to the output screen. This layer also serves as a ground to remove spent electrons from the image tube. If they were not removed, they would accumulate on the output phosphor and build up a negative charge.

The glass tube of the image intensifier is enclosed in a lead-lined metal container that is mounted on the C arm of the fluoroscope in place of the conventional fluoroscopic screen. The lead lining protects the operator from stray radiation, and a lead glass window over the output phosphor absorbs radiation that passes through the intensifier.

The output screen is optically coupled to a viewing system by a tandem lens (Fig. 15–3). The image is viewed either directly through a series of lenses and mirrors, or indirectly through closed-circuit television. A movable mirror, mounted at a 45° angle

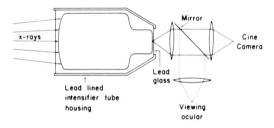

Figure 15–3 Optical coupling between an image intensifier and viewing system

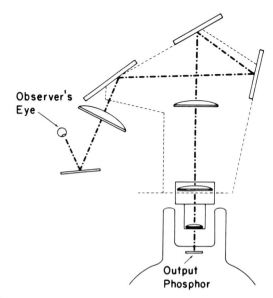

Figure 15–4 Mirror optical system of an image intensifier

between the tandem lenses, allows the operator to switch recording and viewing modes. If the mirror is semitransparent, so that some light is transmitted and the rest reflected, the image can be monitored during cinefluorography.

A mirror optical system is shown in Figure 15–4. As you can see, light travels a long distance, and it is reflected and focused several times. This results in a considerable loss of photons, which is the main disadvantage of any mirror system. The mirror image is only visible in a small viewing angle. If the operator moves his head a few degrees to one side, the image is lost. His freedom of movement is limited by the mirror, making it difficult, if not impossible, to palpate the patient. Also, only one observer can view the image, which is a serious disadvantage in training beginning fluoroscopists.

BRIGHTNESS GAIN

Two methods are used to evaluate the brightness gain of image intensifiers. The first compares the luminance of an intensifier output screen to that of a Patterson-type B-2 fluoroscopy screen when both are exposed to the same quantity of radiation. The brightness gain is the ratio of the two illuminations:

$$\text{Brightness gain} = \frac{\text{intensifier luminance}}{\text{Patterson B-2 luminance}}$$

If the image intensifier is 1000 times brighter, the brightness gain is 1000. The concept is easy to understand, and was readily accepted by radiologists. Patterson-type B-2 fluoroscopic screens, however, vary from one batch to another, and deteriorate at an unpredictable rate with time, so brightness gain measurements are not reproducible. Because of this lack of reproducibility, the International Commission on Radiologic Units and Measurements (ICRU) has recommended a second method of evaluation, called the conversion factor, to supersede the older brightness gain method.[1] The conversion factor is a ratio of the luminance of the output phosphor to the input exposure rate:

$$\text{Conversion factor} = \frac{cd/m^2}{mR/sec}$$

Output screen luminance is measured in candelas (abbreviated cd, and defined as the luminous intensity, in the perpendicular direction, of a surface of a $1/600,000$ m^2 of a black body at the temperature of freezing platinum under a pressure of $101,325$ Nt/m^2... ridiculous to remember). Radiation quality and output luminance are explicitly defined, so the method is accurate and reproducible. **The brightness gain tends to deteriorate as an image intensifier ages.** This means

that the patient dose with an old image intensifier tends to be higher than that with a new intensifier of the same type. Because the deterioration can proceed at a rate of about 10% per year, a periodic check of image intensifier brightness can be valuable. Unfortunately, an accurate check is somewhat complicated. Some indication of image intensifier aging can be obtained by comparing the input dose level required for automatic brightness control operation with the dose level under the same conditions when the intensifier was new.

The brightness gain of an image intensifier comes from two completely unrelated sources, called minification gain and flux gain. We will discuss them separately.

Minification Gain

The brightness gain from minification is produced by a reduction in image size. The quantity of the gain depends on the relative areas of the input and output screens. Because the size of an intensifier is usually indicated by its diameter, it is more convenient to express minification gain in terms of diameter:

$$\text{Minification gain} = \left(\frac{d_i}{d_o}\right)^2$$

where d_i is the diameter of input screen, and d_o is the diameter of output screen. Most x-ray image intensifiers have an input screen from 5 to 9 inches in diameter and an output screen approximately 1 inch in diameter. Recently, image intensifiers with 12- to 14-inch diameter input screens have become routinely available, and larger sizes are in the offing. Of course, these larger sizes are more cumbersome and are still quite expensive compared to a 9-inch intensifier. With a 1-inch output screen, the minification gain is simply the square of the diameter of the input screen; that is, a 9-inch intensifier has a gain of 81.

The brightness gain from minification does not improve the statistical quality of the fluoroscopic image. The same number of light photons make up the image regardless of the size of the output screen. For example, a 6-inch intensifier with a 2-inch output phosphor has a minification gain of 9 ($6^2 \div 2^2 = 36 \div 4 = 9$), while the same intensifier with a 1-inch output phosphor has a gain of 36. The total light output of both units is exactly the same, however, so the same number of photons make up both images. The photons are compressed together on the smaller screen and the image is brighter, but its statistical quality is not improved.

Theoretically, brightness can be increased indefinitely by minification. A 9-inch intensifier with a $\frac{1}{16}$-inch output screen would have a brightness gain from minification alone of over 20,000. Excess minification produces a very small image, though, which has a definite disadvantage. Before the image can be viewed it must be greatly magnified, which not only reduces the brightness but also magnifies the fluoroscopic crystals in the output screen, resulting in a precipitous drop in resolution.

Flux Gain

Flux gain increases the brightness of the fluoroscopic image by a factor of approximately 50. For each light photon from the input screen, 50 light photons are emitted by the output screen. In simplified terms, you may think of one light photon from the input screen as ejecting one electron from the photocathode. The electron is accelerated to the opposite end of the tube, gaining enough energy to produce 50 light photons at the output screen.

The total brightness gain of an image intensifier is the product of the minification and flux gains:

Brightness gain = minification gain × flux gain

For example, with a flux gain of 50 and a minification gain of 81 (9-inch intensifier with a 1-inch output screen), the total brightness gain is 4050 (50 × 81). In general, brightness gains from modern image intensifiers are always over 1000 and frequently as high as 6000.

CESIUM IODIDE IMAGE INTENSIFIERS

Image quality is dramatically better with cesium iodide input screens than it was with the older zinc-cadmium sulfide screens. Two physical characteristics of cesium iodide make it superior; a greater packing density and a more favorable effective atomic number. Cesium iodide can be vacuum-deposited and requires no inert binder, so more active material can be packed into a given space. The packing density of cesium iodide is three times greater than that of zinc-cadmium sulfide. Phosphor thicknesses have been reduced comparably from approximately 0.3 mm with zinc-cadmium sulfide to 0.1 mm with cesium iodide. The principal advantage of the thinner phosphor layer is improved resolution.

Ideally, for maximum photoelectric absorption, the K-absorption edge of a phosphor should be as close to the energy of the x-ray beam as possible, provided the energy of the edge does not exceed that of the beam. An obvious problem arises in attempting to accomplish this ideal. Beam energy is a spectrum, a whole array of energies, while the K edge is a single point or, at most, several points, depending on the number of absorbers in the phosphor. The mean energy of an x-ray beam is approximately one third of its peak energy, depending somewhat on the energy level and filtration. Most fluoroscopy on adults is done at a peak energy of from 100 to 120 kVp, which is a mean energy between 33 and 40 keV. Table 15–1 shows the K edges of elements used as phosphors in various types of screens. The energy of the K edge of cadmium (26.7 keV) is quite good, but its chemical mates, zinc (9.7 keV) and sulfur (2.5 keV) are far from ideal. The K edges of cesium (36 keV) and iodine (33.2 keV) are almost perfect. The more appropriate atomic numbers of cesium and iodine give these screens a substantial advantage over those made of zinc-cadmium

Table 15–1. Atomic Number and K-Absorption Edge of Elements Commonly Used in Intensifying Screens

ELEMENT	ATOMIC NUMBER	K-ABSORPTION EDGE (keV)
Sulfur	16	2.5
Calcium	20	4.0
Zinc	30	9.7
Selenium	34	12.7
Yttrium	39	17.0
Cadmium	48	26.7
Iodine	53	33.2
Cesium	55	36.0
Lanthanum	57	39.0
Gadolinium	64	50.2
Tungsten	74	69.5

sulfide. Cesium iodide input screens absorb approximately two thirds of the incident beam as opposed to less than one third for zinc-cadmium sulfide, even though the cesium iodide screen is only one third as thick.

IMAGE QUALITY

In evaluating image quality with image intensifiers, we must evaluate the same two factors that we considered with conventional fluoroscopy. The first is the statistical quality of the image, and the second is the adequacy of the light level for photopic (cone) vision. If an intensifier does nothing but brighten the image to a level at which it can be seen with photopic vision, it has accomplished a great deal. Remember, photopic visual acuity is 10 times better than scotopic visual acuity. A brightness gain of approximately 1000 will satisfy the light requirements for photopic vision. All modern image intensifiers easily reach this level. The brighter image has several secondary benefits. Dark adaptation is unnecessary. The lights can be turned on in the fluoroscopic room, which relieves patient apprehension and simplifies the examination, especially in children. The image is also bright enough for safe cine-fluorography.

Statistical Image Quality (Quantum Mottle)

The number of absorbed x-ray photons determines the highest possible statistical quality of an imaging system. No form of intensification can improve the image above the statistical level of the absorbed photons. The overall statistical quality of a system is determined by the lowest point, called the **quantum sink.** The quantum sink determines the amount of quantum mottle that we see in the final image. The low point is analogous to the weakest link in a chain. For the same reason that a chain cannot be stronger than its weakest link, the statistical quality of an image cannot be higher than its lowest point. In an image intensifier system, the quantum sink may be either at the input phosphor or at the retina of the eye, depending on the efficiency of optical coupling. If the low point is at the input phosphor, quality can be improved only by the absorption of more x-ray photons. With a mirror optical system, a large number of photons are lost through repeated reflections, and the low point is at the retina. In this case, statistical quality can be improved (i.e., the quantum sink raised) by a higher x-ray-to-light conversion efficiency, but quality can never be raised above that of the absorbed photons.

The number of absorbed photons can be increased in two ways: by increasing the number of photons in the incident beam; and by capturing a higher percentage of the incident photons. Cesium iodide image tubes capture a greater percentage of the incident beam than either conventional fluoroscopic screens or older intensifiers, so statistical quality is superior for any given level of exposure. Statistical fluctuations manifest themselves in the radiographic image as quantum mottle, a sort of grainy appearance. The visibility of mottle is determined by the resolution and contrast levels of the system. Mottle is more visible in a high-resolution, high-contrast image. As we shall see momentarily, cesium iodide image tubes improve both resolution and contrast, so in evaluating overall image quality opposing forces are at work. For any given level of exposure, the image is statistically superior, but the mottle present is easier to see and therefore more distracting.

The mottle level can be adjusted with image intensifiers by changing exposure factors. Increasing exposures increases the number of absorbed photons, which decreases statistical fluctuations. If the image intensifier is used with a cine or spot film camera, where increasing the exposure may overexpose the film, an iris-type diaphragm can be incorporated into the optical system to decrease the light output reaching the film. In Figure 15–5B, the exposure per frame is twice as great as in Figure 15–5A, but both films are exposed to the same density. Balanced film densities are maintained because the diaphragm intercepts half of the light from the output phosphor in Figure 15–5B. At first glance, it looks like the diaphragm cuts the size of the image in half, but such is not the case. The light shown in the optical system all arises from a single point, the center of the output phosphor, and the diaphragm intercepts half the light from this point. The same effect occurs for every point on the output phosphor. The net result of doubling the exposure and halving the light output is an image of unchanged brightness but improved statistical quality.

While image intensifiers were in a developmental stage, it was felt that one of their principal advantages would be greatly reduced patient exposures. Even before the first image intensifier was perfected, however, Sturm and Morgan pointed out an important fact.[2] The number of photons in the x-ray image cannot be decreased indefinitely. Eventually a point is reached at which there are not enough photons to produce an image. The fluoroscopic x-ray image is close to that point. A large decrease in the number of x-ray photons would cause a serious deterioration of image quality. In actual practice, image intensifiers have not significantly decreased patient exposures. Most radiologists are using 2 to 5 mA for adult abdominal fluoroscopy, which is approximately the same as pre-intensifier levels.

Contrast

Contrast can be determined in various ways, and there is no universal agreement as to which is best. The following is a description of the simplest method. A ¼-inch thick lead disc is placed over the center of the input screen. Disc size is selected to cover 10% of the screen; that is, a 0.9-inch diameter disc is used for a 9-inch image intensifier. The input phosphor, with the disc in place, is exposed to a specified quantity of radiation, and brightness is measured at the output phosphor. Contrast is the brightness ratio of the periphery to the center of the output screen. Defined in this way, contrast ratios range from approximately 10:1 to better than 20:1, depending on the manufacturer and intended use. Contrast is definitely better with cesium iodide tubes than it was with the older zinc-cadmium sulfide tubes.

Two factors tend to diminish contrast in image intensifiers. First, the input screen does not absorb all the photons in the x-ray beam. Some are transmitted through the intensifier tube, and a few are eventually absorbed by the output screen. These transmitted photons contribute to the illumination of the output phosphor but not to image formation. They produce a background of fog that reduces image

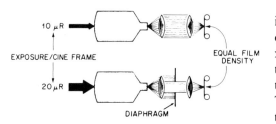

Figure 15–5 Effect of a diaphragm on the brightness of an imaging system

contrast in the same way that scattered x-ray photons produce fog and reduce contrast in a radiographic image. The second reason for reduced contrast in an image intensifier is retrograde light flow from the output screen. Most retrograde light flow is blocked by a thin layer of aluminum on the back of the screen. The aluminum layer must be extremely thin, however, or it would absorb the electrons that convey the fluoroscopic image. Some light photons penetrate through the aluminum, pass back through the image tube, and activate the photocathode. The cathode emits photoelectrons, and their distribution bears no relationship to the principal image. These electrons produce "fog" and further reduce image contrast.

Resolution

The resolution of zinc-cadmium sulfide image tubes is 1 to 2 line pairs per millimeter (lp/mm), which is a little less than the resolution of a conventional fluoroscopic screen. The apparent improvement that the fluoroscopist observes is entirely from the increased visual acuity of photopic vision. The resolution of cesium iodide image tubes is approximately 4 lp/mm, a dramatic improvement over zinc cadmium sulfide. The individual CsI crystals are somewhat aligned and the phosphor layer is thinner, both contributing to improved resolution.

The resolution of an imaging system is usually expressed in terms of its modulation transfer function (MTF). At any given frequency (number of line pairs/mm), the MTF is a specific number that is always less than one. The overall MTF of the system is the product of the component parts. We can use the following series of fractions to demonstrate the effect of the components:

$$0.9 \times 0.1 = 0.09$$
$$0.8 \times 0.2 = 0.16$$
$$0.7 \times 0.3 = 0.21$$
$$0.6 \times 0.4 = 0.24$$
$$0.5 \times 0.5 = 0.25$$

If the numbers were added instead of mul-

tiplied, they would all be equal. When they are multiplied, however, the largest product is obtained when both numbers are equal (i.e., 0.5 × 0.5). If the numbers are a great deal different, their product is much closer to the size of the smaller number. Modulation transfer functions behave in exactly the same way. If the MTF of the glass envelope of an image intensifier is 0.9 and the input phosphor 0.1, at a frequency of 3 lp/mm, their combined MTF is 0.09. Trying to develop a better glass envelope would be a foolish investment. The maximum effort should be directed at improving the input phosphor which is obviously the weaker link in this chain.

Figure 15–6 shows MTF curves for a hypothetical image intensifier. The product of all the component curves yields the curve for the overall system. In this example, the performance of the input and output phosphors are very similar. In older (zinc-cadmium sulfide) tubes the MTF of the input screen was less than the MTF of the output screen. Research and development was directed at input phosphors and now, thanks to the use of cesium iodide, the two are close. The resolution requirements of the output screen are dependent on the size and resolving power of the input screen. A 9-inch input screen with a resolution of 4 lp/mm presents a total of 914 lp to the output screen (9 in. × 25.4 mm/in. × 4 lp/mm = 914 lp). A 15-mm

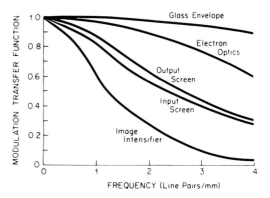

Figure 15–6 Modulation transfer function for an image intensifier and its component parts

output screen, a fairly common size, has to handle 61 lp/mm (914 ÷ 15 mm = 61 lp/mm). A 15-mm output screen with a 6-inch input screen only has to resolve 41 lp/mm (6 × 25.4 × 4 ÷ 15 = 41). Because of this difference, the weakest link in the system may shift from the input phosphor with a 6-inch tube to the output phosphor with a 9-inch tube.

Contrast tends to deteriorate as an image intensifier ages. Again, the strictly objective test just described is somewhat difficult to perform routinely. A comparison of the contrast achievable when the image intensifier was new can help to spot degradation trends (up to 10% per year). Unfortunately, simple tests that depend on observer perception of low-contrast test objects are subjective.

Distortion

In the present state of development, electron focusing is not uniform across the entire width of an image intensifier. Electrons at the center of the unit are more accurately focused than those at the periphery. Peripheral electrons tend to flare out from an ideal course. The result is unequal magnification, which produces peripheral distortion. The amount of distortion is always greater with large intensifiers because, the further an electron is from the center of the intensifier, the more difficult it is to focus. Figure 15–7 shows a cine image of a coarse wire screen taken with a 9-inch intensifier. As you can see, the wires curve out at the periphery. Generally this distortion does not hamper routine fluoroscopy, but it may make it difficult to evaluate straight lines, for example in the reduction of a fracture.

Unequal magnification also causes unequal illumination. The center of the output screen is brighter than the periphery (Fig. 15–7). The peripheral image is displayed over a larger area of the output screen, and thus its brightness gain from minification is less than that in the center. A fall-off in brightness at the periphery of

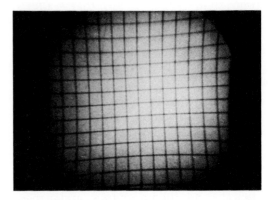

Figure 15–7   Test film of a wire screen (35-mm cine frame) from a 9-inch image intensifier. (Courtesy of Harold Alsobrook, R. T.)

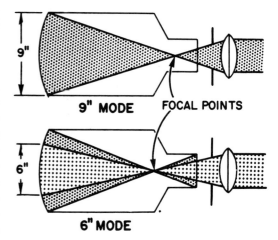

Figure 15–8   Dual-field image intensifier

an image is called **vignetting.** Unequal focusing has another effect on image quality; that is, resolution is better in the center of the screen.

In summary, the center of the image intensifier screen has better resolution, a brighter image, and less geometric distortion. It follows logically that a small image intensifier, which encompasses only the central, more accurately focused electrons, produces a better-quality image than a large unit.

DUAL-FIELD IMAGE INTENSIFIERS

Dual-field, or triple-field, image intensifiers attempt to resolve the conflicts between image size and quality. They can be operated in several modes, including a 4.5-inch, a 6-inch, or 9-inch mode. The 9-inch mode is used when it is necessary to view large anatomic areas. When size is unimportant, the 4.5- or 6-inch mode is used because of better resultant image quality. Larger image intensifiers (12 to 14 inch) frequently have triple-field capability.

Field size is changed by applying a simple electronic principle: the higher the voltage on the electrostatic focusing lens, the more the electron beam is focused. Figure 15–8 shows this principle applied to a dual-field image intensifier. In the 9-inch mode, the electrostatic focusing voltage is decreased. The electrons focus to a point, or cross, close to the output phosphor, and the final image is actually smaller than the phosphor. In the 6-inch mode the electrostatic focusing voltage is increased, and the electrons focus farther away from the output phosphor. After the electrons cross, they diverge, so the image on the output phosphor is larger than in the 9-inch mode. The optical system is preset to cover only the format, or size, of the smaller image of the 9-inch mode. In the 6-inch mode, the optical system "sees" only the central portion of the image, the part derived from the central 6 inches of the input phosphor. Because this image is less minified, it appears to be magnified when viewed through a television monitor or a series of mirrors. The physical size of the input and output screens is the same in both modes; the only thing that changes is the size of the output

image. Obviously, the 6- and 9-inch modes have different minification gains. Exposure factors are automatically increased when the unit is used in the 6-inch mode to compensate for the decreased brightness from minification.

While we are discussing intensifier size, there is another point to consider. A 9-inch image intensifier does not encompass a 9-inch field in the patient. The x-ray image is magnified by divergence of the beam (Fig. 15–9). The intensifier sees a much smaller field than its size would imply, an important point to consider when ordering a unit to perform a particular function.

SUMMARY

An x-ray image intensifier is an electronic vacuum tube consisting of an input phosphor and photocathode, electrostatic focusing lens, accelerating anode, and output phosphor. It converts an x-ray image into a light image, then to an electron image and, finally, back to a light image of diminished size and increased brightness. Electron acceleration produces a flux gain, and size reduction produces a minification gain. The total brightness gain is the product of the gains from flux and minification. Intensifier performance tends to deteriorate with age. Image intensifiers make their most important contribution by increasing screen illumination to the level required for photopic (cone) vision with its superior visual acuity. They have made dark adaptation a thing of the past, and cinefluorography a safe procedure. Lastly, they have brought the television camera into the fluoroscopic room and opened up a whole new world of electron communication.

REFERENCES

1. International Commission on Radiologic Units and Measurements: Methods of Evaluating Radiological Equipment and Materials. Washington, DC, National Bureau of Standards, 1963, ICRU Handbook No. 89.
2. Sturm, R.E., and Morgan, R.H.: Screen intensification systems and their limitations. Am. J. Roentgenol., 62:613, 1949.

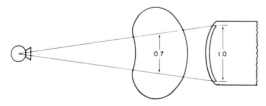

Figure 15–9 Reduction of fluoroscopic field size by an image intensifier

16

Cinefluorography

Cinefluorography is the process of recording fluoroscopic images on movie (cine) film. Before the invention of the image intensifier, cinefluorography required excessively large patient exposures, so it was never widely accepted for clinical radiography. Patient exposures were large for two reasons. First, optical coupling was inefficient, because the cine camera had to be placed a long distance from the fluoroscopic screen to encompass its large size. Most of the available light was lost as a result of the inverse square law, and only a small percentage reached the camera. Second, screen illumination was not bright enough to expose the film without increasing the x-ray exposure factors, which meant more radiation. Thus, because patient exposures were intolerably high, cine techniques were relegated to animal experiments and a few research projects.

The birth of safe, clinically applicable cinefluorography came in the early 1950s after the invention of the image intensifier, which solved the problems that had frustrated earlier attempts. Its image was bright enough to expose the film without exposing the patient excessively, and the image was small enough to couple efficiently to a cine camera.

Two film sizes are currently being used for cinefluorography, 16 and 35 mm. In the United States, 98% of all cine is done on 35-mm film, and 95% of all cine studies involve the heart. Therefore, our major emphasis will be on 35-mm cardiac cinefluorography.

The basic components of a modern cinefluorography system are:

1. camera
2. image intensifier
3. optical system
4. x-ray photon image
5. radiographic equipment
6. film
7. processor
8. projector.

These components can be likened to a length of chain, all tied closely together and all limited by the weakest link. For optimum results, at the lowest possible cost in both dollars and patient exposure, the links should all be of equal strength. Occasionally, an expensive generator is coupled to an expensive image intensifier and then the film is developed in an inexpensive processor of inferior quality. The results are usually unsatisfactory.

Each of the eight basic components in the cinefluorographic system will be discussed separately, in the order listed above. Most of our recommendations are taken from the Report of the Inter-Society Commission for Heart Disease Resources.[2] Because cinefluorography records image-intensified fluoroscopic images onto film, we have taken the opportunity to expand our earlier coverage of some pertinent topics.

CINE CAMERA

Cinefluorography is married to the motion picture industry. We are stuck with their horizontal rectangular format, even though it is not well-suited to our needs. All cine cameras are commercial movie cameras with a few minor modifications. Two film sizes are available, 16 and 35 mm. The basic components of the camera are a lens, iris diaphragm, shutter, aperture, pressure plate, pulldown arm, and film transport mechanism. The lens and iris diaphragm will be discussed in more detail later in the chapter.

Components

Light enters the camera through the lens and is restricted by the **aperture,** a rectangular opening in the front of the camera. The size and shape of the aperture define the configuration of the image reaching the film. Figure 16–1 shows the image sizes as defined by the apertures of 16- and 35-mm cameras. Apertures for 35-mm film are usually 18 × 24 mm.

The **shutter** is a rotating disc with a sec-

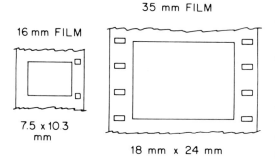

tor cut out of its periphery (Fig. 16–2). It is located in front of the aperture. As the shutter rotates, it interrupts light flow into the camera. The size of the shutter opening is expressed as the number of degrees in the cutout portion of the sector. Openings of 160° to 180° are usually employed for cinefluorography. While the shutter is closed, the **pulldown arm** advances the film to the correct position for the next exposure (Fig. 16–3). The **pressure plate** holds the film against the camera aperture so that it is located in the proper image plane.

An electric drive motor advances the film from the supply reel past the aperture to the takeup reel. A meter attached to the supply reel indicates the amount of unexposed film in the camera. The x-ray pulses and shutter opening are synchronized by an electrical signal from the drive motor. The framing frequency, or number of frames per second, is usually 60, divided or multiplied by a whole number (e.g., $7\frac{1}{2}$, 15, 30, 60 or 120).

The combination of the framing frequency and shutter opening determines the amount of time available for both the exposure and pulldown. For example, with a 180° shutter opening and 60 frames per second, the time available for both the exposure and pulldown is $\frac{1}{120}$ sec. At slower framing frequencies, both are longer. With a smaller shutter opening, the available ex-

Figure 16–1 Film formats as defined by the apertures of 16-mm and 35-mm cameras

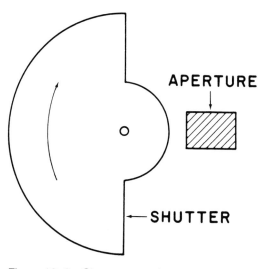

Figure 16–2 Cine camera shutter

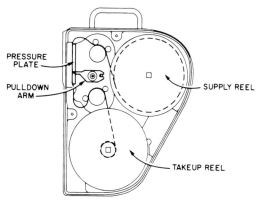

Figure 16–3 Cine camera

posure time is shorter than the pulldown time.

Framing

The output phosphor of the image intensifier and the camera aperture have different shapes, so a portion of either the image or film frame must be discarded. The term "framing" refers to the utilization of the available area on the film (Fig. 16–4). The Report of the Inter-Society Commission for Heart Disease Resources has classified the various degrees of framing for 35-mm film as follows:[2]

Underframing. The maximum dimension of the fluoroscopic image is shorter than the smallest dimension of the frame (not shown in Fig. 16–4). Underframing is caused by a faulty optical system and should be avoided.

Exact Framing. The diameter of the circular intensifier image and shorter dimension of the film (18 mm) are the same. No part of the image is lost, but only 58% of the cine frame is used. Exact framing is recommended when the long axis of the part being examined is vertically oriented, such as the esophagus. It is not generally recommended for cardiac cinefluorography.

Overframing. The diameter of the circular image is greater than the shortest di-

mension of the film, so part of the image is lost.

Mean Diameter Framing. The diameter of the circular image is halfway between the largest and smallest dimensions of the film (24 + 18 = 42 ÷ 2 = 21 mm); 73% of the film area is used and only 4% of the image is wasted (Fig. 16–4).

Equal Area Framing. The area of the circular image, both within and outside the picture frame, is equal to the area of the rectangular frame; 87% of the film area is used and 15% of the image is wasted (not shown in Fig. 16–4). This is the framing type recommended by the International Commission on Radiation Units and Measurements.[1] The diameter of the fluoroscopic image is 23.5 mm, which is almost identical to the diameter of the image from maximum horizontal framing.

Maximum Horizontal Framing. The diameter of the circular image and width of the rectangular field are identical (24 mm). Approximately 12% of the film area is unused and 16% of the image is wasted (Fig. 16–4).

Subtotal Overframing. The diameter of the circular image is midway between the image diameter for maximum horizontal framing and total overframing (24 + 30 = 54 ÷ 2 = 27 mm); 90% of the film area is used and 28% of the image is wasted (Fig. 16–4).

FRAMING MODE	EXACT FRAMING	MEAN DIAMETER FRAMING	MAXIMUM HORIZONTAL FRAMING	SUBTOTAL OVER-FRAMING	TOTAL OVER-FRAMING
ILLUSTRATION	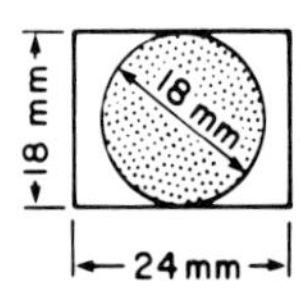 18 mm / 18 mm / 24 mm	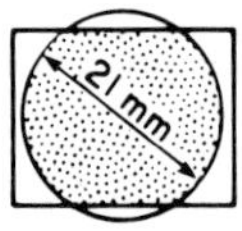 21 mm	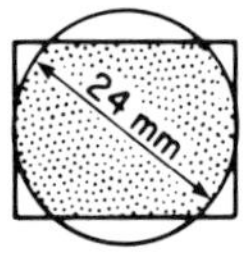 24 mm	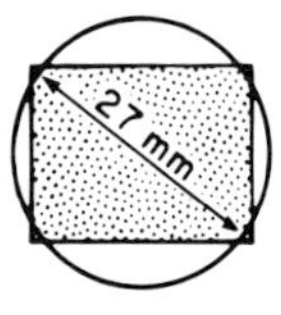 27 mm	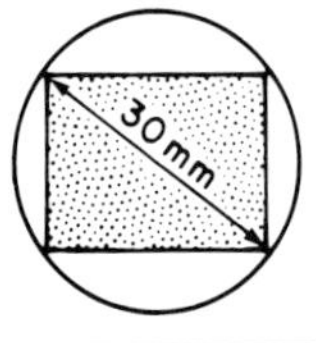 30 mm
FILM AREA USED	58%	73%	88%	96%	100%
IMAGE AREA UNUSED	0%	4%	16%	28%	39%
RELATIVE IMAGE SIZE	1.0	1.17	1.33	1.50	1.67

Figure 16–4   Framing methods. (Modified from Judkins et al.[2])

Total Overframing. The diameter of the circular image is equal to the diagonal measurement of the rectangular aperture (30 mm). All the film is used but 39% of the image is wasted (Fig. 16–4).

Framing and Patient Exposure

The x-ray beam should be restricted to coincide with the framing method. Figure 16–4 shows the percentage of the potential image area that is unused by the various framing methods. If the beam is not correspondingly restricted, these areas of the patient are exposed but the image is never recorded. The problem is actually more complex than Figure 16–4 implies. Most fluoroscopic installations have rectangular field collimators. Figure 16–5 shows the problem diagrammatically. The cine frame is rectangular, with a 4:3 ratio of the horizontal and vertical sides (e.g., 24 × 18 mm), the image intensifier is round, and the x-ray field is either square or rectangular. With this arrangement of shapes, a portion of either the x-ray field or the image intensifier must be wasted with all framing methods except total overframing. With all other framing methods, some portion of the recorded image is lost.

Two examples, one with exact framing and the other with total overframing, will demonstrate the potential magnitude of the patient overexposure. In both examples we will assume that the x-ray field is square and that its sides are tangential to the input phosphor of the image intensifier, as shown in Figure 16–5. With exact framing, none of the image is wasted but the x-ray field is 1.3 times (25 ÷ 20 = 1.3) as large as the image intensifier. The patient exposure (in terms of area) is comparably greater. The only solution is to use a circular field collimator. The second example, total overframing, poses a potentially greater exposure hazard. If the x-ray field is restricted so that its sides are tangential to the image intensifier, a common practice, the exposed patient area is 2.1 times (25 ÷ 12 = 2.1) greater than the recorded area. In this case, the solution is simple: restrict the x-ray beam to the recorded area and not to the image intensifier. With all other framing methods the magnitude of the problem is intermediate between these two extremes, but the solution is more complex in that it demands dual collimation (i.e., both circular and rectangular field collimation).

Framing and Image Size

Framing determines the size of objects in the cine image. Figure 16–6 compares image sizes for exact framing, total overframing, and exaggerated total (plus) overframing. The fluoroscopic image is shown on the left and the recorded, or cine image, is shown on the right. The size of the fluoroscopic image is determined by the size of the anatomic part, shown here as an arrow. The size of the comparable

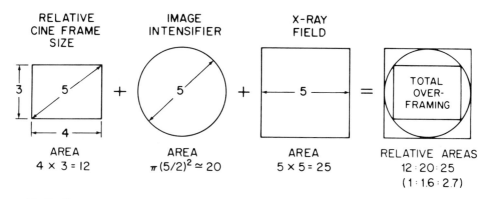

Figure 16–5 Comparison of field shapes for the cine frame, image intensifier, and x-ray field

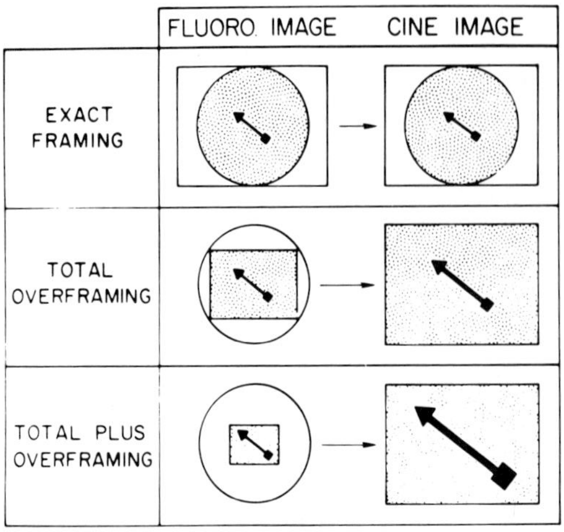

	FLUORO. IMAGE	CINE IMAGE
EXACT FRAMING		
TOTAL OVERFRAMING		
TOTAL PLUS OVERFRAMING		

Figure 16–6 Overframing enlarges the x-ray image

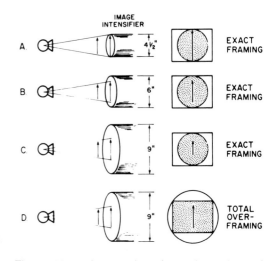

Figure 16–7 Image sizes for various sizes of image intensifiers

cine image is determined by the type of framing, which in turn is determined by the degree of magnification in the optical system. The optical system can be used to record all, or only a small portion of, the output phosphor. When the lens zooms in on a small area of the phosphor, the image enlarges, as shown on the right side of Figure 16–6. In theory, exaggerated overframing could be used to magnify the image indefinitely, but other considerations (see Chap. 20) intervene to destroy image quality and make exaggerated overframing impractical. It is only shown here to illustrate the principle, and is not recommended for routine clinical use.

Figure 16–4 indicates the relative image sizes for the various types of framing, using exact framing as the norm. Image size increases as the degree of framing increases, up to a maximum of 1.67 times for total overframing. Greater degrees of overframing are not recommended for routine clinical use.

Framing and Image Intensifier Size

The size of the object recorded on cine film decreases as the size of the image intensifier increases. This may seem like a paradox at first glance, but the explanation

is quite simple (Fig. 16–7). The illustration shows three different sizes of image intensifiers, all recording the same object (*arrow*) with the same degree of radiographic magnification, with the same framing format, and on the same size of film (Fig. 16–7A, B, and C). With the 4½-inch intensifier (Fig. 16–7A), the image of the arrow fills the cine frame, with the 9-inch intensifier (Fig. 16–7C), the image is only half as large, and with the 6-inch unit (Fig. 16–7B), the image is intermediate in size. The loss in image size with the larger intensifier can be at least partially recouped with overframing (Fig. 16–7D).

Framing Recommendations

The following framing recommendations have been made by the Inter-Society Commission for Heart Disease Resources:

Exact framing is not recommended for angiocardiography. For many angiocardiographic studies mean diameter overframing will provide moderate magnification without serious loss of field size. Maximum horizontal overframing provides more magnification and is desirable for coronary arteriography. More severe overframing can be used with large intensifiers to produce intermediate formats and with small intensifiers for coronary arteriography when marked magnification is desired and panning is not objectionable. When dual mode intensifiers are used, consideration must be given to the effect overframing will have on each mode.[2]

IMAGE INTENSIFIER

Image intensifiers have been described in detail in Chapter 15. We will only review those points that are especially important, or are unique to cinefluorography. The newer cesium iodide tubes have dramatically improved the cine image. They are far superior to the older zinc-cadmium sulfide tubes. Cesium iodide tubes are superior for three reasons: (1) improved quantum detection, (2) better resolution, and (3) better contrast. The improved quantum detection results from a greater packing density (more active material per unit thickness) and a better match between the K-absorption edge of both the cesium and iodine atoms and the mean energy of the x-ray beam. Resolution is better because light diffusion is less in the phosphorescent layer. Diffusion is inherently less in cesium iodide image tubes, and this advantage is accentuated by the fact that the phosphor layer is thinner than in zinc-cadmium sulfide tubes. Resolution is also better because of improvement in the photocathode, electron optics, and output phosphor. The contrast improvement is largely related to increased quantum detection; that is, fewer photons pass through the input phosphor to reach the output phosphor and thus reduce contrast.

The energy conversion factor (see Chap. 15, "Brightness Gain"), an expression of the quantity of light produced per absorbed photon, is lower with cesium iodide image intensifiers than with the older zinc-cadmium sulfide tubes, but this is not of major importance. A higher conversion factor does not improve the statistical quality of the image. Instead, statistical quality deteriorates and quantum mottle becomes more of a problem. (Quantum mottle is discussed in more detail later in this chapter.) If the conversion factor is too high, some of the light gain must be discarded. This is accomplished with an aperture (diaphragm with a small hole) between the two tandem lenses (see Fig. 15–5). Discarding some of the light results in higher patient exposures, but produces a statistically better image.

The optimum size of image intensifier for cinefluorography is the smallest one that will accomplish the job. A 15- to 17-cm intensifer (approximately 6 inches) is appropriate for coronary arteriography and for most pediatric angiography. Larger dual- or triple-mode units are recommended for adult angiography. In general, a single-mode unit can outperform a dual-mode intensifier of any given size. The advantage of the dual mode is versatility.

Wavelength of Light from the Output Phosphor

The output phosphor of both the older and newer image intensifiers is P20, zinc-cadmium sulfide-silver activated (Zn-CdS:Ag). It emits at a peak wavelength of 550 nm, which is in the yellow-green part of the spectrum. About half of the output phosphor's light falls in a rather narrow range of 550 ± 25 nm (5500 Å), as shown in Figure 16–8. Cine film must be selected

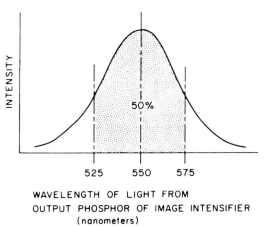

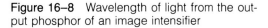

WAVELENGTH OF LIGHT FROM
OUTPUT PHOSPHOR OF IMAGE INTENSIFIER
(nanometers)

Figure 16–8 Wavelength of light from the output phosphor of an image intensifier

to accommodate these wavelengths. Only orthochromatic and panchromatic films make a suitable accommodation. Orthochromatic films are sensitive to wavelengths in the violet, blue, green, and yellow portions of the spectrum. Panchromatic films are sensitive to the entire spectrum, including orange and red.

OPTICAL SYSTEM

The optical system performs the seemingly simple task of conveying an image from the image intensifier, through a tandem lens (two lenses separated by a beamsplitting mirror), to the cine film. In this era of advanced technology this would not seem to be a difficult task. A technology that has produced an instrument as complex as an image intensifier should have no problem with the design of a few pieces of glass. The optical system is more complex than it appears to be at first glance, however, and its design affects the performance of the entire cine system.

Characteristics of a Lens

Before we discuss the optical coupling between the image intensifier and cine film, we must first review several important characteristics of lenses. These are as follows:

1. focal length,
2. magnification,
3. relative aperture,
4. depth of focus,
5. depth of field,
6. resolution,
7. vignetting,
8. chromatic aberrations, and
9. spherical aberrations.

Focal Length

The **optical axis** of a lens is an imaginary line passing perpendicular to the plane of a lens and through its geometric center. When a parallel bundle of light, for instance light from the sun, passes through a biconvex lens, all of its rays except the

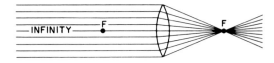

Figure 16–9 Focal point (F) of a lens

central one are bent toward the optical axis (Fig. 16–9). Rays at the periphery are deviated more than those near the center, and the central ray passes through in a straight line. They all converge at a point called the **focal point.** The **focal length** of a lens is the distance between the focal point and the center of the lens. Note in Figure 16–9 that a lens has two focal points (F), one on each side, equidistant from the central plane of the lens. Because light can pass through a lens in either direction, it follows logically that a ray passing through a focal point on one side will emerge on the opposite side in a course parallel to the optical axis.

Magnification

Magnification is defined as the ratio of image size to object size:

$$\text{Magnification} = \frac{\text{image size}}{\text{object size}}$$

The image may be larger than, smaller than, or equal to the object, so magnification can be greater than, equal to, or less than 1. If magnification is less than 1, the image is actually minified, or reduced in size. The degree of magnification depends on three factors: object distance, image distance, and focal length. The importance of each factor is demonstrated in Figure 16–10. The objects are to the left of the lens, and their images are to the right. The images form at the image plane, which is determined by the intersections of two or more light rays originating from the same point. One of the two rays shown in the illustration passes through the near focal point and emerges parallel to the optical axis; the other ray begins parallel to the optical axis and emerges in a course that passes through the far focal point.

The relative size of the object and image for a particular lens depends on the object distance. If the object is located at a distance of two focal lengths from the lens, the object and image are equal in size (Fig. 16–10A). If the object is at a shorter distance, the image is larger. The same focal length lens is shown both in Figure 16–10A and B, but the image is twice as large in Figure 16–10B, because of the shorter object distance.

Figure 16–10B also shows the important relationship between the image distance and object distance. As the illustration is labeled, the image is magnified two times. By simply reversing the light direction, however, or in this case the object and image labels in the drawing, the magnification changes to 0.5.

The third factor that affects magnification is the focal length of a lens. In Figure 16–10B and C, the object distance is the same for both lenses. The image is more magnified in Figure 16–10C, however, because the lens has a longer focal length. For a particular object distance, the degree of magnification is directly proportional to the focal length, that is, the longer the focal length, the greater the magnification. The focal length is a characteristic of the lens

itself. It is the only factor affecting magnification that cannot be changed.

Relative Aperture (Speed)

Relative aperture refers to the speed of a lens, which is probably its most important characteristic. If you find it difficult to think of a lens as being fast, perhaps it will help to think in terms of how fast it can gather enough light to expose a film. Then the concept is easily understood: a fast lens is one that produces a fast (short) exposure.

The speed of a lens is determined by its ability to concentrate light at the image plane. Concentration refers to light intensity per unit area, and depends on both the total quantity of available light and the area over which it is distributed. The total quantity of light is determined by the size of a lens, and the area of distribution by the lens' focal length. A lens is like a window. More light flows through a large window than a small one, and the same thing is true for a lens; that is, a large lens gathers more light than a small one. Focal length is important because it (along with the object distance) determines the degree of magnification and, therefore, the area of the image. A lens with a short focal length causes less magnification, and produces a smaller image than one with a long focal length (assuming equal object distances). Therefore, the available light is more concentrated by a lens with a short focal length. In summary, a fast lens is one with a large diameter (to gather more light) and a short focal length (to concentrate the light into a small area).

The relative aperture (speed) of a lens is indicated by an "f" number, usually written as f/4 or f/8. The lower the f number the faster the lens. The f number is determined by dividing the focal length of a lens by its diameter:

$$\text{f number} = \frac{\text{focal length}}{\text{diameter}}$$

Figure 16–11 shows the relationship between lens diameter, focal length, and rel-

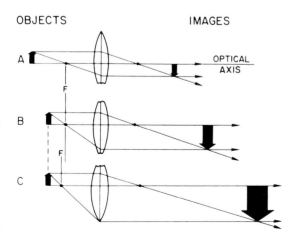

OBJECTS IMAGES

OPTICAL AXIS

Figure 16–10 Magnification

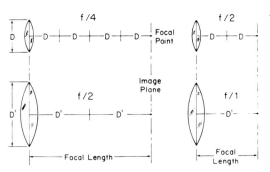

Figure 16–11 Relationship between relative aperture (f number), focal length, and lens diameter

Depth of Field and Depth of Focus

Depth of field and depth of focus are closely related, so we will discuss them together. Depth of focus refers to the range of distances over which the image is in sharp, or relatively sharp, focus. Depth of field is the range of object distances for which the images of objects are in sharp, or relatively sharp focus. They are both similar, but one refers to the object plane (depth of field) and the other to the image plane (depth of focus). Theoretically, for any given object distance, a lens only forms an image at a specific distance from its center (i.e., at the image plane), and the image is out of focus at all other distances. Actually, the image plane is not sharply defined, and there is a range of distances within which the image is reasonably well focused. Both the depth of field and depth of focus are dependent on the f number of the lens. The greater the f number (the slower the lens), the greater the depth of field and focus. As we shall see later, both can be improved by an iris diaphragm that decreases the functional size of the lens. Depth of field is relatively unimportant in cine fluorography because the object (output phosphor image) is flat. Depth of focus is important, however, and cine camera lenses must be accurately positioned to maintain the resolution of the system.

ative aperture. As you can see, focal length and diameter are independent of each other. A large and small lens can both have the same focal length, but they will have different f numbers. Also, two lenses can have the same f number and have different diameters and focal lengths.

F numbers are expressed in the following standard series: 0.70, 1.0, 1.4, 2.0, 2.8, 4.0, 5.6, 8.0, 11, 16, and so forth. (Note: this is the same series as used with film speed class.) Each lower numbered f stop allows twice as much light to reach the image plane as the next higher f number in the series. An f/2.8 lens, then, is twice as fast as an f/4.0 lens and four times as fast as an f/5.6 lens. You can also compare the relative speed of two lenses by comparing the square of their f numbers, and this is the reason this number series is chosen. This is occasionally necessary, because many f numbers fall between the ones in the standard series. The arithmetic is simple. For example, a 16-mm cine camera might have an f/0.9 lens, and 35-mm cameras an f/1.8 lens. Comparing the squares of their f numbers,

$$\frac{(1.8)^2}{(0.9)^2} = \frac{3.24}{0.81} = 4$$

Thus, this 16-mm camera lens is four times as fast as the 35-mm camera lens.

Resolution

The overall resolution of an imaging system is determined by the performance of its individual components. The component with the poorest resolution limits the entire system. In cinefluorography the image intensifier is the limiting factor, because it has the poorest resolution. A well-designed lens system can easily outperform an image intensifier, so optical coupling can be achieved without a significant reduction in the resolving power of the system.

Vignetting

Vignetting is a decrease in light intensity at the periphery of an image. We first

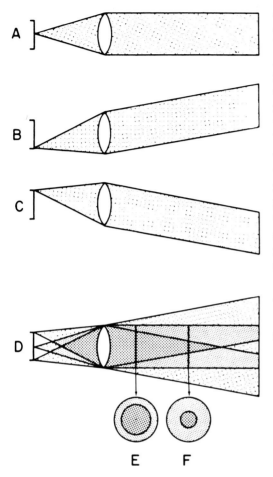

Figure 16–12 Vignetting

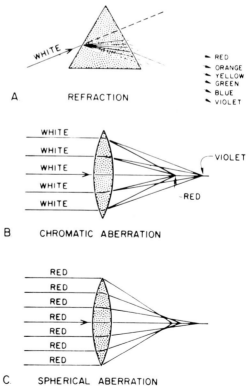

allel bundle, but the bundle is directed along a course oblique to the optical axis. When the three bundles are added together, they produce a central triangle of intense illumination surrounded by areas of lesser illumination (Fig. 16–12D). The illustration only shows a two-dimensional presentation of a three-dimensional light beam. The intensely illuminated central triangle is actually a cone. Cross sections through the center of the beam are shown in Figure 16–12E and F. The size of the maximally illuminated area is larger in Figure 16–12E because the cross section is closer to the lens. Vignetting is least pronounced close to the lens and increases as the distance from the lens increases.

Spherical and Chromatic Aberrations

Spherical aberration is caused by the inability of a lens to bring a monochromatic

Figure 16–13 Refraction (A), chromatic (B), and spherical (C) aberrations

met this phenomenon when we discussed image intensifiers. The cause of vignetting is different with a lens, but the result is the same. Figure 16–12 shows the cause of vignetting. In the illustration, the center of the output phosphor of the image intensifier is located at the focal point of the lens. (Later we will see that the first cine lens is positioned in this manner.) Figures 16–12A, B, and C show bundles of parallel light rays originating from the center, bottom, and top of the output phosphor. The bundle of parallel light rays from the center of the phosphor (Fig. 16–12A) is also parallel to the optical axis of the lens. Light from the bottom (Fig. 16–12B) and top (Fig. 16–12C) of the phosphor is in a par-

bundle of light from all parts of the lens to a point focus. Chromatic aberration is caused by the inability of a lens to bring white light (polychromatic) to sharp focus. These two aberrations are inherent in all lenses. Optical engineers have minimized the aberrations through good design, but the problem can never be completely eliminated.

Figure 16–13 shows both aberrations schematically. In Figure 16–13A, a narrow beam of white light is refracted into its individual components by a prism. Each color, or wavelength, is refracted to a different degree. White light enters the prism and a rainbow of colors emerges. A curved lens behaves in much the same way in that different wavelengths are refracted differently. Figure 16–13B shows the red and violet components of a white (polychromatic) light beam. These two colors are focused to two different points. All other colors (wavelengths) fall between red and violet. The result is a fuzzy image, with a rainbow around it, with poor resolution and contrast. Figure 16–13C shows spherical aberration. All the incident light has the same wavelength (i.e., it is monochromatic; red in the illustration). Because of the curved surface of the lens, refraction is never perfectly balanced at the center and periphery. Even though the light is monochromatic, it is still not brought to point focus. Peripheral refraction is greater than central refraction, so the periphery of the lens has a shorter focal length than the center. The result is a more fuzzy, lower resolution, lower contrast image than an image formed by a lens that has been corrected for spherical aberration.

Auxiliary Apertures

The effective f number of a lens can be changed without changing either the focal length or diameter of the lens. The f number is changed by interposing an iris diaphragm next to the lens (Fig. 16–14). The same lens is shown in both Figure 16–14A

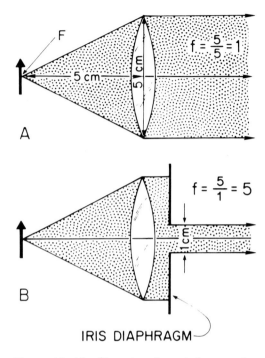

Figure 16–14 Changing the relative aperture with an iris diaphragm

and B. Its diameter (maximum aperture) and focal length are both 5 cm, so its f number is 1 (Fig. 16–14A). When an opaque object with a 1-cm hole (iris diaphragm) is placed next to the lens, the f number changes to 5 (Fig. 16–14B). The technique of changing f numbers with a diaphragm is familiar to all photographers. All but the cheapest cameras are equipped with variable diaphragms.

At first glance, the diaphragm appears to restrict the size of the field and block out part of the picture. Such is not the case. All of the light shown in Figure 16–14A and B originates from one point in the center of the arrow. A similar light bundle could be drawn for any other point. Therefore, the brightness of the image is decreased but its size is not affected. The brightness in the illustration decreases by a factor of 25:

$$\frac{1^2}{5^2} = \frac{1}{25}$$

Placing a small aperture in the light beam produces four desirable effects:

1. Contrast improves.
2. Resolution improves.
3. Spherical aberrations decrease.
4. Depth of field and depth of focus increase.

As a general rule, most lenses perform best at about two f stops above their maximum opening: that is, an f/2 lens usually functions best at f/4 (f/2; f/2.8; f/4 is the second f-stop). If the aperture is made small, in the f/16 to f/32 range, resolution and contrast begin to deteriorate somewhat because of diffraction. Therefore, small apertures should be avoided for cinefluorography. Photographers use these small apertures when a maximum depth of field is needed for esthetic purposes, but a great depth of field is of little value to a radiologist who is recording a nearly flat image.

Lens Selection

Now that we have discussed some characteristics of lenses, we can look into the design of the optical system for a cine camera. To make a lens with high resolution and minimum vignetting, several optical elements are used for each lens, sometimes as many as nine pieces of glass. As you can imagine, the design of such a lens is extremely complex, and it is usually carried out with the aid of a computer. Even though the lens is made up of many elements, however, it still has an f number and focal length of its own.

Figure 16–15 shows a simplified cinefluorographic lens system. The lenses are depicted as single pieces of glass, but each is actually made up of several elements. A large diameter **collector** lens receives the fluoroscopic image from the output phosphor of the image intensifier and collimates the image for the camera lens. The phosphor is positioned at the focal plane of the lens, so the image is transmitted by parallel bundles of light. A smaller diameter **camera lens** receives this light bundle and refocuses it into an image on the cine film. Because the light is transmitted from one lens to the other in a parallel bundle, the amount of separation between the lenses does not affect focusing. It does affect vignetting, however, which produces a serious problem for the lens designer. There are three ways to diminish vignetting:

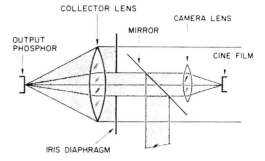

Figure 16–15 Schematic cinefluorographic optical system

1. Make the first lens large to increase the size of the cone that is relatively free of vignetting.
2. Make the second lens small so it fits inside the vignetting free cone.
3. Place the second lens close to the first lens in the larger portion of the cone of maximal illuminations.

The final design of the optical system is always a compromise. A certain amount of vignetting is tolerated. The first lens is always as large as possible (and large lenses are expensive), the second lens is always smaller than the first, and the two lenses are placed as close together as the beam-splitting mirror allows. The mirror deflects a small amount of light (approximately 10%) to a television camera or mirror optical system for image monitoring. Optical coupling would be more efficient if the beam-splitting mirror could be discarded, but at present no other system permits simultaneous image monitoring and recording.

Focal Length of Camera Lens

Previously we pointed out that focal length and object distance determine the degree of magnification. The object distance for cinefluorographic lenses is always the same as their focal lengths. The lenses are purposely positioned with their image planes (output phosphor and cine film) at their focal points. This arrangement accommodates a beam-splitting mirror, because the image is transferred from one lens to the other in a parallel bundle.

Figure 16–16 shows the relationship between the focal length of the two lenses and the size of the output phosphor and cine images. The tandem lenses can be pictured as a pinhole positioned at the junction, or as a crossover of two similar triangles. When any three factors are known, the fourth can be calculated by setting up proportional triangles.

$$L_c = \frac{L_p \cdot D_c}{D_p}$$

L_c = focal length of the camera lens
L_p = focal length of the phosphor (collector) lens
D_c = diameter of the camera (cine) image
D_p = diameter of the output phosphor image

For example, a representative size for an output phosphor is 18 mm and a common focal length for an output phosphor (collector) lens is 65 mm with a 9-in. image intensifier. If we decide to use total overframing, the diameter of the 35-mm cine

image will be 30 mm. The focal length of the camera lens would be

$$L_c = \frac{L_p \cdot D_c}{D_p} = \frac{65 \times 30}{18} = 108 \text{ mm}$$

If we had selected exact framing for the same system, the focal length of the camera lens would be

$$L_c = \frac{L_p \cdot D_c}{D_p} = \frac{65 \cdot 18}{18} = 65 \text{ mm}$$

The focal lengths for camera lenses for 35-mm cinefluorography are usually between 80 and 135 mm, depending on the framing mode selected. Once a particular lens has been selected, it can only be changed at considerable expense. Zoom lenses, usually of lesser quality, have variable focal lengths but are not generally available for cine systems. Consequently the framing mode should be chosen with great care.

Speed of Optical System

A cine optical system is designed to be as fast as reasonable cost and modern technology permit. Collector lenses are exceedingly fast, usually f/0.75. To limit vignetting, the diameter of the camera lens is only half as large as that of the collecting lens. Once the size of the output phosphor, speed of the collector lens, and framing mode have been established, the speed of the system is determined by the maximum aperture, or f number, of the camera lens. As the focal length of the camera lens is increased to cover larger framing formats, the brightness of the cine image will decrease, unless the f number (iris diaphragm) is also changed. If the f number is changed, the brightness change is half or two times for each f stop, depending on whether the iris aperture is made smaller or larger.

Earlier image intensifying tubes used a P20 input phosphor (zinc-cadmium sulfide, silver-activated). The light intensity was somewhat limited. A fast lens and film combination was therefore required to obtain an adequate exposure. The introduc-

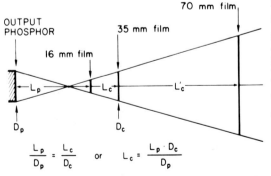

Figure 16–16 Relationship between focal length and image sizes for cinefluorographic lenses

tion of cesium iodide, sodium-activated, as an input phosphor increased light intensity by a factor of about five. Selecting the fastest lens-film combination is thus no longer an absolute necessity. A fast lens is still important to allow stopping down at least two f stops to permit exposure conditions within the critical resolution of the lens. This optimizes the performance of the lens. As long as the film selected can be exposed within this critical resolution range, film speed is of relatively small importance. The main advantage of slower films is a finer grained emulsion.

Regardless of the lens-film combination, a 20-μR/frame input dosage is necessary to minimize quantum mottle.[2]

X-RAY PHOTON IMAGE

The first prerequisite for optimum cinefluorography is a good x-ray photon image. This is the image that exists in space after the x-ray beam has traversed the patient and before the beam has reached the image intensifier. Scatter radiation should be minimized by beam restrictors (collimators) and a radiographic grid. Assuming that scatter radiation is at a minimum, four other factors affect the quality of the x-ray photon image:

1. quantum mottle,
2. motion unsharpness,
3. geometric unsharpness, and
4. contrast.

Quantum Mottle

Quantum mottle is caused by statistical fluctuations in the number of x-ray quanta (photons) absorbed by the input phosphor. The mottle does not become visible until an image is produced, but the statistical fluctuations exist prior to absorption of the photons by the input phosphor.

There must be a certain minimum number of photons to produce a statistically satisfactory image. This minimum, for either 16- or 35-mm film, is 20 μR per frame when viewed at 24 or more frames per second.[2] At lower viewing rates, larger exposures are recommended. Exposures of less than 20 μR per frame generate too much quantum mottle to produce a satisfactory image.

Figure 16–17 shows that the "graininess" on a cine film is primarily caused by quantum mottle rather than by film graininess. The two pictures in the illustration were both made with the same 35-mm film (Kodak CRS Film), the same coarse (1-cm) wire screen, the same magnification, and the same processing system. The only difference between the two films is in the manner in which they were exposed. Film A was exposed by the output phosphor of a 9-inch image intensifier, so it is a picture of a radiographic image. Film B is an ordinary light photograph taken with a 35-mm camera. The mottled appearance of the x-ray image (Fig. 16–17A) is from random statistical fluctuations in the number of x-ray photons, which is quantum mottle by definition. Regardless of the film size, the amount of quantum mottle depends on the number of photons comprising the x-ray image. An image composed of a large number of x-ray photons has less quantum mottle (statistical fluctuation), and is a better quality image (smoother or more uniform in appearance) than one composed of only a small number of photons.

When a cinefluorography system exhibits quantum mottle, the best way to eliminate the mottle is to increase the mAs (milliampere seconds). This will increase the number of x-ray photons absorbed by the

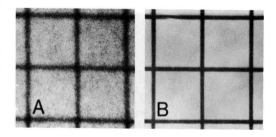

Figure 16–17 Quantum mottle of x-ray image (A) and light image (B)

input phosphor, which is the primary method for decreasing quantum mottle. Increasing the number of absorbed quanta will also increase the overall density of the processed film. Film density can then be decreased by decreasing the kilovoltage, which will also increase contrast. Greater contrast is usually desirable. Another way to compensate for increased mAs is to use a smaller opening in the iris diaphragm— that is, a higher f number.

Motion Unsharpness

Each cine film is a separate picture, exposed with its own individual pulse of radiation. The length of the pulse should be kept as short as possible to stop patient motion without seriously compromising other factors important to image quality. The other important quality factors are contrast and quantum mottle. Exposures of 3 to 5 milliseconds (ms) are recommended. Exposure times can be reduced in several ways, such as higher kVp, more mA current, faster lens, or faster film. In general, all of these, except more mA current, tend to produce more quantum mottle and/or less contrast. For example, halving the exposure with a faster film halves the number of photons in the x-ray image and thus increases quantum mottle. Increasing the kilovoltage shortens the exposure but increases quantum mottle and reduces contrast. With current technology, the heat tolerance of the x-ray tube makes it impractical to produce repetitive exposures below the 3- to 5-msec range.

Geometric Unsharpness

Geometric unsharpness is caused by magnification and the finite size of the focal spot (penumbra). Focal spot sizes for cinefluorography should be as small as practical. An 0.6-mm focal spot is recommended for most situations; 1.0 mm is recommended for large patients, and 0.3 mm for magnification radiography. Industry standards (self-imposed) allow for a 50% tolerance in focal spot sizes. An 0.6-mm

focal spot may actually by 0.9 mm in size and still meet industrial standards. As we shall see later (Chap. 20), this size may increase by more than 200% under peak load. Cine tubes should be special-ordered with actual (based on pinhole or star pattern radiographs) rather than nominal focal spot sizes requested. Manufacturers will meet these requirements at an additional cost.

Magnification is minimized by keeping the image intensifier as close to the patient as possible, and by using a long target-to-tabletop distance. The minimum recommended separation between the x-ray target and patient support (tabletop) is 55 cm.

Contrast

The overall contrast of the cine image is determined by many factors, the first of which is the kVp of the x-ray beam. Optimum contrast is obtained with a voltage between 60 and 90 kVp. Lower voltages (below 60 kVp) subject the patient to excess radiation, while higher voltages produce too little contrast and too much quantum mottle. In general, kVps on the low side of the range are preferred. The higher side of the range should be reserved for large patients. The film type, processing, and viewing conditions also affect image contrast. These factors will be discussed in more detail later.

X-RAY APPARATUS

Many angiocardiographic labs are designed for both serial filming and cinefluorography. The energy demands for cine are generally less than those for serial filming, so the serial filming dictates the energy requirements for the room. The following recommendations pertain to a lab designated exclusively for cinefluorography. They are taken from the Report of the Inter-Society Commission for Heart Disease Resources.[2]

Generator

A 3-phase, 12-pulse, or constant potential generator is recommended. The current (mA) output rating should be three times the cine pulse output to minimize voltage fluctuations during exposures. A 700- to 1000-mA, 100-kVp generator is recommended. However, if the transformer design ensures stable voltages and currents during pulsing (low impedance) a 500-mA generator will suffice. Pulsing and brightness controls are essential, and they will be discussed in more detail after we describe the x-ray tube.

X-Ray Tubes

The instantaneous exposure tolerances of an x-ray tube are determined by the (1) size of the focal spot, (2) diameter of the anode, (3) anode angle, and (4) rotational speed of the anode. The maximum continuous output is determined by (1) the anode's capacity to store heat and by (2) the ability of the anode and housing to dissipate heat into the environment. Individual cine exposures are small by conventional radiographic standards, but they may be repeated 60 times a second for several seconds, so total heat loading is very large. A tube with the following characteristics is recommended for routine 35-mm cardiac cinefluorography.

Focal spot size:	0.6 mm
Heat rating:	60 kW
Anode diameter:	100 mm
Target angle:	6°–12°
Cooling:	Circulatory liquid
Rotational velocity:	10,000 rpm

The optimum target angle is dictated by the size of the image intensifier and distance between the intensifier and x-ray target. Small anode angles (6°) have greater x-ray output, so they are recommended with small image intensifiers in which the field size is not compromised by the heel effect. A 0.3-mm focal spot should be used for magnification techniques, and 1.0-mm size is acceptable for large patients or in cases in which ultrashort exposures are mandatory.

X-Ray Exposure

The timing and intensity of the x-ray exposure are controlled during cinefluorography by two electrical signals that originate from within the cine system. One signal coordinates the x-ray exposure with the open time of the camera shutter (synchronization), and the other maintains a constant level of intensifier illumination by varying the exposure factors for areas of different thickness or density.

Synchronization

When cinefluorographic equipment was in the embryonic stages of its development, x rays were generated continuously throughout a filming sequence, and the patient was needlessly irradiated when the camera shutter was closed. These continuous exposures had two serious disadvantages: patient exposures were large, and they shortened the life expectancy of the x-ray tube. In all modern cinefluorographic systems the x-ray output is intermittent, and the exposure is synchronized with the open time of the camera shutter. Synchronization is controlled by an electrical signal from commutators and brushes of the camera motor. After the motor opens the shutter and advances the film, it signals the generator to make an exposure.

Earlier in the chapter we mentioned that the framing frequency is always a multiple, or fraction, of 60 (e.g., 7½, 15, 30, 60, 120). The choice of the number 60 was not an

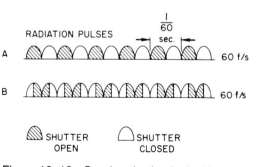

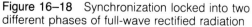

Figure 16–18 Synchronization locked into two different phases of full-wave rectified radiation

arbitrary decision. Thirty-five years ago, when the decision was made, all x-ray circuits in this country operated on 60-cycle alternating current, usually with full-wave rectification. X rays were generated in 120 short bursts each second. Operating the camera shutters at the same frequency as the x-ray pulses ensured a uniform exposure for each frame, regardless of what part of the cycle synchronization locked into. Figure 16–18 shows synchronization locked into the beginning (Fig. 16–18A) and middle (Fig. 16–18B) of the x-ray cycle. In each case, the exposures are exactly the same from frame to frame. The examples shown are for 60 frames per second (f/s), but the results are the same for other frequencies provided they are multiples of 60. With a framing frequency out of phase with the electric supply, consecutive frames would be exposed to a slightly different portion of the x-ray cycle. Some frames would receive more radiation than others, depending on whether they are exposed by the peaks or valleys of the radiation output.

Pulsed Radiation

The newer cinefluorographic units deliver x rays with a completely different wave form than that used for conventional fluoroscopy. Instead of the high ripple pulsations usually generated with full-wave rectification, the x rays are generated in short intense bursts, called pulses. This is achieved with either thyratron or grid-controlled x-ray tubes, both of which allow instantaneous on-off switching of the x-ray pulse. Only the central high-voltage portion of the electrical cycle is used to generate x rays, and the rest of the cycle is discarded. Figure 16–19 shows the wave form from pulsed radiation along with that from full-wave rectification for comparison. The nomenclature is a little confusing, because both wave forms show pulsations. Cine pulses have a wave form that is square, which is completely different from the rounded wave form of full-wave rec-

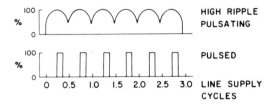

Figure 16–19 Comparison of high-ripple pulsations (full-wave rectification) and cine pulses

tification. A single square pulse is used with three-phase generators. The beginning and termination of the pulse are square, like those shown in Figure 16–19. The length of the pulse is determined by the time required to expose the film. Its height is constant except for ripple pulsations.

The output phosphor of an image intensifier has a certain amount of inherent persistence, which produces an **afterglow** of illumination following the cessation of an x-ray pulse. If synchronization of the shutter opening and x-ray pulse is perfectly timed, the light from afterglow can be utilized for part of the total film exposure with a comparable reduction in the patient's x-ray exposure. Figure 16–20 shows an ideally synchronized cine exposure. The x-ray pulse occurs immediately after the shutter opens, afterglow falls entirely within the open time, and no radiation is generated while the shutter is closed.

Afterglow should not persist beyond its frame of origin. If it is carried into the next frame, the persistent image will be different from the new image and quality will deteriorate. With pulsed radiation, the only function of the camera shutter is to prevent afterglow from reaching the film during its transport time. If an image intensifier discarded an image the instant the burst of radiation terminated, merely pulsing the radiation would be an entirely adequate way of controlling the exposure, and the shutter would be superfluous. The shutter does not control the film exposure in the examples shown in Figure 16–20. Even if the shutter remained open permanently, the film could be transported

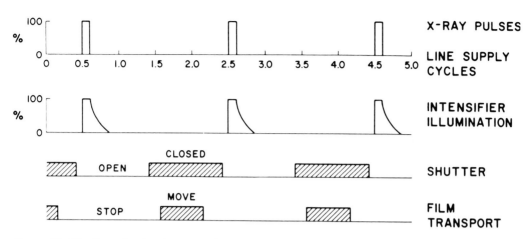

Figure 16–20 Coordination between the x-ray pulse, afterglow, and film transport

without impairing image quality, because the intensifier has already discarded its image. The framing frequency in Figure 16–20, however, is only 30 f/s. At higher frequencies (60 or more f/s), afterglow may persist into the film-transport time, and the shutter intercepts it before it reaches the film, thus performing an important function.

Brightness Control

The brightness of the intensifier image changes constantly as the fluoroscope is moved from one area of the patient to another, and as contrast material enters and leaves the fluoroscopic field. Because cine film does not have enough exposure latitude to encompass the varying intensities coming from the patient, a method of brightness control is needed to ensure proper film density. This is managed in one of two ways, either by measuring the current flowing across the image intensifier or by measuring the brightness of the output phosphor. In both systems, a signal is sent back to the x-ray generator to regulate the intensity of the x-ray pulse. Three basic methods for brightness stabilization are in current use: (1) variable voltage (kVp), (2) variable tube current (mA), and (3) variable pulse width (exposure time).

Variable Voltage (kVp). A motor-driven autotransformer in the primary circuit varies the kVp in response to brightness sensing electrodes in either the image intensifier or optical system. This method has the advantage of covering a very wide range of patient thickness. It has three disadvantages: (1) it is relatively slow; (2) if kVps get too high, contrast decreases; (3) when the kVp goes up, the number of absorbed photons goes down and quantum mottle becomes a problem. The method works well with a large (30- to 50-kW) generator; the mA and time can then be set near optimum levels, and the kilovoltage only has to be adjusted slightly.

Variable Tube Current. With this method the exposure time (pulse width) and voltage are preselected, and brightness is regulated by varying the mA. The method only works well with large generators (30 to 50 kW), and should not be used with generators smaller than 30-kW capacity. A variable tube current has three disadvantages: (1) the response time is slow; (2) it requires considerable expertise to operate satisfactorily; and (3) the brightness range is quite limited. It works best when combined with a variable voltage.

Variable Pulse Width (Time). In this system the mA is set at the maximum heat tolerance level, the kVp is optimized, and the timer regulates the exposure. The system suffers from the same shortcomings as those for variable tube current. It has the advantage of a near instantaneous response time (0.1 ms). Each cine frame can be separately phototimed.

All three systems work best with large generators (30 to 50 kW), and all three require considerable operator experience. The optimum method is a combination of variable kVp and variable time, coupled to a large generator. The kilovoltage is set for optimum contrast, brightness is controlled by varying the exposure time and, if the upper limit of the exposure time is reached, the kVp is automatically raised to provide full exposure control. The system offers the advantages of simplicity and a rapid response time.

All brightness regulators are similar to phototimers. They function empirically, and must be adjusted by trial and error until the image brightness meets the requirements of the particular film-processor system.

CINE EXAMINATION MONITORING

To conduct a cine examination, the radiologist must be able to monitor the cine image. The beam-splitting mirror reflects approximately 10% of the light from the image intensifier for monitoring purposes. Although this percentage is small, it must be remembered that the exposure factors and brightness of the intensifier phosphor are greatly increased during cinefluorography, and the monitoring image brightness is not much different from that used for routine fluoroscopy. At low framing frequencies the image flickers because the x rays are pulsed, but flicker does not interfere with monitoring. The reflected light can be viewed in one of two ways: either directly with a mirror optical system, or indirectly through closed-circuit television.

CINE FILM

The characteristics of radiographic film were discussed in detail in Chapters 10 and 11, so we will only review a few features especially pertinent to cinefluorography.

The film is only one component in a complex system. When the image is unsatisfactory, however, the film is often incorrectly blamed. For example, if contrast is too high, the first inclination is to switch to a lower contrast film. A better choice would be to evaluate the **system contrast,** correct the deficiencies that exist, and then reassess the problem. System contrast is determined by the contrast of the individual components; the more important ones will be discussed next.

Radiographic contrast depends on such variables as kVp, patient thickness, scatter radiation, and contrast materials.

Image intensifier contrast deteriorates with time. This is especially noticeable in the older zinc-cadmium sulfide tubes.

Optical system contrast deteriorates with larger lens openings. Apertures should be used to bring the f number of the system within the critical resolution of the lens, usually two f stops above the maximum aperture.

Processing is one of the most important factors influencing system contrast. Processing time, temperature, agitation, and replenishment are the critical elements of processing that affect film contrast.

Viewing conditions have a profound effect on image contrast. A brightly lit room diminishes contrast. A dirty lens, an inadequately bright bulb, or a dirty screen also diminishes contrast.

Inherent film contrast is the last link in the chain. A high-, medium-, or low-contrast film should not be chosen until all other factors in the imaging system have been optimized. The inherent contrast of the film should then be used to fine-tune the total system contrast using the processing recommendations of the manufacturer.

Types of Film

Table 16–1 shows representative films recommended for cinefluorography. Important characteristics to consider are speed and contrast. In general, faster films

Table 16–1. Representative 35-mm Cinefluorographic Films*

KODAK FILM	DEVELOPMENT TIME (SEC)	RELATIVE SPEED†	AVERAGE GRADIENT‡	FILM BASE TYPE	SPECTRAL SENSITIVITY
CFC	90	100	1.5	ESTAR	Orthochromatic
CFR	90	120	1.2	Acetate	Panchromatic
CFS	60	250	1.5	ESTAR	Panchromatic
CFX	90	800	1.4	Acetate	Panchromatic
CFH	60	300	1.8	Acetate	Panchromatic

*Exposure was 1/50 sec to a source that simulates the spectral distribution of the P-20 phosphor. Films were processed in a cinefluorographic film processor. Processing chemicals were KODAK CINEFLURE developer and replenisher, and KODAK CINEFLURE fixer and replenisher at 85° F (30° C), mixed according to instructions packaged with the chemicals.
†Measured at a density of 0.85 above gross fog. The CFC film has been arbitrarily assigned a value of 100.
‡Measured as the slope of the line between densities of 0.15 above gross fog and 1.5 above gross fog.
Note: Data courtesy of the Eastman Kodak Company. These data were obtained without the introduction of the many variables of cinefluorography and can only be used as a starting point.

tend to be grainier than slow films. The graininess of a fast film may contribute to the "noise" seen in the projected image, but this contribution is usually minor relative to the increase in quantum mottle that occurs with faster films. Quantum mottle increases because fewer x-ray photons are needed to produce an image.

Film should not be selected until all the components of the system have been evaluated. A film should then be chosen to have the appropriate contrast for the system. This film should be as slow as the exposure factors permit. After the film is selected, it should be tested on a phantom and processed as recommended. The phantom tests should include a series of exposures made with different sizes of iris diaphragm openings (f numbers). This f-stop series will allow the selection of the proper aperture to match film density with the other established parameters. The processed films should be analyzed in a projector to duplicate the viewing conditions that will exist for later clinical studies. A patient should not be examined until the system has been thoroughly analyzed by phantom studies.

PROCESSING

Improper processing and excessive quantum mottle are the two most important factors that degrade cine image quality. We have already discussed quantum mottle, and now we will discuss processing.

The first rule is that a cine lab should have its own cine film processor. Automatic processors designed for motion picture processing are preferable, because they are designed to control the factors that regulate cine film quality rigidly. Good cine processors are expensive. Many desirable features of cine processors have been presented in the Report of the Inter-Society Commission for Heart Disease Resources.[2]

Processing should be kept in the hands of skilled professionals, and not turned over to the least skilled and lowest paid member of the angiographic team. The following six factors are involved in successful processing.

Temperature Control. Temperature is a critical element in cine processing. Ideally, developer temperature should be controlled to ±0.25° F (±0.14° C); variations of greater than ±0.5° F (±0.28° C) are unacceptable. Other temperatures should be kept within 1 or 2° F of their recommended values.

Machine Speed. Processing time is controlled by the film transport speed. The actual transport speed, not that shown on the controls, should not exceed ±5% of the speed required for acceptable processing.

Agitation. Good agitation is desirable. Agitation must be uniform throughout the developer tank, but especially at the beginning of the cycle. Uneven agitation causes mottle and irregular streaks. Proper agitation (1) helps to produce the film's inherent speed and contrast, (2) ensures uniform processing from frame to frame, and (3) prevents exhaustion products of development from inducing artifacts.

Replenishment. Both the developer and fixer must be replenished to ensure optimum processing. Recommended replenishment rates should be obtained from the manufacturer and followed as starting points. Replenishment should accomplish the following three objectives: (1) restore the used developer and fixer agents to maintain the sensitometric characteristics of the film; (2) dilute the solutions to prevent the buildup of reaction products; and (3) maintain the solutions at the proper level in the tanks. Improper replenishment of the developer will affect film density, contrast, and fog. Overreplenishment of the fixer is wasteful. Underreplenishment may affect washing, drying, and storage life of the processed film. Too high a developer temperature produces the same effect as overreplenishing, while too low a temperature has an effect comparable to that for underreplenishing.

Filtration. Particulate matter from the developing and fixing solutions tends to cling to film during processing. These particles produce minus density spots on the film. They are then greatly magnified when the film is projected. A filter should be used to remove particles larger than 25 μ.

Film Drying. Relative humidity and temperature are the most important factors in film drying, because they control the physical characteristics of the film. Insufficient drying leaves the film soft and tacky. Overdrying causes excess curl and brittleness. In general, film should be dried at the lowest temperature consistent with adequate drying, and in relation to the ambient relative humidity. Most processors are set for 125° F. If the film does not have the proper physical characteristics, it may break or jam in the projector.

Quality Control

Cine processors should be monitored on a daily basis to ensure consistency of performance. Records should be kept of solution temperatures, developer immersion times, developer and fixer replenishment rates, and solution changes. When an angiographic suite is first installed, a complete H & D curve should be plotted to serve as a standard for future comparisons. These curves should be reconstructed whenever any component in the processing system is changed or whenever a spot check of daily performance falls outside accepted norms.

The heart of a quality control program is a short pre-exposed film strip, similar to the one shown in Figure 16–21. The film strip was exposed to precisely controlled steps of increasing light intensity by an instrument called a **sensitometer.** Several manufacturers produce commercial units designed specifically for this purpose. They all vary somewhat in design. The one used to expose the strips shown in Figure 16–21 was a Du Pont Cine Sensitometer. With this unit, the film is only exposed on the emulsion side. Sensitometers for x-ray film expose from both sides because x-ray film has a double emulsion. The light source in the cine sensitometer is green to match the yellow-green light of the inten-

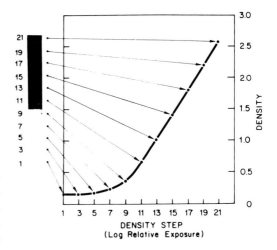

Figure 16–21 Characteristic (H & D) curve of a typical cine film

sifier output phosphor. The exposure is made through a step wedge of neutral density filters. Successive steps in the filter differ in density by the square root of 2. Thus, every other step (i.e., two steps) doubles, or halves (depending on the direction), the quantity of light reaching the film. The log relative exposure difference between every other step is 0.3, and the total range of exposure is 3.

The density of the steps in the test film is read with a densitometer and plotted on graph paper to construct an H & D curve similar to those shown in Figures 16–21 and 16–22. Both of these show the same curve, but the numbers on the x-axes have been changed from density steps in Figure 16–21 to log relative exposures in Figure 16–22. The average gradient of the film was determined by first selecting two points on the H & D curve and then by connecting these points with a straight line (Fig. 16–22). Densities of 0.15 and 1.5 above gross fog were used to define the points. The gross fog density was 0.16. Densities of 0.31 (0.15 + 0.16) and 1.66 (1.5 + 0.16) were used to define the average gradient, which turned out to be 1.13 on our test film. This value is quite low compared to

that of x-ray film, but the Inter-Society Commission has recommended a low average gradient for cine film.[2] (Log relative exposures and average gradients were described in more detail in Chapter 11.)

The construction of H & D curves is too time-consuming to use as a daily check of system performance. Lawrence has described a much quicker and more practical method.[3] Instead of measuring the density of the whole film strip, he only measured a few preselected steps. The density of these steps quantitates three important film characteristics: gross fog, speed, and contrast. Gross fog is the density of an unexposed portion of the film. The density of the unexposed film is the sum of base fog (the density of the film base plus emulsion) and processor or darkroom fog. Film speed (called the **speed index** by Lawrence) is the density of one preselected step. Film contrast (called the **contrast index**) is the difference in the density between two preselected steps. These three parameters are then plotted on a **processor control chart,** such as the one shown in Figure 16–23. The density of step 13 was used for the speed index in this chart; the contrast index was the difference in density between steps 14 and 10. Upper and lower limits were then set to define the range of acceptable variation.

If any parameter slips out of the acceptable range, an investigation is undertaken to determine the cause. The first step is always to repeat the test; that is, expose another film strip and repeat the measurements. If the error persists, then a systematic search is begun, guided in part by the particular parameter(s) that has changed. For example, suppose that gross fog and the speed index go up, and the contrast index goes down. Gross fog is not particularly sensitive to changes in replenishment rates or developer temperature. Consequently, a light leak is a more likely cause for the problem. One common source of a light leak is a defective safe light (x-ray film safe lights are unsatisfactory for cine film).

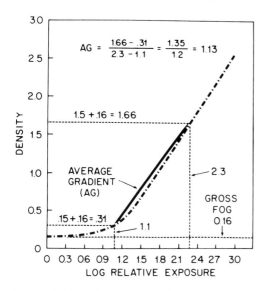

Figure 16–22 Average gradients of the film shown in Figure 16–21

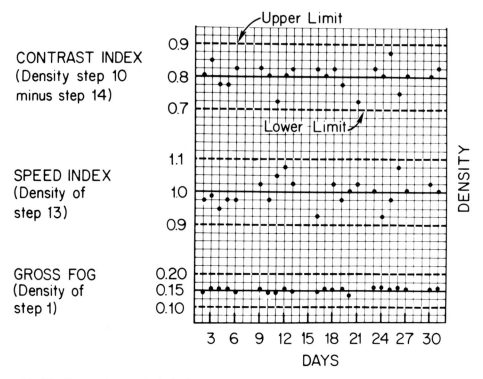

Figure 16–23   Processing control chart

If the gross fog in our example had been normal and the speed index had risen while the contrast fell, then an error in replenishment or developer temperature would have been a more likely cause.

PROJECTORS

Projectors have not kept pace with the other components in the cine system, at least not for 35-mm film. With few exceptions, commercial projectors tend to be either prohibitively expensive or poorly suited for cinefluorography.

Projectors have three functioning components: a film transport mechanism, a light source and condenser optics, and an imaging optics. The film transport mechanism should conveniently accept large rolls of any standard polyester- or acetate-based film, have a continuously variable forward and reverse transport at frame rates from 1 to 50 frames/second, and not damage the film with repeated viewing.

The transport should also be quiet, flickerless, and hold the film motionless for single framing. The condenser optics focus the filament of the light source into the aperture of the projection lens. The condenser has a heat-absorbing glass to reduce the heat of the projector beam so as not to burn the film. The imaging optics projects and focuses the cine image onto the built-in screen or to a small conference room screen. The optical system should produce a bright, high-contrast, critically focused image with uniform resolution across the entire width of the image. The projector lamp should also have a variable brightness control.

FRAMING FREQUENCY

The optimum framing frequency for a cine examination should be determined by the speed of the physiologic motion being recorded. The exposures should be frequent enough to record only a slight difference between consecutive frames. Too few pictures produce a jerky motion, and too many needlessly irradiate the patient. For example, 7.5 frames/sec (f/s) are adequate for the stomach and duodenum, while 30 to 60 f/s are required for coronary angiography.

A cine film should be projected at a speed of at least 16 f/s in order for the eye to perceive a smoothly flowing motion. If the film was recorded at a slower frequency, the image will appear to be moving faster than it actually is; if recording was faster, motion will be slowed down. In either case, the picture will flow smoothly. If the projector is operated at a frequency of less than 16 f/s, the eye recognizes individual cine frames, and it cannot integrate from one frame to the next. The result is the kind of jerky motion usually associated with old Charlie Chaplin movies.

Stop-Action versus Motion Pictures

With pulsed radiation, individual cine frames are exposed by a single, short-duration pulse, short enough to stop most physiologic motion. Each frame contains a sharp image that is ideal for stop-action viewing, that is, for examining the frames individually. These sharp images, however, do not necessarily produce the best motion pictures. In fact, some degree of blurring is desirable to help convey the sense of motion.

Most cinefluorographic films are viewed as both stop-action and motion pictures. As a general rule, blurring distracts more from stop-action pictures than sharp images do from motion pictures, which is why cinefluorographic exposures are as short as possible. The quality of a cine image may be improved by showing it as a motion picture because of an averaging out of quantum mottle. Fortunately, the eye does not "see" the individual frames of a motion picture. Instead, the eye sees several frames. It integrates these images, adds them together, and smooths out the information voids left by quantum mottle. The resulting movie image is visually superior to the image of any individual frame. When cine film is projected at a frequency lower than 24 f/s, the number of integrated frames is too small to significantly improve image quality. If the film is meant to be shown at fewer than 24 f/s, it may be necessary to increase the x-ray exposure above the recommended 20 μR/f to compensate for the resulting loss in image quality.

Flicker

Flicker is a completely different and more difficult problem to eliminate than jerky motion. Flicker persists up to approximately 50 f/s, while jerky motion is eliminated at 16 f/s. Physiologists measure the eye's ability to detect flicker by rotating a partial disc, similar to the camera shutter, in front of a light source. The eye recognizes individual flashes up to approximately 50 per second, depending on the brightness of the light. At higher flash frequencies, the light appears to be continuous, and flicker disappears. For example, an ordinary incandescent lamp flickers 120 times/sec with alternating current, but the eye perceives a continuous light. Radiologists usually accept flicker, and it does not seriously interfere with perception. Interestingly, the movie industry has devised an ingenious method of eliminating flicker. The projector shutter is run twice as fast as the film, and each frame is shown twice. Because movie film is normally made at 24 f/s, by showing each frame twice, the number of light pulses is increased to 48, which is sufficient to eliminate flicker.

PATIENT EXPOSURE

The amount of radiation that a patient receives during a cinefluoroscopic examination depends on many factors (mA, kVp, distance, patient thickness, grids, intensifier size, camera f number, and processing), but the following three are more important than the others:

1. synchronization
2. framing frequency

3. f number of the optical system.

Fortunately, all modern equipment is synchronized, which decreases patient exposures by at least 50%. The framing frequency is usually dictated by the nature of the examination, but it is fairly obvious that the more frames exposed per second, the greater the patient's exposure. Filming should be performed within the critical resolution of the cine lens. This is generally about two f numbers smaller than the maximum lens aperture.

The Inter-Society Commission for Heart Disease Resources has recommended a minimum exposure of 20 μR/f, measured at the front of the image intensifier. Before we can compare the recommended exposures with those in the literature, we must have comparable units of measurement. Because skin (or tabletop) exposure rates are usually reported in the literature, we will convert the 20 μR/f into skin exposures. For an example, we will consider a 60-f/s cine examination of the heart. Assuming the patient to be large, up to 99% of the initial beam may be absorbed by the patient and grid, or lost by the inverse square law. Thus, the skin exposure is 100 times as large as the image intensifier exposure. The patient receives a per frame exposure of

$$100 \times 20 \ \mu R/f = 2000 \ \mu R/f \text{ (or 2 mR/f)}$$

This 2-mR/f skin exposure can be converted to mR/min by multiplying it by the number of f/s and sec/min:

$$2 \text{ mR/f} \times 60 \text{ f/s} \times 60 \text{ s/m} = 7200 \text{ mR/min}$$

In this example, the patient's skin received an exposure of 7.2 R/min at 60 f/sec. If the framing frequency were halved, the exposure would also be halved, to 3.6 R/min.

Table 16–2 shows some exposure rates reported in the literature. They are generally higher than those in the examples above. All these exposures were measured, however, during the era of zinc-cadmium sulfide image intensifiers. We would anticipate that the exposures would be lower with cesium iodide image tubes.

SPOT FILM CAMERAS

Spot film cameras are almost identical to cine cameras. Film sizes are larger and framing rates slower, but optical coupling is the same with tandem lenses and a beam-splitting mirror. Spot film cameras require a lens with a longer focal length to cover the larger film formats. Four sizes are commercially available at present: 70-, 90-, and 105-mm roll film, and 100-mm cut film. The optimum size is a matter of personal preference, but everyone agrees that the image must be large enough to view without magnification.

Spot film cameras are used in two different clinical settings. Initially their use was limited to gastrointestinal fluoroscopy, because the resolution and contrast of the older zinc-cadmium sulfide image tubes were inadequate for more intricate structures. GI barium studies did not require a high-resolution imaging system, and the barium provided excellent inherent contrast. In this setting, spot film cameras were merely used as a substitute for conventional spot films. After cesium iodide image tubes were developed, a second application became apparent. Spot film cameras could be used for serial filming in various kinds of angiography. The limiting factors in this application is the relatively small size of the image intensifier compared to cut film changers. The problem can be partially offset by panning, that is, moving the image tube during the procedure to increase the area of coverage.

Advantages and Disadvantages

The principal advantage of spot film cameras over direct filming methods is a substantial reduction in patient exposure. A rough idea of the degree of reduction is shown in Table 16–3. The recommended per frame exposure for spot film cameras is 100 microroentgens (μR). The exposure for a comparable serial film is 300 μR,

Table 16–2. Exposure Rates for Cinefluorography

AUTHOR	YEAR	ANATOMIC AREA	FILM SIZE (mm)	FRAMES PER SECOND	EXPOSURE RATE (R/min)
Feddema	1960	Stomach	35	16	6–20
Speyer	1960	Stomach	16	16	7–45
Tristan	1960	Esophagus	35	15	21
Chérigie	1961	Stomach	16	25	20–25
Nunnally	1970	Heart	35	60	28–64

(Summarized from Kaude, J.: Integral dose in 35-mm cinefluorography of the gastrointestinal tract. Acta Radiol. [Diagn.] (Stockh.), 7:1970, 1968.)

Table 16–3. Recommended per Frame (or Film) Exposures for Various Imaging Systems[2]

IMAGING SYSTEM	FILM SIZE	EXPOSURE/FRAME
Cinefluorography	16–35 mm	20 μR
Spot film camera	70–105 mm	100 μR
Serial radiography	35 × 35 cm (14 × 14 in.)	300 μR

three times as much. The disadvantages and other advantages of spot film cameras relate to convenience, economics, and the clinical setting. For gastroenterology, cameras are more convenient than conventional spot films. The film does not have to be changed between exposures, and the delay between initiation and completion of an exposure is shorter, because no cassette has to be moved into position for a spot film camera. The only part that moves to start an exposure is the small beam-splitting mirror. Exposure times are shorter, so motion is less likely to be a problem. In addition, films can be taken more rapidly. Most commercial units are designed to function at a maximum framing frequency of 6 to 12 frames/second.

The **advantages** of spot film cameras for serial angiography are as follows:

1. Reduction in procedure time.
2. Ease of performance.
3. Constant monitoring of the images during performance of a study.
4. Reduced patient exposure.
5. Shorter exposure times.
6. Reduced equipment wear.
7. Cheaper film and processing.
8. Reduced film storage problems.

The **disadvantages** of spot film cameras for serial angiography are as follows:

1. Limited film coverage, which prevents application in certain areas. For example, in peripheral angiography each extremity must be studied separately.
2. More experience is required to learn panning techniques.
3. Medical personnel in the angiography suite receive additional radiation exposure.
4. Not applicable to studies of some neoplasms because of reduced resolution of image intensifier.

Framing Methods

Spot film cameras have a square image that simplifies framing compared to cinefluorography. Remember, cine film has a 4 × 3 ratio (24 × 18 mm) format, and the image can be framed to either film dimension. Only four framing formats are recommended for spot film cameras compared to six (or more) for cine film. The four formats are shown in Figure 16–24, and may be summarized as follows.

Exact Framing. The entire circular intensifier image is included in the useable square film frame. The word **useable** refers to the fact that part of the film is lost to the transport system (i.e., perforations along the edge of the film). The exact

FRAMING MODE	EXACT FRAMING	EQUAL AREA FRAMING	MEAN DIAMETER FRAMING	TOTAL OVERFRAMING
ILLUSTRATION	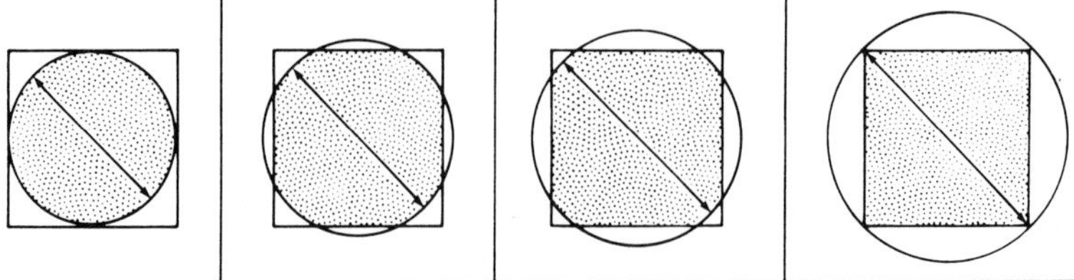			
FILM AREA USED	79 %	91 %	96 %	100 %
IMAGE AREA UNUSED	0 %	9 %	16 %	36 %
RELATIVE IMAGE SIZE	1.0	1.13	1.21	1.41

Figure 16–24   Framing formats for spot film cameras

amount lost depends on the film size and design of the transport system, and varies somewhat from one manufacturer to another. With exact framing, no part of the image is lost but 21% of the film is wasted.

Equal Area Framing. The area of the intensifier image is equal to the useable square film area. Approximately 9% of both the image and film are lost.

Mean Diameter Framing. The diameter of the intensifier is equal to the mean of the transverse and diagonal dimensions of the useful square film area; 16% of the image is lost but only 4% of the film is unused.

Total Overframing. The diameter of the image intensifier is equal to the diagonal dimension of the useful square film area. The entire film is used, but 36% of the image is unused.

The optimum frame format depends on several factors: (1) the size of the image intensifier; (2) the size of the film; and (3) the clinical application for which the imaging system is intended. For any given system, the size of the recorded image enlarges as the diameter of the format increases (Fig. 16–24). Note in the illustration that the arrow increases in size as the framing format increases. For this reason, more overframing is recommended for small formats (70 mm) than for larger formats (105 mm). In general, exact framing is not recommended for any clinical application. It is especially undesirable for 70-mm film, because the final image is too small. Total overframing is not recommended, except possibly for 70-mm film in which maximum magnification is desirable. Either equal area or mean diameter framing is recommended for most clinical situations.[2] Total overframing is impractical with larger film sizes (100 and 105 mm) because the required focal length of the camera lens becomes prohibitively long. As a general rule, a focal length of greater than 400 mm is not recommended. Longer focal length lenses are impractical because of their large physical size and weight.

The film for spot film cameras should have a relatively low contrast. An average gradient between 1.0 and 1.6 has been recommended by the Inter-Society Commission for Heart Disease Resources.[2] A minimum exposure of 100 μR/film is required to minimize quantum mottle. This is the exposure at the input phosphor of the image tube after the x-ray beam has traversed the patient and grid. Remember that quantum mottle originates in the fluorescent screen so it is not affected by the size of the recorded image. Therefore, the same exposures are recommended for both 70- and 105-mm films.

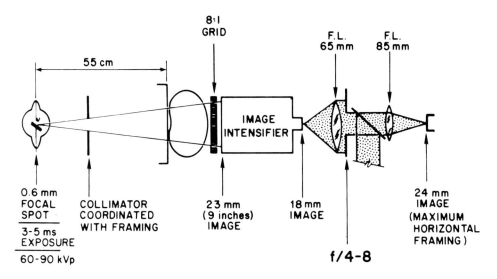

Figure 16–25 Summary of recommendations for a cinefluorographic system

SUMMARY

The emergence of cinefluorography came about as a byproduct of the development of the x-ray image intensifier. The intensifier is prerequisite for efficient optical coupling and for an image bright enough to expose the film without excessively exposing the patient. Figure 16–25 summarizes the various components of a typical cine system. Beginning on the left side, a 0.6-mm focal spot is recommended. Exposures should be kept in the 3- to 5-ms range, with beam energies between 60 and 90 kVp. At least 55 cm should separate the target from the tabletop or patient support. The beam should be collimated to the framing mode selected. The image intensifier should be chosen for the particular clinical situation and, in general, should be as small as practical. The collector lens should be as fast as cost and technology permit. The framing mode should be selected and the camera lens designed to produce the appropriate frame size. Lens performance is improved with iris diaphragms. Resolution, contrast, depth of field, and spherical aberrations are all improved with an iris diaphragm. An aperture about two f numbers less than maximum is recommended.

Cine film should have a wide latitude, low contrast, and low-base fog, and be processed to an average gradient in the 1.0 to 1.6 range. An input phosphor exposure of 20 μR per frame is recommended to minimize quantum mottle. The temperature, replenishment rates, and transport times of cine processors must be precisely controlled, and processor performance should be monitored daily. Sensitometric studies should include spot checks of gross fog, speed, and contrast. Other components of the cine system should also be monitored on a regular basis.

Spot film cameras are similar to cine cameras in design but not in function. They are used to produce static images either for GI type radiography in place of conventional spot films or for serial angiography. Film sizes of 70, 90, 100, and 105 mm are in current usage. An exposure of 100 μR/frame is recommended, regardless of film size. The principal advantage of spot film cameras over screen-film radiography is a substantial reduction in patient exposures. The major disadvantages are a relatively small size of radiographic field and some loss of resolution in the image intensifier.

REFERENCES

1. International Commission on Radiation Units and Measurements: Cameras for image intensifier fluoroscopy. Washington, DC, International Commission on Radiation Units and Measurements, 1969, Report 15.
2. Judkins, M.P., Abrams, H.L., Bristow J.D., et al.: Report of the Inter-Society Commission for Heart Disease Resources. Circulation, 53:No. 2, February, 1976.
3. Lawrence, D.J.: A simple method of processor control. Med. Radiogr. Photogr., 49:2, 1973.

17

Television

Before the invention of the x-ray image intensifier, attempts at displaying the fluoroscopic image on television were only partially successful. The large fluoroscopic screen required an elaborate optical system, and suboptimal screen brightness produced a weak video signal. The development of the image intensifier solved both these problems. Its small output phosphor simplifies optical coupling, and a brightness gain of 3000 to 6000 produces a strong video signal. Two types of television cameras have been used for fluoroscopy, image-orthicon and vidicon cameras. Initially, the image-orthicon camera was the only one sensitive enough to record the limited brightness gains of early image intensifiers. Recently brightness gains have increased and vidicon cameras have improved, so that now they have completely replaced image-orthicon cameras in fluoroscopy.

CLOSED-CIRCUIT TELEVISION

The components of a television system are a camera, camera control unit, and monitor (Fig. 17–1). To avoid confusion in

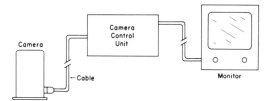

Figure 17–1 Components of a television system

nomenclature, we will use the terms "television" and "video" interchangeably. Fluoroscopic television systems are always closed-circuit systems; that is, the video signal is transmitted from one component to the next through cables rather than through the air, as in broadcast television. A lens system conveys the fluoroscopic image from the output phosphor of the image intensifier to the video camera, where it is converted into a series of electrical pulses called the **video signal.** This signal is transmitted through a cable to the camera control unit, where it is amplified, and then forwarded through another cable to the television monitor. The monitor converts the video signal back into the original image for direct viewing by the fluoroscopist.

Before discussing the individual components of a television system, we will move a little ahead of ourselves and describe the nature of the video picture. An appreciation of this will make the design of both the camera and monitor easier to understand. The television image is similar to the screened print shown in Figure 17–2. It is made up of a mosaic of hundreds of thousands of tiny dots with different brightness, each contributing a minute bit to the total picture. When viewed from a distance the individual dots disappear but, at close range, or with magnification, they are clearly visible. The dot distribution is not random or haphazard in a television picture. Instead, the dots are arranged in a specific pattern along horizontal lines,

229

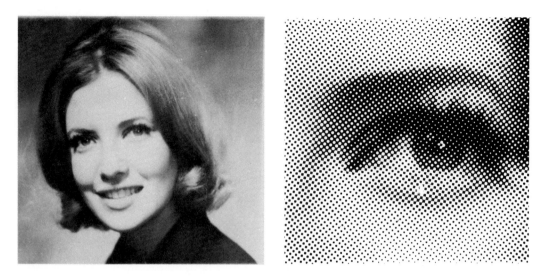

Figure 17–2 Dot picture and enlargement of a screened print

called **horizontal scan lines.** The number of lines varies from one television system to another but, in the United States, most fluoroscopy and all commercial television use 525 scan lines. To avoid confusion we must clarify the meaning of television lines. When a radiologist thinks of lines, it is usually in terms of lines per unit length. For example, if a grid has 80 lines, the unit is "lines per inch." Television lines have only the unit of "lines," and no unit of length. The 525 lines in most television systems represent the total number in the entire picture, regardless of its size. The lines are close together in a small picture tube and spread apart in a large tube, but in both the total number is the same. The television camera converts the features present in the fluoroscopic image into a series of dots because it can only transmit one dot at a time.

Television Camera

The vidicon camera is the one usually employed for fluoroscopy, and is the only one that we will discuss in any detail. It is a relatively inexpensive, compact unit (5 inches in diameter, 9 inches long) that weighs approximately 6 lb. The essential parts of a vidicon camera are shown in Figure 17–3. The most important part is the vidicon tube, a small electronic vacuum tube that measures only 1 inch in diameter and 6 inches in length. The tube is surrounded by two pairs of coils, electromagnetic focusing coils and electrostatic deflecting coils.

The fluoroscopic image from the image intensifier is focused onto the target assembly, which consists of three layers: (1) a glass faceplate; (2) a signal plate; and (3) a target. The only function of the glass faceplate is to maintain the vacuum in the tube. Light merely passes through the faceplate on its way to the target. The signal plate is a thin transparent film of graphite located on the inner surface of the faceplate. It is an electrical conductor with a positive potential of approximately 25 volts. The signal plate is so named because it transmits the video signal.

The vidicon target is functionally the most important element in the tube. It is a thin film of photoconductive material, usually antimony trisulfite suspended as globules in a mica matrix. Each globule measures 0.001 inch in diameter and is insulated from its neighbors and from the signal plate by the mica matrix. The globules form a mosaic of tiny light-sensitive elements, and they form the dot picture that

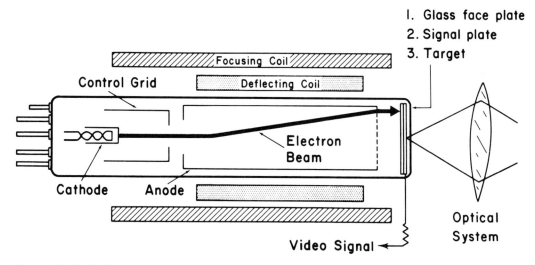

Figure 17–3   Vidicon camera

we described earlier. Their function is very complex, but they behave like tiny capacitors. After reviewing the other elements in the camera, we will return to these globules and discuss them in more detail.

The cathode is located at the opposite end of the vidicon tube from the target and is heated indirectly by an internal electric coil. The cathode-heating coil assembly is called an **electron gun.** The heating coil boils electrons from the cathode (thermionic emission), creating an electron cloud. These electrons are immediately formed into a beam by the control grid, which also initiates their acceleration toward the target. As the electron beam progresses down the tube, it moves beyond the influence of the control grid and into the electrostatic field of the anode. The anode has a positive potential of approximately 250 volts with respect to the cathode, and it accelerates the electron beam to a relatively high velocity. The anode extends across the target end of the tube as a fine wire mesh. The wire mesh and signal plate form a uniform decelerating field adjacent to the target. The signal plate (+25 volts) has a potential of 225 volts less than that of the wire mesh (+250 volts), so electrons should flow from the signal plate to the wire mesh. The electrons from the cathode are accelerated to

relatively high velocities, however, and they coast through the decelerating field like a roller coaster going uphill. By the time they reach the target, they have been slowed to a near standstill. The decelerating field also performs a second function: it straightens the final path of the electron beam so that it strikes the target perpendicularly.

Because the electron beam scans a dot picture, it must be focused to a point the size of the dots. This is accomplished by two pairs of electromagnetic focusing coils that wrap around the vidicon tube (Fig. 17–4A). These coils extend almost the entire length of the tube and create a constant magnetic field that forces the beam of electrons into a narrow bundle. As the electrons are forced together, they repel each other and diverge, only to be brought back together by the focusing coil. They progress down the tube in a series of oscillating spirals, and strike the target while they are focused at a point (Fig. 17–4B).

The electron beam is steered by variable electrostatic fields produced by two pairs of deflecting coils that wrap around the vidicon tube in a manner similar to that of the focusing coils. Vertical deflecting coils are shown in Figure 17–4C. By alternating the current on the coils, the focused elec-

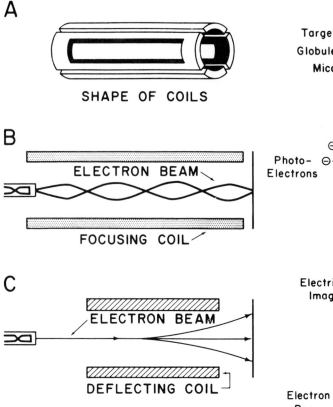

Figure 17–4   Focusing and deflecting coils

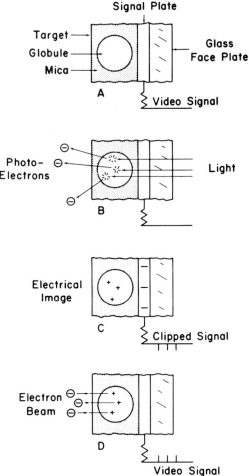

Figure 17–5   Formation of the video signal

tron beam is moved up and down to scan the target. The other pair of coils moves the beam from side to side along a horizontal line. All four coils, working together, move the electron beam almost instantaneously over the target in a repetitive scanning motion.

Video Signal

Now that we have discussed the physical makeup of the camera, we can return to the critical target end of the tube and the formation of the video signal (Fig. 17–5A). When a globule absorbs light, it emits electrons (Fig. 17–5B). The electrons are immediately attracted to the anode and removed from the tube. The globule, having lost electrons, becomes positively charged. It is insulated from its surroundings so that it behaves like half of a tiny capacitor, and draws a current into the conductive signal plate. The current that flows into the signal plate is ignored, or clipped, and is not recorded (Fig. 17–5C). Similar events occur over the entire surface of the target. A brighter area in the light image emits more photoelectrons than a dim area, and produces a stronger charge on the tiny capacitors. The result is a mosaic of charged globules that store an electrical image that is an exact replica of the light image focused onto the target.

The electron beam scans the electrical image stored on the target, and fills in the holes left by the emitted photoelectrons, thus discharging the tiny globule capacitors. Excess electrons from the scanning beam drift back to the anode and are removed from the tube. At the instant of discharge, a current flows through the conductive signal plate, and this current forms the video signal (Fig. 17–5D). The globules are not all discharged at the same time. Only a small cluster, a dot, is discharged each instant in time. Then the electron beam moves on to the next dot in an orderly sequence but, moving at an enormous speed, it discharges all the globules on the target. The result is a series of video pulses, all originating from the same signal plate but separated in time. Each pulse corresponds to an exact location on the target. Reassembling these pulses back into a visible image is done by the camera control unit and the television monitor.

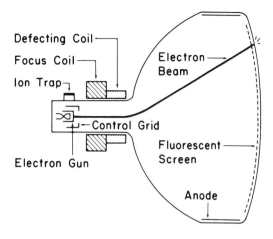

Figure 17–6   Television monitor

Camera Control Unit

The power supply and all the controls that regulate the camera are located within the camera control unit. It amplifies the video signal (after preamplification in the camera), regulates the focusing and deflecting coils, and synchronizes the video signal between the camera and monitor.

Television Monitor

The last link in the television chain is the monitor. It contains the picture tube and the controls for regulating brightness and contrast.

A picture tube is similar to a vidicon camera tube (Fig. 17–6). Both are vacuum tubes and both contain an electron gun, control grid, anode, focusing coils, and deflecting coils. A picture tube, however, is much larger. The focusing and deflecting coils are wrapped around the neck of the tube, and they control the electron beam in exact synchrony with the camera tube. The brightness of the individual dots in the picture is regulated by the control grid. It receives the video signal from the television camera, and uses this signal to regulate the number of electrons in the electron beam. To produce a bright area in the television picture, it allows a large number of electrons to reach the fluorescent screen. To produce a dark area, it cuts off the electron flow almost completely.

The anode is plated onto the inside surface of the picture tube near the fluorescent screen. It carries a much higher positive potential (10,000 V) than the anode of the camera tube (250 V), so it accelerates the electron beam to a much higher velocity. The electrons strike the fluorescent screen at the flared end of the tube and emit a large number of light photons, which form the visible television image. Many secondary electrons are set free by the impact of the electron beam with the screen, and they are attracted to the anode and conducted out of the picture tube.

A large tube, like a television picture tube, can never be completely evacuated. Some residual gas is always present, and "outgassing" (release of adsorbed gas) from the components of the monitor adds to the problem. These gas molecules are eventually ionized and removed from the tube by an ion trap located in the end of the monitor (Fig. 17–6).

TELEVISION SCANNING

The television image is stored as an electrical image on the target of the vidicon tube, and it is scanned along 525 lines by a narrow electron beam 30 times per sec-

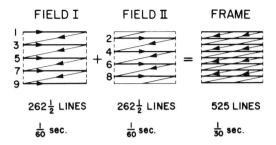

FIELD I   FIELD II   FRAME

262½ LINES   262½ LINES   525 LINES

$\frac{1}{60}$ sec. $\frac{1}{60}$ sec. $\frac{1}{30}$ sec.

Figure 17–7   Interlaced horizontal scanning

ond. Each scan of the entire target is called a frame. The electron beam scans the target in much the same manner that we read a page in a book. Beginning at the top left corner, it drifts across a line, sending out a video signal as it moves, and then rapidly returns to the left margin and repeats the process over and over until all 525 lines have been read. When we reach the last line of a page, we move on to the top line of the next page and continue reading. The electron beam does exactly the same thing, only it does not have to turn pages. Instead, as the beam reads, it also erases. As the electron beam discharges the globule capacitors, it erases their image. As soon as a line is read and erased, it is ready to record a new image, and it begins immediately. When the electron beam returns it sees a different image than it saw the time before. Because the electron beam scans the target 30 times each second, the change in the image from one scan to the next is slight, and our eyes perceive a continuous motion in exactly the same way that we see motion in a cine film.

In the discussion of cinefluorography we mentioned that the eye can detect individual flashes of light, or flicker, up to 50 pulses per second (see Chap. 16). A television monitor only displays 30 frames per second, so an electronic trick, called **interlaced horizontal scanning** is employed to avoid flicker. Instead of scanning all 525 lines consecutively each frame, only the even-numbered lines are scanned in the first half of the frame, and only the odd-numbered lines are scanned during the

second half (Fig. 17–7). Each pass of the electron beam over the video target is called a field, and consists of 262½ lines. Even though only 30 frames are displayed each second, they are displayed in 60 flashes of light (fields), and flicker disappears.

Video Signal Frequency (Bandpass)

Bandpass, also called bandwidth, is the frequency range that the electronic components of the video system must be designed to transmit. An analogy with sound will simplify the explanation. Sound is audible at frequencies from about 16 Hertz (cycles/sec) to 30,000 Hz. Sound equipment (e.g., recorders, amplifiers, speakers) is designed to transmit this range of frequencies. The range from the lowest to the highest frequency is called the bandpass (Fig. 17–8). The electronic components are engineered to transmit all the frequencies in this range as accurately as possible. The cutoffs are not sharply defined at the two frequency extremes, and not all frequencies are transmitted with the same quality. Thinking in terms of music, bandpass is the frequency range that the electronic components must "pass" from the "band" to the listener. A video signal is exactly the same as an audio signal, except that the video signal covers a wider range of frequencies.

As the electronic beam moves along a horizontal scan line, a video signal is transmitted to the camera control unit and then forwarded to the TV monitor. The frequency of the video signal will fluctuate from moment to moment, depending on the nature of the television image. Figure 17–9 shows one scan line of an image containing four equally spaced black and white lines, or four line pairs. As the electron beam moves across the image, the video signal increases and decreases in voltage in a cyclic fashion. Like alternating current, one cycle (the shaded area in the illustration) includes one up limb and one down limb and represents two lines, or one line pair. The scanning process is repeated over

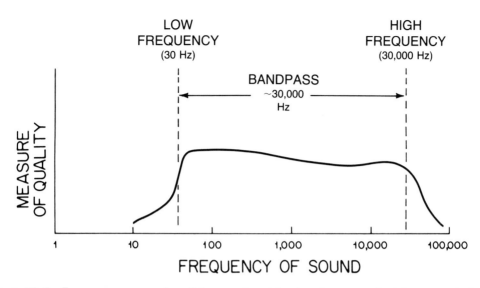

LOW
FREQUENCY
(30 Hz)

HIGH
FREQUENCY
(30,000 Hz)

BANDPASS
~30,000
Hz

MEASURE
OF QUALITY

FREQUENCY OF SOUND

Figure 17–8 Frequency range of audible sound and the bandpass required for accurate transmission

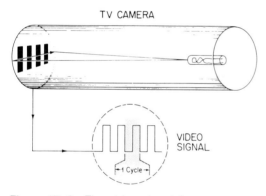

TV CAMERA

VIDEO
SIGNAL

1 Cycle

Figure 17–9 The video signal from one scan line of a line pair phantom

and over 525 times per frame and 30 frames per second. We can calculate the frequency, or number of cycles per second of the video signal generated by the four line pair image by multiplying the number of cycles per scan line (four in this case) by the number of scan lines per frame by the number of frames per second:

$$\frac{cycles}{scan\ line} \times \frac{scan\ lines}{frame} \times \frac{frames}{seconds} = cycles/sec$$
$$4 \times 525 \times 30 = 63,000$$

When the number of line pairs in the image changes, the frequency of the video

signal also changes. The lowest frequency signal occurs with an image of one line pair, (i.e., a screen that is half black and half white). The highest frequency signal is determined by the amount of money that one is willing to pay for electronic equipment. A reasonable compromise is a system with equal vertical and horizontal resolution. This is accomplished in a 525-line system with 525 vertical lines, or $262\frac{1}{2}$ line pairs. In this case the lowest and highest frequency signals will be as follows:

$$\frac{cycles}{scan\ line} \times \frac{scan\ lines}{frame} \times \frac{frames}{second} = cycles/sec$$

Minimum			
1 $\times$	525 $\times$	30 =	15,750
Maximum			
$262\frac{1}{2}$ $\times$	525 $\times$	30 $\simeq$	4,130,000

The frequency of the video signal will fluctuate between a minimum of 15,750 Hz and a maximum of 4,130,000 Hz. To transmit the signal accurately, the electronic components should have a bandpass of 4.13 to 0.016 MHz, or approximately 4.1 MHz. Actually, a little higher bandpass is required. About 10% of the scan time is lost in retracing from one line to another. This additional 10% increases the required bandpass to approximately 4.5 MHz for a

525-line system. At this bandpass, vertical and horizontal resolution are equal.

Synchronization

It is necessary to synchronize or coordinate the video signal between the camera and monitor; that is, keep them in phase with each other. The camera control unit adds synchronization pulses to the video signal at the end of each scan line and scan field. Appropriately, they are called horizontal and vertical synchronization pulses. They are generated during the retrace time of the electron beam, while no video signal is being transmitted. First, the picture screen is blackened by a blanking pulse, and the synchronization signal is added to the blanking pulse. If the synchronization pulses were added to the video signal while the screen was white they would generate noise in the form of white streaks, but no visible noise is produced by synchronization on a black screen.

TELEVISION IMAGE QUALITY

Resolution

The number of scan lines and the bandpass of a television system impose an absolute ceiling on resolution. Obviously, a dot picture cannot display an image smaller than the individual dots. The only way that television resolution can be improved is with more and smaller dots, which means more scan lines, and a greater bandpass. A greater dot concentration improves resolution but does not remove the ceiling. Regardless of the quality of the x-ray image, the television image has this absolute ceiling on quality.

Television resolution is measured on the face of the TV monitor and expressed in total lines. A resolution of 370 lines means that 370 separate lines, or 185 line pairs (lp), are visible on the entire TV monitor. If the bandpass is properly selected, horizontal and vertical resolution are equal. The ratio between the vertical resolution and the number of horizontal scan lines is

called the **Kell factor.** Kell factors are determined experimentally by measuring the maximum number of lines that can be seen with a line pair imaging system. The Kell factor for a 525-line TV system is 0.7. The vertical resolution of this system is

$$\text{Kell factor} = \frac{\text{resolution}}{\text{number of scan lines}}$$
$$0.7 = \frac{\text{resolution}}{525}$$
$$\text{Resolution} = 525 \times 0.7 \approx 370$$

This is the maximum vertical resolution that can be attained with a 525-line system, regardless of the size of the monitor. A resolution of 370 total lines represents 185 black lines separated by 185 equal thickness white lines, or 185 line pairs. Monitor resolution can only be improved by employing more scan lines and a higher bandpass. Such systems are available but have numerous disadvantages, including increased cost and incompatibility with the commercial systems currently used in most hospitals. Also, the higher bandpass is usually associated with more electrical noise, and noise diminishes the detectability of subtle contrast differences.

The overall resolution of the imaging system (i.e., the image intensifier-lens-TV system) depends on the size of the input image. If the TV monitor resolution of 185 lp is used to show a large picture, resolution will be poor. For example, suppose we use television to display the image from a 9-inch image intensifier. Converting to millimeters, a 9-inch image intensifier is 229 mm in diameter (9 inch × 25.4 mm/inch). The system resolution in lp/mm is as follows:

$$\frac{185 \text{ lp}}{229 \text{ mm}} = 0.8 \text{ lp/mm}$$

Table 17–1 shows system resolution for three different-sized image intensifiers. The same numbers would apply to a triple-model (4.5-, 6-, and 9-inches) image intensifier. The television monitor always displays the same 185 lp but, when supplied with the image from a 4.5-inch image in-

Table 17–1. Resolution of a TV Imaging System for Various-Sized Image Intensifiers

SIZE OF IMAGE INTENSIFIER		TELEVISION RESOLUTION
in.	mm	(lp/mm)
4.5	114	1.6
6	152	1.2
9	229	0.8

*Based on a 525-line TV system with a total resolution of 185 lp.

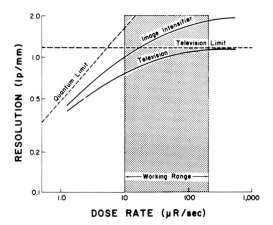

Figure 17–10   Image intensifier and television resolution during fluoroscopy. (Modified from Gebauer, et al.: Roentgen Television. New York, Grune & Stratton, 1967)

tensifier, this 185 lp represents a resolution of 1.6 lp/mm, twice as good as the 0.8 lp/mm of the 9-in. image intensifier. Even though a resolution of 1.6 lp/mm is a considerable improvement, it falls far short of displaying the entire resolution of the newer cesium iodide image intensifiers. These tubes have a resolution of up to 4 lp/mm, and some are available in 12- to 14-inch sizes. The only way that this resolution can be adequately displayed at the present time is with a film system such as a 35-mm cine, or 105-mm spot films.

With the appropriate optical system, the 185 lp of television resolution can transmit any desired degree of system resolution, provided the size of the initial image is reduced proportionately. For example, if we start by looking at a radiograph of a whole hand, then gradually zoom in (with the appropriate lens) to look at one phalanx, and finally only a small portion of one cortex, the system resolution increases tremendously. If, in the end, we are looking at an area 10 mm in diameter, the system resolution could be as high as 18.5 lp/mm (185 lp ÷ 10 mm). In this case, system resolution would be limited by the input phosphor of the image intensifer and not by the television image.

Figure 17–10 compares the resolution of an older zinc-cadmium sulfide image intensifier and television fluoroscopy in terms of dose rate (μR/sec). At low radiation dosages, there are too few x-ray photons to produce a good image, and resolution is quantum-limited in both systems. At higher dose rates television resolution continues to be limited, but at a higher level, by the dot composition of the image. A transmitted radiation level of 20 μR/sec produces a good quality image without excessively exposing the patient. A television camera cannot improve image quality beyond that of an image intensifier, because it receives its image from the intensifier.

Contrast

Both the camera and monitor affect the contrast of a television image. A vidicon camera reduces contrast by a factor of approximately 0.8, and the monitor enhances contrast by a factor of 2. The net result is a definite improvement in contrast beyond that of the image intensifier alone. Furthermore, both the brightness and contrast levels can be regulated with the monitor, so the optimum combination can be selected to show a point of interest best.

Lag

An undesirable property of most vidicon tubes is lag, or stickiness, which becomes apparent when the camera is moved rapidly during fluoroscopy (i.e., the image blurs). Lag occurs because it takes a certain amount of time for the image to build up and decay on the vidicon target. In one respect a certain amount of lag is actually advantageous. It averages out the statistical fluctuations that normally occur with low-dose fluoroscopy, and minimizes the annoying effects of quantum mottle.

Brightness

The brightness of the image changes constantly in all fluoroscopic systems as the fluoroscope is moved from one area of the patient to another. Usually this does not cause any serious problem, and both the chest and abdomen can be examined with preset exposure factors. With television fluoroscopy, however, changes in image brightness seriously affect image quality. As the fluoroscope is moved from the abdomen to the chest a sudden surge of brightness floods the system, the image becomes chalky, and all detail is lost. Therefore, the brightness level of the television monitor must be controlled within rather narrow limits. This is usually accomplished by varying the x-ray exposure factors. A photocell located between the image intensifier and television camera measures the brightness of the fluoroscopic image, and it transmits a signal back to the x-ray control unit to adjust the exposure factors.

The brightness level of the television monitor can be increased indefinitely, but this does not improve image quality. At low levels of radiation, image quality is limited by quantum mottle, and at high levels it is limited by the inherent ceiling imposed on resolution by a dot image. Usually brightness and contrast are adjusted in combination. Contrast is brought to a near maximum level, and brightness is adjusted to produce a satisfactory level of illumination.

Plumbicon and Image-Orthicon Cameras

We have delayed mentioning plumbicon and image-orthicon cameras because we will discuss them only on the basis of their performance, and will not attempt to describe their mode of operation.

A plumbicon camera is simply a vidicon camera with a lead monoxide photocon-ductor for its target. Its tube is usually a little larger than a standard vidicon tube, and some do not fit into a conventional vidicon housing. Plumbicon tubes have two advantages over other vidicon tubes: (1) contrast is not diminished, and (2) lag is considerably less. Motion blurring is almost completely eliminated but, with diminished lag, quantum mottle becomes a problem. In general, plumbicon tubes have considerably more mottle than other vidicon tubes.

Image-orthicon cameras are much larger than vidicon cameras, and they have a completely different electronic design. They are extremely sensitive to light and function well with low levels of illumination. In the early days of television fluoroscopy, image-orthicon tubes were the only ones sensitive enough to transmit a good image with the limited light gain of early image intensifiers. The other advantages are superior resolution and a complete freedom from lag.

Image-orthicon cameras, though, have serious disadvantages. To begin with, they are too expensive for most radiologists, and their large size makes them cumbersome to operate. Even more important, they are extremely sensitive to temperature changes and require a long warm-up time (up to 20 min). Recently vidicon cameras have completely replaced image-orthicon cameras for fluoroscopy.

MAGNETIC RECORDERS

The commercial television industry has been storing programs on tape recorders for many years. When magnetic recorders were first developed, their prohibitive cost severely limited their availability for clinical radiology. Less expensive models have recently been developed, and now video tape is commonly used to store fluoroscopic images. A second type of magnetic recorder, a video disc, is also being used in fluoroscopy. The physical principles are exactly the same for tape and disc recorders. We will start by describing tape recorders as a prototype and then briefly point out a few characteristics of disc recorders.

Video Tape Recorders

The same unit is used for both recording and playback. As a recorder, it receives a video signal from the camera control unit and, for playback, transmits the signal to one or several television monitors. Both these transmissions are conducted through cables, so it is a closed-circuit television system. The image is stored on either 1- or 2-inch wide Mylar tape, coated on one side with a magnetic film. Two-inch video tape records a better quality image, but costs considerably more, so most fluoroscopy is recorded on 1-inch tape.

A schematic presentation of a tape recorder is shown in Figure 17–11. The three essential components, besides the electronic circuitry, are a magnetic tape, a recording and/or reading head, and a tape transport system. Exactly the same type of head is used for both recording and playback, and we will call it a writing head. The writing head converts an electrical signal into a fluctuating magnetic field for recording, and converts a magnetic signal into an electrical signal for replay. Some recorders have separate recording and playback heads, while in others one head performs both functions. The drive spindle moves the tape past the writing head at a constant velocity. The tape is kept in physical contact with the writing head at all times during both recording and playback.

The writing head of a video tape recorder is shown in Figure 17–12. The head is similar to a transformer (see Chap. 3) in that it consists of a magnetic core, such as an iron-nickel alloy wrapped with two coils of wire, but the writing head is different in two ways. First, a narrow segment, or gap, is cut from the core, as shown in Figure 17–12. Second, the two coils are wired together so that their magnetic fields reinforce each other. As a changing electric field moves through the coils, a changing magnetic field is produced in the gap. When the current in the illustration moves from left to right, the magnetic field is in the direction of the arrows. The field reverses when the current changes directions. The magnetic field extends out beyond the gap in the writing head (Fig. 17–13). This extended magnetic field is the critical portion that interacts with the magnetic tape.

The magnetic layer of video tape is composed of oxides of magnetic materials. The molecules of this material behave like tiny bar magnets, called **dipoles.** Each dipole aligns itself in a magnetic field like the needle of a compass. They are randomly arranged on unrecorded tape (Fig. 17–13A). As the tape moves past the writing head gap, the alignment of the dipoles is changed to coincide with the magnetic

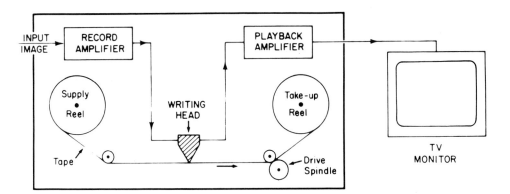

Figure 17–11   Components of a video tape recorder

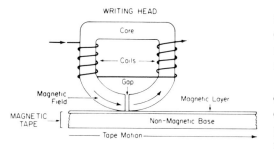

Figure 17–12   Video writing head

field impressed on them while they are passing the gap (Fig. 17–13B). When the video signal (sine curve in Fig. 17–13) is negative, the dipoles are aligned toward the left; when the signal is positive, alignment is in the opposite direction. At the zero points in the video signal, no magnetic field exists in the gap, and dipole alignment is random. The degree of alignment is exaggerated in the illustration to demonstrate the point. The actual alignment is proportional to the strength of the magnetic field. Complete alignment is prevented by the neighboring molecules, which offer some resistance to dipole movement, and by the inertia of the dipoles

themselves. Once the tiny magnetic particles leave the magnetic field in the gap, they retain their orientation until some other magnetic force causes them to change.

Playback is exactly the reverse of the recording process, except that the magnetic dipoles are not unaligned in playback. The partially aligned magnetic dipoles have a magnetic field of their own. As this field moves past the gap in the writing head, it induces a magnetic field in the core, which in turn induces an electrical signal in the wire coils. This is the video signal that is forwarded to the display monitor.

Every component of the video signal must be recorded on a different portion of the magnetic tape. The transport system must move fast enough to keep a fresh supply of tape at the writing heads. If the tape moves too slowly, the dipole alignment of one cycle is unaligned by the magnetic field of the next cycle. To record a frequency of several million cycles per second, the tape must move at a very high velocity. This is accomplished by moving both the tape and writing heads (Fig. 17–14). The tape moves diagonally past paired writing heads

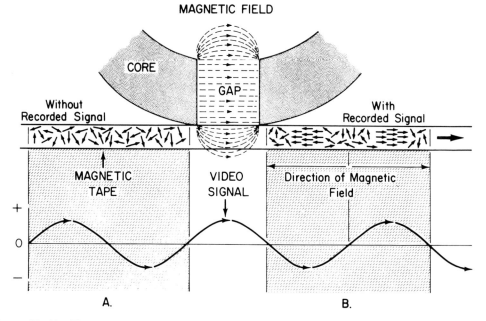

Figure 17–13   The magnetic signal on video tape

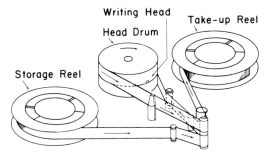

Figure 17–14 Video tape recorder. (Modified from Operating Manual for Ampex Model VR-6000 Videotape Recorder. Elk Grove Village, IL: Ampex Corporation, 1966)

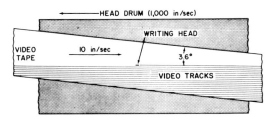

Figure 17–15 Video tracks on video tape

mounted on either side of a rapidly revolving drum. The tape moves in one direction at a speed of 10 inch/sec and the writing heads move in the opposite direction at 1000 inch/sec, for an effective writing speed of 1010 inch/sec. While one head is recording the other is away from the tape, so only one writing head is recording at any particular time. Each writing head records one video frame as it passes diagonally across the tape. The signal is laid down in separate tracks approximately 0.006 inch wide (Fig. 17–15). The tape moves just fast enough to separate the tracks of the two heads. Consecutive lines are always written by different heads. Video tracks are separated by a narrow guard band. Each 10 inches of video tape stores approximately 1000 inches of magnetic tracks. A reel of tape (3000 feet) plays for approximately 1 hour and, if handled carefully, it can be reused more than 100 times.

Image quality is a little better with direct (live) television than with video tape, but the difference is not large. The Ampex Model VR-6000 shown in Figure 17–14 has a bandpass of 3.5 MHz, and its resolution is reported by the manufacturer to be 350 lines (175 lp), nearly the same as the 370 lines (185 lp) of direct television.

Cassette tape recorders are now increasing in popularity. They have only one advantage over other systems, ease of loading and unloading the tape. Otherwise cassette recorders are exactly the same as other tape recorders.

Video Disc Recorders

Video disc and video tape recorders operate on exactly the same physical principle, but they have completely different functions. Tape recorders are designed to show motion, comparable to a movie camera. Disc recorders are designed to show stationary images, more like a spot-film camera. A tape recorder can be used to show a single frame by stopping the tape against the revolving drum, but this subjects the tape to considerable physical wear. Video disc recorders are designed for stop action. The discs themselves look like phonograph records. The video tracks are laid down in preset grooves. Each groove in a video disc is a completely separate track. The tracks are not continuous from groove to groove. One picture frame is recorded in each track. When a particular frame is selected for replay, exactly the same picture is shown over and over 30 times a second for as long as the operator desires. Most disc recorders can only store a few hundred frames.

Video discs have several advantages over tape. The most important one is **random access.** The video grooves are numbered, and the recorder can go directly to any desired number without playing the intervening numbers. This instantaneous access is considerably different than a tape recorder, which may take several minutes to reach a specific frame, even with a rapid wind mode. Another advantage of discs is that they are not subjected to physical wear in the stop action mode. Actually, they are designed to operate in this mode. Only the disc moves during both recording and playback, so it is not subjected to the physical wear of a rotating drum. In a clinical setting, video disc recorders are used as a substitute for spot films, and the x-ray exposure factors are frequently increased, just as they would be for spot films. This exposure increase improves the quality of the disc image by decreasing quantum mottle. Primarily because of this exposure increase, image quality is generally better with video discs than with video tape. Resolution is best with the smallest image intensifier mode consistent with the clinical situation.

Comparison of Video Tape and Cine Film

Video tape recorders have two advantages over cinefluorography: the image is available for instant replay without any intermediate processing system, and the patient's exposure to radiation is not increased. Both of these are important. Instant replay allows the radiologist to examine the record before the patient leaves the room, so that inadequacies in a study can be corrected immediately. Because exposure factors are not increased, the whole fluoroscopic examination can be recorded if so desired. If nothing of permanent value is found, the tape is erased and used again for another patient.

Video tape also has disadvantages, the most important being poor image quality. Cine film (either 16 or 35 mm) produces an image of superior quality. Whether or not this difference is significant depends on the importance of image quality for the particular examination. For a study such as coronary angiography, which requires a high-quality image, cine film is preferable, but for most gastrointestinal examinations video tape is entirely adequate. Another disadvantage of video tape is its fixed frame speed (e.g., 30 frames/sec in the United States). Cine cameras can be operated at several different speeds, but a frequency of 30 frames/sec is adequate for most fluoroscopic needs.

In summary, video tape recording offers more convenience with instant playback and decreased patient exposures. Cine film produces a better quality image and a greater variety of shutter speeds. Medical needs dictate the preference.

REFERENCE

1. Templeton, A.W., Dwyer, S.J., et al.: Standard and high-scan-line television systems. Radiology, 91:725, 1968.

18

Body Section Radiography

Body section radiography is a special x-ray technique that blurs out the shadows of superimposed structures to show more clearly the principal structures being examined. We must point out immediately that it is not a method of improving the sharpness of any part of a radiographic image. On the contrary, it is a process of controlled blurring that merely leaves some parts of the image less blurred than others. Various names have been used to describe body section radiography. Most were initially applied to a specifically designed unit. Over the years considerable confusion has developed over nomenclature. In 1962 the International Commission on Radiologic Units and Measurements adopted the term **tomography** to describe all types of body section techniques,[3] and we will use this term synonymously with body section radiography. Some commonly used names are

1. tomography (tomogram) preferred
2. planigraphy (planigram)
3. stratigraphy (stratigram)
4. laminography (laminogram).

A revolutionary new technique, called computed tomography (CT), was developed in England in 1972. Computed tomography differs from conventional tomography in almost every way. In fact, about the only point the two have in common is that they both display a thin layer, or slice, of tissue. Because the two tomographic systems are completely different, we will discuss them separately. This chapter will be devoted entirely to conventional tomography, and CT will be discussed in Chapter 24.

BASIC METHOD OF TOMOGRAPHY

Many ingenious tomographic methods have been devised. We will begin by describing the simplest (Fig. 18–1A). The essential ingredients are an x-ray tube, an x-ray film, and a rigid connecting rod that rotates about a fixed fulcrum. When the tube moves in one direction, the film moves in the opposite direction. The film is placed in a tray under the x-ray table so that it is free to move without disturbing the patient. The fulcrum is the only point in the system that remains stationary. The amplitude of tube travel is measured in degrees, and is called the tomographic angle (arc). The plane of interest within the patient is positioned at the level of the fulcrum, and it is the only plane that remains in sharp

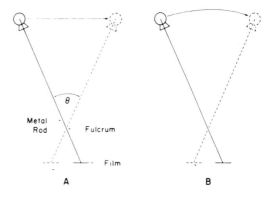

Figure 18–1   Tomographic method

243

focus. All points above and below this plane are blurred.

A second type of tube motion is illustrated in Figure 18–1*B*. Both the x-ray tube and film move along an arc instead of in a straight line as they did in Figure 18–1*A*. Both methods give similar results. The primary advantage of a straight line motion is that it can be easily adapted to a standard x-ray table and requires no expensive equipment. It has more moving parts, however, including slip joints at both ends of the connecting rod, which eventually wear and get out of adjustment. A tomographic system that moves the tube and film in an arc has fewer moving parts and is less likely to get out of adjustment, but it requires a special table and tube stand built specifically for tomography, so it is more expensive.

All points that are parallel to the x-ray film and on the same plane as the fulcrum are displayed in sharp focus on the tomogram. A whole plane is in focus, not just a point. In Figure 18–2, points A, B, and C are several centimeters apart on the same plane and their images all move exactly the same distance as the x-ray film; therefore, they are not blurred. When the tube moves to the left, the distance from point C to its image on the film is greater than the comparable distance of points B and A. The ratio of the object-tube and object-film distance for all three points is the same, and there is no difference in magnification of objects on the same plane.

Tomographic techniques blur all points that are outside (above or below) the focal plane. In Figure 18–3, point A is above and point C below the focal plane. As the x-ray tube moves, only the image of point B, which is on the focal plane, remains in sharp focus, because it is the only image that moves exactly the same distance as the film. The image of point A moves more than the film, and the image of point C less than the film, so both are blurred. The further an object is from the plane of the fulcrum, the more its image is blurred.

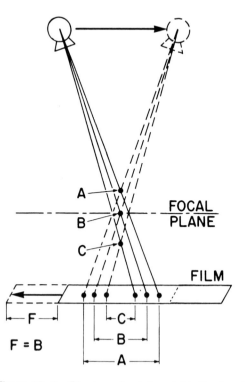

Figure 18–3   Blurring of points outside the focal plane

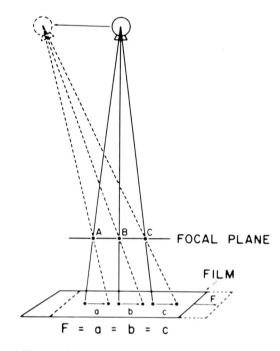

Figure 18–2   Focal plane

Types of Tube Motion

If we look down from the ceiling at the system we have just described, the x-ray tube and film move in a straight line. Appropriately, this is referred to as linear tomography. Many other types of tube motion have been devised. Most of them circumscribe some sort of arc (not to be confused with the arc shown in Figure 18–1B, which is a side view). The six basic types of tube motion in common usage are shown in Figure 18–4. Remember that these are patterns of tube and film motion as seen from above.

TERMINOLOGY

Before going further with our discussion of tomography, it will be helpful to define a few of the terms we have used. **Blurring** is the distortion of definition of objects outside the focal plane. The **fulcrum** is the pivot point about which the lever arm rotates. It determines the plane that will be in focus. Two mechanically different types of fulcrums are in common use. In the first, the relationship between the x-ray tube, fulcrum, and film is fixed. The patient is moved up and down on an adjustable table to bring the level of interest to the plane of the fulcrum. The second type has an adjustable fulcrum that is moved to the height of the desired plane, while the patient remains stationary on the table. The **focal plane** is the plane of maximal focus, and represents the axis (fulcrum) about

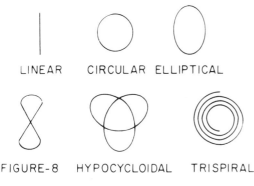

LINEAR CIRCULAR ELLIPTICAL

FIGURE-8 HYPOCYCLOIDAL TRISPIRAL

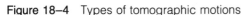

Figure 18–4 Types of tomographic motions

which the x-ray tube and film rotate. The **focal plane level** is the height of the focal plane above the tabletop. The **tomographic angle** (arc) is the amplitude of tube travel expressed in degrees (Fig. 18–1A). The **exposure angle** is the angle through which the x-ray beam (or central ray) moves during the exposure. The tomographic angle and exposure angle are not always equal. Occasionally, x rays are not emitted during part of the tube travel, in which case the tomographic angle is greater than the exposure angle. Sometimes this is intentional, but usually it is the result of an equipment malfunction.

BLURRING

The whole purpose of tomography is to distort, or blur, the objects that might interfere with our perception of a particular radiographic image. To use our equipment to best advantage, we must understand the factors that control blurring. In tomography, the term "blurring" is used only with reference to objects outside the focal plane, and the same term should not be used to describe the image unsharpness inherent in all tomographic systems.

Width of the Blur

The width of the blue refers to the distance over which the image of an object is spread out on the film. It is determined by four factors:

1. amplitude of tube travel
2. distance from the focal plane
3. distance from the film
4. orientation of tube travel.

Each of these will be discussed separately.
Amplitude of Tube Travel. The width of the blur is a direct linear function of the number of degrees of tube travel. As the amplitude of tube travel increases, the width of the blur increases. When the number of degrees of tube motion is doubled, the amount of blurring doubles.
Distance from Focal Plane. The farther an object is from the focal plane, the more

it is blurred. Unfortunately, we have no control over this distance in diagnostic radiology. The relationships between anatomic parts and pathologic lesions are fixed in the patient, and we cannot change them.

Distance from Film. Objects far away from the film are blurred more than objects close to the film (assuming they are both the same distance from the focal plane). The patient should be positioned so that the objects we want to blur are as far from the film as possible.

Orientation of Tube Travel. Many body parts are long and narrow and have a longitudinal axis. When the longitudinal axis of an object is oriented in the same direction that the x-ray tube travels, the image of the object is not blurred, even though it lies outside of the focal plane. Figure 18–5 shows a conventional radiograph (Fig. 18–5A) and a linear tomographic film (Fig. 18–5B) taken on a phantom consisting of multiple crossed and curved wires. The wires are located 1 cm below the focal plane on the tomogram. As you can see, the image of one of the wires is not blurred, and the unblurred wire is the one oriented in the direction of x-ray tube motion. Increasing the tomographic arc will not blur this wire but will merely elongate its image.

Maximum blurring occurs when the long axis of the part to be blurred is perpendicular to the direction of tube travel.

Blur Margin

The edge of a blurred image is called the blur margin. Figure 18–6 shows linear (Fig. 18–6A) and circular (Fig. 18–6B) tomograms of the same test phantom shown in Figure 18–5. As you can see, the blur margins are different with these two types of tube motions. With linear tomography the entire image is uniformly blurred and fades off gradually at its edge. With a circular tube motion, however, the blurred image is not uniform. The margin appears whiter and more sharply defined on the film than the rest of the blur pattern. The reason for the sharply defined border is shown in Figure 18–7. The tube moves both across and parallel to the axis of the wire during different portions of its travel. Maximum blurring occurs as the tube moves across the axis of the wire (a), and this portion of the exposure produces the center of the blur pattern. Little blurring occurs while the tube is moving parallel to the wire's axis (b), and it is during this por-

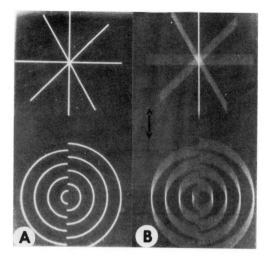

Figure 18–5 Blur patterns with linear tomography. (Courtesy of Dr. J. T. Littleton)

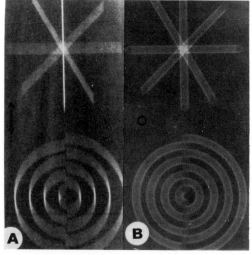

Figure 18–6 Character of blur margins for linear and circular tomography. (Courtesy of Dr. J. T. Littleton)

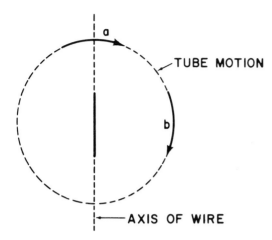

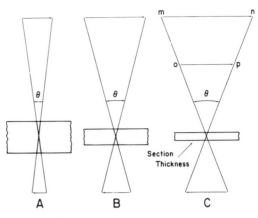

Figure 18–8   Section thickness

Figure 18–7   Circular tomographic motion superimposed on test wire (*top view*)

SECTION THICKNESS

tion of the exposure that the incompletely blurred image is projected to the edge of the blur pattern. This sharply defined blur margin is important in phantom image formation, which we will discuss later in the chapter.

There is no accurate way of defining section thickness. It means the thickness of the section that is in sharp focus on a tomogram. In theory, the focal plane is indeed a "plane" and has no thickness. The image that we see is actually made up of many thin planes superimposed on one another. The closer these planes are to the true focal plane, the sharper they are in focus. There is no abrupt cutoff in sharpness, just a gradual progressive deterioration of image quality as we move away from the focal plane. The point at which the image is no longer considered in focus is subjective. It varies from one observer to another.

Section thickness is inversely proportional to the amplitude of x-ray tube travel (in degrees), as shown in Figure 18–8. The larger the tomographic angle, the thinner the section. In Figure 18–8C, you can see the length of tube travel does not determine the number of degrees in the tomographic arc. The tube moves the same

number of degrees going from point **m** to **n** as it does from point **o** to **p**, although it travels a greater distance between **m** and **n**. With greater target-film distances, the tube must move a greater distance to subscribe the same angle.

Although it is always desirable to have objects outside the focal plane maximally blurred, it is not always desirable to have the section as thin as possible. In fact, if we could cut an infinitely thin section, we would not be able to see it. Imagine a coronal section through the human body only one micron thick. If we could take this section out of the body and x ray it, we could not produce an x-ray image. There would be no contrast. Contrast depends on both the density and thickness of adjacent parts. Without some thickness, there is no contrast and, without contrast, there is no image.

Figure 18–9 shows section thicknesses for various tomographic angles and, as you can see, there is little change with angles larger than 10°. Even though the section thickness does not change with large tomographic arcs, the blurring of objects outside the focal plane does change. Blurring continues to increase as the amplitude of tube travel increases, which is why a film taken with a 10° angle looks a great deal different than one taken with a 50° angle.

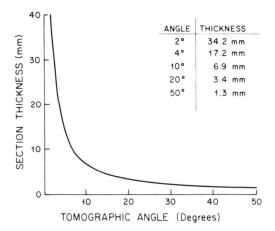

ANGLE	THICKNESS
2°	34.2 mm
4°	17.2 mm
10°	6.9 mm
20°	3.4 mm
50°	1.3 mm

Figure 18–9 Section thickness for various tomographic angles

NARROW- VERSUS WIDE-ANGLE TOMOGRAPHY

We can use tomography to approach a diagnostic problem in two different ways. One system uses a wide tomographic arc, and strives for maximal blurring of obscuring shadows. The other system, usually called zonography, uses a narrow tomographic arc, and attempts to present a view of the whole object, undistorted and sharply defined. The choice depends primarily on the type of tissue we are examining and the nature of the problem. At times the two systems are in conflict, but basically each is designed to do its own particular job.

Wide-Angle Tomography

The purpose of wide-angle tomography is to extend the limits of Roentgen visibility to enable us to see objects that are completely obscured by overlying shadows on conventional roentgenograms. Figure 18–10 illustrates this principle. A series of lead letters are stacked on plastic shelves (*top*). On a standard roentgenogram all the letters are superimposed and obscure each other (*center*), but on the wide-angle tomogram (*bottom*) the letter C becomes clearly visible.

One disadvantage of wide-angle tomography is that it decreases contrast. Adjacent

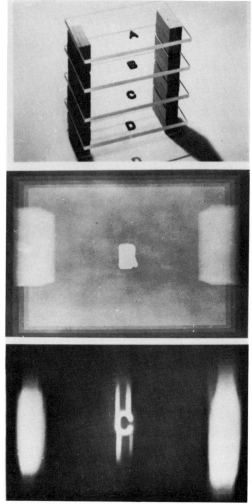

Figure 18–10 Extended visibility with wide-angle tomography. (The Fundamentals of Radiology. Rochester, NY, Eastman Kodak, Radiography Markets Division)

thick parts produce greater image contrast than thin parts of the same radiographic density, and because wide-angle tomography produces thin sections, it reduces image contrast. It is most effective in studying tissues that have a great deal of natural contrast, such as bone. It has been used extensively to examine the inner ear, in which there is still enough contrast to produce good images, even though the section thickness is very thin.

The sharpness of all images is decreased by wide-angle techniques, including those originating from the focal plane; the wider the tomographic arc, the more unsharp the images become. Theoretically, images from the focal plane should be in sharp focus, but in actual practice it is impossible to coordinate the motions of the x-ray tube and film perfectly. Minor vibrations cause unsharpness of the focal plane image, but the newer tomographic units are superbly engineered and unsharpness is minimal.

Narrow-Angle Tomography (Zonography)

Narrow-angle tomography refers to body section roentgenography employing an arc of less than 10°. Zonography is not efficient with linear tomography, and requires a multidirectional tube motion, which in practice is usually circular. Narrow-angle tomography produces undistorted, sharply defined images of the objects on the focal plane. An entire structure is displayed in sharp focus against a background of slight blurring. Our eyes tend to ignore the blurred images. The quality of the primary image is almost as good as it is with conventional roentgenograms, and interference from overlying shadows is diminished.

Zonography is especially useful when the tissues being examined have little natural contrast. Wide-angle techniques diminish contrast, while narrow-angle techniques retain all the natural contrast that is present. Contrast is usually minimal in soft tissue radiography, and zonography is the preferred tomographic method. The lung offers an ideal medium for this technique. Contrast is low, and the interfering ribs are usually several centimeters from our plane of interest. Rib blurring is sufficient to prevent them from interfering with visualization of the primary image.

One of the main objections to narrow-angle tomography is its tendency to produce phantom images. Both the narrow angle and circular motion contribute to phantom image formation. These images will be discussed in more detail later.

Table 18–1 summarizes the differences between wide- and narrow-angle tomography.

CIRCULAR TOMOGRAPHY

The more a tomographic motion differs from the shape of the object being examined, the less likely it is to produce phantom images, so tomographic units have been designed to operate with a wide variety of curvilinear tube motions, including circles, ellipses, hypocycloidals, sinusoids, spirals, and even a random motion. We will limit our discussion to circular tomog-

Table 18–1. A Comparison of Wide- and Narrow-Angle Tomography

WIDE-ANGLE TOMOGRAPHY	NARROW-ANGLE TOMOGRAPHY
1. Tomographic arc of more than 10° (usually 30° to 50°)	1. Tomographic arc of less than 10°
2. Less section thickness	2. Greater section thickness
3. Considerable unsharpness of focal plane images	3. Very little unsharpness of focal plane images
4. Maximum blurring of objects outside focal plane	4. Minimum blurring of objects outside focal plane
5. Best for tissues with high contrast (bone)	5. Best for tissues with low contrast (lung)
6. Can be done with either linear or circular motion	6. Usually done with circular tomographic motion
7. Unlikely to cause phantom images	7. Frequently causes phantom images
8. Long exposure times	8. Short exposure times (with properly designed equipment)

raphy, although the same principles apply to all pluridirectional motions.

The movement of the x-ray tube, film, and grid for circular tomography is shown in Figure 18–11A. The x-ray tube and film are located at opposite ends of a rigid connecting rod. The tube moves in a circular motion, and the film follows at the opposite end of the rod. The film does not revolve as it moves. Point a in Figure 18–11A identifies one side of the film and, as you can see, it remains in the same relative position as the film moves through a 360° circle. The grid must revolve to avoid cutoff, however, because the entire exposure is made with the x-ray tube angled toward the grid. The only way cutoff can be avoided is to revolve the grid to keep the grid lines pointed toward the tube (Fig. 18–11B).

Point a on the grid changes its position as the grid revolves, so that the lead strips of the grid maintain a constant orientation with the target of the x-ray tube. By examining Figure 18–11A and B together, you can see that the grid gradually rotates over the film throughout the 360° cycle. Grid lines are obscured by the relative motion of the x-ray tube and film, and no Bucky mechanism is necessary.

Advantages

The primary advantage of circular tomography is that it produces a uniform section thickness. Figure 18–6 shows the blur pattern of a test phantom obtained with both linear and circular tomographic motions. With a circular motion all portions of the phantom are uniformly blurred, no

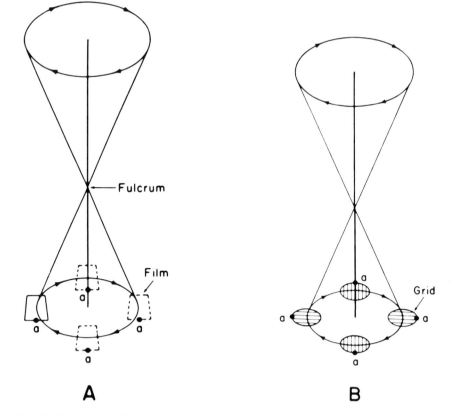

A   **B**

Figure 18–11 Position of film with circular tomography (A) and position of grid with circular tomography (B)

matter how they are oriented in space. Linear tomography does not produce a true section thickness. The amount of blurring is completely dependent on the orientation of the part with reference to tube motion. The only wire in the illustration that is maximally blurred is the one perpendicular to the direction of tube travel. Because linear tomography does not blur all parts uniformly, it frequently produces streaking or "parasite" lines that remain in sharp focus even though they are several centimeters from the focal plane. These lines represent the edges of linear objects oriented along the line of tube motion. They do not occur with circular tomography.

Disadvantages

To most radiologists the principal disadvantage of circular tomography is the high cost of the equipment. Circular tomographic units are much more expensive than linear units, which can usually be adapted to existing equipment. Another disadvantage is the length of time it takes to obtain an exposure. For a standard radiograph, the exposure time is determined primarily by the thickness and density of the part being examined. Tomographic exposure times, however, are determined by the length of time that it takes the tube to complete its arc, which is almost always considerably longer than the time that is needed to expose the film. One of the more popular tomographic units takes 3 seconds to complete a circular motion and 6 seconds for a hypocycloidal motion.* These long exposure times are a great disadvantage, especially for chest radiography, in which there is considerable involuntary motion.

Another disadvantage of circular tomography is the sharp cutoff of the blur patterns, which is conducive to phantom image formation.

Table 18–2 summarizes the differences between linear and circular tomography.

*Polytome, manufactured by Phillips.

COMPLEX TOMOGRAPHIC MOTIONS

The tomographic objective is to blur images of objects outside of the focal plane as much as possible and as uniformly as possible. This can only by fully accomplished with a linear tube motion oriented at right angles to a linear structure. Figure 18–12B shows such an arrangement with three wires displaced 1 cm from the focal plane. The blur pattern of the wire oriented perpendicular to the tomographic motion is perfectly uniform. The blur pattern of the diagonal wire is also uniform, but not maximum. With a circular motion all the wires are blurred to the same degree, and all are maximally blurred, but the blurring is not uniform; that is, the blur margin is more sharply defined than the rest of the blur pattern (Fig. 18–12D). Because no anatomic part is shaped like a wire, the ideal can never be fully accomplished in a clinical setting. The more complex tomographic motions (e.g., ellipses, circles, trispirals, figure 8s, and hypocycloidals) are all designed to improve the uniformity of blurring.

Figure 18–13 demonstrates how the size of the tomographic arc is determined for complex motions. The number of degrees is measured from the extremes of tube motion. In the illustration, the arc is 35° from all four types of tube motion.

Table 18–3 compares the relative length of tube travel for four different tomographic motions. The numbers are only theoretic, because no manufacturer produces a unit that can perform all these motions with a 48° arc. As the type of motion becomes more complex, the length of tube travel increases. Using the 92-cm linear motion as the norm, the relative length of tube travel increases about five times for the hypocycloidal motion. The result is a considerable improvement in the uniformity of blurring. Figure 18–12 shows the blur patterns for several different tomographic motions. As you can see, blurring is more uniform for the more complex mo-

Table 18–2. A Comparison of Linear and Circular Tomography

LINEAR TOMOGRAPHY	CIRCULAR TOMOGRAPHY
1. Equipment is inexpensive	1. Equipment is very expensive
2. Section thickness is dependent on orientation of body parts (no true section thickness)	2. Section thickness is independent of orientation of parts (produces a uniform section thickness)
3. Blur margins are tapered and indistinct	3. Blur margins are abrupt and sharply defined
4. Objects outside the focal plane may be incompletely blurred, producing "parasite" streaks	4. Objects outside the focal plane are uniformly blurred (no "parasite" streaks)
5. Does not produce phantom images	5. Likely to produce phantom images (with narrow-angle tomography)

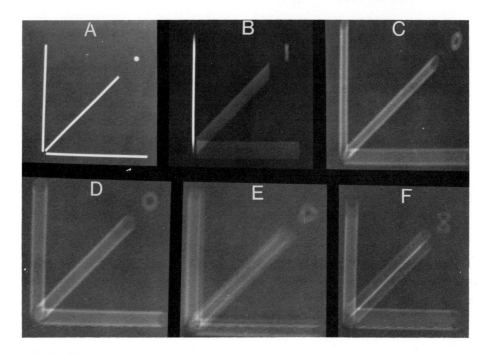

Figure 18–12 Three wire phantoms *(A)* and blur patterns for linear *(B)*, elliptic *(C)*, circular *(D)*, hypocycloidal *(E)*, and figure 8 tomographic motions *(F)*

tions. Increasing the length of tube travel, however, does not necessarily improve blurring. The tomographic motion must be efficiently designed to be effective. For example, running the tube back and forth in a linear motion lengthens tube travel but does not improve the blur pattern. Section thickness is determined solely by the number of degrees in the tomographic arc, and is not affected by the complexity of the tube motion. Note in Table 18–3 that the section thickness is 1.3 mm for all four tomographic movements.

PHANTOM IMAGES

Phantom is defined by Webster as "something that appears to the sight but has no physical existence." Phantom images appear on tomograms, but they do not actually exist. These unreal images are always a little less dense and a little less sharp than real images, but they can still cause considerable difficulty in film interpretation.

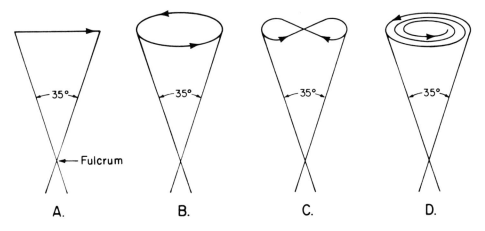

Figure 18–13 Method of determining the tomographic arc for complex motions

Table 18–3. Approximate Length of Tube Travel for Various Tomographic Motions

TYPE OF MOTION	TOMOGRAPHIC ARC (°)	LENGTH OF TUBE TRAVEL (cm)	SECTION THICKNESS (mm)	RELATIVE LENGTH OF TUBE TRAVEL
Linear	48°	92	1.3	1.0
Elliptic	48°	222	1.3	2.4
Circular	48°	292	1.3	3.9
Hypocycloidal*	48°	450	1.3	4.9

*Polytome, Medical Systems Division, North American Phillips Corporation, Shelton, CT; 45″ FFD.

Phantom images are produced by the blurred margins of structures outside of the focal plane, and they are most likely to occur with circular tomography and narrow-angle techniques. With a narrow-angle tube motion, objects outside the focal plane are only minimally blurred. The margins are still fairly distinct, and they tend to produce phantom images. Blurring is so complete with wide-angle tomography that phantom images are unlikely.

Phantom images are formed by two different mechanisms, which we will discuss separately. We should emphasize, however, that the parasite lines that occur in linear tomography are not phantom images. These lines represent the unblurred margins of structures oriented in the same direction as the x-ray tube motion. The images are real and represent structures that do exist.

The first type of phantom image is produced by narrow-angle tomograms of regularly recurring objects, such as the wires shown in Figure 18–14. Three wires are equally spaced a short distance above the focal plane. Figure 18–14A represents a standard radiograph, and Figure 18–14B and C represent tomograms taken with two different arcs. In Figure 18–14A the images of the wires appear as dots. In Figure 18–14B the images are blurred but still separate. In Figure 18–14C the blur margins overlap slightly, and the overlapping edges produce the phantom images. These images are not real and, as you can see, it takes three wires to produce two phantom wires. Bony trabeculae, teeth, ribs, and dye-filled vessels are several of the anatomic parts that are apt to cause phantom image formation.

The second type of phantom image is formed by the displacement of the blurred image from an object outside the focal plane to simulate a less dense structure within the focal plane. Frequently, the

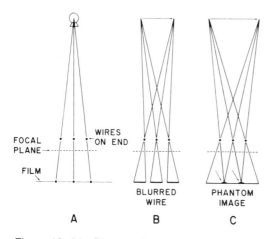

Figure 18–14   Phantom image formation

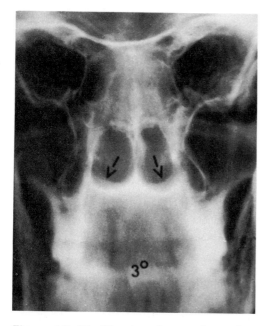

Figure 18–15 Phantom image formation. (Courtesy of Dr. J. T. Littleton)

blurred image of a bone will simulate a soft tissue structure. Figure 18–15 shows a narrow-angle tomogram of a dried skull. The apparent mucosal thickening along the floor of the nasal cavities represents the blurred images of the bone in front of the focal plane. The films were taken with a circular tomographic motion, so the blur

margins are fairly sharp. Because the images are from a dried skull, the apparent mucosal thickening must represent a phantom image. Bone is quite dense and, when it is minimally blurred by narrow-angle tomography, it retains enough density to simulate soft tissue. This type of phantom image formation is most likely to occur when the shape of the part being examined is similar to that of the x-ray tube motion, so it is common with circular tomography about the skull. The same mechanism, however, may produce phantom images in other anatomic areas. For example, a densely calcified granuloma in the chest, when incompletely blurred, may appear on a tomogram as a somewhat larger soft tissue nodule. The density of the calcification is spread out over a larger area so it becomes that of soft tissue, and the margins are sharply defined because of the circular tube motion.

Figure 18–16 shows a conventional radiograph of a nickel (Fig. 18–16A) and three circular tomograms taken with the same coin at slightly different distances from the image plane. One side of the coin is marked with a line that identifies the position of the same edge on all four films. The coin's image is blurred to exactly twice its original diameter in Figure 18–16C, a little less than twice its diameter in Figure 18–16B, and a little more in Figure 18–16D. If the original coin had represented a densely calcified pulmonary granuloma, then the exactly doubled image (Fig. 18–16C) would look like a larger, less dense soft tissue nodule, the less than doubled image (Fig. 18–16B) would look like a nodule with a calcific center, and the more than doubled image would exactly mimic a thick-walled cavitary lesion (Fig. 18–16D). Interpretive errors of this type can be avoided by carefully correlating the tomograms with the plain films.

In summary, phantom images are produced in two ways, by the superimposition of the blur margins of regularly recurring structures, and by displacement of the blur

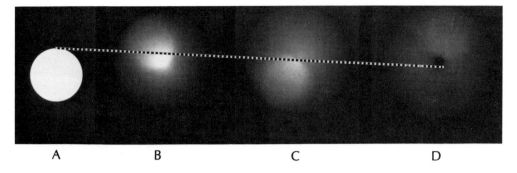

A   B   C   D

Figure 18–16 Plain film of a coin (*A*) and three circular tomograms taken with the coin at different distances from the focal plane (*B–D*)

margins of dense objects to simulate less dense objects. They are most likely to occur with narrow-angle circular tomography, and they are never as dense or as sharply defined as real images.

SIMULTANEOUS MULTIFILM TOMOGRAPHY

The basic principle of simultaneous multifilm tomography is very simple. Several layers of x-ray films are placed in a special "book cassette," and all the films are exposed simultaneously during a single tomographic sweep. The only difference between multifilm and single-film tomography is in the cassette. Figure 18–17 illustrates the principle diagrammatically. There is one mechanical fulcrum (point A) for the top film in the book cassette, and a virtual axis (points B and C) for every other film. The virtual axis is a point in space about which the x-ray film and tube rotate. Its position is determined by the spacing of the films in the cassette. When the films are spaced 1 cm apart the virtual axes are 1 cm apart and each object layer has its own separate fulcrum level. As you can see in Figure 18–17, the top and bottom layers are equally magnified. Even though the lower films are farther from the mechanical fulcrum, the ratio of the tube-fulcrum (real or virtual) distance to the fulcrum-film distance is the same for all levels.

Book Cassette

Simultaneous multifilm tomography is done with a specially designed film holder called a book cassette. Books are usually made up of from three to five sets of x-ray screens separated by x-ray transparent spacers. The spacers are composed of polyurethane sponge, the thickness of which can be varied from $\frac{1}{2}$ to 2 cm. Figure 18–18 shows a five-film cassette with 1-cm spacers. The total thickness of the cassette is 4 cm. The resiliency of the sponge helps to maintain good screen-film contact.

As x rays pass through the book cassette, their intensity decreases because of absorption by the screens and films, and to a lesser extent because of the inverse square law. If all of the screens in a book were of the same speed, the first film would be properly exposed, and the succeeding films would become progressively lighter. To produce a series of equally exposed films, we must "balance the book," by increasing the speed of the screens in each successive layer. The first layer of screens is very slow, the next layer is a little faster, and the last layer is very fast. In this way, all the films are exposed to the same degree of blackness, even though they receive different quantities of radiation. No serious loss in film quality results from the use of the faster screens, because tomographic image quality is not good to begin with.

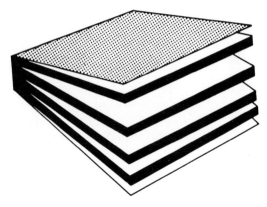

Figure 18–18   Book cassette

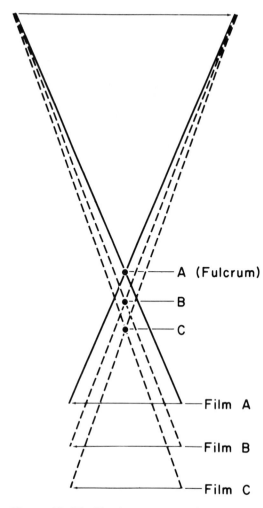

Figure 18–17   Simultaneous multifilm tomography

Advantages

One obvious advantage of simultaneous multifilm tomography is a saving in technologist time and equipment load, but this should only be a secondary consideration. Patients receive smaller doses of radiation with multifilm tomography, and this is its greatest advantage. When five films are produced with a single exposure, there is a definite decrease in the patient's radiation dose. The saving is not as great, however, as the 5:1 film-production ratio suggests. Remember, the first pair of screens in a book cassette is slow, so the exposure factors must be increased over those required for a single-film technique. The patient's exposure dose per film is approximately half as much with simultaneous multifilm tomography. This means that two films can be exposed with the same amount of radiation that would be required to expose a single film with conventional tomography. The exact figure will vary somewhat, depending on the thickness of the book cassette. Another advantage of the book cassette is that it allows us to obtain tomograms at various levels during one physiologic cycle. We can be sure that the difference between films represents a real change in the structure that we are examining, and not merely a change in position that took place in the interval between exposures.

Plesiosectional tomography refers to a somewhat different multifilm system that is used to obtain tomograms at 1-mm intervals. No spacers are used in the book cassette. A pair of screens is about 1 mm thick, so they serve as their own spacers.

A properly balanced book only functions effectively in a limited kVp range. Most books are balanced to produce films of uniform density at about 80 kVp and, if you use them at much lower or higher energies, they are likely to be out of balance. At lower energies, the lower films in the cassette become progressively lighter.

Disadvantage

The one serious problem that plagues simultaneous multifilm tomography is uncontrolled scatter radiation. Film quality is never as good as it is with a single-film technique. The lower films in the book cassette are fogged by scattered photons from the upper layers, and the amount of scatter radiation increases as the thickness of the book cassette and energy of the radiation increase. Because of the poor image quality associated with multifilm techniques, most radiologists prefer single-film tomography.

DETERMINATION OF TOMOGRAPHIC ANGLE

Hundreds of different phantoms and multiple ingenious methods have been devised to study the characteristics of tomographic units. We will only discuss one, the pinhole camera technique described by Hodes and coworkers.[1] Figure 18–19 illustrates the principle. The only special equipment you need, in addition to the tomographic unit, is a sheet of lead with a small hole in its center. The lead is positioned at the level of the focal plane, and a film is placed on the x-ray table directly under the center of the pinhole. The film remains stationary throughout the test. It is exposed twice, the first time with the x-ray tube perpendicular to the center of the film to mark the center of the tomographic arc, and the second time while the tube swings through its arc to record a series of superimposed dots that are a record of the tomographic motion. The line of dots produced on the film by the pinhole technique gives us the following information:

1. It is a geometric presentation of the type of tube motion (e.g., linear, circular, hypocycloidal, etc.).
2. It makes it possible for us to calculate the length of the exposure angle, which is the number of degrees of tube motion during which x rays are emitted. We only need to know two sides of a triangle for the calculation. The first side is the distance between

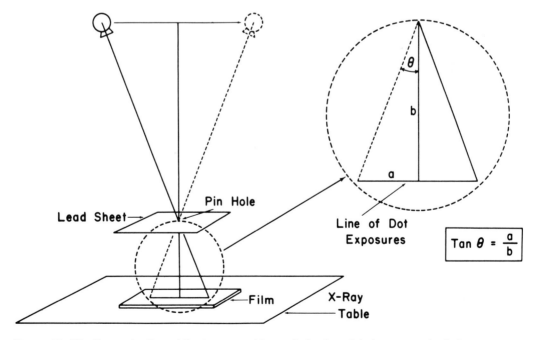

$$\text{Tan } \theta = \frac{a}{b}$$

Figure 18–19 Determination of the tomographic angle by the pinhole camera technique

the pinhole and the film, and the second side is recorded on the film as shown in Figure 18–19 (*insert*). We can calculate the tomographic angle from the formula given in the illustration.

3. It shows us the symmetry of the exposure angle. With a properly functioning unit, the exposed dotted line will be equal in length on either side of the center of the tomographic arc. If the line is asymmetric, each side must be calculated separately, and then the two sides added to find the true exposure angle.

SPECIAL TOMOGRAPHIC TECHNIQUES

Axial Transverse Tomography

In all the tomographic techniques that we have described, tomographic sections are cut through the coronal plane of the patient. In axial transverse tomography the plane of the section runs through the patient transversely (Fig. 18–20). The patient sits in a special rotating chair in an upright position. The x-ray film lies flat on a rotating horizontal table beside the patient (Fig. 18–21). The table is positioned a little below the desired focal plane. X rays are directed obliquely through the patient and onto the film. The x-ray tube remains stationary throughout the exposure. The pa-

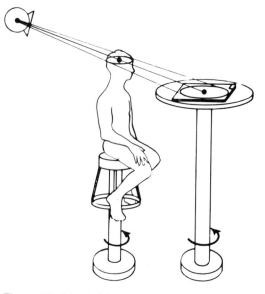

Figure 18–21   Axial transverse tomography

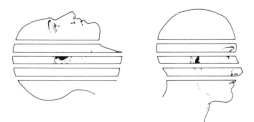

CONVENTIONAL TOMOGRAPHY   **AXIAL TRANSVERSE TOMOGRAPHY**

Figure 18–20   Orientation of the focal plane with conventional (A) and axial transverse tomography (B)

tient and film both rotate in the same direction and at the same velocity. Only those points actually on the focal plane remain in sharp focus throughout a rotation. Points above and below the focal plane are blurred. The section thickness is determined by the angle between the x-ray tube and film. The more obliquely the central ray is directed toward the film, the thinner is the tomographic section. Because the x-ray beam passes through a considerable thickness of tissue, it is usually necessary to use an x-ray grid. The grid is placed as close to the x-ray film as possible, and it remains stationary while the film rotates. Grid lines are blurred by the relative motion between the film and grid.

Axial transverse tomography does not distort the radiographic image. Distortion is produced by unequal magnification. When one portion of an object is more magnified than another portion, its image is distorted. In axial transverse tomography, however, points close to the film are also close to the x-ray target, and points far from the film are far from the target, so the object-film to object-target ratios are all the same. Because all points are equally magnified, the image is not distorted.

"Skip" Tomography

"Skip" tomography is a tomographic method that stops the exposure through a portion of the tube's motion. Occasionally the object of interest is completely obscured during the central portion of the tomographic arc by dense superimposed structures. Because no useful image is produced on the film during this portion of the exposure, if it is omitted, the overall tomographic effect is improved. Figure 18–22 illustrates the principle. The exposure is skipped during the central portion of the tomographic arc, when the dense vertebral structures are superimposed over our point of interest. The method is only applicable to wide-angle techniques in which the goal is to broaden the limits of visualization. Usually about 20° of the tomographic angle is skipped. The technique only works well when there is a fairly large distance between the object of interest and the object to be blurred.

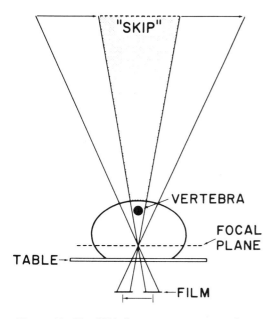

Figure 18–22 "Skip" exposure tomography

Autotomography

Autotomography is a technique designed to show the midline structures of the brain stem (aqueduct and fourth ventricle) during pneumoencephalography (Fig. 18–23). The x-ray tube and film both remain stationary while the head is rotated back and forth through an angle of approximately 10°. The only structures that remain in focus are those located along the axis of rotation. Other structures are blurred, including the dense petrous portion of the temporal bone, which tends to obscure the delicate architecture of the brain stem.

Pantomography

Pantomography is a special radiographic technique that produces a panoramic roentgenogram of a curved surface. The patient sits in a chair and remains stationary through the examination (Fig. 18–24). The x-ray tube and film holder both rotate during the exposure. The film holder has a protective lead front, and is considerably longer than the film. The film is exposed through a narrow slit in its holder. The film moves across this slit as the x-ray tube rotates, and the radiographic image is "laid out" as the film passes by the slit, in much the same way that paint is applied to a wall with a roller. The resultant roentgenogram is a flattened out image of a curved surface. The rounded configuration of the mandible and teeth are especially well suited to pantomography, and it is widely used in dentistry. Pantomograms of the jaw show

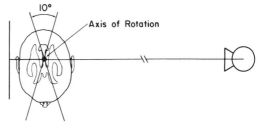
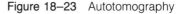

Figure 18–23 Autotomography

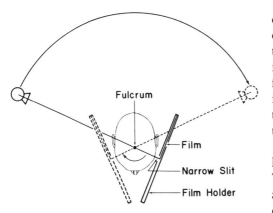

Figure 18–24   Pantomography

the temporomandibular joints on either side of the film with the teeth laid out between them (Fig. 18–25).

SUMMARY

Body section radiography is a special x-ray technique that blurs out the shadow of superimposed structures to show more clearly the principal structures being examined. The x-ray tube and film are connected by a rigid rod, which rotates about a fulcrum. When the tube moves in one direction, the film moves in the opposite direction. The level of the fulcrum is called the focal plane. Images originating at the focal plane level are in sharp focus on the film. The thickness of the section that is in focus depends on the amplitude of tube travel (in degrees). The larger the amplitude, the thinner the section.

If an object is located above or below the level of the focal plane, its image is blurred. The amount of blurring depends on the amplitude of tube travel, distance of the object from the focal plane and film and, in linear tomography, the orientation of the long axis of the part in relation to the direction of tube travel.

Pluridirectional tube motions (e.g., circles, ellipses, hypocycloidals, and spirals) are superior to linear motion because they produce a uniform section thickness, that is, one that is independent of the orientation of the long axis of the part to be blurred. Pluridirectional motions produce a sharply defined blur margin, however, and they are more likely to produce phantom images, especially with small tomographic angles.

Simultaneous multifilm tomography,

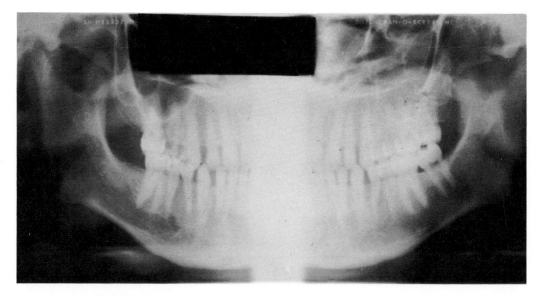

Figure 18–25   Pantomogram of the mandible

employing a book cassettte, exposes more than one film with a single tomographic exposure. These techniques diminish the patient's radiation exposure, but they produce poorer quality tomograms. Recently most radiologists have abandoned simultaneous multifilm techniques.

Axial transverse tomography is a special technique that produces a cross-sectional tomogram. Autotomography, in which the patient is rotated along his central axis, produces a linear image plane in which all points are blurred except those along the axis of rotation. Pantomography is a special x-ray technique that produces a panoramic roentgenogram of a curved surface.

REFERENCES

1. Hodes, P.J., De Moor, J., and Ernst, R.: Body section radiography: Fundamentals. Radiol. Clin. North Am., 6:229, 1963.
2. Littleton, J.T.: A phantom method to evaluate the clinical effectiveness of tomographic devices. Am. J. Roentgenol., 108:847, 1970.
3. National Bureau of Standards: Methods of Evaluating Radiological Equipment and Materials. Washington, DC, National Bureau of Standards, 1963, Handbook 89.

19

Stereoscopy

J. MacKenzie Davidson introduced stereoscopy to radiology in 1898, and it won immediate and widespread acceptance. Stereoscopy grew in popularity, and by 1930 most radiographs were taken stereoscopically. You can gain some insight into its popularity from a statement made by Jarre and Teschendorf in 1933:

> A discussion of roentgen stereoscopy and some of its phases may seem rather unnecessary; no American roentgenologist doubts the advantages to be derived from the study of stereo-roentgenograms. To the well-informed observer it is even apparent that frequently overemphasis is placed upon the esthetic satisfaction of the tridimensional image, especially by many a young clinician using roentgenograms rather casually to the point of refusal of any non-stereo projection no matter how instructive it may be.[4]

Stereoscopy had reached the height of its popularity. Then, gradually, the pendulum began to swing.

The first step in the decline of stereoscopy was probably the result of its earlier overemphasis. When we expect too much we are frequently disappointed, and stereoscopy was no exception to this dictum. In addition, routine stereoscopy is expensive and time-consuming. The death blow came with the discovery that radiation causes mutations. The popularity of stereoscopy dropped precipitously, and the pendulum made its full swing. Unfortunately, stereoscopy is no longer used by many radiologists. Throughout the country stereoscopes are collecting dust, being placed in x-ray museums along with gas x-ray tubes as a remembrance of the past or, even more humiliating, serving as stands for coffee pots.

Although we agree that stereoscopy was overemphasized in the past, this does not justify its present abandonment. Stereoscopic roentgenograms can give information that cannot be obtained in any other way, or at least not as easily in any other way. When properly used, it is still a valuable tool, and worthy of the attention of all radiologists.

PHYSIOLOGY OF DEPTH PERCEPTION

A basic knowledge of the physiology of depth perception is essential to an understanding of the principles behind stereoscopic filming and viewing systems. Depth perception is extremely complex and has some serious limitations. It depends on two completely independent mechanisms: the first, monocular or photographic depth perception, requires only one eye; the second, stereopsis, requires binocular vision. We will discuss each mechanism separately.

Monocular Depth Perception

Monocular depth perception is familiar to all accomplished artists. The artist depicts depth the same way we see depth with one eye. The mechanisms are as follows.

Size. Near objects are larger than distant objects.

Overlapping Contours. Near objects overlap distant objects.

Perspective. We see objects from a particular vantage point, or perspective. By following lines and contours we gain a sense of depth.

Shading. A sphere has the contour of a circle, but with proper shading we perceive its true shape.

Air Haze. Water vapor, dust, and smoke in the atmosphere absorb and reflect light, casting a veil over distant objects and causing them to appear farther away and less sharp.

These monocular mechanisms of depth perception are of little value in interpreting radiographs. Object size may occasionally give us some concept of depth, provided that two objects known to be the same size are both visible on one film. Perspective is of some value in determining depth, but only after we have become thoroughly familiar with anatomy. In a crude sort of way, unsharpness from penumbra is comparable to air haze; that is, objects close to the film are sharper than objects far from the film. Overlapping contours and shading contribute nothing to depth perception in radiography. In general, there is little that allows us to see depth on a single radiograph.

Stereopsis

Binocular depth perception, called stereopsis, is a unique characteristic of man and other primates. It is dependent on the brain's ability to receive slightly different images from each eye, **discrepant images,** and then to fuse them into a single image that has depth. Discrepant images are the heart of stereopsis, and fusion occurs in the brain. The degree of discrepancy is of vital importance. If the images are too different, the brain cannot fuse them, and the stereoscopic effect is lost. If the difference is too small, the fused images appear flat.

Accommodation and Convergence

In the past, physiologists thought that accommodation and convergence were responsible for stereoscopic depth perception, but now it is known that they play only a passive role. Accommodation is the ability to change the curvature of the lens with a change in visual distance. Convergence is a turning in of the optical axes so that both eyes can see the same object. The ciliary muscles, which regulate the curvature of the lens, and the internal rectus muscles, which converge the eys, do not send the impulses that allow us to perceive depth. They are responsible for the mechanical changes, however, that produce discrepant images from the two eyes, so they play a major role in stereopsis, but only in a subservient manner. They are involved in the mechanism of image formation, but not in the actual perception of depth.

Relative and Absolute Depth Perception

There are two types of depth perception: one relative, the other absolute. Relative depth perception is the ability to distinguish which of two objects is closer to the observer. Absolute depth perception is the ability to judge how far away an object is, or the distance between two objects. One is qualitative and the other quantitative. Stereopsis is relative. It only allows us to distinguish which of two objects is closer to us. To judge the distance between them accurately, we rely exclusively on monocular depth perception. Because monocular depth perception is of no value in interpreting radiographs, x-ray stereoscopy is only relative. It is a rank order type of depth perception. We can accurately rank objects in their order of closeness, but we cannot accurately judge the distance between them. A failure to appreciate this fact is one reason why some radiologists have been disappointed in stereoscopy.

Parallax

Parallax is the apparent displacement of an object when viewed from two different vantage points. In Figure 19–1, point A moves with respect to point B as the view shifts from one eye to the other eye. The convergent angle, α, is larger from A than

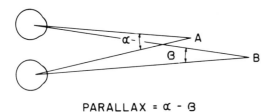

PARALLAX = α - β

Figure 19–1   Parallax

from B (β), and the difference is called the angle of instantaneous parallax. As points A and B are moved closer together, eventually the angle of instantaneous parallax becomes so small that the brain can no longer recognize a difference between the images from the two eyes. The smallest recognizable angle has been found experimentally to be between 1.6 and 24 seconds of arc, depending on the investigator.[2] We can use this information to calculate the in-depth resolution of a stereoscopic filming system. If we use the largest reported angle of instantaneous parallax (24 sec), a 40-inch filming distance, and a 4-inch stereo tube shift, we should be able to recognize a difference in depth between two adjacent objects of slightly less than $\frac{1}{16}$ inch, which is sufficiently accurate to meet most of our radiologic needs.

STEREOSCOPIC FILMING

Stereoscopic filming techniques are simple, and usually require no special equipment. Two films are exposed, one for each eye. Figure 19–2 shows the relationship between the x-ray tube, patient, and film. The film is changed between exposures. The second film should be placed in exactly the same position as the first film. The tube is shifted from the left to the right eye position between exposures, and it is the only part that moves. The patient must remain absolutely still. Usually the film is placed in a Bucky tray under the grid so that it can be changed without disturbing the patient. If the examination does not require a grid, the film is placed in a flat box with an open

end (stereo tunnel), as shown in Figure 19–2.

Magnitude of Tube Shift

In the past, radiologists thought that the stereoscopic tube shift had to be equal to the interpupillary distance (2.6 inches), but now we know that this is neither necessary nor desirable. The optimal quantity of tube shift is empiric. We have learned by trial and error that a tube shift equal to 10% of the target-film distance produces satisfactory results. A 10% shift is simple to apply and produces discrepant images, which is the only prerequisite to stereoscopic image formation. For example, if the filming distance is 40 inches, the tube shift will be 4 inches.

In some radiographic units, especially head units, the x-ray tube and film are mounted on rigid connecting rods, so that the tube moves in an arc. With these units it is easier to shift the tube a certain number of degrees rather than a specific distance. Referring to Figure 19–3, and applying the 10% rule, you can see that a 10% tube shift is equal to an angle (θ) of approximately 6°. This angle will always be the same, regardless of the filming distance. The entire 4 inches (or .6°) tube shift in Figure 19–3

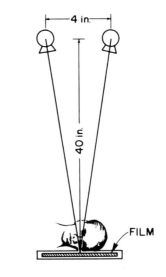

Figure 19–2   Stereoscopic filming

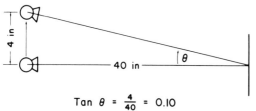

$$\text{Tan } \theta = \frac{4}{40} = 0.10$$

$$\theta \backsim 6°$$

Figure 19–3 Stereoscopic tube shift

is in one direction, which is perfectly acceptable, although it is more customary to shift 2 inches on either side of center.

Direction of Tube Shift

The direction of tube shift is important for two reasons. First, many stereoscopic examinations are done with grid techniques, and it is undesirable to shift across the long axis of a grid because of grid cutoff from lateral decentering (see Chap. 8). In general, all grid-type techniques should be done with a longitudinal tube shift (i.e., along the long axis of the grid). If there is a compelling reason for using a cross shift, then you should use a low-ratio grid. Usually you can expect satisfactory films with a 10% cross shift on an 8:1 or lower ratio grid, but at the expense of increased patient exposure. Both exposures should be made with exactly the same tube shift to either side of grid center. If the shift is greater to one side, the films will not be equally exposed. Under no circumstances should you attempt a cross shift with a 12:1 or higher ratio grid. The chances of obtaining a satisfactory study are slight, and patient exposures are excessive because of grid cutoff from lateral decentering.

The direction of tube shift is important for a second reason. The objective in stereoscopic filming is to produce discrepant images. The tube shift should be in the direction that produces maximum discrepancy. In Figure 19–4, the tube was shifted across the axes of the lines to produce maximum image discrepancy. If the tube had been shifted along the longitudinal axes of

the lines, the difference between the two images would be less, and the stereoscopic effect would be correspondingly less. In this respect, stereoscopy is closely related to tomography. Both use a tube shift, and both yield best results when the tube is shifted across the long axis of the part being examined. You can think of the lines in Figure 19–4 as the tibia and fibula, the anterior and posterior ribs, or the front and back cortices of a joint. In each case the stereoscopic effect is greatest when the tube is shifted across the lines of interest.

STEREOSCOPIC VIEWING

The stereoscope is an optical instrument used to superimpose two pictures taken from slightly different vantage points. It was invented by Wheatstone in 1838, long before Roentgen discovered x rays. Since that time, many different designs have been described.

Preliminary Steps

Before we can view films stereoscopically, there are three preliminary steps we must follow to determine how the films should be oriented for stereoscopic viewing.

The first step is to **identify the tube side of the film,** that is, the side that is closer to the patient and thus facing the x-ray tube during the exposure. Usually we read x-ray films as if the patient were facing us. For example, frontal films of the skull are usually taken PA (i.e., with the patient facing the film). Most radiologists, however, read the films as if the patient were facing them. For stereoscopic viewing, we should think of our eyes as the tube, and view the patient as if he were standing between us and the film. If we do not do this, the left and right sides are likely to be reversed.

The next step is to **determine the direction of the x-ray tube shift.** In Figure 19–5, the films in the upper illustration were obtained with a cross shift, and those in the lower illustration with a longitudinal shift. The films must be viewed as shown to pre-

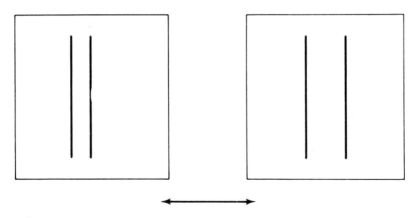

Figure 19–4 Stereoscopic images

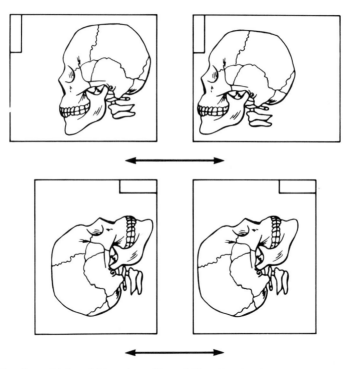

Figure 19–5 Direction of tube shift and position of films for viewing

sent the eyes with discrepant images. If the films are viewed in any other way, there will be no stereoscopic effect. Usually the direction of tube shift is determined by superimposing the images on the films (Fig. 19–6). The two edges of the film that superimpose (*upper* and *lower* in the illustration) represent the axis along which the x-ray tube shifted.

The last preliminary step is to **determine which film is to be viewed by the left eye, and which by the right eye.** Each eye must view its appropriate film. The whole concept of film placement is simplified if we merely think of ourselves as the x-ray tube. Our right eye represents the tube when it is on the right side, and our left eye represents the tube from the left side. Now, if

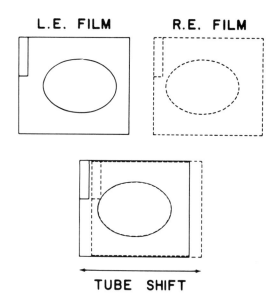

Figure 19–6   Right and left eye films

we place the patient between us and the film, we are duplicating the manner in which the films were taken, and this is exactly the manner in which they must be viewed. Referring again to Figure 19–6, when the two films are superimposed, the right eye film will project out on the right side. If you just think of how they are taken, you can usually tell by inspection which is the right eye film. When the exposure is made from the right eye side, the image is projected over toward the left side of the film, and vice versa for the left eye exposure.

If you superimpose the images on a pair of stereo films, the two edges of the films do not superimpose, then one (or more) of three things went wrong: (1) the patient moved, and the stereoscopic effect was lost; (2) the second film was put in a different position than the first film, in which case the study is still perfectly satisfactory, but the films must ve viewed a little askew, with one film higher in the view box than the other (Fig. 19–7A); or (3) the tube moved in two directions during the stereo shift. Again, the study is usually salvageable, but the films must be viewed diagonally so that our eyes converge along the true direction

of tube shift (Fig. 19–7B). The only way of determining which of the three errors actually occurred is to put the films up in various positions and attempt to view them stereoscopically.

In summary, to keep the image of the patient properly oriented with regard to left and right, we must view stereoscopic films from the tube side, with our eyes converging along the direction of tube shift, and with each eye viewing its appropriate film.

Viewing Systems

Formerly, it was felt that the filming and viewing distances had to be the same or the distance between objects would be distorted. Before discussing individual viewing systems, we must clarify this point. Stereopsis, or binocular depth perception, is only qualitative. **With stereoscopic radiographs we are incapable of judging the absolute distance between objects.** All we can appreciate is which of two objects is closer to us (i.e., a rank order type of depth perception). All we need for stereopsis are discrepant images, and the degree of discrepancy must be sufficiently great to permit an appreciation of depth, and yet not

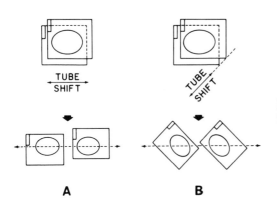

TUBE
SHIFT

TUBE SHIFT

A   B

Figure 19–7 Stereoscopic viewing of films taken improperly

so great that the brain cannot fuse the images. With this fact in mind, we can understand why the film reading distance is not important. Whatever distance is convenient and comfortable is perfectly adequate. The same stereoscope can be used to interpret all stereoscopic films, no matter what distance was used for the exposure.

Cross-Eyed Stereoscopy

In the routine interpretation of roentgenograms, both eyes are focused at a single area of interest, accommodation and convergence are coordinated, and both eyes see identical structures in sharp focus. With cross-eyed stereoscopy, two films are interpreted at the same time (Fig. 19–8). Accommodation and convergence must be dissociated. Our eyes cross so the right eye sees the film on the left side, and both eyes converge to point C in the illustration. If our eyes also accommodated for point C, the films would be out of focus because they are much farther away. Therefore we must converge on a point considerably in front of the films and still accommodate to the plane of the films. This dissociation requires a lot of practice, causes eye strain, and for many people, produces an image that is reduced in size or out of focus.

In spite of all these difficulties, many radiologists have become quite proficient at cross-eyed stereoscopy. You can test your own ability on Figure 19–4. Hold a finger between your eyes and the illustration, and focus both eyes on your finger. In the background you will see three images. The image in the center is formed by the fusion of the left and right eye images, and it has depth. Concentrate on it. If you are seeing stereoscopically, the right line will be suspended in space above the page. It takes a lot of practice to become proficient, but with enough effort you can master it.

Because no special equipment is needed, cross-eyed stereoscopy has two advantages over any other system. It costs nothing, and it is always available. It is certainly the most convenient system to use.

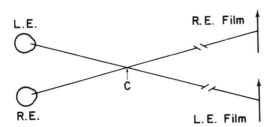

L.E.   R.E. Film

C

R.E.   L.E. Film

Figure 19–8 Cross-eyed stereoscopy

Wheatstone Stereoscope

The principal disadvantage of cross-eyed stereoscopy is that it requires a dissociation of accommodation and convergence. All other stereoscopic systems are designed to overcome this disadvantage. The Wheatstone stereoscope will be used to illustrate how they function. With a Wheatstone unit, convergence is assisted by a pair of mirrors that are located halfway between the films (Fig. 19–9). We accommodate to the plane of the films and view reflected mirror images. The mirrors are adjusted to superimpose the right and left eye films without changing our convergent effort from what it would normally be for the viewing distance. We see a stereoscopic image hanging in space behind the mirrors and, because accommodation and convergence are coordinated to the same distance, our eyes feel no strain. All other stereoscopes operate on the same principle using either mirrors or prisms to assist the eye in convergence. In stereoscopes containing mirrors, the mirrors reverse the left and right sides of the patient's image; that is, they produce mirror images. To compensate for the reversal, the films must be turned over, so that they are viewed from the side away from the x-ray tube. This reverses the image again and brings it back into proper orientation.

Many other stereoscopes have been designed, but we will mention only a few of them. Figure 19–10 shows a stereoscope designed by Caldwell in 1906.[1] It consists of a pair of prisms mounted into binoculars. The unit is compact and convenient to use. Gass and Hatchett have described a similar system, in which they mounted a pair of thin prisms into eyeglasses.[3] The simplest stereoscope, described by Kerekes, requires only a small pocket mirror and a steady hand.[5] The mirror is held against the side of the nose and both eyes focus on the left eye film (Fig. 19–11). The mirror is adjusted to interrupt the view of the right eye, which then sees a mirror image of the right eye film. The mirror is carefully adjusted until the left and right eye images superimpose and are fused into a combined image having depth. Because the right eye sees a mirror image, the film must be reversed so that both images are seen in the same orientation. The mirror should be silvered on its front surface because of the high angle of reflection. The primary disadvantage of this system is that it is difficult to hold the mirror steady.

Many other stereoscopes have been designed, most of them using two or more mirrors to assist the eyes in convergence.

Figure 19–9   Wheatstone stereoscope

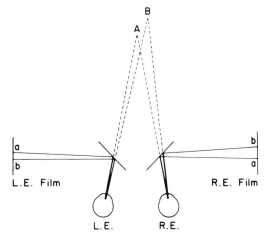

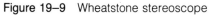

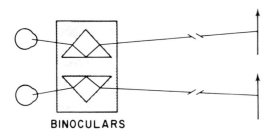

BINOCULARS

Figure 19–10 Binocular prism stereoscope

They all work well, but they have one disadvantage in common. They greatly limit the number of viewers. In fact, most of them allow only one person to see the films. Two other systems have been devised that at least partially overcome this difficulty. One system uses polarized light,[6] and the other colored filters.[7] They will be discussed under stereofluoroscopy.

ADVANTAGES AND DISADVANTAGES
Advantages

The advantages (or perhaps **uses** is a better term) of stereoscopy depend on the skill of the stereoscopist. We will discuss only a few of the situations in which we have found stereoscopy to be helpful. The list could be extended considerably.

Education. The teaching of normal anatomy is simplified with stereoscopic images. Lines that are superimposed into a confusing array for the novice migrate to their true position in depth, and they create a perspective that is not possible on a single film.

Foreign Body Localization. Stereoscopy cannot compete with a pair of right-angle radiographs for localization of a single foreign body. Stereoscopy is superior for the localization of many foreign bodies, such as multiple pellets from a shotgun wound. It allows us to localize each object from a single vantage point. With two right-angle films, it is not always possible to identify one particular foreign body on both films, because they all look alike.

Localization of Intracranial Calcifications. Some intracranial calcifications are so small that they can only be seen on the lateral view, and the only way they can be localized is with stereoscopic films. In fact, some calcifications can only be recognized stereoscopically.

Unimposing Confusing Shadows. The more confusing a radiograph is, the more likely stereoscopy is to be helpful. For example, a collection of gas in the colon may be impossible to differentiate from a destructive lesion in the pelvis on a single film. A good stereoscopist can recognize the true situation with ease. You can argue that a repeat film the next day would solve the problem, and you are correct. Almost all problems can be solved without resorting to stereoscopic films, but frequently stereoscopy offers the simplest solution.

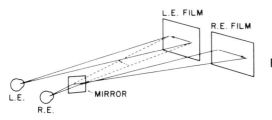

L.E. FILM

R.E. FILM

L.E.

R.E.

MIRROR

Figure 19–11 Single-mirror stereoscope

Disadvantages

The disadvantages of stereoscopy are much better defined than the advantages.

Expense. Stereoscopy requires two films, which adds to the cost of an examination. It requires more technician time, is wearing on the equipment, and doubles the cost of films and processing.

Patient Exposure. The principal disadvantage of stereoscopy, the reason it should not be used routinely, is the increased patient exposure required to produce two films.

Need for Patient Cooperation. Because the patient must remain perfectly still between exposures, stereoscopy cannot be used on patients who are unable to cooperate.

Need for Practice. To become and remain a good stereoscopist, you must practice. The more stereoscopy you do, the better you will become. Most of us only dust off our stereoscopes when we have a problem and, in the long interval between examinations, we become rusty and lose our confidence. Stereoscopy should be practiced daily; routine lateral skull films are probably the most satisfactory study to use, because they frequently give information that cannot be obtained in any other way.

STEREOFLUOROSCOPY

Researchers have been working on stereofluoroscopy for almost 70 years, but have not developed a system that has gained widespread clinical acceptance. Stauffer and coworkers have reported on two different methods. The first employs two x-ray tubes and two image-orthicon television cameras (Fig. 19–12).[8] The x-ray tubes fire alternately, and the cameras are synchronized with the tubes. One camera records a right and the other a left eye image. The images are displayed on two television monitors mounted at right angles to each other. A semitransparent beam-splitting mirror permits observation of both monitors at the same time. The light from the monitors is polarized, and

is viewed through polarized eyeglasses. One image is polarized vertically, the other horizontally, and the glasses are similarly oriented. If you follow the light waves in Figure 19–13, you can see that after light is polarized vertically, it can only be seen with a vertically oriented polarized lens. Similarly, the other eye sees the light that is polarized horizontally. The beam-splitting mirror reflects and transmits equal quantities of light, which permits superimposition of the slightly different, or discrepant, images.

A second more compact system has been described by Stauffer et al.[7] This system employs a twin-target stereoscopic x-ray tube, one image intensifier, and one image-orthicon color camera. The x-ray tube and color television camera are synchronized so that the camera records both a right and a left eye image alternately 30 times per second. Both images are displayed on a single television monitor, one image in red and the other in green. Each second the monitor alternately flashes 30 red and 30 green images, which are viewed by an observer wearing red and green glasses. Each eye sees a slightly different image from a single monitor; the fusion of these two images produces a stereoscopic picture.

Polarized light and colored filters can also be used to view standard stereoscopic radiographs. The polarized system is set up exactly as shown in the right-hand side of Figure 19–12. Conventional view boxes are used in place of the television monitors, one holding the left and the other the right eye film. With a color system the view boxes are arranged in the same manner, but the polarizing material is replaced with colored filters. Each eye sees its appropriate film through colored glasses with the aid of a semitransparent beam-splitting mirror.

SUMMARY

Stereoscopic filming techniques are simple and require no special equipment. Two films are exposed, one for each eye. Between exposures, the x-ray tube is shifted

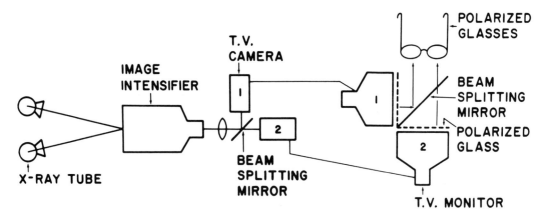

Figure 19–12   Stereofluoroscopy. (Modified from Stauffer et al.[7])

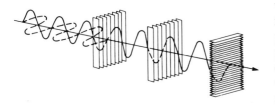

Figure 19–13   Polarized light

10% of the target-film distance (6°); the films are changed, taking care to position the second film in exactly the same position as the first film. The films of the stereoscopic pair present the eye with slightly different, or discrepant, images. Many viewing systems are available, but all accomplish the same purpose. They assist the eyes in coordinating accommodation and convergence. Stereoscopic depth perception is only relative, a rank order type of depth perception, which ranks objects in their order of closeness but does not disclose the distance between them. A failure to appreciate this fact is one reason why some radiologists have been disappointed in stereoscopy.

Stereoscopy has several serious disad-vantages. The examination requires two films, so that it is costly and doubles the patient's radiation exposure. Because the patient must remain perfectly still between exposures, it cannot be used on patients who are unable to cooperate. In spite of these disadvantages, stereoscopy is still a valuable tool, and frequently offers the simplest solution to a difficult radiologic problem.

REFERENCES

1. Caldwell, E.W.: The stereoscope in roentgenology. Am. J. Roentgenol., 5:554, 1918.
2. Davson, H.: The Physiology of the Eye. 2nd Ed. Boston, Little, Brown and Company, 1963.
3. Gass, C.C., and Hatchett, C.S.: A simple inexpensive set of prisms for viewing stereoscopic roentgenograms. Am. J. Roentgenol., 61:715, 1949.
4. Jarre, H.A., and Teschendorf, O.E.W.: Roentgen stereoscopy: A review of its present status. Radiology, 21:139, 1933.
5. Kerekes, E.S.: A simple device for stereoscopic viewing of films. Am. J. Roentgenol., 75:140, 1956.
6. Stamm, R.W.: The polaroid stereoscope. Am. J. Roentgenol., 45:744, 1941.
7. Stauffer, H.M., Haas, C., and Blackstone, A.W.: Progress in stereofluoroscopy "transmissions." Radiology, 82:125, 1964.
8. Stauffer, H.M., Henny, G.C., and Blackstone, A.W.: Stereoscopic television fluoroscopy. Radiology, 79:30, 1962.

20

Magnification Radiography

We have previously discussed the geometric principles of direct x-ray magnification. If the distance between the x-ray tube and the film (focus-film distance) remains constant, magnification of the image of an object will increase as the object is moved away from the film and closer to the tube. The degree of magnification is the ratio of the focus-film distance and focus-object distance:

$$\text{Magnification} = \frac{\text{focus-film distance}}{\text{focus-object distance}}$$

The standard focus-film distance is 40 inches. If a magnification of 2 is desired, the object is placed halfway between the x-ray tube and film (focus-object distance = 20 inches):

$$M = \frac{40}{20} = 2$$

Using a focus-film distance of 40 inches, what will the focus-object distance be if magnification of 1.5 is desired?

$$1.5 = \frac{40}{x}$$
$$x = \frac{40}{1.5} = 26.6, \text{ or about 27 in.}$$

Remember, 27 inches is the focus-object distance. The object-film distance will be 40 minus 27, or 13 inches.

TRUE VERSUS GEOMETRIC MAGNIFICATION

If x rays were generated from a point source, the preceding discussion of magnification would be correct, and true magnification (M) and geometric magnification (m) would be the same. Figure 20–1 diagrams this situation. If a represents focus-object and b represents object-film distance, then the equation for both true (sometimes termed total) magnification and geometric (sometimes termed nominal) magnification is the same (i.e., we are using a point source focal spot):

$$M = m = \frac{a + b}{a}$$

Unfortunately, real focal spots have a finite size. If we assume that x-ray production is of uniform intensity across the focal spot (that this is often untrue will be emphasized subsequently), and that the object is about the same size or smaller than the focal spot, the image of the object will be formed as diagrammed in Figure 20–2. Notice that the total image size (I) now contains a central (U) region and two areas of edge gradient (E). (The term edge gradient, rather than penumbra, is preferred.) Derivation of the equation that must be used to calculate true magnification in this situation is an interesting exercise, but we will be content to record the equation that relates total magnification (M) to geometric magnification (m)

$$M = m + (m - 1)\left(\frac{f}{d}\right)$$

M = true magnification
m = geometric magnification
$$\left(\text{calculated from } m = \frac{a + b}{a}\right)$$
d = object size
f = focal spot size

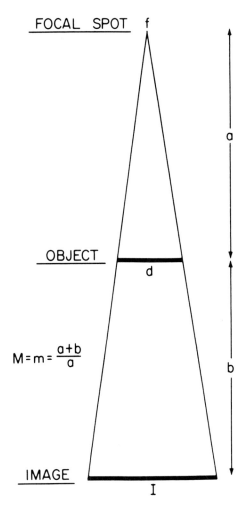

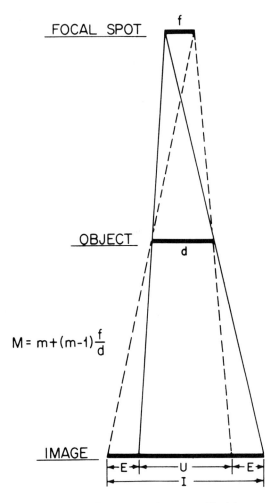

Figure 20–1 Geometry of a magnified image produced by a point source focal spot

Figure 20–2 Geometry of a magnified image produced by a focal spot with finite size

Note that as objects become smaller than the focal spot, the term $\frac{f}{d}$ becomes large, and true magnification becomes much greater than geometric magnification. Conversely, if an object is large compared to focal spot size (i.e., radiography of the femur with a 1.2-mm focal spot tube), the term $\frac{f}{d}$ becomes small and, for practical purposes, we may conclude that M and m are identical.

To summarize, **true magnification (M)** is a function of the ratio of focal spot size to object size $\left(\frac{f}{d}\right)$.

An example will help in understanding this concept of true versus geometric magnification. Assume you are filming a renal angiogram using a 40-inch target-film distance and an 0.6-mm focal spot. What will be the size of the image of a 200-micron (0.2 mm) renal artery located 4 inches from the film? First we must calculate geometric magnification (m). Refer to Figure 20–3A.

$$m = \frac{a + b}{a} = \frac{36 + 4}{36}$$
$$m = 1.11$$

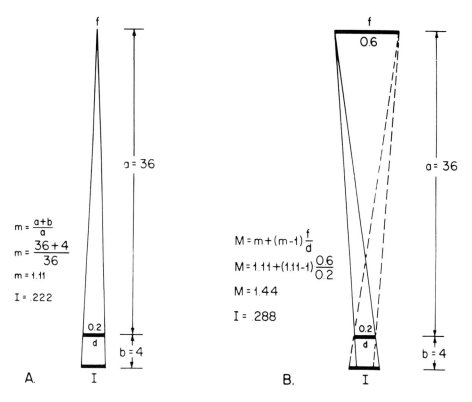

Figure 20–3   Calculation of geometric magnification (m) and true magnification (M)

With a punctiform focal spot image size would be 0.222 mm or 222 microns (200 × 1.11 = 222). But, because the object is small compared to the focal spot (0.2 mm vs. 0.6 mm), the term $\frac{f}{d}$ will be large and we must calculate how the term $(m - 1)\frac{f}{d}$ will affect true image size (Fig. 20–3B):

$$M = m + (m - 1)\frac{f}{d}$$
$$M = (1.11) + (1.11 - 1)\frac{0.6}{0.2}$$
$$M = 1.11 + (0.11)(3) = 1.44$$

Thus, true magnification is 44% versus geometric magnification of only 11%, and true image size will be 0.288 mm or 288 microns (200 × 1.44 = 288). Keep in mind that the various causes of unsharpness (i.e., screen, geometric, absorption, and motion) will make the precise boundaries of the image of our hypothetical vessel difficult to identify.

X-RAY TUBE FOCAL SPOTS

Magnification radiography demands use of the smallest practical focal spot because geometric unsharpness must be reduced as much as possible. A focal spot size of 0.3 mm or less is required for magnification, but simply purchasing a standard 0.3-mm focal spot tube may not get the job done. We must examine the following:

1. What does focal spot size mean?
2. How is focal spot size measured, and how are the measurements useful?
3. How does focal spot size vary with change in tube operating conditions (mA and kVp)?

Focal Spot Size

In the United States, the National Electrical Manufacturers Association (NEMA) has established a standard method for measuring focal spot size and has specified the amount that a focal spot can vary from its stated size.* The 1970 NEMA standards for measurement of focal spot size are shown in Table 20–1. These standards allow measurement of focal spot size at significantly lower mA settings than those usually used in clinical applications. It is important to recognize that focal spot size changes with different kVp and mA settings (focal spot blooming at high mA), so the 1970 NEMA standards allow focal spot measurements to be compared but often do not define the size of the focal spot under normal use. In recognition of this, the NEMA 1974 standard differs from that shown in Table 20–1 as follows: "spots are to be taken at one-half the maximum allowable current for 0.1 second exposure."[3] We will discuss focal spot size variation under different operating conditions later.

NEMA standards also define the tolerance limits by which a focal spot can vary from its stated size (Table 20–2). Because tolerance limits for a 0.3-mm focal spot are 50%, such a focal spot may measure 0.45 mm and meet specifications. When purchasing a small focal spot tube for use in

Table 20–1. 1970 NEMA Recommendations for Proper kVp and mA Settings Used to Measure Focal Spot Size*

FOCAL SPOT SIZE (mm)	MILLIAMPERES
0.4 and less	15
0.5 to 0.9	50
1.0 to 1.4	100
1.5 to 1.9	200
2.0 and greater	300

*Measurements were made at 85 kVp with rotating anode tubes and single-phase full-wave rectification.

*NEMA Standards Publication No. XR5-1974, Measurement of Dimensions of Focal Spots of Diagnostic X-Ray Tubes, 155 East 44th Street, New York, NY, 10017.

Table 20–2. NEMA Tolerance Limits for Focal Spot Variation

FOCAL SPOT SIZE (mm)	TOLERANCE (%)	
	MINUS	PLUS
Less than 0.8	0	50
0.8 through 1.5	0	40
Greater than 1.5	0	30

magnification radiography, one should consider specifying a true 0.3-mm focal spot in the contract (and expect to pay more for this special consideration). For routine radiography the tolerance standards are generally considered acceptable.

Measurement

After the tube is installed, it is necessary to measure focal spot size under conditions of clinical use. NEMA specifications call for focal spots 0.3 mm or smaller to be measured with a line pair resolution test pattern (such as a star test pattern), and those greater than 0.3 mm to be measured with a pinhole camera. There are significant differences in interpreting focal spot "size" as determined by these two methods, and we must understand both the measurement techniques and the appropriate application of the data to clinical magnification radiography.

Pinhole Camera. The pinhole technique measures the physical size of the focal spot and demonstrates the intensity distribution of radiation from the focal spot. The pinhole consists of a small hole in a sheet of lead. The pinhole assembly is placed between the x-ray tube and a sheet (no intensifying screens) of x-ray film, and an exposure is made that produces a density of 0.6 to 1.0 on the film (Fig. 20–4). If the pinhole is placed exactly halfway between the focal spot and film, as in Figure 20–4, the image of the focal spot will be the same size as the actual physical dimensions of the focal spot. The pinhole technique will also demonstrate the intensity distribution of radiation from the focal spot.

Figure 20–5 is a photographically mag-

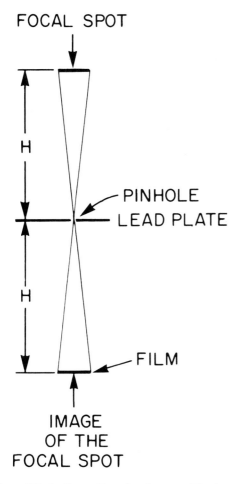

FOCAL SPOT

H

PINHOLE
LEAD PLATE

H

FILM

IMAGE
OF THE
FOCAL SPOT

Figure 20–4 Formation of an image of the focal spot by a pinhole camera

nified pinhole image of a focal spot showing that x-ray intensity is much greater along the edges of a focal spot than in its central area.[4] This is termed edge-band distribution and, although it is the most common type of intensity distribution, it is the least desirable, as we will discuss later. There are several problems with the pinhole technique of measuring focal spots:

1. The size of the pinhole must be small with respect to the size of the focal spot. Recommended pinhole diameters are

   0.03 mm for focal spots below 1 mm

   0.075 mm for focal spots from 1.0 to 2.5 mm

The 0.03-mm pinhole transmits so little radiation that producing a film image of the focal spot requires multiple exposures at high mA values.

2. The size of the image of a 0.3-mm focal spot is so small that accurate measurement without special equipment is difficult.

3. Accurate measurement of the length of the focal spot is difficult. X-ray intensity along the cathode-anode axis (length) peaks near the center of the focal spot and fades toward each extremity. To compensate for this uneven distribution, it is recommended that the measured length of the focal spot (cathode-anode axis) be reduced by multiplying it by 0.7. The accuracy of this correction factor is questionable.

4. It is important to align the pinhole to the central beam of the x-ray tube accurately. This location is difficult to determine.

The pinhole technique provides a measurement of the size of the focal spot and its intensity distribution. Focal spot size measured by this technique is used to calculate anode heat-loading characteristics of the x-ray tube and is the measurement (f) used in the formula to calculate true radiographic magnification (M). We will return later to the importance of intensity distribution.

Line Pair Resolution Test Patterns. Because of the problems associated with use of a small pinhole, line pair resolution test patterns are now recommended for imaging focal spots of 0.3 mm or less. Commonly, a star test pattern is used (Fig. 20–6). This pattern consists of a circular sheet of lead 50 microns thick, with a diameter of 45 mm, divided into 180 spokes, of which 90 are lead and 90 are blank. Each spoke subtends an angle of 2°. A star test pattern can be viewed as consisting of many line pair test patterns, with each diameter

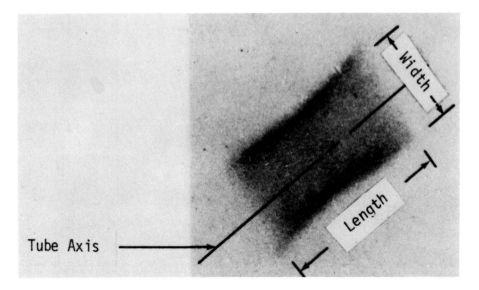

Figure 20–5   Pinhole image of a focal spot with edge band distribution. (Bull, K.W.: The effects of the x-ray focal spot on primary beam magnification of small vessels. Master's thesis, the University of Texas Health Science Center at Dallas, May 1973)

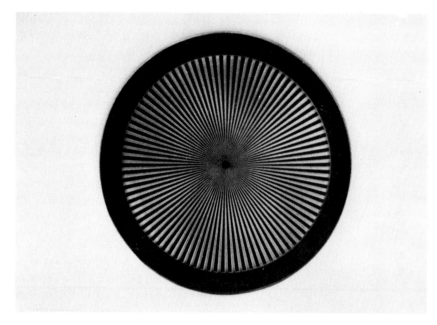

Figure 20–6   Photograph of a star resolution pattern. Notice inability of the camera lens to record the inner spokes

of the star corresponding to a line pair of a different size. To measure focal spot size, the star test pattern is positioned about midway between the focal spot and film (do not use screens), exactly parallel to the film, and in the central axis of the x-ray beam. Figure 20–7 is a diagram of this technique, and Figure 20–8 is a picture of an actual star test pattern. As one moves toward the center of the image, an area is encountered at which the image of the rays of the star gradually disappears (D, Fig. 20–7). This is termed the area of failure of resolution, and the diameter (D) of the blurred image is measured both parallel and perpendic-

ular to the cathode-anode axis of the tube. It must be noted that D is measured perpendicularly to the desired dimension of the focal spot (in Figure 20–8 one would measure D for the cathode-anode axis of the focal spot in the dimension perpendicular to the cathode-anode alignment of the tube when the exposure was made). Focal spot size is then calculated by the formula

$$f = \frac{\theta D}{57.3 (M - 1)}$$

f = focal spot size
θ = angle of one of the lead spokes
D = diameter of the blurred image of the star phantom parallel or perpendicular to the tube axis (cathode-anode axis)
M = magnification (true)

Because θ = 2° in the star phantom, the equation used with this phantom reduces to

$$f = \frac{D}{28.65 (M - 1)}$$

M is easily measured. The diameter of the star pattern is always known (the one illustrated has a diameter of 45 mm), and the diameter of the image of the pattern is quickly measured. Magnification is calculated:

$$M = \frac{\text{image size}}{\text{object size}}$$

Note in Figure 20–7 that continuing inward from the region of failure of resolution the image of the test pattern reappears, but the light and dark lines will have shifted 180° in their alignment (called a phase shift). This is the area of spurious resolution that is seen with focal spots with edge band intensity distribution, and corresponds to spatial frequencies where the modulation transfer function (MTF) of the focal spot is negative. Milne has described this phenomenon in detail, so we will not further consider phase shift and spurious resolution.[10] Focal spot size measured with a star phantom depends on two characteristics of the focal spot,

1. focal spot size and

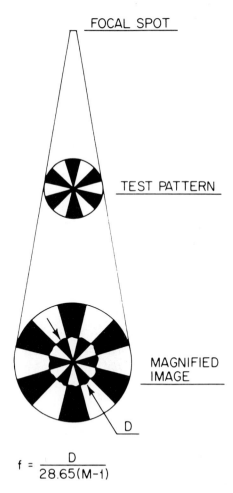

FOCAL SPOT

TEST PATTERN

MAGNIFIED IMAGE

D

$$f = \frac{D}{28.65(M-1)}$$

Figure 20–7 Using a star resolution pattern to determine focal spot size (not drawn with correct perspective)

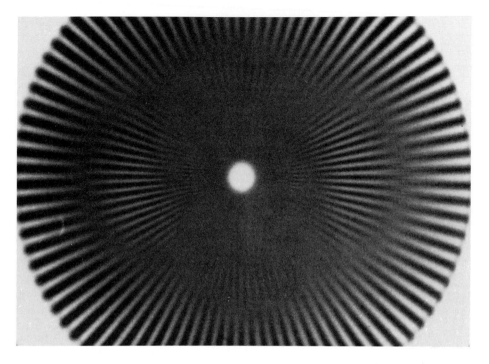

Figure 20–8   Appearance of a star test pattern image used to calculate focal spot size

2. radiation intensity distribution within the focal spot.

Thus, **this technique does not measure the actual physical size of a focal spot** (size is measured with the pinhole camera), but measures the **resolving capacity of the focal spot,** which is a function of both size and radiation intensity distribution.

The effect of the intensity distribution of a focal spot has been discussed by Milne.[9] There are three types of intensity distribution encountered in focal spots (we will not consider the ring distribution of a field emission x-ray tube):

1. Edge band distribution (Fig. 20–5).
2. Homogeneous distribution, in which radiation intensity is uniform throughout the focal spot.
3. Centrally peaked distribution, in which radiation intensity is peaked in the central portion of the focal spot and tapers toward the margin (i.e., the "opposite" of edge band distri-

bution); also termed Gaussian distribution.

The type of intensity distribution has an important influence on the resolving capacity of a focal spot. Milne has advised that the term **effective** focal spot size be used to describe the physical size of a focal spot as measured with a pinhole camera.[9] To this is added another measurement: the **equivalent** focal spot size (the size measured with a star pattern). The definition of equivalent size is "The equivalent size (F_{eq}) of a focal spot F with any type of intensity distribution is equal to that size of homogeneous focal spot which has the same resolving power as F."[9] The focal spot with the best resolving power has a peaked intensity distribution, next best is homogeneous, and worst is edge band distribution.

Table 20–3 illustrates the difference in equivalent (star test pattern) focal spot size that results from differences in radiation intensity distribution in three focal spots that have identical effective (pinhole) focal

Table 20–3. Comparison of Effective and Equivalent Focal Spot Sizes for Various Radiation Intensity Distribution

EFFECTIVE (Pinhole) FOCAL SPOT SIZE (mm)	RADIATION INTENSITY DISTRIBUTION	EQUIVALENT (Star Test Pattern) FOCAL SPOT SIZE (mm)
1.0	Homogeneous	1.0
1.0	Edge band	2.0
1.0	Centrally peaked	0.5

spot size measurements. Note that the focal spot with edge band distribution has an equivalent size twice that of the one with homogeneous distribution, while the centrally peaked focal spot has an effective size only half that of the homogeneous one. Many measurements of focal spot resolving power have been made that assumed a homogeneous intensity distribution. Obviously, such measurements will not be accurate if applied to focal spots with other types of intensity distribution.

Let us digress a moment to emphasize that the star pattern measurement of focal spot size gives information about resolving power, which is the ability of the focal spot to record separate images of small objects placed close together (i.e., a series of 100-μ interlobular vessels in the renal cortex). The ability of the focal spot to image a single, isolated 100-μ vessel is determined by the physical size of the focal spot (pinhole size), although the intensity distribution will influence the shape of the edge gradient (i.e., how sharp the edge of the vessel will appear). If one wishes to calculate true magnification (M) of a small object, the focal spot size (f) used in the equation must be that determined by the pinhole camera. If one wishes to determine the resolving power of a particular focal spot, the size determined from a star pattern may be used, or the size measured with a pinhole may be adjusted for the type of intensity distribution (this usually requires photographic enlargement of the tiny pinhole image or use of a microdensitometer, both of which are not usually available in clinical situations).

Variation of Focal Spot Size with Changes in Tube Operating Conditions (mA and kVp)

Two articles by Chaney and Hendee have nicely documented the fact that focal spot size varies depending on tube operating conditions.[5,7]

Focal spot size increases in direct proportion to tube current. This is called **blooming** of the focal spot, and is much more marked at low kVp and high mAs techniques. Weaver has reported the effect of the current on focal spot bloom at 40 and 80 kVp to be as shown in Table 20–4.[14] Focal spot bloom is much more marked parallel to the tube axis. Focal spot bloom perpendicular to the cathode-anode tube axis depends on the accuracy of the focusing of the electron beam, and measurements with a star pattern show wide variation between identical models of tubes.

Focal spot size will decrease slightly with increasing kVp. As measured by Chaney and Hendee, this change was approximately proportional to $\frac{1}{f_0 V^{3/2}}$, where f_0 = focal spot size for a small tube mA and V = tube kVp.[5] Weaver has illustrated decreasing focal spot size with increasing kVp, as shown in Table 20–5.[14] There is no industry standard regarding focal spot

Table 20–4. Measured Sizes of a Typical Focal Spot at Various Exposure Factors

TUBE (kVp)	TUBE (mA)	FOCAL SPOT SIZE
40 kVp	100 mA	2.0 mm
40	300	2.3
80	100	1.7
80	300	1.8

Table 20–5. Measured Size of a Typical Focal Spot at Various kVp Settings, mAs Constant

TUBE (kVp)	TUBE (mA)	FOCAL SPOT SIZE
40 kVp	100 mA	2.0 mm
60	100	1.8
80	100	1.7
150	100	1.7

blooming. Because blooming will vary significantly between supposedly identical tubes, the acceptable amount of focal spot blooming may need to be specified when purchasing a tube to be used for magnification radiography. As an alternate approach, the tube mA and kVp that must be used to produce a star pattern equivalent to a 0.3-mm focal spot in both parallel and perpendicular dimensions relative to the tube axis may have to be specified.

Off-Axis Variation

Focal spot measurements must be made in the central part of the x-ray beam. As one moves away from the central ray, the apparent size of the focal spot will change. **The projected focal spot length is much shorter in the heel (anode side) of the beam than at the cathode side.** Figure 20–9 illustrates the marked variation in focal spot length as one moves from the beam center to 10° toward the anode and 10° toward the cathode on the cathode-anode tube axis. Focal spot changes are less significant in the cross-axis direction, where focal spot shape may become more diamond-shaped but the width and length remain almost constant. The pinhole camera or resolution test pattern must always be accurately aligned with the x-ray beam center if focal spot measurements are to be reliable.

Let us conclude this short review of focal spots by emphasizing what is now an obvious fact: the radiologist who hopes to make successful use of magnification radiography must use great care in selecting an appropriate x-ray tube.

QUANTITATIVE EVALUATION OF RESOLUTION

With magnification techniques it is necessary to combine the most appropriate film-screen combination with the correct focal spot, and then to determine which amount of magnification is optimum. The serious problem of object motion must also be considered. In this respect, it is useful to study the resolution properties of the components of the entire radiographic system with the aid of the modulation transfer function (MTF) of the individual and combined components. To review briefly, an MTF is a curve that describes the ability of an imaging system, or any part of the system, to reproduce (or record) information. An MTF of 1.0 is perfect, indicating that the system can record all the information it has received. An MTF of 0 indicates that none of the information has been reproduced. We shall use the MTF curves to compare various system components. Precise data about how the curves are derived and detailed analyses will not be considered, but these are available in the literature.[11,12]

Figure 20–10 depicts the MTF curves of three imaginary x-ray tube focal spots up to an object frequency of 10 line pairs per mm. Focal spot 1 images perfectly (MTF = 1) at all frequencies. Focal spot 2 is not nearly as good, with its MTF dropping to 0.5 at 5 line pairs per mm., and focal spot 3 is lousy, with an MTF of 0 at 6 line pairs/ mm. Obviously, one need not know much about MTF curves to be able to glance at Figure 20–10 and determine that curve 1 is the best, 2 is next best, and 3 is the worst. We will use the following MTF curves to make quick graphic comparisons.

There is one additional use we must make of the MTF. If one knows the MTF of each of several components of an imaging system (i.e., film, intensifying screen and focal spot), the MTF of the entire system is calculated by multiplying the MTF

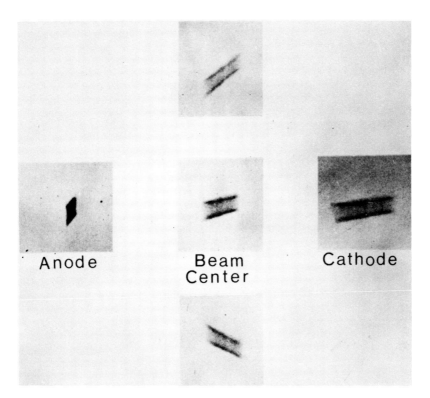

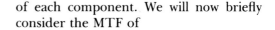

Anode   Beam Center   Cathode

Figure 20–9 Pinhole images showing variation of focal spot size and shape at various positions in the x-ray beam. (Bull, K.W.: The effects of the x-ray focal spot on primary beam magnification of small vessels. Master's thesis, the University of Texas Health Science Center at Dallas, May 1973)

of each component. We will now briefly consider the MTF of

Film
Focal spots
High-speed intensifying screens
Object motion

and show how magnification influences the MTF of film, focal spots, and screens.

Film

The ability of x-ray film to image objects with a frequency of 10 to 20 line pairs per mm is so good that we may consider film to have an MTF of 1.0 for all clinical applications of magnification radiography.

Focal Spots

We will assume focal spots of uniform intensity distribution. Figure 20–11A is a set of calculated MTF curves of a 0.3-mm

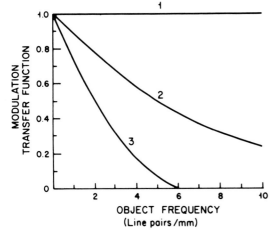

Figure 20–10 Illustrative MTF curves

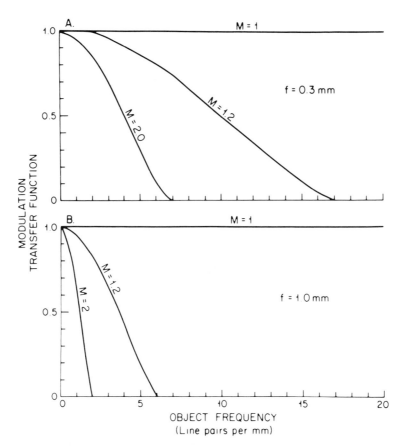

Figure 20–11 Calculated MTF curves for a 0.3-mm *(A),* and 1.0-mm *(B)* focal spot (f) at magnifications of 1, 1.2, and 2

focal spot for magnification factors of 1.0 (contact radiography, not possible clinically), 1.2, and 2.0. **Notice how rapidly the MTF deteriorates as the magnification factor increases,** even in the case of this small focal spot. Figure 20–11*B* shows similar data for a 1.0-mm focal spot, emphasizing that the larger the focal spot the more drastic the deterioration of MTF produced by magnification. **Focal spot MTF is adversely affected by magnification.**

Intensifying Screens

We will consider only high-speed screens, because they are the ones usually employed for magnification angiography. Figure 20–12 diagrams the approximate MTF curves of the Du Pont Quanta II (barium fluorochloride) screens at magnifica-

tions of 1.0, 1.2, and 2.0. It is clear from Figure 20–12 that **screen MTF improves with magnification.** In fact, the worse the MTF curve of the screen, the more improvement one sees with magnification, which is fortunate because we are usually using high-speed screens in clinical situations in which magnification is attempted. It is quite easy to understand why screen MTF improves with magnification when one considers what magnification does to the frequency (line pairs per mm) of information in the image presented to the intensifying screen. Assume that a test object has a frequency of 4 line pairs/mm (Fig. 20–13). When the object is magnified by a factor of 2, the 4 lines pairs are presented to the intensifying screens over an area of 2 mm, thus reducing the frequency of the

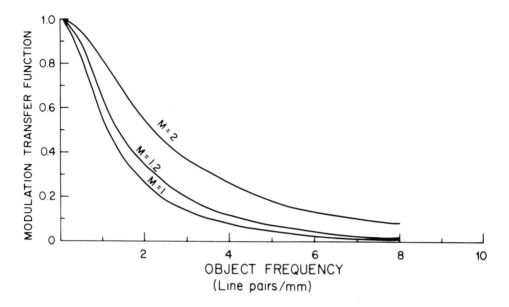

Figure 20–12 Approximate MTF curve of a Quanta II intensifying screen at magnifications of 1.0, 1.2, and 2.0. (Courtesy of E.I. du Pont de Nemours and Company, Inc.)

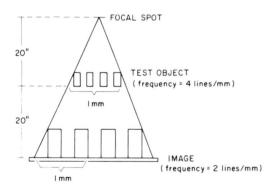

Figure 20–13 Resolution demanded at the level of the screen decreases as magnification increases

image presented to the screen to 2 line pairs per mm. The frequency of the image is less than the frequency of the object, and is calculated by dividing object frequency by the magnification factor. For example, assume a test object has 6 line pairs per mm. When the object is magnified by a factor of 1.5, the 6 lines will cover 1.5 mm at the level of the intensifying screens, corresponding to an image frequency of $\frac{6}{1.5}$,

or 4 line pairs per mm. Similarly, at a magnification factor of 2, the object frequency of 6 line pairs/mm is reduced to an image frequency of 3 line pairs per mm. Because magnification reduces the frequency (i.e., line pairs per mm) of information that must be resolved by the intensifying screen, the screen is able to do a better job.

Focal Spot and Screens

Because focal spot MTF gets worse with magnification, and screen MTF improves, what degree of magnification is best when only focal spot and screen are considered (assume film MTF of 1.0 in all situations)? Under these conditions (no object motion), the best resolution (MTF) is obtained by using detail screens and as little magnification as possible. In the clinical situation object motion must be considered, and this changes all the answers.

Object Motion

The amount of unsharpness caused by motion of an object is independent of the amount of magnification. Motion unsharpness depends only on

Velocity of motion
Exposure time.

Velocity (v) is expressed in mm per second, and exposure time (t) is expressed in seconds. The product vt can be used to determine the MTF caused by object motion. For example, if an object is moving at a rate of 10 mm per second (such as a pulmonary artery), and an exposure time of 0.025 seconds is used, the product vt will be $10 \times 0.025 = 0.25$. Assume an object frequency of 2 line pairs/mm (i.e., an opacified pulmonary artery 0.250 mm in diameter, giving two arteries and two spaces of 0.250 mm each per 1 mm), Table 20–6 shows that the MTF caused by motion will be 0.64. Table 20–6 lists the MTF caused by object motion for an object frequency of 2, 3, 5, 8, and 10 line pairs per mm at vt values of 0.1, 0.25, 0.5, and 1.0. The equation used to calculate these MTF values is terrifying, but is available to those able to deal with such matters.[12] From Table 20–6, it can be appreciated that knowledge of object motion is required if the optimal exposure factors in the case of moving objects are to be evaluated seriously.

As a general rule, if it is determined that the product of object motion (v) and exposure time (t) is less than 0.1, motion unsharpness will be minimal. If the value of vt is large (1.0 or greater), motion unsharpness becomes the dominant factor in total imaging system MTF. One will sacrifice any other component of the imaging system to make the exposure time shorter (i.e., use the fastest available film and screen regardless of quantum mottle and screen unsharpness). If the product of vt is greater than 0.1 but less than 0.5, a compromise is usually best: use a fast (but not the fastest) film-screen system, which will keep quantum mottle and screen unsharpness as favorable as possible and still allow reasonably short exposure times. Because magnification is useful when fast screen-film systems are used, the MTF of angiographic studies of moving vessels can usually be improved with magnification if the focal spot is of the correct size and shape. For example, consider an abdominal angiogram in which vessel motion is about 3 mm per second. Assume one uses Quanta II screens (Fig. 20–12), a 0.3-mm focal spot with uniform intensity distribution (Fig. 20–11A) and an exposure time of 0.033 seconds (vt = $3 \times 0.033 = 0.1$). At an information content of 4 line pairs per mm (i.e., blood vessels 0.125 mm in diameter), will system MTF be better at a magnification factor of 1.0, 1.2, 1.5, 2.0, or 3.0? The appropriate calculations are shown in Table 20–7, which shows system MTF to be best at a magnification factor of 2. Although calculation of MTF values does not tell the entire story of useful information content of the radiographic image, it does provide us with a means of beginning an objective analysis of a complex subjective problem (for example, this treatment neglects system noise, or quantum mottle).

HOW MUCH MAGNIFICATION IS BEST?

With a 0.3-mm focal spot there is a rather narrow range of magnification that will re-

Table 20–6. Calculated MTF Caused by Object Motion

OBJECT MOTION (vt) (mm)	MOTION MTF (line pairs/mm)				
	2	3	5	8	10
0.1	0.94	0.85	0.64	0.24	0
0.25	0.64	0.30	0	0	0
0.5	0	0	0	0	0
1.0	0	0	0	0	0

Table 20–7. Sample Calculations of MTF Values of Various Components of a Magnification Radiographic System*

MAGNIFICATION	SCREEN MTF	FOCAL SPOT MTF	MOTION MTF	TOTAL SYSTEM MTF
1.0	0.08	1.0	0.76	0.06
1.2	0.12	0.91	0.76	0.08
1.5	0.16	0.76	0.76	0.09
2.0	0.27	0.51	0.76	0.10
3.0	0.44	0.24	0.76	0.08

*Focal spot size: 0.3 × 0.3 mm; object motion: 3 mm/sec; exposure time: 0.033 sec; image frequency: 4 line pairs/mm; very fast screens: Du Pont Quanta II.

sult in improvement in resolution. No significant improvement greater than a magnification of about 2 is possible, so 2× magnification is the upper limit with a 0.3-mm focal spot. This amount of magnification is calculated for structures inside the body, so magnification as calculated from the skin surface of the body nearest the tube will be about 1.6 to 1.8. Because the correct magnification factor will vary between tubes (i.e., focal spots are not the same), Milne has suggested that some experiments should be performed before clinical work is done.[8] For example, place a resolving power target in an appropriate phantom and then make a series of exposures at different degrees of magnification, using the same mA as will be used with patients. The degree of magnification that gives the best resolution is then determined. With small focal spots, information content will increase over much higher ranges of magnification (up to 8.0× with a 0.1-mm focal spot).

QUANTUM MOTTLE

Quantum mottle is statistical fluctuation in the number of x-ray photons used by the imaging system to form the image. With magnification radiography, the number of x-ray photons per square millimeter required to produce the image is the same (if film density is the same) for any degree of magnification. That is, **quantum mottle does not change with radiographic magnification.** If a radiograph is photographically enlarged there is a change in quantum mottle. If 40,000 photons per mm²

were used to form the radiographic image, photographic magnification of 2× will increase the area from 1 to 4 mm² and reduce the number of x-ray photons to 10,000 per mm². Thus, photographic enlargement increases quantum mottle in the magnified image by a factor of $\frac{N}{m^2}$, in which

$$N = \text{number of photons used}$$
$$m = \text{magnification}$$

How does quantum mottle (noise) affect the radiographic image? Quantum mottle influences the perception of low-contrast objects with poorly defined borders. By comparison, system MTF largely defines the ability to record small objects with sharp borders and high contrast. Therefore, radiographic magnification (as opposed to photographic or optical magnification) may improve visualization of low-contrast images because it does not increase noise.

PATIENT EXPOSURE

If 2× magnification radiography requires that the patient's body surface be twice as close to the x-ray tube as in non-magnification radiography, one would conclude that exposure to the skin would be increased by a factor of 2^2 or 4 (inverse square law). This is incorrect for the following reasons.

First, in routine radiography there is always some amount of magnification, usually by about 1.1 to 1.2 at the skin on the tube side of the body. The inverse square law calculated with these values shows skin exposure to increase by

$$\frac{2^2}{1.1^2} = 3.31, \text{ or } \frac{2^2}{1.2^2} = 2.78$$

Second, with magnification radiography a smaller portion of the body is exposed to x rays because a smaller body area now covers the film. With magnification only relatively small anatomic areas can be recorded. Because of the limited area that can be encompassed, careful collimation of the x-ray beam and accurate alignment of the part being examined with the central beam are mandatory. This improves image quality and decreases patient exposure.

Third, with magnification high-speed or ultrahigh-speed screens are used, and a grid is not needed.

Because of these considerations, the increase in patient exposure with magnification is less than that anticipated by application of the inverse square law, and in some cases there might even be no increase or an actual decrease in skin exposure.

SUMMARY

Because x rays do not originate from a point source, calculations dealing with magnification of objects that are small compared to the size of the focal spot require an understanding of the relationship between geometric magnification (m) and true magnification (M). True magnification is a function of the ratio between focal spot size and object size $\left(\dfrac{f}{d}\right)$.

Specifications and measurements of focal spot size raise many issues. Industry standards define acceptable tolerance limits in focal spot size. Focal spot size varies with tube operating conditions, with the most marked variation being blooming with high mA low-kVp techniques. The intensity distribution of radiation from the focal spot is important in determining the resolving power of the focal spot. The pinhole technique measures the physical size

of the focal spot, and this measurement is used to calculate heat loading of the tube and magnification of small objects. Resolution chart (star pattern) measurements do not measure the physical size of a focal spot, but indicate the resolving power of the focal spot.

The resolution characteristics of magnification radiography may be studied in terms of the MTF of the various components of the imaging system. Film MTF is considered to be 1.0. Intensifying screen MTF improves with magnification while focal spot MTF deteriorates rapidly with magnification. Magnification represents a compromise wherein deterioration of focal spot MTF and improvement in screen MTF combine to produce maximum MTF of the entire imaging system. Magnification offers advantages when high-speed screens are used and object motion is present. The amount of unsharpness caused by object motion is unrelated to magnification, and depends on the velocity of motion and the exposure time. The optimum magnification for any system must be determined experimentally; with a 0.3-mm focal spot this will vary from about 1.6 to 2.0. Quantum mottle (noise) is not increased with radiographic magnification. Patient skin dose is usually increased with magnification, but the increase is less than the inverse square law would indicate.

REFERENCES

1. Bergeron, R.T.: Manufacturers' designation of diagnostic x-ray tube focal spot size: A time for candor. Radiology, 3:487, 1974.
2. Bernstein, H., Bergeron, R.T., and Klein, D.J.: Routine evaluation of focal spots. Radiology, 3:421, 1974.
3. Bernstein, F.: Specifications of focal spots and factors affecting their size. SPIE, 56:159, 1975.
4. Bull, K.W.: The effects of the x-ray focal spot on primary beam magnification of small vessels. Master's thesis, the University of Texas Health Science Center at Dallas, May 1973.
5. Chaney, E.L., and Hendee, W.R.: Effects of x-ray tube current and voltage on effective focal-spot size. Med. Phys., 1:141, 1974.
6. Dunisch, O., Pfeiler, M., and Kuhn, H.: Problems and aspects of the radiological magnification technique. Siemens Electro Medica, 3:114, 1971.

7. Hendee, W.R., and Chaney, E.L.: X-ray focal spots: Practical considerations. Appl. Radiol., 3:25, 1974.
8. Milne, E.N.C.: Magnification radiography. Appl. Radiol. Nucl. Med., 5:12, 1976.
9. Milne, E.N.C.: Characterizing focal spot performance. Radiology, 3:483, 1974.
10. Milne, E.N.C.: The role and performance of minute focal spots in roentgenology with special reference to magnification. CRC Crit. Rev. Radiol. Sci., 2:269, 1971.
11. Rao, G.U.V., Clark, R.L., and Gayler, B.W.: Radiographic magnification: A critical, theoretical and practical analysis. Part I. Appl. Radiol., 1:37, 1973.
12. Rao, G.U.V., Clark, R.L., and Gayler, B.W.: Radiographic magnification: A critical, theoretical and practical analysis. Part II. Appl. Radiol., 2:25, 1973.
13. Spiegler, P., and Breckindidge, W.C.: Imaging of focal spots by means of the star test pattern. Radiology, 102:679, 1972.
14. Weaver, K.E.: X-ray tube focal spots. Contained in the Syllabus of the AAPM 1975 Summer School, The Expanding Role of the Diagnostic Radiologic Physicist. Rice University, Houston, July 27–August 1, 1975.

21

The Subtraction Technique

The subtraction technique is a photographic method used to eliminate unwanted images from a radiograph. The method does not add any information; its purpose is to make diagnostically important information easier to see. The radiographic applications of the subtraction technique were first described by a Dutch radiologist, Ziedes des Plantes, in 1935.

When two radiographs differ in only certain details, subtraction can be used to accentuate the difference. This is illustrated in Figure 21–1. Films A and B are radiographs of an assortment of lead numbers and letters. The two films are almost identical, the only difference being the addition of two letters to Film B. Because there is so much information on both films, it is difficult to identify this difference. If all the information contained in film A could be subtracted from film B, the two letters added to film B would become obvious. To accomplish this, a negative of film A is prepared (A reversed in Fig. 21–1). Note that the images of the letters and numbers are black in the negative. When these negative (black) images are exactly superimposed on the positive images in film B, the images of the subtracted letters and numbers fuse with the background density. The negative (A reversed) does not contain a reversed image of the two letters that were not present in film A; therefore, only these two letters remain visible in the final subtraction film. The subtraction technique is easily applied to angiography, in which a series of films are available which differ only in the pattern of contrast material in blood vessels. We will use cerebral angiography as an example.

Three conditions are required for the subtraction technique: a **scout film,** an **angiogram film with contrast material** in vessels, and **no motion** of the head between the exposure of the scout film and subsequent angiogram films. Usually the first film of a cerebral angiogram series is exposed before the bolus of contrast medium has been injected; this first film is used as a scout film. Slight patient motion is almost always present, prompted by the sensation produced by the injection of contrast material, so perfect subtraction is seldom obtained in clinical practice.

The principles of subtraction are based on the following. The scout film shows the structural details of the skull and of the adjacent soft tissue. The angiogram film contains exactly the same anatomic detail, if the patient did not move, plus the opacified blood vessels. If all the information in the scout film could be subtracted from the angiogram film, only the opacified vessel pattern would remain visible. Figure 21–2 illustrates the subtraction technique.

Let us consider how information can be subtracted from a radiograph. It will be recalled that a radiograph provides diagnostically important information because of contrast, or density differences, between areas of the film. No contrast means no information. A lateral skull film usually has a density range of about 0.3 (mastoids) to 1.7 (frontal sinuses). The subtraction tech-

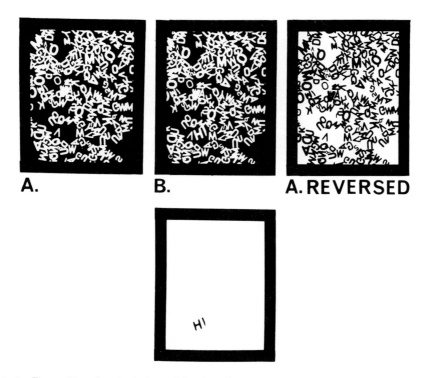

Figure 21–1   The subtraction technique (simulated)

nique destroys this density difference by adding density to the film in a carefully controlled manner. Consider the typical lateral skull. If a density of 1.7 were added to the mastoid area, and density 0.3 added to the frontal sinus region, both would then have a density of 2. The loss of contrast would make it impossible to see any difference between the image of the mastoids and sinuses. Thus, if the correct density were added to each part of the film, all contrast would be destroyed and the image of the skull would disappear.

SUBTRACTION MASK

The addition of the proper amount of density to the film is accomplished by exactly superimposing a second film, termed the **subtraction mask,** over the original radiograph. The subtraction mask is a negative of the scout film. Where the scout film is white, the mask is black (see mask, Fig. 21–2). The mask is a contact print made from the scout film. Commercially avail-

able printers, such as the Du Pont Cronex Printer, are designed for use in copying radiographs and in preparing subtraction masks and prints. Because of ease of use and uniformity of results, these printers have almost completely replaced glass-fronted printing frames (discussed in previous editions). Both subtraction and subtraction print films require exposure to a white light source. (The special films used for duplicating radiographs must be exposed with ultraviolet light, so commercial printers have both a white and an ultraviolet light source.) We will now deal with the question of the type of film used to make the subtraction mask.

The subtraction mask is a negative of the scout film (look at mask, Figure 21–2 again). It is a special type of negative. The density differences present on the negative must correspond exactly to the density differences of the scout film. In the scout film of Figure 21–2, assume the density of the mastoid area to be 0.3, the frontal sinuses

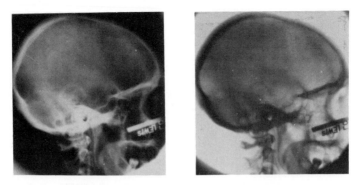

SCOUT   **MASK**

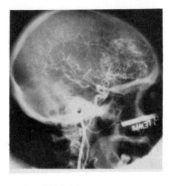   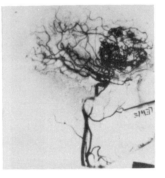

ANGIOGRAM   **SUBTRACTION**

Figure 21–2 The subtraction technique

1.7, and the midportion of the skull 1.0. If the image on the scout film is to be completely destroyed by superimposition of the subtraction mask, the density on each part of the subtraction mask must be exactly correct. For example, assume that it is determined that the final density of the subtracted image will be 2.0 (that is, all densities will be 2.0, so no image will be seen because there is no contrast). This will require densities on the subtraction mask to be as shown in Table 21–1.

These requirements can be met only if the film used to produce the subtraction mask has a gamma of 1. Gamma 1 means that the film will not exaggerate or lessen density differences found in the scout film, but will produce a negative whose contrast is exactly complementary to the contrast of the scout film. Subtraction film (Du Pont Cronex Subtraction Film and Kodak X-Omat Subtraction Masking Film) now available will produce an excellent mask when developed in an automatic x-ray film processor. These film emulsions have been designed to yield a gamma of 1 over the

Table 21–1. Sample Calculation of Subtraction Mask Density

	DENSITY		
	MASTOID	MIDSKULL	FRONTAL SINUS
Scout film	0.3	1.0	1.7
Subtraction mask	1.7	1.0	0.3
Scout + mask	2.0	2.0	2.0

wide range of developing conditions that exist in the various x-ray film processors. They are single-emulsion films, and their use makes the production of a subtraction mask very easy.

SUBTRACTION PRINT

The subtraction mask can be used in several ways. It may be superimposed in exact registration on an angiogram film and the result examined directly. When the mask and angiogram film are superimposed, the resulting film density will be very high (about 2.0 or greater). An ordinary view box does not produce enough light to allow direct viewing of this type of subtraction. A spotlight, or special view box with brighter illumination, must be used. With direct viewing the opacified blood vessels will, of course, be seen as light (low-density) structures. It is also obvious that if the patient moved between the exposure of the scout film and subsequent angiogram films, exact superimposition of the mask and angiogram will not be possible.

To produce a permanent record of the subtraction or to prepare illustrations, a print of the subtraction must be made. This is very easy to do. The same commercial printer used to produce the mask is used to make the subtraction print. The radiograph and subtraction mask are merely superimposed, and a contact print is produced on the desired film. Technical matters concerning exposure time and light intensity are easily determined from manufacturer recommendations and a few trial runs.

There are basically two types of film used to produce the subtraction print. The print can be made on a gamma 1 film (the same film used to produce the mask) or, for higher contrast, on subtraction print film. Both Kodak and Du Pont produce a single-emulsion film designed to produce subtraction prints (Kodak X-Omat Subtraction Print Film, and Du Pont Cronex Subtraction Print Film). Figure 21–3 is copied from the Du Pont product information

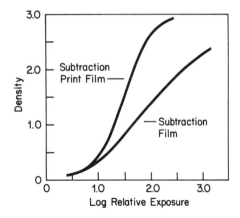

Figure 21–3 Comparison of the characteristic curves of subtraction film and subtraction print film. (Courtesy of E. I. du Pont de Nemours and Company, Inc.)

sheet E-23360, and shows graphically the difference in contrast between the use of Du Pont Cronex Subtraction Film and Du Pont Cronex Subtraction Print Film. In general, the angiographer is interested in obtaining maximum contrast between opaque blood vessels and background tissue densities. There are circumstances that require recording wide ranges of contrast, and this can be accomplished by making the print on the lower contrast subtraction mask film. For example, an angiogram film covering the aortic arch and great vessels in the neck might require that a subtraction print be made on low-contrast (wide latitude) film if all opacified arteries are to be satisfactorily recorded.

All the films mentioned for printing the final subtraction are transparencies. If desired, the final print can be made on photographic paper to be viewed as an ordinary photograph. Except for the preparation of illustrations for publication, this application is seldom employed.

The principle of the subtraction technique can be used to show a change in position of a structure occurring between the taking of the first and second radiographs. For example, a faintly opaque foreign body in the eye might be identified if the head were absolutely immobilized and the direction of gaze changed between two otherwise identical exposures. Because of its movement, the foreign body would theoretically be the only structure not subtracted. Successful use of the subtraction technique for foreign body identification requires that absolutely no unwanted patient motion occur between exposures.

FILM-SCREEN INTRAVENOUS SUBTRACTION ANGIOGRAPHY

The recent application of digital equipment to intravenous angiography (digital subtraction angiography, or DSA) has also stimulated interest in applying film-screen techniques to intravenous subtraction angiography.[1] The subtraction technique (whether electronic or photographic) allows visualization of vessels with much lower concentrations of contrast media than is present with conventional arteriography. A recent Du Pont publication has reviewed the technical considerations of film-screen subtraction angiography.[6]

SUMMARY

The subtraction technique is a photographic method of eliminating (or subtracting) the unwanted images from a radiograph. Development of subtraction and subtraction print films that can be developed in an automatic x-ray film processor has made use of the technique easy, fast, and inexpensive.

REFERENCES

1. Ducos de Lahitte, M., Mare-Vergues, J.P., Rascol, A., et al.: Intravenous angiography of the extracranial cerebral arteries. Radiology, *137*:705, 1980.
2. Hanafee, W., and Shinno, J.M.: Second-order subtraction and simultaneous bilateral carotid, internal carotid injections. Radiology, *86*:334, 1966.
3. Joyce, J.W., et al.: Improved contrast in subtraction technique. Radiology, *94*:157, 1970.
4. Oldendorf, W.H.: A modified subtraction technique for extreme enhancement of angiographic detail. Neurology, 15:336, 1965.
5. Oldendorf, W.H.: Subtraction and autosubtraction techniques for reproducing radiographs. J. Biol. Photogr. Assoc., *32*:65, 1964.
6. Schwenker, R.P., and Wayrynen, R.E.: Film-screen intravenous subtraction angiography. Wilmington, DE, E. I. du Pont de Nemours and Company, Photo Products Department, Pamphlet 347-10.

22

Copying Radiographs

Making full-sized copies of radiographs is now a routine procedure. Radiograph duplicating film is familiar to radiologists and offers a fast, simple, and relatively inexpensive way to copy radiographs. We will briefly examine the photographic principle (solarization) utilized in radiograph duplicating film.

Equally important to the radiologist is the ability to produce 35-mm slides of radiographs. A number of techniques have been proposed. Several of the best methods have been presented in Copying Radiographs.[1] In this chapter we will discuss a method with which the authors have had considerable personal experience, that we feel is highly satisfactory for producing large numbers of good quality slides quickly and inexpensively. The method employs a direct positive film that, like radiograph copy film, utilizes the principle of solarization.

SOLARIZATION

We have previously discussed (Chap. 11) the fact that as light (or x-ray) exposure increases, so does the resulting developed density of the film, up to a maximum limit. If the exposure is increased considerably beyond what produces the maximum density, a decrease in density occurs. The phenomenon responsible for this decrease in density with very high exposures is called solarization. From the standpoint of individual grains in the film emulsion, solarization means that the increased exposure has actually destroyed the developable

state that had been induced by the earlier part of the exposure. Figure 22–1 shows the zones of a film's characteristic curve (toe, straight line portion, and shoulder); this curve extends into the region of solarization in which increased log relative exposure produces decreased density. Remember, the exposure scale is logarithmic, so reaching the solarization region of the curve requires a high exposure as compared to that commonly used in photography.

The physical process responsible for solarization is still subject to debate. Current evidence favors the **rebromination hypothesis**, which we will discuss briefly.

In discussing latent image formation, we examined in some detail the way in which metallic silver is deposited at latent image centers. We also mentioned that bromine is formed when silver bromide decomposes in the photolytic process. The bromine passes from the silver halide crystal into the surrounding gelatin. Gelatin is able to neu-

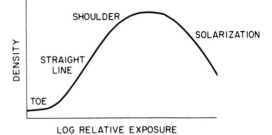

Figure 22–1 Characteristic curve extended into the region of solarization

295

tralize the small quantities of bromine formed in normal latent image formation. Gelatin, however, is easily saturated with bromine. The amount of bromine liberated during the large exposures of the solarization region cannot be destroyed by the gelatin. During such exposures, large quantities of bromine build up in the spaces between emulsion grains. When the exposure is completed, this excess bromine reacts with metallic silver at the latent image centers on the surface of the grain. This coats the latent image center with a layer of silver bromide, which effectively isolates it from the action of the developing solution. Thus, the grain, even though it contains one or more latent image centers, will not be developed.

The important fact about the solarization process is that more light exposure produces less film density. This is just the opposite of standard photographic exposures.

The two films we are going to discuss (radiograph copy film and 35-mm direct positive film) have an emulsion that has been solarized. The emulsion may be solarized before or after it is coated on the film. The solarizing process may be done with light, but chemical treatment of the emulsion will also cause solarization. The exact processes are trade secrets. Several years ago it was possible to solarize the emulsion of routine x-ray film. After prolonged exposure to light, the x-ray film could be used to produce a direct positive copy of a radiograph. The emulsions now used in x-ray film cannot be solarized satisfactorily.

RADIOGRAPH DUPLICATING FILM

Radiograph duplicating film has a solarized emulsion coated on one side of a blue-tinted polyester film base. An antihalation coating is on the opposite side of the base.

Halation

When image-forming light passes through a film and into the air beyond it, some light is reflected back into the film. This reflected light spreads out beyond the boundaries of the image and causes unsharp edges. Halation may be prevented by coating the back side of the film base with a layer of gelatin containing a dye that absorbs the reflected light to which the emulsion is sensitive. The dye used is decolorized or washed away during film processing.

Solarized Emulsion

The emulsion of radiograph duplicating film is a solarized emulsion. It is designed to be exposed with an ultraviolet light source, such as a BLB ultraviolet fluorescent lamp. A commercially available duplicating printer may be used. These printers are simple to operate and provide copies of uniform quality.

Commercially available printers are now routinely used to prepare full-sized copies of radiographs. The glass front cassette we described in previous editions has met about the same fate as the intravenous cholangiogram. Duplicating film is available coated on a blue-tinted base for copying routine radiographs. Also available is duplicating film coated on a clear base, designed for copying images on clear-based films commonly used with computed tomography, ultrasound, and nuclear medicine.

Because the emulsion of the copy film is solarized, light passing through the radiograph and reaching the copy film will produce a copy that looks like the orginal radiograph. Remember, the more light that reaches the solarized film, the less the density that is produced. Areas of low density in the original radiograph allow more light to reach the copy film and are, therefore, reproduced as areas of low density on the copy.

Densities of the duplicate may be made to differ from those of the original. If the original is too dark (too much density), a longer exposure will produce a copy with less density. Similarly, the density of the copy may be increased by decreasing the exposure.

Radiograph duplicating film is available in several sizes.

35-MM SLIDES

Camera

Most 35-mm slides are exposed with a single-lens reflex camera. This means that the exact area being photographed is seen through the view finder of the camera. An expensive camera is not necessary. Usually the camera should be mounted on a copying stand directly above a view box. These stands can be obtained at most photo supply stores. A standard illuminator used for routine radiograph viewing provides a satisfactory light source. The standard lens on most 35-mm cameras works well, but this lens will not allow the close-up work that is important in many illustrations. The use of extension tubes or positive diopter supplementary lenses provides an inexpensive means of achieving close-up capabilities. A more utilitarian lens is one that will allow both close-up and standard distance work. Purchase of these special macro lenses is not necessary unless large volumes of work are anticipated. Positive diopter supplementary lenses simply attach to the front of the regular lens. They are easy to use, but the results are not of such good quality as those achieved with extension tubes. Extension tubes are more costly and are less convenient to use, but they produce a better quality close-up. We are using a high-quality single-lens reflex camera with a lens that allows focusing from about 4 inches to infinity.

Film

Three types of film are used to produce 35-mm slides of radiographs: reversal color film; negative film used with reversal processing (Kodak Panatomic-X); and direct positive film. Each has its own advantages and disadvantages.

Color Reversal Film

Details of using this type of film have been adequately described.[1] The film is widely available. Because short exposures are possible with some color films (such as high-speed Ektachrome), the camera can be handheld, an important feature when photographing scientific exhibits. The major disadvantage is that the slides may exhibit an abnormal tint, ususlly a pale green or blue, a problem that can be remedied with the proper filter. In addition, these slides are relatively expensive compared to those made with black-and-white films. In general, color films offer the advantage of convenience.

Reversal Processing

By a modification of the development process, called reversal processing, a normal emulsion can be made to yield a positive rather than a negative image. In this process, after the negative is developed, the metallic silver in the negative image is dissolved away. The film is reexposed to light, which makes the residual silver halide developable. The film is then redeveloped, producing a positive image.

The black-and-white film most commonly used for reversal processing in preparing slides of radiographs is Kodak Panatomic-X film.[1] It is available in cassettes of 20 and 36 exposures, and may be bought in bulk form. It has a wide exposure latitude, and we have had good results using a standard x-ray view box light source with an exposure time of 2 to 5 sec. at f/16. A dark film may require an exposure time of 10 to 20 sec.

The major disadvantage of this film is the intricate processing required. There is a direct positive developing kit available, but it requires considerable time to develop your own slides, and few commercial film processors are willing to develop Panatomic-X as a direct positive. In most areas the film must be mailed to a processor, and the delay in receiving the finished product can be most inconvenient when the material is needed promptly. In our experience, Panatomic-X produces good slides.

Direct Positive Film

Direct positive, or direct reversal, film contains a solarized emulsion. Therefore, it produces a direct black-and-white duplicate of a radiograph when processed in a conventional manner (reversal processing is not needed).

Eastman Direct MP Film 5360 (MP stands for motion picture) is such a film.[3] It is a fine-grain, high resolving power film of medium contrast. It was designed to be used for editing purposes in the motion picture industry. Herein lies its major disadvantage for those who wish to use it for making 35-mm slides, because it requires repackaging by the user. It is not available in the handy 20- and 36-exposure cassettes to which we have become accustomed. Instead, the film must be specially ordered in 1000-ft rolls. Empty 35-mm film cassettes are readily available, however, and it is quite easy to cut appropriate lengths and "roll your own" from the 1000-ft roll. Obviously, 1000 ft of film will produce several thousand 35-mm slides. Storage of this film for over 6 months requires refrigeration at subfreezing temperatures. In currently available quantities, some film will usually be wasted. Perhaps this or a similar film will become available in a length better suited to the needs of the amateur photographer.

The film has several outstanding advantages. Exposure latitude is extremely large, so exposure times are not critical. Using a standard view box for a light source, exposure time varies between 10 and 30 sec with the lens aperture set at f/3.5. A roentgenogram of average density requires an exposure of 10 to 15 sec. Copying drawings, charts, pictures of radiographs, and so forth is also easy. We use a light source provided by four 75-W photoflood bulbs mounted on the copying stand (such units are commercially available). A satisfactory exposure for such prints is 12 sec at f/3.5.

Exposure latitude is so great that a change in exposure time of 2 or 3 sec will produce no visible difference in the final product.

The other great virtue of this film is the ease with which it can be developed. Temperature and solution concentrations need not be precisely regulated. This is fortunate, because it is necessary to do your own developing. The mechanics of development can be learned in a few minutes from personnel in any photographic supply store. The exposures suggested above require the following development technique:

1. Develop in Kodak D-19 developer (diluted stock solution 1:1) for 10 min at normal room temperature.
2. Change the developing solution after each 36-exposure roll of film is developed.
3. In fixing, use Kodak Rapid fixer, full strength, for 5 min.

The techniques suggested have evolved through trial and error in our department. The extreme latitude of exposure and processing is especially attractive in a large department in which many persons are involved in producing slides, because the job does not require an expert. The processing technique is not only simple, but fast, and it is possible to produce a completed slide in about an hour. The cost per slide is low: the cardboard mount costs more than the photograph.

Our experience with Eastman Direct MP Film 5360 has been gratifying. Preparation of large numbers of slides (up to 25,000 per year) has become relatively simple, and slides are routinely available in 24 hours. All processing is done in the radiology department. This method of preparing 35-mm slides can be recommended for use in any department in which many slides are needed promptly.

Eastman Kodak has available a 35-mm film designed to permit production of 2- × 2-inch slides of good quality, from radiographs or printed material, with a minimum of time and effort. The film is Kodak Rapid Process Copy Film 2064. RPC/2064 is a slow, fine-grain, direct positive film.[3] It is available in convenient 36-exposure magazines, and may also be obtained in 150-feet rolls. Exposure techniques and factors are roughly the same as described for Eastman Direct MP Film 5360.[3] Exposure latitude is great, but some experimenting and several rolls of poor slides will always be required as one first begins using these films.

The great convenience of this film is that it can be processed in a 90-second x-ray film automatic processor to obtain a dry film as quickly and almost as easily as routine radiographs are obtained. The exposed film must be taped to a film leader 8 × 10 inches or larger. The leader and film (emulsion side up) are then simply fed into the automatic processor. After processing, the film is easily cut to size and mounted as slides in one of several types of slide mounts available from almost any photographic supply dealer. Using these copy films it is possible to produce a slide ready for projection in about 10 minutes (a phenomenon that can become a nuisance when one's colleagues develop the bad habit of asking for "a little help" in preparing conferences and lectures at the last minute). A recent Kodak publication contains many helpful suggestions.[2] It is possible to process this film manually. Manual processing may be used to change the gamma and maximum density of the film, but such manipulation is rarely necessary

unless one's hobby compels experimentation. Our continued use of MP Film 5360 and RPC/2064 shows both films to produce excellent slides. Film #5360 has a clear base and RPC/2064 has a blue base. This difference produces differences of opinion as to which film produces the "best" slides of radiographs.

SUMMARY

Duplicating radiographs with radiograph duplicating film is a routine procedure requiring almost no extra equipment. The phenomenon of solarization makes this process possible.

Producing 35-mm slides of radiographs requires choice of the proper film to fit the circumstances. Reversal color film is acceptable when only a few slides are needed, and the short exposure time required by some color films offers a method of copying material when the camera must be handheld. Reversal processing of black-and-white film will also produce good slides. This film is convenient to use, but film processing is intricate. Direct positive 35-mm film is now available that is so convenient to use that this method should be considered to be the manner in which slides of radiographs are routinely prepared.

REFERENCES

1. Copying Radiographs. Rochester, NY, Eastman Kodak Company, Radiography Markets Division.
2. Kodak Rapid Process Copy Film/2064. Rochester, NY, Eastman Kodak Company, Radiography Markets Division. Publ. No. M3-148, 12-79.
3. Technical Data Sheet, Eastman Direct MP Film 5360 (35-mm), Rochester, NY, Eastman Kodak Company.

23

Xeroradiography

Xeroradiography is the production of a visible image utilizing the charged surface of a photoconductor (amorphous selenium) as the detecting medium, partially dissipating the charge by exposure to x rays to form a latent image, and making the latent image visible by xerographic processing. Xerography was invented by a physicist, Chester F. Carlson, in 1937. In 1944 the Battelle Memorial Institute, and in 1947 the Haloid Company (now Xerox Corporation), began laboratory investigations of this process and its potential application to industrial and medical radiographic procedures. The Xerox Corporation has developed a highly automated xeroradiographic system that has allowed radiologists to make practical clinical use of this type of x-ray imaging. It is interesting to note that medical uses of xeroradiography were investigated as early as 1952 by Dr. John F. Roach of Albany Medical College, New York.

GENERAL PRINCIPLES

Xeroradiography is a complex electrostatic process based on a special material called a photoconductor. A **photoconductor** will not conduct an electric current when shielded from radiation, but becomes conductive when exposed to radiation such as visible light or x rays. The photoconductor used in xeroradiography is **amorphous selenium**. The selenium is deposited as a thin layer onto a sheet of aluminum to form the xeroradiographic plate, which is analogous to film used in conventional radiography. The plate is enclosed in a light-tight cassette.

The xeroradiographic imaging process consists of several steps:

1. A uniform charge is deposited onto the surface of the selenium. This sensitizes the plate before exposure to x rays.
2. The charged plate is placed in a light-tight cassette and exposed to x rays, just like a film-screen cassette. X rays reaching the plate cause the photoconductor layer to lose its charge in an amount corresponding to the intensity of the x-ray beam. The uniform charge is thus partly dissipated, and the remaining charge pattern forms the latent electrostatic image.
3. The latent electrostatic image is developed (made visible) by exposing the surface of the plate to fine-charged powder particles (called "toner") that are attracted to the plate surface in proportion to the intensity of the remaining charge.
4. The powder image is transferred to paper by placing suitable paper in contact with the plate and using an electrostatic charge to attract toner away from the plate and onto the paper.
5. The powder image is fused to the paper by exposure to heat to make a permanent record.
6. The plate is cleaned of all remaining powder (toner) and prepared for

reuse. The plate is not charged during storage.

PHOTOCONDUCTION

Solid materials may be classified as **conductors, semiconductors** (of which photoconductors are a special class), and **insulators**. This classification depends on whether or not the solid is capable of sustaining a current (moving electrons) if a voltage is applied. A brief review of the structure of an atom is necessary to understand why amorphous selenium, which is a photoconductor, is capable of forming the electrostatic latent image that is the basic physical phenomenon on which xeroradiography is based. (An introduction to atomic structure will be found in Chapter 2, "Interaction of Electron Beam with X-Ray Tube Target.")

The atom is made up of a nucleus around which electrons are spinning in orbits. The forces existing within the atom are electrostatic forces (neglecting nuclear forces) that always exist between two electrical charges. Electron orbits represent precisely defined energy levels for the electrons, and no electron may exist at any level (or orbit) other than one of these permissible levels. Groups of permissible orbits are combined into electron shells. The number of electrons in the outer energy shells determines the chemical and electrical properties of the atom. The atomic number of selenium is 34, which means that selenium has 34 electrons: 2 in the K shell, 8 in the L shell, 18 in the M shell, and 6 in the N shell, which is the outermost occupied shell for selenium. The electrons in the outermost shell are called valence (from the Latin *valere*, to have power) electrons because they determine the action of the atom when it reacts with atoms of another element to form compounds (chemical reaction).

Electrons move in a curved orbit around the nucleus because of the electrostatic force of attraction provided by the nucleus. If the electron is provided with more energy, the orbit of the electron must change. The electron must obey structural laws, however, and move into a permissible higher energy (farther from the nucleus) orbit. **Electrons cannot exist between permissible orbits**. One way that the energy of an electron is increased is by the absorption of electromagnetic radiation.

Atoms are bound together to form solids by the interaction of valence electrons. The interactions not only bond the atoms together, but also slightly change the value of permissible energy that the valence electrons may have. The energy of the valence electrons in an isolated atom is defined by the discrete energy levels. **In solids the outer discrete energy levels are replaced by energy bands, and the electrons may have any energy within the energy band (a narrow range of energies).** Inner shells may remain undisturbed by the bonding. In the isolated atom, the discrete energy levels are separated by nonpermissible energy values, and electrons may not exist with nonpermissible energy. The energy bands in solids may be separated by nonpermissible energy values or by forbidden energy bands.

In isolated atoms, the energy levels are filled to particular levels. Higher levels exist, but normally there are no electrons in these levels. Similarly, the energy bands in solids are filled to a particular level. The band with the highest energy that also has electrons is called the **valence band**. The next higher band is called the **conduction band**. The two bands may be separated by the **forbidden gap**. In considering electrical properties of solids, only these two bands are of interest. Figure 23–1 shows the relationships of the conduction and valence bands for semiconductors.

The conduction band always has more energy states than electrons, and the electrons may move from one energy state to another. Therefore, the electrons are fairly free to move when influenced by an external field in the form of a voltage (i.e., an electric current will flow). Solids that have

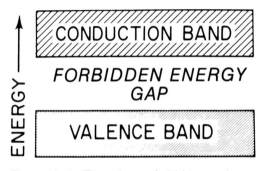

Figure 23–1 The valence, forbidden and conduction energy bands of a semiconductor

many electrons in the conduction level are known as conductors, of which silver and copper are good examples.

The valence band is the highest energy band in which electrons normally exist. The electrons in the valence level are not free to move because nearly all the available energy states already are occupied by electrons, so an electron having no place to go must stay in the state it is in. With proper addition of energy, however, electrons in the valence band may be elevated to the conduction band. To do this, the electron must acquire sufficient energy to bridge the gap between the valence and conduction bands. This gap is known as the forbidden energy band. It is the energy difference across this forbidden energy band that determines whether a solid acts as a conductor, an insulator, or a semiconductor.

In a conductor there is no forbidden region between the valence band and the conduction band. Insulators are those solids in which the forbidden gap is so large that electrons seldom absorb enough energy to bridge the gap.

A semiconductor is a solid that contains a small forbidden gap. Addition of the appropriate quantity of energy will allow some electrons to bridge the forbidden gap and enter the conduction band. In a **photoconductor** the energy is provided by absorption of visible electromagnetic radiation (light). Energy added to a semiconductor will cause electrons in the valence band to enter the conduction band, and the semiconductor will then be able to conduct an electric current if an external force (voltage) is applied.

When an electron leaves the selenium atom, the atom has an excess positive charge (the atom is ionized). The area of the absent negative charge (electron) in the valence band is termed a positive hole. Thus, the action of the energy of an absorbed light photon in selenium produces an electron and a positive hole, usually termed an electron-hole pair. When an electron-hole pair is subjected to an electrical field, the two members of the pair migrate in opposite directions. The electron moves toward the positive electrode. The atom containing the positive hole does not actually move. Instead, the hole is transferred from one atom to another and the result is that the hole moves toward the negative electrode. Later in this chapter we will discuss the migration of the electron to the positively charged selenium surface of the xeroradiographic plate, and migration of the positive hole through the selenium toward the induced negative charge on the aluminum substrate of the plate.

XERORADIOGRAPHIC PLATE

The xeroradiographic plate is a sheet of aluminum approximately $9\frac{1}{2} \times 14$ inches in size on which a layer of amorphous (vitreous) selenium has been deposited. In addition, there is an interface layer between the selenium and aluminum, and an overcoating protecting the selenium surface (Fig. 23–2).

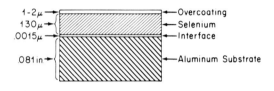

Figure 23–2 Cross section of a xeroradiographic plate

Aluminum Substrate

The aluminum plate on which the selenium is deposited is made of meticulously cleaned aluminum with an exceedingly smooth surface. Xeroradiographic sensitivity to any defect in the aluminum substrate is extremely high. Defects produce changes in the electrostatic charge in the selenium that may become visible during xerographic developing.

Interface Layer

Heat treatment of the surface of the aluminum substrate serves to form a thin layer of aluminum oxide. Although aluminum is a conductor, aluminum oxide is an insulator. The thickness of the aluminum oxide layer is not critical; a layer about 1.5 nm (.0015 microns) thick has been shown to be satisfactory. The purpose of this interface between the selenium and the aluminum substrate is to prevent negative charges induced in the aluminum from migrating into the selenium and dissipating the positive charge induced on the selenium surface. We will examine the nature of these induced charges shortly.

Selenium Coating

The photoconductive layer of the xeroradiographic plate is highly purified selenium in the amorphous, also called vitreous (i.e., not selenium crystals), form. It is deposited onto the aluminum substrate by condensation of vaporized liquid selenium in a high vacuum. The thickness of the selenium layer is 130 microns.

Protective Overcoating

The selenium surface of xeroradiographic plates is protected by an overcoating (most other xerographic plates and drums do not have an overcoating). The material used for the overcoating is cellulose acetate, applied by dip-coating from solution to form a layer about 1 to 2 microns thick. Cellulose acetate bonds well to selenium. It has a resistance high enough to prevent lateral conduction of charges, which would degrade the electrostatic latent image. Overcoating extends the life of a xeroradiographic plate by a factor of about 10.

Photoconductive Layer

There are three properties required of the photoconductor used in xeroradiography. First, the electrical conductivity in the dark must be that of a good insulator so that a charge pattern present on the surface will be retained long enough to complete the steps of development. Second, the material must become electrically conducting during exposure to x rays so that an electrostatic image pattern can be formed on its surface by the exposure. Third, it must have mechanical properties of durability and ease of fabrication. The only photoconductor that presently fulfills these criteria for commercial use is selenium. Practically all selenium is derived as a by-product of the electrolytic refinement of copper sulfide ores, either as gaseous SeO_2 or water-soluble Na_2SeO_3. Purification of selenium is very difficult, and any residual impurity may have a significant effect on its photoconductive properties.

The most stable form of selenium is its crystalline structure. This form is not used in xeroradiography because it has relatively high electrical conductivity. Crystalline selenium is used in selenium rectifiers. In addition to its crystalline structure, selenium also exists in an amorphous form, and it is this form that is used as the photoreceptor in xeroradiography. The amorphous form may be considered to be the super-cooled form of liquid selenium. It is formed by cooling the liquid suddenly so that crystals do not have time to form (the melting point of selenium is 216° C). In practice, amorphous selenium is deposited onto the aluminum plate by condensation of vaporized liquid selenium in a high vacuum. Pure amorphous selenium is mandatory as the presence of any impurity increases the dark decay rate. **Dark decay is**

the reduction of plate voltage while the plate remains in darkness. For xeroradiography this rate should not exceed 5% per minute.

The selenium layer is 130 microns thick. **Sensitivity of the plate to x rays depends on selenium thickness and on the energy (kVp) of the x-ray beam**. For x rays in the energy range usually used in medical diagnostic xeroradiography, a selenium plate about 130 microns thick has been shown to exhibit maximum sensitivity. We will define sensitivity as the reciprocal of the exposure in Roentgens required to reduce the charge on the plate to half its initial value.

Plate Charging

The first step in the xeroradiographic process is to sensitize the photoconductor by applying a uniform electrostatic charge to its surface in the dark. Because selenium is an insulator in the dark, during charging the xeroradiographic plate can be considered to be a parallel plate capacitor in which the outer (adjacent to protective coating) selenium surface and the aluminum backing (substrate) act as the parallel plates, and the selenium itself acts as the dielectric (see Fig. 23–4). The device used to produce a charge on the surface of the selenium operates on the principle of corona discharge in a gas. A brief review of capacitance and corona discharge is necessary.

Capacitance

A capacitor, or condenser, consists of two sheets of conducting material, with a sheet of insulating material between them. An electrical charge is placed on each plate (one plate is positive and the other negative); therefore, a potential difference, or voltage, exists between the two plates. The material between the plates has a strong influence on the amount of charge that can be placed on the plates. This material is an insulator, and is known as the dielectric. When influenced by the electric field between the plates, the atoms of the dielectric become distorted into a configuration known as an induced dipole. Consider Figure 23–3, in which a negatively charged rod is placed near an atom. The normal atom has its electron cloud centered on its nucleus (Fig. 23–3 A). The presence of the negative rod near the atom attracts the nucleus and repels the electrons so that the center of the electron cloud falls on the far side of the nucleus (Fig. 23–3 B). The atom now appears to have a positive side and a negative side; hence, it has become an induced dipole. Similar distortion exists in the atoms of the dielectric material between the charged plates of a capacitor.

Now consider the xeroradiographic plate. The outer surface of the selenium layer behaves like one plate of a capacitor, the aluminum backing (substrate) behaves like the other plate, and the photoconductor (selenium) acts as the dielectric (Fig. 23–4). If a positive charge is deposited onto the surface of the selenium, the remainder of the selenium atoms are distorted into the configuration of induced dipoles. The negative pole of each atom is attracted toward the positive charge, causing the atomic layer adjacent to the aluminum substrate to present a positive charge at the selenium-aluminum interface. Polarization of selenium atoms will attract negative charges (electrons) in the aluminum substrate toward the back of the selenium

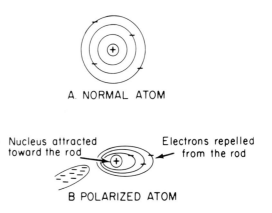

A. NORMAL ATOM

Nucleus attracted toward the rod   Electrons repelled from the rod

B POLARIZED ATOM

Figure 23–3 Polarization of an atom in an electric field

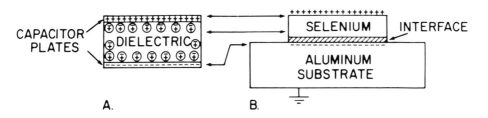

Figure 23–4 Charging of a parallel plate capacitor (A) and a xeroradiographic plate (B) is similar

layer. In other words, a negative charge has been induced in the aluminum susbstrate by the presence of the positive charge on the free surface of the selenium. It is obvious that these induced negative charges cannot be allowed to enter the selenium if the positive charge on the selenium surface is to be retained. It is now easier to understand the function of the interface layer between the selenium and the aluminum. The interface layer (aluminum oxide) reduces negative charge leakage from the substrate into the selenium.

Corona

If a sufficiently high potential difference (called the corona threshold voltage) is applied between a fine wire and ground, the air near the wire becomes ionized. If the voltage is positive, free electrons in the gas near the wire will move toward the wire. These electrons will be of high energy and instead of going straight to the wire, they will interact with many molecules or atoms in the air and create many additional ions. The positive ions thus created will move outward from the wire. This movement of ions is called corona current. The corona around a wire with a positive voltage has the appearance of a uniform bluish-white sheath over the entire surface of the wire. When such a wire is placed close to the surface of the xeroradiographic plate (the distance is about $\frac{11}{16}$ inch) some positive ions repelled from the wire will be deposited onto the surface of the plate. The corona threshold voltage is quite high compared with the needed positive voltage on the surface of the plate. The wire is cor-

rosion-resistant (commonly stainless steel or aluminum), and about 3.5 mils in diameter.

Corona threshold voltage for such a wire is about 4400 volts. By comparison, the positive voltage desired on the surface of the plate ranges from about 1000 to 1600 volts. This creates two problems. First, overcharging the surface of the plate must be prevented, suggesting that the potential difference (voltage) on the charging wire should be kept as low as possible. Second, small variations in wire diameter or dirt on the wire will affect the threshold voltage at different points along the wire and cause nonuniformity of corona current. These variations can be minimized if the wire is operated considerably above the corona threshold voltage, at about 7500 volts. Two devices have been developed to control the amount and uniformity of plate charging, the scorotron and the corotron.

Charging Devices

The **scorotron** involves use of a control screen, or grid, that acts somewhat like the grid in a thyratron tube. This device consists of the corona-emitting wire (or wires) and a grounded backing plate. In addition, a grid of parallel wires about $\frac{3}{32}$ inch apart is placed between the corona wire and the surface of the xeroradiographic plate (Fig. 23–5). If the grid wires are operated at a positive potential, they will suppress the flow of positive ions from the corona wire to the surface of the plate (i.e., the positive charge on the grid will partially repel positive ions in the air attempting to reach the plate). The grid may be operated from

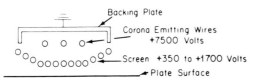

Figure 23–5 Cross-sectional schematic diagram of a grid-controlled corona-charging device (scorotron)

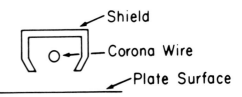

Figure 23–6 Cross-sectional schematic diagram of a corotron

about 350 to 1700 volts positive potential relative to the grounded plate.

Assume that the grid is operated at +1000 volts. Initially, with no voltage on the plate surface, the entire 1000-volt potential difference will repel positive air ions from the grid to the selenium surface. As a positive voltage begins to accumulate on the plate surface, the potential difference between the grid and plate will decrease. When the voltage on the plate surface reaches 1000 volts, no potential difference will exist between the grid and plate, and the movement of positive air ions will stop. The grid allows more precise control of plate charging. Also, because it is now grid voltage rather than voltage on the corona wire (wires) that controls plate charging, the corona wire may be operated at a voltage that produces a more uniform corona current (flow of ions). This corona voltage is usually about 7500 volts DC, and is not under the control of the operator of the unit. The grid voltage can be regulated by local maintenance personnel to produce the contrast desired by the individual using the apparatus. The influence of initial plate voltage on the developed xeroradiographic image will be discussed later.

The **corotron** is a simpler device that has the same function as the scorotron. The corotron consists of a long U-shaped channel (called the shield) with inwardly bent lips and a single corona wire. A cross section of a corotron is illustrated in Figure 23–6. The shield is usually maintained at ground potential. The corona current to the plate is controlled by the corona wire voltage, the configuration of the shield,

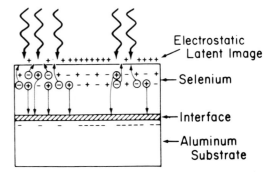

Figure 23–7 Exposure of the charged xeroradiographic plate to x rays creates an electrostatic latent image

and the location of the wire within the shield.

The plate is charged by causing it to move at a uniform rate under the stationary charging device, which may be a scorotron or corotron. Because the charged photoconductor is sensitive to light as well as to x rays, plate charging and all subsequent operations leading to obtaining a developed xeroradiographic image must be carried out with the plate completely shielded from light.

EXPOSURE OF CHARGED PLATE

After the plate is sensitized by corona charging it must be enclosed in a cassette that is light-tight and rigid enough to provide mechanical protection for the fragile plate. The plate-cassette combination is then used just as an x-ray film in its cassette would be used.

When the charged selenium plate is exposed to x rays (or light), **electron-hole pairs** are created (Fig. 23–7). These charged particles come under the influence of the corona-induced positive charge on the surface of the selenium, and the induced negative charge in the aluminum substrate. The electrons migrate to the plate surface and discharge the positive charge originally laid down. The positive holes "migrate" through the selenium toward the substrate, where they are neutralized by the induced negative charges. The amount of discharge of the positive charges on the surface of the plate is proportional to the intensity of x rays that penetrated the patient, so the variation of charge pattern remaining on the plate accurately reflects the pattern of attenuation of x rays caused by the patient. The remaining charge pattern on the plate is called the **electrostatic latent image**.

Conductivity Induced by X Rays

The energy gap between the valence band and conduction band (i.e., the forbidden energy band) in amorphous selenium is about 2.3 eV (electron volts). This corresponds to a wavelength of about 5400 Å which is visible light in the green-yellow range:

$$E = \frac{12,400}{\lambda}$$

$$2.3 = \frac{12,400}{\lambda}$$

$$\lambda = \frac{12,400}{2.3} \text{ or } 5348 \text{ Å } (534.8 \text{ nm})$$

E = photon energy in eV
λ = wavelength in Angstroms (Å)

This calculation is a rough estimate used to illustrate the principle leading to creation of photoconductivity induced in selenium by light. Stated in another way, an electron in the valence band of amorphous selenium must absorb all the energy of a light photon of wavelength 5400 Å (540 nm) to be elevated into the conduction band, where it will be able to move when influenced by the positive voltage on the surface of the plate. Obviously, light is absorbed very near the surface of the selenium, with 63% of attenuation occurring within 0.125 μ of the incident surface.

Photoconductivity induced in amorphous selenium by x rays differs in two important ways from photoconductivity induced by light. First, the x-ray photons can penetrate further into the selenium, and their absorption may be almost uniform throughout the selenium layer. Second, the energy of an absorbed or scattered x-ray photon is transferred to a photoelectron or a recoil electron (Compton scattering), and each of these electrons will usually have enough kinetic energy to produce many more charge carrier (electron-hole) pairs along its track. The sensitivity of selenium plates of different thicknesses of selenium can be calculated by measuring the x-ray exposure required to reduce plate voltage to half its original value. This sensitivity will also vary with the quality (kVp) of the x rays. Figure 23–8 is a drawing taken from a series of curves in the literature, and shows the relative sensitivity of selenium plates of varying thickness to a 40-kVp x-ray beam.[2] The significantly greater sensitivity of plates in the 130- to 160-μ range explains the choice of 130 μ as the thickness of commercially available xeroradiographic plates. Although **plate sensitivity is largely a function of the thickness of the selenium layer and the kVp** at which the exposure is made, it is also true that plate sensitivity can depend on the x-ray

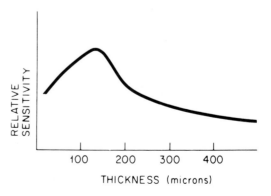

Figure 23–8 Sensitivity of a selenium plate to 40-kVp x rays as a function of selenium thickness. (Modified from Boag[2])

tube type, wave form of the x-ray generator, and amount of filtration.

Electrostatic Latent Image

After exposure by x rays there remains on the xeroradiographic plate surface a latent image composed of variations in the positive charge that represent the structure of the object examined. This is called the electrostatic latent image, and it is accompanied by an electric field. The character of this electric field distribution above the latent image has a strong influence on the visible image formed when the image is developed. Because xeromammography is a well-established clinical application of xeroradiography, we will use this examination as a prototype to illustrate some basic principles. Typically, a xeroradiographic plate used for mammography will be charged to a positive potential of about 1625 volts. After exposure, some areas of the plate will be almost completely discharged (e.g., areas outside the breast tissue), while other areas will retain almost all the 1625 volts (e.g., under a large calcified fibroadenoma).

Electric Field Distribution Above Latent Image

Because the development of the electrostatic latent image depends on the attraction of charged toner particles to the surface of the plate, knowledge of local electric field strengths is necessary to understand the development process. This subject is highly complex, but for practical purposes we will confine our attention to two aspects of the electric fields existing above the latent image. First, the field has both a vertical and a horizontal component. Second, the field strength declines rapidly as one moves away from the charged surface.

Consider a plate that has been exposed so that a narrow strip retains its full initial charge (i.e., no x rays have reached the plate in that area), and the area on each side of the strip has been completely discharged. The lines of force existing above

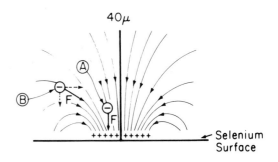

Figure 23–9   Electric field configuration above a narrow charged strip. (Modified from Boag[2])

the plate will be similar to those shown in Figure 23–9, in which lines drawn close together represent stronger electrical fields. Note that the lines of force become further apart rapidly as distance from the plate surface increases by only a few microns. A negative charge at A, which is placed directly above the charged strip, will be attracted to the plate surface only by a nearly vertical force pulling it straight down to the surface of the plate. If the negative charge were located directly over the discharged portion of the plate, but near the charged area (B), both a vertical and a horizontal force act on the particle and cause it to pursue a curved path as it is attracted to the edge of the charged area. Because of this horizontal force component, negatively charged particles will be "stolen" from the area adjacent to a charged zone on the plate. We will use this concept to explain the phenomena of edge enhancement and deletion that are encountered in the developed xeroradiographic image.

Sensitometry

Xeroradiography is unique in that the response of the plate to x-ray exposure can be measured independently of the development process. To do this, the plate is usually exposed using an aluminum step wedge, just as film sensitometry is done. For measurements in the mammographic range, a nine-step aluminum test object with thicknesses ranging from 0 to 0.4 inch

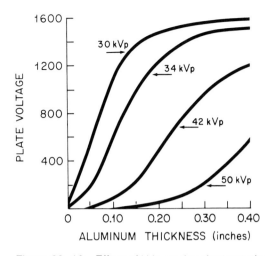

Figure 23–10   Effect of kVp on the electrostatic latent image. (Modified from Thourson[7])

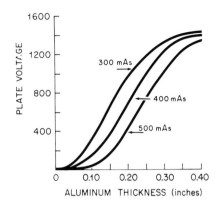

Figure 23–11   Effect of mAs on the electrostatic latent image. (Modified from Thourson[7])

is used. Then an electrometer is positioned over the plate and the voltage remaining on the plate under the center of each step of the wedge is measured (this must be done in the dark). The results are plotted as a discharge curve, giving the voltage remaining on a plate after exposure through a given thickness of the aluminum step wedge. Such a curve is illustrated in Figure 23–10, in which response for variation in x-ray tube kVp is plotted. In this illustration plate voltage may be considered to be the equivalent of film density in the more familiar film characteristic curve. Note that these curves have a toe, straight line portion, and shoulder, similar to x-ray film characteristic curves. Also note that **the effect of increasing kVp is to decrease the slope of the straight-line portion of the curve (decrease contrast)**. This is an important difference compared to an x-ray film characteristic curve. The characteristic curve of a film is established by the manufacturer; inherent film contrast cannot be changed by the radiologist.

The effect of changing mAs (kVp constant) is illustrated in Figure 23–11. **Increasing exposure shifts the curve to the right** (i.e., greater exposure more completely discharges the plate under each step of the wedge) without making any significant change in the slope of the straight-line portion of the curve. This result should be easily understood based on knowledge of the effect of mAs and x-ray film exposure.

Xeroradiographic Undercutting

Xeroradiographic undercutting is caused by ionization of the air in the space between the selenium surface of the xeroradiographic plate and the lid of the cassette. This ionization can be caused by interaction of x rays directly with air molecules, or it may be caused by high-speed electrons being able to escape from the selenium and enter the air space. This results in the presence of positive and negative air ions in the dark space between the selenium surface and the cassette lid. At the same time these air ions are being created, the x-ray exposure has caused some areas of the selenium plate to be discharged more than others (i.e., the electrostatic latent image has been formed).

Assume that a test exposure has been made in which part of the cassette has been covered by a lead bar that prevents any x rays from reaching the selenium plate (Fig. 23–12A). This will cause an abrupt step in charge density on the plate surface, with charge varying from virtually zero to almost the initial voltage on the plate. Across this step strong electrostatic fields will exist in the air space immediately above

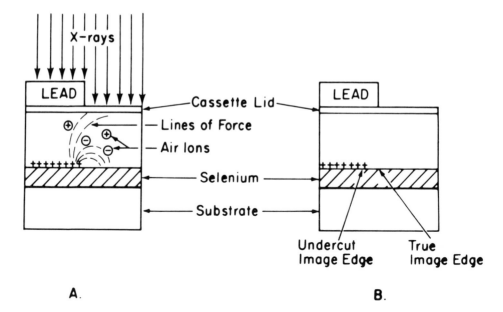

Figure 23–12   Xeroradiographic undercutting

the plate. Because the initial charge on the plate surface is positive, the electrostatic forces will cause negative air ions to be deposited on the edge of the high plate charge and tend to neutralize the charge. This **deposition of negative ions would tend to "move" the edge of the electrostatic image toward the shielded side of the plate** (Fig. 23–12*B*) and, in extreme cases, could actually **cause the image to become considerably smaller** than the object being imaged. To eliminate this problem, a DC voltage is applied between the cassette lid and the aluminum backing of the plate. This will cause any air ions formed to move in a direction perpendicular to the plate so that they cannot be pulled from any area into the charge field at the edge of an image. If the cassette lid is made positive, negative air ions can be attracted away from the plate surface. In practice, the potential difference (voltage) applied between the cassette lid and aluminum plate substrate is about 450 volts. The problem of xeroradiographic undercutting is rarely serious in medical xeroradiography, but can occur frequently in industrial radiog-

raphy at the border of totally absorbing metal parts.

Because of the highly localized nature of the electrostatic fields at the edge of a sharp charge difference, the results of xeroradiographic undercutting tend to move the charge pattern toward the center of the more highly charged area. Note that this differs from the more familiar concept of edge unsharpness on film radiographs, which causes a sharp edge to become less sharp but does not move the position of the edge.

DEVELOPMENT

Development of the xeroradiographic image may be defined as the selective deposition of imaging material onto a surface in response to electrostatic forces. Development consists of attracting small charged dust particles, called **toner**, to the electrostatic latent image on the selenium surface of the plate. The most commonly used toner in xerographic copy machines is charcoal, with a particle size of about 1 micron. Xeroradiography, however, requires use of a pigmented thermoplastic material of dark blue (called Type 5B by Xerox Corporation) or blue-green (Type 5) color. Mean diameter of the particle is in the general range of a few microns.

Powder Cloud Development

The terms powder cloud development and aerosol development are synonyms. This is the form of development used in xeroradiography. It is fast, relatively simple, and **provides the edge enhancement** that is so characteristic and desirable in the developed image. Also, the powder cloud method is the form of development that is least damaging to the selenium surface.

The exposed xeroradiographic plate is placed on top of a dark box into which an aerosol of charged toner particles is sprayed through a nozzle (Fig. 23–13).

Aerosol Generation and Toner Charging

If pressurized gas (commonly nitrogen gas) is used to force toner through a small bore tube, an aerosol of toner particles is created. An aerosol is a suspension of small liquid or solid particles in a gaseous medium. Aerosol particles have random movement. It has been found that a conventional paint spray gun will produce satisfactory aerosols from dry powders. Agglomeration of toner into unacceptably large particles is prevented because of the turbulent flow produced when the aerosol passes through the small bore nozzle.

The electric charge on the toner particles is produced by friction between the toner and the wall of the nozzle. This process is called triboelectrification (from the Greek *tribein* meaning "to rub"), or contact electrification. Charging particles by contact electrification involves complex processes, and a discussion of the physics involved is beyond the scope of this text. Toner particles with both a positive and a negative charge are produced in roughly equal numbers, and it is possible to attract either the positive or negative particles to the surface of the selenium. "Positive" developing involves attracting negatively charged toner particles to the remaining positive charge on the surface of the selenium.

Development Process

Xeroradiographic development consists of attracting the charged toner particles to the configuration of residual positive electrostatic charges on the selenium surface. The plate containing the electrostatic latent image is clamped onto the top of a powder cloud chamber, and toner is introduced into the chamber as an aerosol (Fig. 23–13). Diffusion air is also introduced into the chamber to create air turbulence. The toner cloud contains both positive and

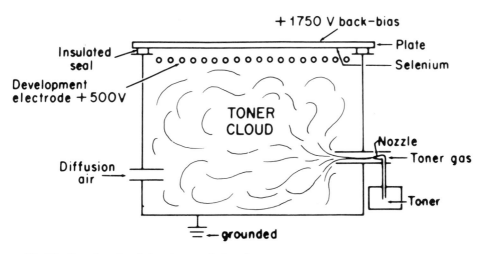

Figure 23–13 Powder cloud development chamber

negative particles of pigmented thermo-plastic, but particles of only one polarity are used to form the image. To get a "positive" image a positive voltage is applied to the aluminum backing of the plate to attract only negatively charged toner. It is necessary to use this positive voltage applied to the plate back (termed the back-bias voltage) to attract negatively charged toner particles close enough to the plate to allow the electrostatic forces of the latent image to act on the toner. There are now two electrostatic forces influencing the motion of the particles: the uniform electric field of the back-bias voltage, and the non-uniform field caused by the latent image. For typical positive development the back-bias potential is +1750 volts DC. Conversely, a "negative" image can be produced by applying a negative bias voltage to the back (−2750 volts DC is a typical value) and attracting positive toner to the plate. This is done by moving one switch in the development processor. In the positive mode, positive toner particles are repelled by the positive potential on the plate and are directed to the grounded bottom of the powder cloud chamber.

We must now examine what happens to the negatively charged toner particles (all examples will be for positive development) as they approach the surface of the selenium in the region of an image representing a high-contrast edge. For example, we might consider a step wedge image in which an abrupt change in charge on the selenium surface of 100 volts is produced (e.g., +900 versus +1000 volts) by the abrupt change in x-ray exposure at one step. Examination of this high-contrast edge will help in understanding the concepts of edge enhancement and deletion.

Edge enhancement arises from the electric field pattern associated with any abrupt change in charge density on the surface of the plate. The negatively charged toner particle in the powder cloud moves toward the plate under the influence of both the back-bias voltage and the latent image elec-

tric field. Although a uniform flow of toner approaches the plate, the electrostatic latent image electric field will cause significant change in "flow" as toner gets very near (e.g., 100 microns) the plate surface. Near an abrupt step in charge the electrostatic lines of force actually form closed loops, and charged toner particles moving along these lines of force are thrown toward the side of highest charge and excluded from the other side. The increase in toner deposited on the more highly charged side of the edge will be at the expense of toner deposition on the lower charge side. At some distance from the edge, in either direction, the influence of the edge gradient is greatly diminished, and the uniform back-bias field dominates to cause even more deposition of toner.

Deletions can also be explained in terms of the electric field distribution. In Figure 23–14 it can be seen that if toner particles strictly followed the lines of force, no toner would be deposited in the region marked "X". Air turbulence in the development chamber, however, causes some toner to break through the "shield" formed by the lines of force, but toner that does penetrate will be attracted only to the highly charged side of the edge. This causes development to occur completely to the edge of the area

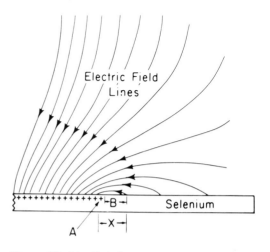

Figure 23–14   Deletions are caused by electric field lines of force

of higher charge (A, Fig 23–14), but still leaves the region immediately adjacent to the edge (B, Fig. 23–14) undeveloped. This undeveloped region is called a deletion. Although small deletions may sometimes be desirable, a large deletion may result in loss of information in the deletion zone.

There is a relationship between edge enhancement (or edge contrast), initial xeroradiographic plate voltage, the back-bias voltage, and the size of a deletion. The size of a deletion depends on the voltage contrast (voltage difference) at an edge and on the magnitude of the back-bias voltage. Large contrasts lead to large deletions, while increasing the bias voltage reduces deletion width. If the back-bias voltage is too high, low contrast detail in other parts of the image may be obscured. A lower initial plate voltage will reduce overall image contrast, and this will also reduce deletion width. For the low contrast encountered in mammography, however, higher initial plate voltage is usually used.

To review,

	CONTRAST	DELETION WIDTH
High back-bias	Low	Small
High plate voltage	High	Large
High contrast image	High	Large
Low contrast image	Low	Small

Development Electrode

The development electrode is an electrode placed in front of the plate during powder cloud development, and is given a voltage of appropriate sign (+ voltage for "positive" development) to superimpose a uniform helping field in the direction of the plate for the toner particles of desired charge (Fig. 23–13). **One major effect of the development electrode is to cause a visible image to be developed in uniformly exposed regions of the electrostatic latent image**. Otherwise these areas would go undeveloped. For example, use of a development electrode with xeromammography will make possible imaging of skin and large soft tissue areas of the

breast. Additionally, the development electrode can be used to influence edge enhancement and the width of deletions, such as those that surround dense breast calcifications. The developing electrode is actually a grid (series of wires) placed close (1.5 to 2.5 mm) to the surface of the plate. The potential applied to the grid is usually +500 volts DC.

We will use a specific example to explain the way in which a development electrode influences the electrostatic field of the latent image. Assume a selenium plate with an initial surface charge of +1625 volts has been exposed so that a large area (e.g., a 2-cm^2 area of normal dense breast tissue) retains a uniform charge of +1200 volts. Close to this large area there is a small area (e.g., a 50-μ^2 area under a breast calcification) in which the plate receives little x-ray exposure and retains a +1500-volts charge. Figure 23–15A diagrams the electric field that exists above both these areas (it is assumed that the space between these two areas has been completely discharged). Above the small area there is a strong electric field, but the electric field strength and potential have decreased significantly at a distance of 1.5 mm from the surface of the plate (we will assume that +600 volts remain). Above the broad area the electric field is weak, and the potential drop is minimal, so that at 1.5 mm most of the original potential persists. The voltage above each area must fall to zero volts at the opposite side of the development chamber (this side of the chamber is grounded to keep it at zero volts potential; see Fig. 23–13), but the potential drop over the small charged area is very rapid near the plate while the potential over the large area drops rather evenly from the plate to the grounded development chamber bottom.

To summarize, (1) the electric field strength above the small area is strong and drops rapidly with distance from the plate, and (2) the electric field strength above the large area is weak, and drops slowly. Charged toner particles approaching the

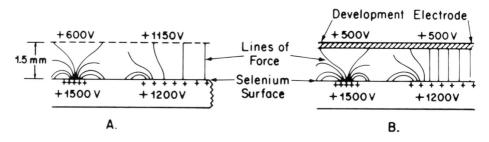

Figure 23–15 Effect of the development electrode

surface of the plate in Figure 23–15*A* would be strongly attracted to the narrow area, and to the edge of the broad area, but would have little attraction to the central part of the broad area. Thus, edge enhancement and deletions would be maximal, but there would be little visualization of structures in broad areas of relatively uniform exposure (e.g., normal breast tissue or skin).

Now, let us place a development electrode 1.5 mm from the surface of the plate, and place a potential of +500 volts on the development electrode. What effect does this electrode have on the electric field above the 50-μ^2 and the 2-cm² areas of the plate? Above the small area (50 μ^2), almost no effect. Above the large area (2 cm²) there will be a marked increase in strength of the electric field, shown by the increased number of lines of force drawn in Figure 23–14*B*. We must explain why this happens.

The electric field (E) between two parallel plates is equal to the voltage (V) divided by the distance (d) between the plates, provided d is small compared to the area of the plates:

$$E = \frac{V}{d}$$

If the distance (d) can be made smaller, the electric field (E) will increase if voltages are the same. Without the development electrode in place, the potential above the 2-cm² field falls to zero across the entire distance from the surface of the plate to the grounded bottom of the development chamber (i.e., d is large, so $\frac{V}{d}$ is small). The addition of a development electrode with a +500-volt potential, 1.5 mm from the surface of the plate, will force the voltage above the 2-cm² field to drop from +1200 to +500 volts over a small (1.5-mm) distance. This causes a large potential difference (V) to occur in a short distance (d), so the expression $\frac{V}{d}$ is now large, and the electric field (E) between the plate and development electrode has become much stronger. Conversely, the strength of the electric field above the small (50-μ^2) area is minimally affected because a strong electric field (E) associated with a rapid potential drop (V) existed without the development electrode being present.

The important concept is the change the development electrode has caused in the electric field above each area. The development electrode has little effect on the field near fine detail, but greatly increases the strength of the electric field over more uniformly charged areas. Properly used, **the development electrode allows satisfactory detail to be developed in broad exposure areas without sacrificing information in areas of fine detail.**

SENSITOMETRY OF DEVELOPED IMAGE

We have previously explored the way in which kVp affects the contrast present in the electrostatic latent image. It is now nec-

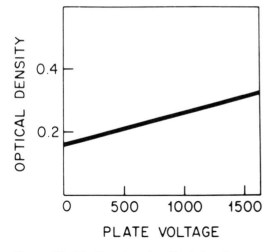

Figure 23–16 Developed optical density as a function of plate voltage (positive development)

essary to consider the characteristics of the developed optical density of the xeroradiographic print. Figure 23–16 shows developed optical density as a function of plate voltage, using positive development and a plate initially charged to + 1625 volts. Note that there is little change in developed optical density, or contrast, across the entire range of voltage in the electrostatic latent image. This provides a system with **great latitude**, in that all variations in plate voltage can be developed, but the resulting image would have so little contrast that it would be of almost no diagnostic value. More important than this total density range is the **contrast** (change in optical density) **across an image edge**. Because of the edge enhancement inherent in xeroradiography, the developed optical density on the high-voltage side of the edge falls above the general density level of the plate (positive development), while the density on the low-voltage side of the edge falls below the general density level. A density peak and valley exist at the edge. The perceptibility of an edge depends on the difference in optical density (contrast between the high-density peak and low-density valley) that exists at an edge. This density difference is a function of the voltage contrast

that exists at the edge of the electrostatic latent image with more voltage contrast resulting in greater density difference.

Figure 23–17 shows examples of densitometer scans across step edges of various voltage contrasts. You will recall that it is possible to measure voltages on the selenium plate before the electrostatic latent image is developed. In Figure 23–17 the average optical density is about 0.5, and at edge gradients developed optical density falls above and below the average density. Because of edge enhancement, a voltage difference of only 1 volt across an edge can be detected in the developed image.

QUALITY OF XERORADIOGRAPHIC IMAGE

The quality of the developed xeroradiograph may be evaluated by its resolving power (line pairs per mm) and by its modulation transfer function (MTF).

The inherent resolution of the latent image on the surface of a selenium plate is high, with resolution as high as 2000 line pairs per millimeter being reported in laboratory experiments using liquid developer. When powder cloud development is used, the size of the toner particles sets a limit on resolving power. For toner with a mean particle diameter of 5 microns, this limit is thought to be about 50 line pairs per mm. Other factors, such as the charge on the toner particles and the thickness of

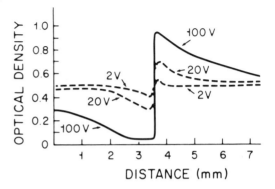

Figure 23–17 Densitometer scans across step edges of different voltage contrast

the selenium layer, have some influence on resolution. The inherent resolving power of both the selenium plate and the powder cloud development process are not limiting factors in resolution in the xeroradiographic image as it is used for medical diagnosis. Limitations imposed by the focal spot of the x-ray tube and by patient motion are the two major factors in limiting resolving power.

The modulation transfer function of xeroradiography is quite different from that of film. Curves comparing the MTF of xeroradiography and film have been published, and such a diagram is presented in Figure 23–18.[4] Notice that for xeroradiography, the low spatial frequencies are poorly reproduced, while frequencies near 1 line pair per mm are greatly accentuated. Film has its best response at lower spatial frequencies (i.e., the less information to be recorded, the better job film can do). The upper limit of both film and xeroradiography MTF curves is about the same because this represents a limit imposed by factors other than the film or xeroradiographic plate (e.g., x-ray tube focal spot and patient motion). The unusual shape of the MTF curve of a xeroradiograph is compatible with clinical observations that large homogeneous structures, such as areas of

normal dense breast tissue, are difficult to image. Stated another way, **xeroradiography may be said to exhibit enhanced fine structure contrast and subdued broad area contrast.**

Exposure Latitude

Xeroradiography exhibits broad exposure latitude compared to x-ray film exposure. Experimental data show that xeroradiography will produce satisfactory image resolution over a wider range of kVp selections than will film. In other words, it may be said that with xeroradiography the resolution capability is less sensitive to exposure, and a single exposure will produce good image resolution in all portions of a breast (thick and thin areas). Using film, obtaining good resolving power of the image under thin breast areas often requires a significantly different kVp than that required to produce a similar image under thick breast areas. With xeroradiography an appropriate kVp that produces satisfactory resolution in all portions of the image is more easily found. Another illustration of this concept of broad exposure latitude of xeroradiography is that objects such as blood vessels will exhibit equal contrast over wide variations in breast thickness.

IMAGE TRANSFER AND FIXING

It is necessary for the powder image on the surface of the xeroradiographic plate to be transferred to paper and fixed there to form a permanent image. An electrostatic transfer process is used. The paper is coated with a slightly deformable layer of plastic, such as a low-molecular weight polyethylene material. When this paper is pushed against the powder image under relatively high pressure, the toner particles become slightly embedded in the plastic.

After development, the plate is removed from the development chamber and prepared for this transfer process by being passed over a pretransfer corotron that has a negative charge. This negative corona

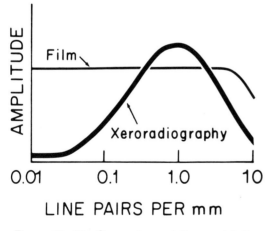

Figure 23–18 Comparison of the modulation transfer function of film and xeroradiography. (Modified from Kilgore et al.[4])

loosens the attraction between toner particles and the selenium surface of the plate, and gives the toner a negative charge to prepare it for the transfer process. The plate then comes in contact with the paper over a transfer corotron, and the image is transferred to the paper. The transfer corotron has a positive charge that attracts the negatively charged toner to the paper. The paper is also mechanically pressed against the powder image. After the image is transferred, the paper is peeled off the plate, and the loosely held powder image is made into a permanent bonded image by heating the paper to about 475° F. The heat softens the plastic coating on the paper and allows toner particles to sink into and become bonded to the plastic. The toner particles do not melt or flow.

After fixing, also called fusing, the imaging portion of the xeroradiographic process is complete, and the completed image is delivered from the processor ready for viewing. With positive development, areas that received little x-ray exposure (such as dense breast calcification) will appear dark blue on the print, and areas receiving heavy x-ray exposure will appear light blue. If a charged plate is inadvertently exposed to room light and then developed (positive), the paper will be almost devoid of toner. Conversely, a charged but unexposed plate will produce a uniformly deep blue print if it is subjected to positive development.

PLATE CLEANING AND STORAGE

After transfer of the toner to paper, some toner remains on the plate surface. All toner must be removed before the plate can be used again. After the transfer process is completed, the plate is exposed to a light source (electroluminescent strip) that reduces the bond holding residual toner to the plate. Next, a preclean corotron exposes the plate to an alternating current that serves to neutralize the electrostatic forces holding toner to the plate. A clean-ing brush then mechanically brushes the residual toner from the plate.

Relaxation (Plate Fatigue)

Relaxation is done to prevent faint "ghost" images from appearing (this phenomenon is sometimes called plate fatigue). Absorption of x rays in the selenium produces an alteration in the physical state of the selenium atoms that causes some photoconductivity to persist for as long as several hours after exposure. If the plate were charged for a new exposure without allowing it to rest for several hours, this residual photoconductivity would cause some discharge in the dark and create a faint "ghost" image of the previous exposure to appear when the plate was developed. This rest period can be reduced to only 2 or 3 minutes if the plate is relaxed by heating it to 140° F for 150 seconds. The cleaned and relaxed plate is then held in the storage compartment of the conditioner module of the xeroradiographic system at 89° F until needed for another exposure.

The life of a xeroradiographic plate is of the order of several thousand exposures. Exposure to x rays or to light does not shorten the life span. The main cause of plate failure is physical damage caused by handling and the cleaning process.

AUTOMATIC XERORADIOGRAPHIC SYSTEM

Processing of a xeroradiographic plate takes place in two units that have been termed the conditioner (prepares the plates for exposure) and the processor. (Fig. 23–19).[5] Following processing, cleaned plates are stored in a box (1) in the processor unit. The box can hold as many as six plates. When this storage box is inserted into the input station of the conditioner, the plates are extracted one at a time and transported to the relaxing oven (2). The relaxed plates are stored in the storage unit (3) for an indefinite period of time. When a sensitized plate is needed, an

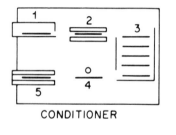

CONDITIONER

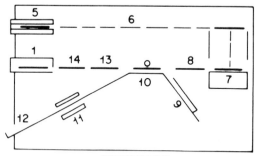

PROCESSOR

1. Plate storage box
2. Relaxation oven
3. Plate storage compartment
4. Plate charging
5. Cassette
6. Plate transport mechanism
7. Development chamber
8. Pre-transfer station
9. Paper storage and feeder
10. Transfer station
11. Fusing oven
12. Paper print tray
13. Pre-cleaning station
14. Plate cleaning station

Figure 23–19 Diagram of the automatic xero-radiographic processing system. (Modified from McMaster and Hoyt[5])

empty cassette is inserted into the cassette station of the conditioner (5). This causes a plate to be removed from the storage area and passed under the charging device (4). Immediately after charging, the plate is moved into the cassette (5), and is ready for use. The conditioner requires about 15 seconds to charge a stored plate and place the plate in a cassette.

After exposure, the cassette (5) is placed in the processor where development trans-

fer, and cleaning take place. The exposed plate is extracted from the cassette and transported (6) to the back of the processor unit, where it is sealed to the top of the development chamber (7). During development, a sheet of paper is transported from the paper storage tray (9) to the transfer station (10). The developed plate passes the pretransfer station (8) and then proceeds to the transfer station (10), where the image is transferred from the plate to the paper. The paper is then pulled away from the plate and into the fusing oven (11), where the image is fixed to form a permanent image. The paper then proceeds to the output tray (12). At the same time the paper is being processed, the plate passes through the precleaning (13) and cleaning (14) stations. The clean plates may be stored in the storage box (1) until six plates have accumulated, or transferred back to the conditioner before the box is full. The processor is able to produce a completed print in about 2 minutes. In many processors it is possible to begin transport of a plate to the developing chamber while another plate is in the transfer and cleaning areas, thus speeding the rate of processing of multiple plates.

The front of the conditioner of the Xerox 125 conditioner has a control knob labeled "B", "C", and "D". This control changes the initial plate voltage, and corresponds to approximately 975 volts (B), 1300 volts (C), and 1625 volts (D). The D setting is generally used in xeromammography because high contrast is desirable.

The front of the Xerox 125 processor has two control knobs, labeled "Mode" and "Density." The mode knob determines whether a positive or negative print is obtained. The density knob is used only with the negative mode, and determines the number of powder bursts that will be introduced into the development chamber during plate development. The stations on the density knob are labeled "B", "C", and "D," and correspond to 10 (B), 18 (C) and 26 (D) powder bursts. In the positive mode, development is accomplished with 10 powder bursts.

PATIENT EXPOSURE FROM FILM-SCREEN AND XERORADIOGRAPHIC MAMMOGRAPHY

Several years ago the radiation dose received during mammography was measured as the entrance dose to the skin of the breast.[7] Recent studies indicate that the amount of radiation absorbed by the glandular tissue below the skin surface is a more important measurement.[4] It is presumed that it is the glandular tissue which is at risk of developing cancer in the future. Accurate estimates of this midbreast dose must take into account many factors, including the ratio of glandular to fatty tissue, beam quality, the area of the breast irradiated, and the dose to the skin of the breast. The average of a typical midbreast dose for xeroradiography is about 0.74 rad for a two-view examination (using a molybdenum target x-ray tube).[4] The average for a typical film-screen examination, using a tungsten-target x-ray tube, is 0.08 rad for two views.[4]

SUMMARY

The summary is contained in the beginning of this chapter under the heading "General Principles."

Xeroradiography is a radiographic method that has imaging characteristics different from those of film, which include:

1. edge enhancement
2. subdued broad area response
3. deletions
4. broad exposure latitude.

This system is useful for imaging low-contrast objects defined by sharp edges. Because of subdued broad area response and edge enhancement, object latitude is large, and a single image can contain useful information over a wide range of object thicknesses.

REFERENCES

1. Boag, J.W.: Electrostatic imaging. Contained in the syllabus of the AAPM, 1975 Summer School, The Expanding Role of the Diagnostic Radiologic Physicist, Rice University, Houston, July–August 1, 1975, p. 159.
2. Boag, J.W.: Xeroradiography. Phys. Med. Biol., *18*: 3, 1973.
3. Dessaver, J.H., and Clark, H.E.: Xerography and Related Processes. London, Focal Press, 1965.
4. Hammerstein, G.R., Miller, D.W., White, D.R., et al.: Absorbed radiation dose in mammography. Radiology, *130*:485, 1979.
5. Kilgore, R.A., Gregg, E.C., and Rao, P.S.: Transfer functions for xeroradiographs and electronic image enhancement systems. Opt. Eng., *13*:130, 1974.
6. McMaster, R.C., and Hoyt, H.L.: Xeroradiography in the 1970's. Mater. Eval., *29*:265, 1971.
7. Rothenberg, L.N., Kirch, R.L.A., and Snyder, R.E.: Patient exposures from film and xeroradiographic mammographic techniques. Radiology, *117*:701, 1975.
8. Thourson, T.L.: Xeroradiography. Proc. Soc. Photo-Opt. Eng., *56*:225, 1974.
9. Wolfe, J.N.: Xeroradiography of the Breast, Springfield, IL, Charles C Thomas, 1972, pp. 3–17.

24

Computed Tomography

At the Annual Congress of the British Institute of Radiology, in April of 1972, G.N. Hounsfield, a senior research scientist at EMI Limited in Middlesex, England, announced the invention of a revolutionary new imaging technique, which he called computerized axial transverse scanning.[7] The basic concept was quite simple: a thin cross section of the head, a tomographic slice, was examined from multiple angles with a pencillike x-ray beam. The transmitted radiation was counted by a scintillation detector, fed into a computer for analysis by a mathematical algorithm, and reconstructed as a tomographic image. The image had a remarkable characteristic, one never before seen in an x-ray image: it demonstrated a radiographic difference in the various soft tissues; blood clots, gray matter, white matter, cerebrospinal fluid, tumors, and cerebral edema all appeared as separate entities. The soft tissues could no longer be assigned the physical characteristics of water. The computer had changed that concept.

Computed tomography has had many names, each referring to at least one aspect of the technique. Two of the more popular names are computerized axial tomography (CAT) and computed (computerized) tomography (CT). Computed (computerized) tomography (CT) is currently the preferred name and the one we will use in this text.

Like most great discoveries, CT was the end product of years of work by numerous investigators. An Austrian mathematician, J. Radon, working with gravitational theory, proved in 1917 that a two- or three-dimensional object could be reproduced from an infinite set of all its projections.[17] Thus, the mathematical concept was established 55 years before the production of a commercial CT scanner. Workers in several unrelated fields (i.e., electron microscopy, astronomy, optics) were all struggling with a similar problem. In 1956, Bracewell, working in radioastronomy, constructed a solar map from ray projections.[1] Oldendorf in 1961 and Cormack in 1963 understood the concept of computed tomography and built laboratory models, but both lacked either the foresight or resources to develop a production unit.[3,14] Kuhl and Edwards in 1968 built a successful mechanical scanner for nuclear imaging, but did not extend their work into diagnostic radiology.[8] It remained for Hounsfield to put a CT system together and demonstrate its remarkable ability.

The field of computed tomography is changing rapidly. The hardware and computer programs are changing from day to day. These constant changes make it difficult to describe CT in a way that will still be meaningful after several years. The description is made more difficult by the fact that the mathematical principles are beyond the scope of this text. To avoid the problem of constant change, we will use the one unit that will never change, the original EMI scanner as the prototype to describe the basic principle. By necessity the discussion of the software, or mathematics, will be exceedingly superficial.

BASIC PRINCIPLE

The basic principle behind CT is that **the internal structure of an object can be reconstructed from multiple projections of the object.** The principle is illustrated in Figure 24–1. The object is made up of multiple square blocks, five of which have been removed to form a central cross (Fig. 24–1A). Projections could be obtained by passing an x-ray beam through the blocks and measuring the transmitted radiation. For the sake of simplicity, we will represent the ray projections by the number of blocks in each row. The horizontal sums (called ray projections) are shown on the right, while the vertical ray sums are shown below the object. All the horizontal and vertical ray sums are added, like the two shown in

Figure 24–1B, to produce a numerical reconstruction of the object (Fig. 24–1C). The numbers included in the reconstruction are 4, 6, 7, 8, 9, and 10. A gray scale value is then assigned to the numbers to produce an image like the one shown in Figure 24–1D. The image can be manipulated to highlight certain areas; that is, contrast can be adjusted. For example, the gray scale can be narrowed to include only black and white, and applied at any point along the numerical sequence. In Figure 24–1E, the scale is centered at the 9–10 level. Blocks with the number 10 are white and all other blocks are black. A perfect reproduction is achieved in Figure 24–1F by centering the black-white scale at the 6–7 level. This simple method of reconstructing an object may illustrate the basic idea, but unfortunately will not work in practice.

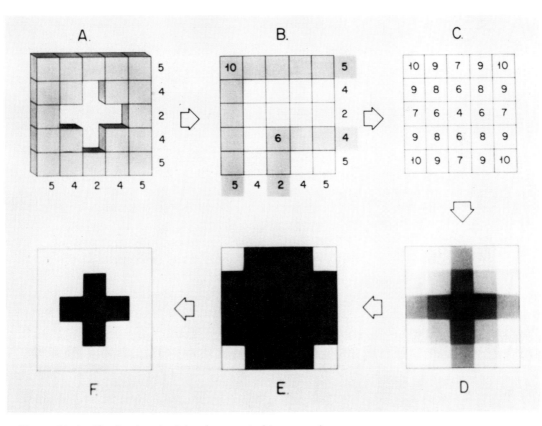

Figure 24–1 The basic principle of computed tomography

In x-ray CT the method of forming the ray projections is different than in our illustration, and the number of projections and picture elements is much greater, but the principle is exactly the same. The ray projections are formed by scanning a thin cross section of the body with a narrow x-ray beam and measuring the transmitted radiation with a sensitive radiation detector, the same as those used to detect the distintegrations of radionuclides. The detector does not form the image. It merely adds up the energy of all the transmitted photons. The numerical data from multiple ray sums are then computer-processed to reconstruct an image.

DATA ACCUMULATION

Data-gathering techniques have progressed through four distinct stages, called generations, in the first 5 years of clinical CT scanning. In a human society, a generation lasts between 20 and 30 years, and those in the younger generations tend to care for their elders. Computed tomographic units reproduce much more rapidly than humans, and younger generations have little regard for their elders. Each new generation of scanner has pushed the older ones into relative obsolescence. In view of the staggering cost of CT scanners, this is a frightening situation. Obviously, future designs must be engineered for easy updating to accommodate technologic advances. Before going through the various generations, the original EMI scanner will be used as the prototype to show how data are accumulated.

Original EMI Scanner

The original EMI scanner was designed specifically for evaluation of the brain. In this unit, the head was enclosed in a water bath between the x-ray tube above and a pair of detectors below (Fig. 24–2). A third, a reference detector, intercepted a portion of the beam before it reached the patient. A rigid scanner gantry maintained the relative position of the x-ray tube and detec-

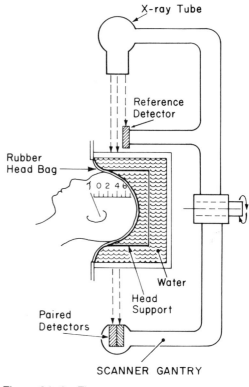

Figure 24–2 The scanner gantry

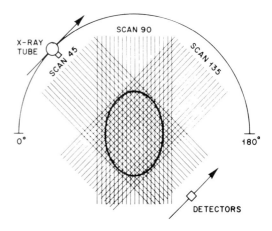

Figure 24–3 First-generation scanner (the original EMI unit)

tors and ensured their proper alignment. The x-ray beam was collimated to the exact size of the two side-by-side detectors.

The patient remained in one position throughout the scan. The gantry moved through two different types of motion, one linear and the other rotary (Fig. 24–3). The linear motion was repeated over and over 180 times. Between each of these 180 linear movements, the gantry rotated 1°. Thus, the total rotary motion encompassed a 180° semicircle. The axis of rotation passed through the center of the patient's head. In Figure 24–3 the linear motions are called "scans." Only 3 of the 180 linear motions are shown (i.e., numbers 45, 90, and 135). The x-ray beam was "on" throughout the linear movement and "off" during the rotary movements. The transmitted radiation was measured 160 times during each linear movement. The total number of transmission measurements was the product of the number of linear measurements (160) and rotary steps (180), which was 28,800 in the original EMI scanner. The total scan time was between 4.5 and 5 minutes. Each scan pass simultaneously examined two tomographic sections, one for each of the paired detectors. Multiple tomographic sections were required for most patients, frequently as many as ten. Each pair of tomographic sections took 5 minutes, so the total scan time for a clinical study was approximately 25 minutes (5 minutes × $^{10}\!/_2$ tomographic sections), plus a few minutes to reposition the patient in the gantry between sections.

The x-ray tube and paired detectors moved continuously and in unison during the linear scanning movement. They did not stop for the 160 transmission readings. The transmission readings represented a composite of the absorption characteristics of all the elements in the path of the beam. In the original EMI scanner, the CT image was reconstructed and then displayed on an 80 × 80 matrix in two different formats: a paper printout of CT numbers and a visual image on a cathode ray tube. The CT numbers were proportional to the linear attenuation coefficient. (They will be discussed in more detail later.) Each square in the image matrix was called a **pixel,** and it represented a tiny elongated block of tissue called a **voxel.** Figure 24–4 shows the

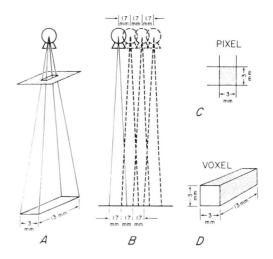

Figure 24–4 Comparison of the width of the x-ray beam (A), distance between detectors (B), pixel size (C), and voxel size (D) of the original EMI scanner

sizes of the x-ray field (Fig. 24–4A), distance between transmission readings (Fig. 24–4B), and sizes of the pixel and voxel (Fig. 24–4C and D) for the original EMI scanner. The x-ray field (Fig. 24–4A) was collimated to 3 × 13 mm (the actual length was 26 mm, which produced two parallel slices per scan, one for each of the paired detectors). This field moved across the 27-cm wide water bath making 160 transmission measurements, one every 1.7 mm (270 mm ÷ 160). The data from these measurements were computer-processed and presented in multiple little squares (pixels), each representing 3 × 3 mm of patient cross section. The CT number for each pixel represented the average attenuation coefficient for all the elements in a block of tissue (voxel) 3 × 3 × 13 mm in size. The size of the pixel was determined by the computer program and not by the dimensions of the x-ray beam. The same transmission data could be computer-processed for any pixel size. With a modified program, the original EMI data could be displayed with either 1.5- or 3-mm pixels. The length of the voxel, 13 mm in Figure 24–4, was determined by the width of the x-ray beam. This dimension could not be changed once the transmission data had been collected. It could only be changed by recollimating the x-ray beam and repeating the scan.

An oil-cooled stationary anode tube was used in the original EMI scanner. Its nominal focal spot size was 2.25 × 12 mm. The tube was operated by a three-phase generator at 120 kVp and 33 mA. The x-ray beam was heavily filtered with a half-value layer of 6 mm of aluminum (0.22 mm of copper).[10] The mean, or effective, energy of the 120-kVp beam when it reached the detectors was 70 keV.[15] Beam size was restricted by a pair of slitlike collimators, one near the tube and the other near the detectors. The detectors were sodium iodide scintillation crystals coupled to photomultiplier tubes. The reference detector furnished an exposure factor to compensate for moment-to-moment variations in x-ray output.

A large difference in attenuation between adjacent areas, such as air surrounding the head, makes computations more difficult, so the patient's head was incorporated into a boxlike water bath in the original EMI unit to facilitate data analysis within the computer. A slip ring between the rubber head cap and water bath allowed the bath to rotate independently of the head.

Scanning Motions

Like human generations, CT generations are not accurately defined. The most agreed on standard is probably the type of motion that is used to gather the transmission readings. At the time this original chapter was written (fall of 1977), four generations had been clearly defined and a fifth was in the planning stages. By the spring of 1983, only the third- and fourth-generation scanners were in widespread use, and a new candidate for the fifth-generation scanner may soon be available.

First Generation

The original EMI unit was a first-generation scanner. It employed a pencillike x-ray beam and a single detector, that is one detector per tomographic section. The x-ray tube-detector movements were both linear and rotary.

Second Generation

One major objective of second-generation scanners, and of all later generations, was to shorten the scanning time for each tomographic section. Faster scanning times facilitate patient handling and improve equipment utilization. If a CT unit is sufficiently fast, a whole scan can be accomplished while the patient holds his breath, a necessity for body scanning, in which respiratory motion tends to destroy image quality. The increased speed was accomplished by abandoning the single detector and pencil beam of the original EMI scanner and adopting a fan-shaped beam and multiple detectors (Figs. 24–5 to 24–7). The fan beam is a cross between a conventional x-ray beam and the pencil beam of the original EMI unit. As viewed from the side, the fan beam looks like a conventional x-ray beam. In the other view, parallel to the page in the illustration, the beam is collimated to the width of the detectors, so it actually has the shape of an open fan.

Figure 24–5 shows the physical makeup and movements of a typical second-generation scanner. The number of detectors in the fan beam array varies from one manufacturer to another. Only a few detectors are shown in the illustration, but there may be as many as 30. The movements of the x-ray tube-detector array are both linear and rotary, just like a first-generation scanner, but the rotary steps are larger. The 30 detectors gather more data per linear scan, so fewer linear movements are needed to gather an adequate data base. Instead of moving 1° at the end of each linear scan, the gantry rotates through a greater arc, up to 30°, and the process is repeated at greater than 1° intervals. The number of

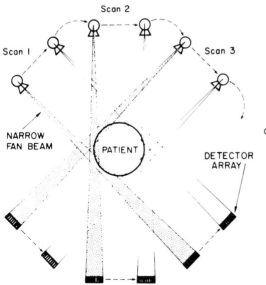

Figure 24–5 Second-generation scanner

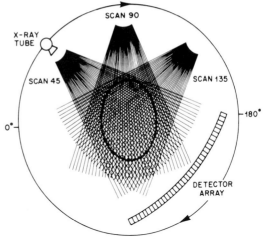

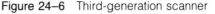

Figure 24–6 Third-generation scanner

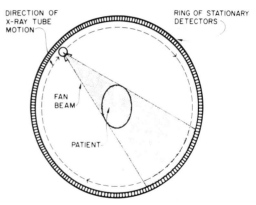

Figure 24–7 Fourth-generation scanner

repetitions is determined by the number of detectors in the detector array. With 30 detectors, the linear movements only have to be repeated six times rather than the 180 linear movements of the original EMI unit. Second-generation scanners produce a tomographic section in between 10 and 90 sec, depending on the manufacturer.

Third Generation

Third-generation scanners employ a much wider fan beam and many more detectors than a second-generation unit. A typical configuration for a third-generation scanner is shown in Figure 24–6. The fan beam is wide enough to encompass the entire width of the patient. The number of detectors may be in the 300 range (quite variable with different manufacturers). The x-ray beam is shown in three different positions in Figure 24–6, but the gantry actually rotates through a complete 360° circular movement. There are no linear-type movements with third-generation scanners. Each rotation completes one tomographic section. The scanning gantry does not stop to make readings. The gantry moves continuously, and the computer program is designed to compensate for this movement. Scan times for third-generation scanners range from 2 to 10 seconds.

Fourth Generation

Figure 24–7 shows the configuration of a fourth-generation scanner. A ring of detectors completely surrounds the patient. Only the x-ray tube moves and the detectors remain stationary. The tube rotates through a 360° arc with a wide fan beam. As the fan beam revolves, it activates the detectors that fall in its path. Fourth-generation scanners are not faster in principle than third-generation units. Their major advantage is easier detector calibration, a subject that we will discuss later.

At the time this chapter was first written, the fall of 1977, the fastest scan times were about 2 seconds. This represented a reduction in time by a factor of over 100, from 4 to 5 minutes in 1972 to 2 seconds in 1977. If the next 5 years had been as fruitful, the CT scan times would have been the same as the exposure times used in conventional radiography. That seemed unlikely, however, because of the massive size of the scanning gantry. Future progress seemed more likely to come from a fifth-generation scanner, probably one with multiple x-ray tubes surrounding the patient. A scanner of this type would have had no moving parts. The x-ray tubes would be fired sequentially at a ring of fixed detectors, and tomographic sections would be complete in a few milliseconds. As of the spring of 1983, a scanner with a single, large x-ray target that surrounds the patient and scans the x-ray beam about the patient (with a fixed array of detectors and no moving parts) has been announced.

The advantage of a fan beam-multiple detector array is speed. Obviously, multiple detectors can gather data faster than a single detector. One principal disadvantage of the fan beam is an increased amount of scattered radiation. At the high energies used for CT, usually 120 kVp, Compton scattering is a common basic interaction. The total number of Compton reactions is nearly the same for pencil beam and fan beam scanners, but the scattered photons are more likely to be recorded by a fan beam unit. Figure 24–8 shows the comparison diagrammatically. Two scattered photons are generated by a narrow pencil beam, but both miss the detector and go unrecognized (Fig. 24–8A). In the fan beam scanner the same two scattered photons, generated from the same volume of tissue, strike a detector and are recorded as noise (Fig. 24–8B). The problem of scatter radiation is exaggerated by the illustration for two reasons. First, the likelihood

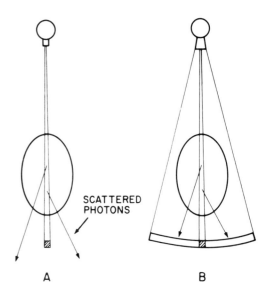

Figure 24–8 Pencil beam scanner (A) is less likely to record scattered radiation than fan beam scanner (B)

of a photon striking the detectors depends on the solid angle between the point of origin of the scatter radiation and the detectors. The scattered photons shown in Figure 24–8 may have been scattered into or out of the page, and thus they would go undetected. Secondly, the detectors in a fan beam array have their own individual collimators. Most scattered photons are absorbed by these collimators.

X-Ray Tubes

Ideally, the radiation source for CT would supply a monochromatic x-ray beam (i.e., one made up of photons all having the same wavelength). With a monochromatic beam, image reconstruction is simpler and more accurate. Early experimental models used radionuclides to supply such a beam, but radiation intensities were too low to be clinically useful. Conventional x-ray tubes are currently being used in all commercial scanners. Earlier models used oil-cooled, fixed-anode, relatively large (2 × 16 mm) focal spot tubes at energies of about 120 kilovolts (constant potential) and 30 mA.[11] The beam was heavily filtered to remove low-energy photons and to increase the mean energy of the radiation.

Most newer fan beam units have a diagnostic-type x-ray tube with a rotating anode and a much smaller focal spot, in some units down to 0.6 mm, and generate x rays in short bursts, or pulses. These tubes are air-cooled and operate at much higher currents, up to 600 mA. They are oriented in the gantry with their long axis (cathode-anode) perpendicular to the fan beam to avoid asymmetry in x-ray output because of the heel effect.

Recently, special types of x-ray tubes have been developed for CT. These tubes are designed to withstand the very high heat loads generated when multiple slices are acquired in rapid sequence. Cylindric targets (rather than disk-shaped) and other modifications to the basic x-ray tube geometry have been tried. No single type of x-ray tube has been proven to be clearly superior for CT application as yet.

In a third-generation scanner, more than 300 separate radiation pulses may be delivered during the circular motion required to produce one tomographic section. The tube moves continuously, even though the radiation is pulsed. The computer is programmed to compensate for the motion. Each pulse lasts 2 to 3 msec, so the tube is actually producing radiation for a little less than 1 sec for each scan (3 msec/pulse × 300 pulses = 0.9 sec). With a 5-sec scan time, the actual exposure occupies approximately 20% of the total time. The advantages of a pulsed system are the following:

1. Much larger quantities of radiation can be delivered in a short time, so scan times are less.
2. Smaller focal spots allow much more accurate collimation, which results in lower patient exposures, especially with multiple slices (discussed in more detail later).
3. The electronic circuitry can be recal-

ibrated between pulses so that x-ray output is more accurately controlled.
4. The pulse length can be accurately regulated to optimize counting statistics and detector response.

Collimators

The x-ray beam is collimated at two points, one close to the x-ray tube and the other at the detector(s). Perfect alignment between the two is essential. The collimator at the detector is the sole means of controlling scatter radiation. Each detector has its own collimator. The collimators also regulate the thickness of the tomographic section (i.e., the voxel length). Most units employ section thicknesses of 3 to 13 mm. Some have provisions for variable thickness. For example, in the original EMI scanner you could select a section thickness of either 8 or 13 mm. Pixel size is determined by the computer program and not by the collimator. The computer can use the input data to print out an image on any size matrix.

Detectors

CT detectors measure the energy deposited in them. As you will recall from Chapter 5, the energy in a beam is the product of the number and energy of the individual photons. The detectors are the same as those used to detect radionuclide scintillations. Radionuclide detectors usually use "energy discrimination" windows to detect only a narrow range of photon energies. More or less energetic photons, those falling outside the window, are ignored. When all primary photons have the same energy (a monochromatic beam), energy discrimination is an excellent way of ignoring scatter radiation, because the scattered photons are all less energetic than the primary photons. Energy discrimination, however, is impractical for CT detectors. To begin with, the beam is heterochromatic (polychromatic), so it contains a whole spectrum of energies, and the window would have to be quite wide. Secondly, photons only lose a small amount of energy during a Compton scattering in the CT energy range. A 75-keV photon, which is near the mean energy of most CT beams, only loses 0.7 keV when it undergoes a 30° scattering. At 74.3 keV it would still fall within the window and would be erroneously recorded as a primary photon. Consequently, the detector collimator is used as the sole means of controlling scatter radiation. The tube collimator decreases the overall size of the scattering medium and thus the number of scattered photons. The detector collimator eliminates most of the small residuum.

Characteristics

The most important characteristics of detectors are their cost, efficiency, stability, and responsiveness.[11]

Cost. Detector costs are a major reason for the high cost of CT scanners, especially fan beam units, which may have as many as 600 detectors.

Efficiency. Efficiency refers to the percentage of the energy absorbed from the beam. Ideally, detector efficiency should be 100%. Then the entire beam would be captured, which would improve counting statistics and minimize patient exposure. Later we will see that the computer must correct for the heterochromatic nature of the beam. The correction is more difficult with less than 100% efficiency, because many of the higher energy photons go through the sensor undetected.

Stability. Stability refers to the consistency and reproducibility of detector response from moment to moment. Detectors are constantly recalibrated to ensure their stability. In first-generation linear scanners, detectors are calibrated at the end of each linear run, or 180 times for each tomographic section. Second-generation scanners are also calibrated at the end of each linear movement. Third-generation scanners may only be calibrated once per day, so detector stability is much more important with these units. When the response of one third-generation detector strays from the norm, ringlike artifacts are produced in the tomographic image. Fourth-generation scanners are calibrated twice during one rotation: first along the leading edge of the moving fan beam, and later along the trailing edge.

Responsiveness. Response time refers to the length of time it takes for a detector to receive, record, and discard a signal. A detector should respond instantaneously to a signal and then just as quickly discard that signal and be ready for the next one. Afterglow, or phosphorescence after the signal has passed, is a serious problem with some detectors. It is most pronounced when an unattenuated portion of the beam strikes the detector. The water bath was incorporated into the original EMI scanner to cope with this problem.

Other desirable features are a linear response over a wide range of beam intensities and energy levels, freedom from noise, and compact size.

Types

Two types of detectors are currently being used in CT scanners, scintillation crystals coupled to photomultiplier tubes or to other light detectors and gas-filled ionization chambers. Figure 24–9 shows a **scintillation crystal-photomultiplier tube detector.** The crystal in the illustration is sodium iodide, which we will use as a prototype. When a scintillation crystal absorbs an x-ray photon, the interaction produces

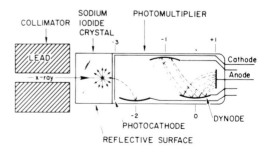

Figure 24–9 Scintillation crystal-photomultiplier tube detector

light (a scintillation). The amount of light is proportional to the energy of the x-ray photon; that is, high-energy photons produce more light than low-energy photons. The surface of the scintillation crystal is coated with a highly reflective material so that most of the light from a scintillation eventually reaches the immediately adjacent photomultiplier tube.

We described photomultipliers in Chapter 3, so we will only briefly review them at this time. A photomultiplier tube consists of an evacuated glass envelope containing an anode, cathode, and several intermediate electrodes called dynodes. The cathode is coated with a photoemissive surface, so it is called a photocathode. When the photoemissive surface is struck by light from the scintillation crystal, the surface emits electrons in numbers proportional to the intensity of the light. The electrons are called photoelectrons, but they are no different than any other electrons (the "photo" simply refers to the manner in which they were liberated). The dynodes are coated with a material that emits secondary electrons when struck by another electron. The first dynode has a higher voltage than the photocathode, and each subsequent dynode has a higher voltage (less negative) than the preceding one. Thus, electrons are propagated down the tube in a step-wise fashion from one dynode to another. At each step the number of electrons is multiplied. Only a single light photon and photoelectron are shown in Figure 24–9, but the actual numbers are much greater. Many light photons are produced with each scintillation, and each light photon produces one or more photoelectrons. Only three dynodes are shown, but there may be as many as ten. At each dynode the number of electrons is multiplied, and the degree of multiplication is the same for every electron. Therefore, the strength of the output signal (an electric current) is proportional to the strength of the input signal (light from scintillations), but the output signal is greatly amplified.

The principal advantage of scintillation crystal detectors is their efficiency. A 2.5-cm thick sodium iodide crystal is almost 100% efficient in the diagnostic energy range, but sodium iodide crystals have an important disadvantage. The disadvantage is afterglow, or phosphorescence, after encountering high-radiation intensities. Afterglow used to be an especially serious problem in scanners that did not have a water bath surrounding the patient. Partly because of this problem with afterglow, other crystals are now being used. For instance, bismuth germinate combines the desirable features of high efficiency and no afterglow. All scintillation crystal-photomultiplier detectors have a nonlinear response for different radiation intensities. This limits the range of x-ray intensities over which they can be used.

The second type of radiation detector is a **gas-filled ionization chamber** (Fig. 24–10). It is much simpler than a scintillation-type detector. An ionization chamber has only two electrodes, an anode, and a cathode. The cathode is plated onto the inner wall of the chamber. The anode is a wire running through the center of the chamber. Gas molecules in the chamber are ionized by interactions with the x-ray beam. The ions are then attracted to the appropriate electrodes by a voltage between the electrodes. The magnitude of the voltage is adjusted so that the number of ionizations is proportional to the intensity of the x-ray beam. The voltage is not as high as that of a Geiger counter. The voltage in a Geiger counter is high enough to produce an avalanche effect; that is, the ions from one interaction acquire enough energy as they move toward the electrodes to produce other ionizations and completely discharge the chamber. The voltage in CT ionization chambers is accurately adjusted so that the resultant current is proportional to the energy of the absorbed x rays.

The principal disadvantage of ionization chambers is their inefficiency. Because of the relatively low density of gases as com-

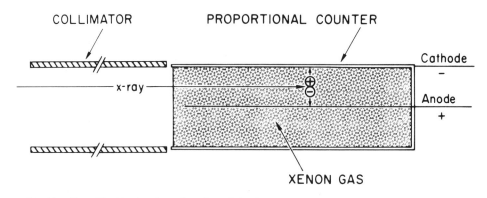

Figure 24–10 Gas-filled ionization chamber detector

pared to solids, many x-ray photons pass through the chamber undetected. This problem is at least partially overcome in three ways: (1) by using xenon, the heaviest of the inert gases; (2) by compressing the xenon to 25 atmospheres to increase its density; and (3) by using a long chamber to increase the number of molecules along the path of the beam. The voltage between the electrodes must be high enough to remove ion pairs instantaneously before they can recombine and be lost to the detector system. The principal advantage of gas detectors is a linear response unaffected by changes in beam intensity (no afterglow) over a wide range of energies. They are also easier to manufacture in small sizes. The disadvantages of gas chambers are reduced efficiency and some problems with stability.

IMAGE RECONSTRUCTION

In computed tomography a cross-sectional layer of the body is divided into many tiny blocks such as the ones shown in Figure 24–11, and then each block is assigned a number proportional to the degree that the block attenuated the x-ray beam. The individual blocks are called voxels. Their composition and thickness, along with the quality of the beam, determine the degree of attenuation. The linear attenuation coefficient (μ) is used to quantitate attenuation. The mathematics are really quite simple. We will start by describing the simplest case, a single block of homogeneous tissue (an isolated voxel) and a monochromatic beam of x rays:

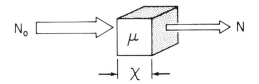

The value of μ, the linear attenuation coefficient, can be calculated with the equation for exponential attenuation described earlier in Chapter 5:

$$N = N_0 e^{-\mu x}$$

In this equation, e is the base of the natural logarithm (2.718). The number of initial photons (N_0), transmitted photons (N), and thickness (x) can all be measured. The linear attenuation coefficient (μ) is the only unknown in the equation.

If two blocks of tissue with different linear attenuation coefficients are placed in the path of the beam, the problem immediately becomes more complex:

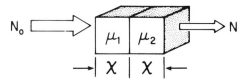

TISSUE SECTION
REPRESENTED IN
COMPUTER MATRIX

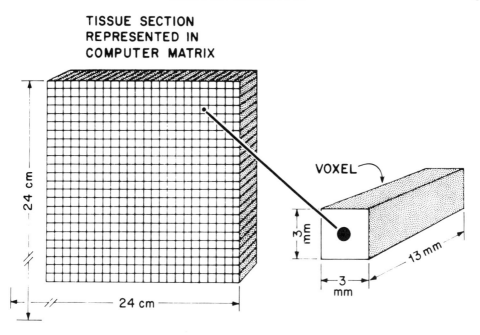

Figure 24–11 The tissue section represented in the computer matrix

Now the equation has two unknowns, μ_1 and μ_2, and is written as

$$N = N_0e^{-(\mu_1 + \mu_2)x}$$

The values of μ_1 and μ_2 cannot be determined without additional information. At least one additional equation is required, and the equation must contain the same two unknowns. Additional equations can be obtained by examining the blocks from different directions. In this case we will also increase the number of blocks in our example to four, so that each reading represents the composite of two blocks:

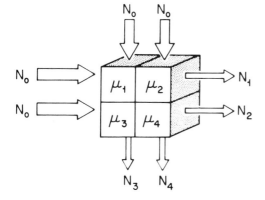

We have gone from two to four unknowns, but we can now construct four different equations:

$$N_1 = N_0e^{-(\mu_1 + \mu_2)x}$$
$$N_2 = N_0e^{-(\mu_3 + \mu_4)x}$$
$$N_3 = N_0e^{-(\mu_1 + \mu_3)x}$$
$$N_4 = N_0e^{-(\mu_2 + \mu_4)x}$$

This array looks formidable, but the equations can all be simultaneously solved for the value of the linear attenuation coefficient with the aid of a computer. Exactly the same principle applies to computed tomography, but the number of unknowns is much larger. For example, in the original EMI scanner, the matrix in the computer contained 80 × 80, or 6400, separate picture elements. Each transmission measurement records the composite of 80 separate linear attenuation coefficients:

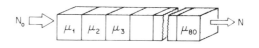

The equation is longer and looks more

awesome, but is has exactly the same format:

$$N = N_0 e^{-(\mu_1 + \mu_2 + \mu_3 + \cdots \mu_{80})x}$$

To solve this equation, we must have transmission readings taken from at least two different directions, just as we did for the simple example above. The number of separate equations and unknowns now becomes 6400. The original EMI unit took 28,800 readings (160 linear readings × 180°), and a fan beam scanner may take as many as 90,000 readings (300 pulses × 300 detectors). An equation like the one shown above can be reconstructed for each of these readings. Even though Radon understood the mathematical principles in 1917, he could not put his knowledge to practical use. The mathematics were so tediously long that before computers it would have taken years to construct a single image.

Two correction factors are incorporated into the CT program. The first is a correction for the heterochromatic (polychromatic) nature of the beam. As heterochromatic radiation passes through an absorber, filtration increases its mean energy. The linear attenuation coefficient changes with energy, as shown in Figure 24–12. The illustration compares the linear attenuation coefficients of water for 70-keV monochromatic and 120-kVp heterochromatic beams. The initial mean energy of the heterochromatic beam is 70 keV. The monochromatic linear attenuation coefficient (μ) is constant, but the heterochromatic μ strays down on the graph as filtration increases its mean energy from 70 to 75 keV. The CT program must be written to compensate for this stray and bring the calculated μ back to a straight line.

The second program correction is a weighting factor to compensate for the differences between the size and shape of the scanning beam and the picture matrix. Figure 24–13 shows the problem geometrically. In Figure 24–13A, the parallel rays of a linear-type scanning motion exactly co-

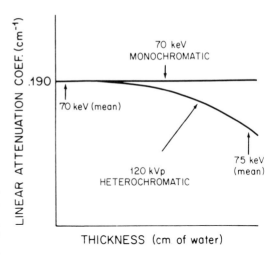

Figure 24–12   The linear attenuation coefficient of a heterochromatic beam decreases as filtration increases its mean energy

incide with the size and square shape of the picture elements. In Figure 24–13B, the scanning rays cross the picture elements obliquely. A weighting factor (WF) is used to compensate for the difference in size between the actual elements and that seen by the beam. In these examples, the weighting factor would be 1 in Figure 24–13A and less than 1 in Figure 24–13B.

Algorithms for Image Reconstruction

An algorithm is a mathematical method for solving a problem. Thousands of equations must be solved to determine the linear attenuation coefficients of all the pixels in the image matrix. Several different methods, or algorithms, are in current use. They all attempt to solve the equations as rapidly as possible without compromising accuracy. The original EMI scanner took 4 to 5 minutes to process the data for a single CT section. This long processing time seriously limited the number of patients that could be handled in a working day. More recent algorithms are much faster and can display a picture immediately after the tomographic section is completed. We have tried to make the discussion more pictorial than mathematical, because the actual mathe-

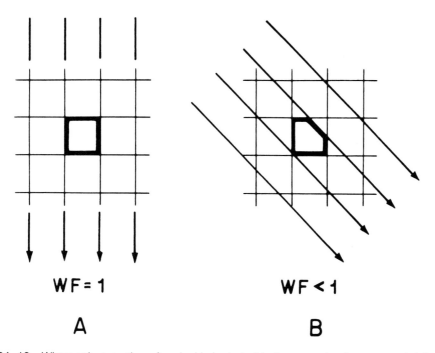

WF = 1

A

WF < 1

B

Figure 24–13 When only a portion of a pixel is included in the scanning beam, a weighting factor (WF) is used in the mathematical reconstruction

matics go beyond the intended scope of this text. Most of our description of mathematical principles is taken from an excellent article by Brooks and DiChiro.[2] The following three mathematical methods of image reconstruction will be described:

1. Back-projection
2. Iterative methods
3. Analytical methods

The object of all the methods is to produce an accurate cross-sectional display of the linear attenuation coefficients of each element in the image matrix.

Back-Projection

Back-projection, sometimes called the summation method, is the oldest means of image reconstruction. None of the commercial CT scanners use back-projection, but it is the simplest method to describe so we will use it as a prototype. The principle is shown schematically in Figure 24–14, which demonstrates a two-dimensional re-

construction of a cross cut from the center of a solid block. The block is scanned (Figure 24–14A) from both the top and left sides by a moving x-ray beam to produce the image profile shown in Figure 24–14B. The image profiles look like steps. The height of the steps is proportional to the amount of radiation that passed through the block. The center transmitted the most radiation, so it is the highest step in the image profile. The steps are then assigned to a gray scale density that is proportional to their height. These densities are arranged in rows, called rays (Fig. 24–14C). The width of the rays is the same as the width of the steps in the profile. In the illustration the ray length is equal to the height of the original object, but in an actual clinical situation, in which the image is displayed on a television monitor, these heights and widths could be any convenient size. When the rays from the two projections are superimposed, or back-projected, they produce a crude reproduction of the original object (Fig. 24–14D). In practice

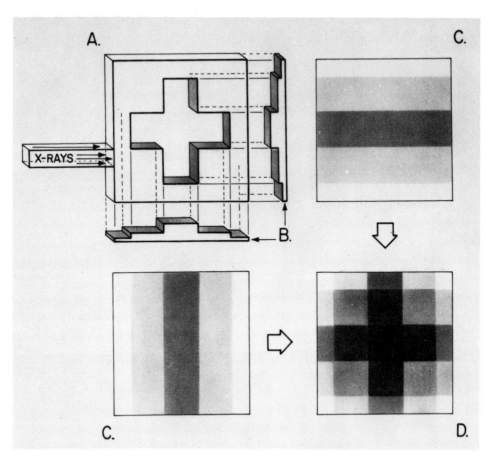

Figure 24–14 Image reconstruction by back-projection

many more projections would be added to improve image quality, but the principle is the same.

All points in the back-projected image receive density contributions from neighboring structures. The result of these contributions is dramatized in Figure 24–15. The black dot in Figure 24–15A represents a radiodense material, such as a drop of Pantopaque. The radiodense material severely attenuates the beam and produces localized spikes in the image profiles. Back-projection of the rays from these spikes produces a star pattern like the one shown in Figure 24–15B. A great number of projections will obscure the star pattern, but the background density remains as noise to deteriorate the quality of the CT image.

Iterative Methods

An iterative reconstruction starts with an assumption (for example, that all points in the matrix have the same value) and compares this assumption with measured values, makes corrections to bring the two into agreement, and then repeats the process over and over until the assumed and measured values are the same or within acceptable limits. There are three variations of iterative reconstructions, depending on whether the correction sequence involves the whole matrix, one ray, or a single point.

Simultaneous Reconstruction. All projections for the entire matrix are calculated at the beginning of the iteration, and all corrections are made simultaneously for each iteration.

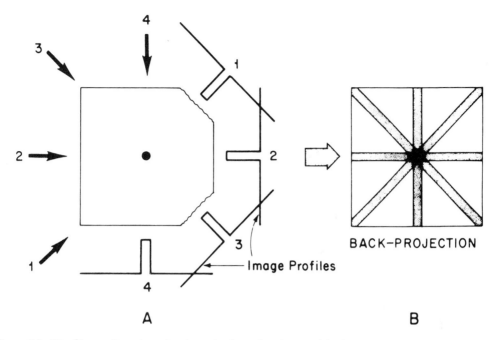

Figure 24–15 Star pattern from back-projection of a dense object

Ray-by-Ray Correction. One ray sum is calculated and corrected, and these corrections are incorporated into future ray sums, with the process being repeated for every ray in each iteration.

Point-by-Point Correction. The calculations and corrections are made for all rays passing through one point, and these corrections are used in ensuing calculations, again with the process being repeated for every point.

Figure 24–16 illustrates a ray-by-ray iterative reconstruction for a four-element square. Horizontal, vertical, and diagonal ray sums are shown in the adjacent blocks. In the first step, the two horizontal ray sums (16 and 6 in the hatched blocks) are divided equally among the two elements in the ray. If the ray sums had represented ten elements, the sum would have been divided equally among all ten elements. Next, the new numbers in the vertical row are added to produce the new ray sums (11 and 11 in the shaded blocks) and compared with the original measured ray sums (also in shaded blocks). The difference between

the original and new ray sums ($10 - 11 = -1$ and $12 - 11 = +1$) is divided by the number of elements in the ray ($-1 \div 2 = -0.5$ and $+1 \div 2 = +0.5$). These differences are algebraically added to each element ($8 - 0.5 = 7.5$, $3 - 0.5 = 2.5$, $8 + 0.5 = 8.5$, and $3 + 0.5 = 3.5$). The process is repeated for diagonal ray sums to complete the first iteration. In this example, the first iteration produces a perfect reconstruction. With more complex data, iterations may have to be repeated six to twelve times to reach an acceptable level of agreement between the calculated and measured values. The first 80 × 80 matrix EMI scanner used an iterative reconstruction, but most manufacturers are now using one of the analytic methods.

Analytic Methods

Analytic methods are used in almost all x-ray CT today. These algorithms differ from iterative methods in that exact formulas are utilized for the analytical reconstructions. These formulas are frighteningly complex to most radiologists,

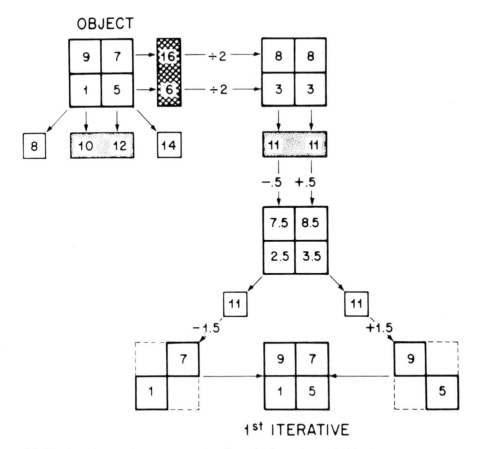

Figure 24–16   Iterative ray-by-ray reconstruction of a four-element object

although mathematicians say they are really quite simple. We will only attempt a pictorial explanation of the two popular analytic methods, two-dimensional Fourier analysis and filtered back-projection.

Two-Dimensional Fourier Analysis. The basis of Fourier analysis is that any function of time or space can be represented by the sum of various frequencies and amplitudes of sine and cosine waves. Figure 24–17 shows three functions: projections of a phantom skull containing bone, air, and calcium. The ray projections are shown with squared edges, which is the most difficult wave form to reproduce. The actual projected images would be more rounded than those shown, which would simplify a Fourier reconstruction.

Figure 24–18 shows progressively improving Fourier reconstructions. A single

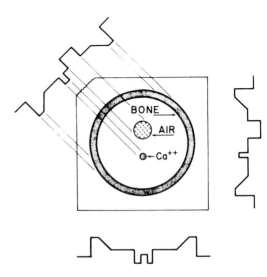

Figure 24–17   Projections of a skull phantom

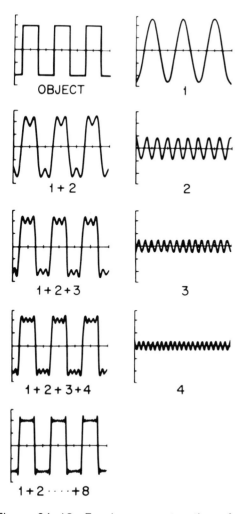

Figure 24–18   Fourier reconstruction of a square wave form

to exactly counterbalance the effect of sudden density changes, which causes blurring (the star pattern) in simple back-projection. The projected information is filtered much like light is filtered by a polarizing lens. Those frequencies responsible for blurring are eliminated to enhance more desirable frequencies. Figure 24–19 is a two-dimensional filtered back-projection of a square object. The density of the projected rays is adjusted to compensate for the star effect; that is, the inside margins of dense areas are enhanced while the centers and immediately adjacent areas are repressed. The net effect is an image more closely resembling the original object than could have been achieved with back-projection alone. Image quality is further improved with each additional projection. Most CT units use a Fourier reconstruction or filtered back-projection.

Comparison of Mathematical Methods

No general agreement exists as to which mathematical method is superior and, indeed, a system's superiority under one set of circumstances may disappear under new circumstances. In terms of speed, analytical

cosine wave of the appropriate height (amplitude) and length (frequency) makes a first approximation of the square wave, and each subsequent addition improves the reproduction. The last reconstruction represents the sum of eight cosine waves, but only the first four steps are shown. This type of mathematical manipulation is easily and quickly processed in a computer. The reconstruction is a little more complex for a two-dimensional image such as a CT section, but the basic principle is the same.

Filtered Back-Projection. Filtered back-projection is similar to back-projection except that the image is filtered, or modified,

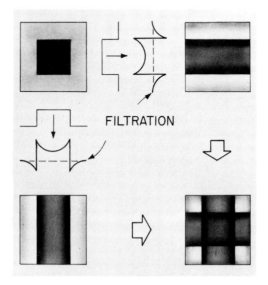

Figure 24–19   Filtered back-projection of a square object

reconstructions are clearly faster than iterative methods. A projection can be processed immediately after recording, so the entire reconstruction can be displayed seconds after completion of the last projection. Iterative reconstructions may take several minutes to process after scan completion. Both methods are equally accurate if the projection data are complete. With incomplete data (i.e., insufficient to determine the image fully) iterative methods are superior. Analytic methods must do time-consuming interpolations to fill in missing data, while iterative methods simply average adjacent points. Thus, with incomplete data, analytical methods are slowed while iterative methods are actually made faster than they would be with complete data.

CT Numbers

Ideally, linear attenuation coefficient calculations should be precisely correct, both in absolute and in relative value from pixel to pixel. Computers are designed for maximum relative accuracy, which is the more important of the two for imaging purposes. The relative accuracy of the original EMI scanner was 1 part in 200, or ± 0.5%. As we shall see later, the degree of accuracy is limited primarily by patient exposure and pixel size, and not by equipment design. Therefore, accuracy is approximately the same in the newer generations of scanners as it was in the original EMI unit.

After the CT computer calculates a relative linear attenuation coefficient for each pixel, the number is normalized to a reference material (water), magnified to a larger whole number (integer), and reported as a new number, called a CT number. The densest body tissue, compact bone, and the least dense body tissue, air, are assigned the values of +1 and −1, times a magnifying constant. The size of this constant was 500 in the original EMI scanner, but it could be any number large enough to express the accuracy of the scanner in whole numbers. Because the original EMI accuracy was 1 part in 200, a magni-

fying constant of 500 left a generous margin for technical improvements. Nevertheless, newer units have an even more expanded scale employing a magnifying constant of 2000 or more. The mathematical manipulations involved in the derivation of a CT number are shown in the following equation:

$$CT \text{ number} = K \frac{\mu_p - \mu_w}{\mu_w}$$

K = magnifying constant
μ_p = linear attenuation coefficient of the pixel in question
μ_w = linear attenuation coefficient of water.

You can see from this equation that the CT number of water is 0, regardless of the size of the magnifying constant. With a magnifying constant of 500, the CT number of dense bone is +500 and air is −500. All other tissues are intermediate in value, as shown in Table 24–1. The computer will print out the CT numbers for any or all elements in the matrix on request. Knowing the magnifying constant of the computer, the linear attenuation coefficient can be calculated from the above equation. Magnifying the scale does not improve the accuracy of a scanner. An accuracy of 1 part in 200 (±0.5%) is ±2.5 CT numbers with a magnifying constant of 500 and ±10 CT numbers with a magnifying constant of 2000. All three of these plus-or-minus numbers represent exactly the same degree of accuracy.

Table 24–1. CT Numbers and Linear Attenuation Coefficients for Various Body Tissues with a Magnifying Constant of 500 (120 kVp; effective 70 keV)

ABSORBER	CT NUMBER	LINEAR ATTENUATION COEFFICIENT (cm^{-1})*
Bone (dense)	+500	0.380
Intracranial	+25	0.200
soft	to	to
tissues	+5	0.192
Water	0	0.190
Fat	−50	0.171
Air	−500	0

*These linear attenuation coefficients were calculated from the CT numbers, except for water, which was taken to be 0.190.

An actual improvement in CT accuracy has occurred, partly because of the optimization of reconstruction algorithms to make more efficient utilization of dose, and partly because more efficient detectors with wider dynamic range (the ability to handle both very small and very large values) have been developed. Modern CT scanners have accuracies on the order of 0.2%, and are capable of seeing relatively small structures embedded within bone.

Image Display

A CT image can be displayed in two basic modes: as a paper printout of CT numbers, or as a gray scale image on a cathode ray tube or television monitor (Fig. 24–20). The paper printout is time-consuming, and is used primarily to evaluate scanner performance, and not as an image method. Figure 24–21 shows the type of gray scale used to construct the visual image. The CT numbers in the illustration are for a unit with a magnification constant of 500. At full scale, dense bone with a CT number of +500 is assigned a gray scale level of peak white and air at −500 the level of black. The contrast difference between the intermediate structures, such as brain and cerebrospinal fluid, may be too small to demonstrate at full scale because the CT numbers of these structures are so close together. The contrast of the video image, however, can be adjusted to augment minor differences in specific areas, the one capability that sets CT apart from every other radiographic imaging technique.

As a general rule, conventional roentgenograms cannot show a density difference of less than 10%. The CT numbers for intracranial soft tissues range from +5 to +25 (Table 24–1), a total of 20 CT numbers on a scale of 500. This represents a difference between the least dense and most dense of 4% (20 ÷ 500 = 0.04 × 100% = 4%). This difference can be demonstrated by coning down to a narrow portion of the CT scale (Fig. 24–21). In this figure, the gray scale is adjusted so that the CT numbers between −5 and +55, a total of 60 numbers, cover the whole range of gray from black to white. Viewed in this way, −5 and all lower numbers are black, while +55 and all higher numbers are white. The result is greatly increased contrast within the preselected range. In this example, the contrast difference between the most dense and least dense intracranial soft tissue structures changes from 4% to 33% (20 ÷ 60 = 0.33 × 100% = 33%).

The range of CT numbers selected for gray scale amplification is called the window width (60 CT numbers in Fig. 24–21). Window width can be adjusted in various increments from full scale to a single unit. The size and number of the increments is determined by the manufacturer. For example, the options on a theoretical unit may include the following window widths: 1, 8, 16, 32, 64, 128, 256, 512. The operator could select one of these widths and center it to a specific level, called the window level. In the example shown in Figure 24–21, the window level is +25 (halfway between −5 and +55). When the window width is set at 1, all points in the image matrix are either black or white.

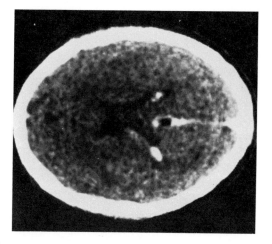

Figure 24–20 Gray scale CT television image (Courtesy of Dr. Kenneth R. Maravilla, University of Texas Health Science Center at Dallas)

IMAGE QUALITY

Image quality is not accurately defined for computed tomography. We will attempt to use the same terms and definitions described in Chapter 13 for the radiographic image. Image quality (clarity) is the visibility of diagnostically important structures in the CT image. The factors that affect quality are all interrelated, so when we discuss one we will frequently refer to the others. The more important factors are defined below under three separate headings:

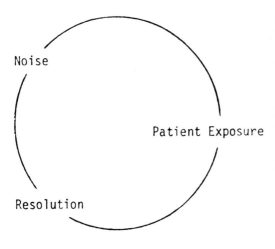

These three factors are intimately tied together, but we will discuss them separately. All other factors affecting image quality will be included under these three headings.

Quantum Mottle

Precision in computed tomography is a measure of background, or matrix uniformity. If is perfectly homogeneous object such as a water bath is examined with a CT scanner, all elements in the picture matrix should have exactly the same CT number. Deviations from uniformity represent statistical fluctuations, called quantum mottle. We will use the terms quantum mottle and noise interchangeably. **A lack of precision, or the presence of mottle, is the limiting factor in CT performance at the present time.** The number of photons for each ray projection is precariously close to the statistical limit of acceptability for an intracranial scan in which subject contrast is minimal. Figure 24–22 shows anticipated

statistical fluctuations as a function of the number of counts in a ray projection. Counts of 100, 1000, 10,000, and 100,000 are shown as paired bar graphs, with each bar in the pair representing 1 standard deviation (SD) above and below the anticipated value. The counts are normalized to demonstrate the decrease in percentage fluctuation. At 100 counts, the statistical fluctuation is $\pm 10\%$, or from 90 to 110 counts. As the number of counts increases, the percent fluctuation decreases. At 10,000 counts, 1 SD is 100 counts ($10,000^{1/2} = 100$), which is a percentage fluctuation of $\pm 1\%$ ($100 \div 10,000 = 1\%$). The advertised accuracy of the original EMI scanner was $\pm 0.5\%$. With a 4.5-minute scan time, approximately 100,000 photons were recorded for each ray in the projection.[13] The illustration shows a statistical fluctuation of $\pm 0.3\%$ at 100,000 counts, which is consistent with the claims of the manufacturer. If the number of counts is decreased to any significant degree, however, there must be a concomitant decrease in precision and increase in mottle.

Precision cannot be improved by a more accurate mathematical reconstruction. In fact, mottle becomes more visible as the accuracy of the reconstruction improves. This principle is shown diagrammatically in Figure 24–23, a bar graph similar to the one shown earlier in Figure 24–22. The heights of the shaded bars depict the actual number of counts in two adjacent ray projections of a water phantom. Because the phantom is homogeneous, the difference in the counts between the two bars represents noise (statistical fluctuations). Employing an iterative algorithm after the first iteration, the two bars are almost the same height and, if the image were displayed at this time, the noise would be smoothed out and the image would appear quite homogeneous. Each iteration more closely approximates the reconstructed image to the original data until finally, after many iterations, the two are nearly identical. The image will then show the noise more ac-

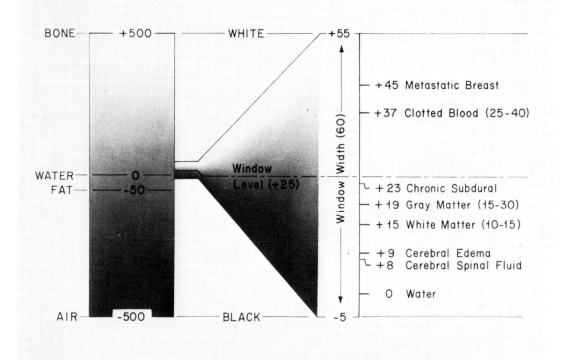

Figure 24-21 EMI gray scale display with adjustable window width and level

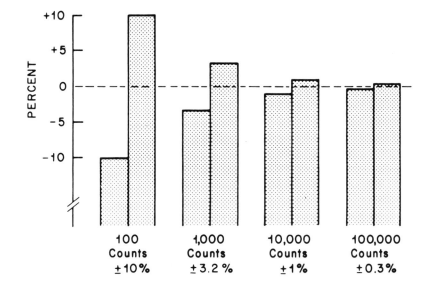

Figure 24-22 Decreasing statistical fluctuations with increasing count rates

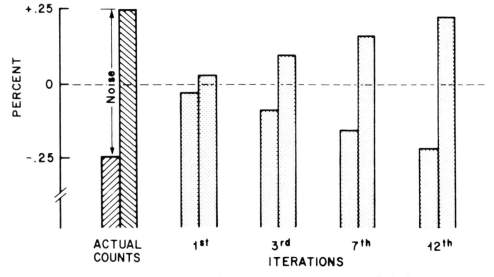

Figure 24–23   Accurate reconstructions bring out statistical fluctuations (noise)

curately than the earlier reconstruction. **Most of the noise in current CT images is a result of statistical fluctuations and is not related to the mathematical reconstruction.**

The number of counts per picture element is determined by numerous factors, including the quantity and quality of the x-ray beam, the number and efficiency of the detectors, the amount of absorber in the path of the beam, the number and volume of the picture element, and the scan time. Motion has a devastating effect on image quality in CT, so shorter scan times are a noble objective, especially in body work in which respiratory motion is a problem. For any given scanner and voxel size, however, scan times can only be shortened at the expense of precision. When high-quality images are essential, scan times may have to be lengthened to produce a statistically more accurate reconstruction.

Counting statistics are intimately related to voxel size. **A voxel is a volume element, as opposed to a pixel, which is a picture element.** A pixel is a flat surface without thickness. The image is displayed on a television monitor as thousands of tiny pixels, each representing a specific tiny cross-sec-

tional area in the patient. The stated size of a pixel, such as 3×3 mm, refers to their size in the patient. Their actual size in a video image is determined by the size of the television monitor. A given size of pixel will appear larger on a large TV monitor than it would on a smaller monitor, but in both cases it would represent the same area in the patient. A voxel adds the third dimension to the area represented by the pixel, so the voxel is a volume element. A 1-mm square pixel might represent a 5- or 10-mm thick section; the first would be a 5-mm³ and the second a 10-mm³ voxel. Diminishing voxel size decreases the number of counts per each element, assuming that other factors remain constant. Table 24–2 shows the size of some EMI voxels with volume factors and patient exposure factors normalized to the original 3- × 3-mm pixel (80 × 80 matrix) and the 13-mm thick section of the original EMI scanner. Assuming that the counting statistics (precision) are kept constant, the superior resolution of the smallest sized (18-mm³) voxel can only be realized with a 6.4-fold increase in patient exposure. An important point to keep in mind when selecting techniques is that precision is better (and noise is less)

Table 24–2. Relationship Between Voxel Size and Patient Exposure

VOXEL SIZE (mm)	VOLUME (mm³)	VOLUME FACTOR	PATIENT EXPOSURE FACTOR*
3 × 3 × 13	117	1.0	1.0
3 × 3 × 8	72	0.62	1.6
1.5 × 1.5 × 13	29.3	0.25	4.0
1.5 × 1.5 × 8	18	0.15	6.4

*For comparable counting statistics.

with an 80 × 80 matrix than with a 160 × 160 matrix for any given patient exposure.

Matrix size, field size, and pixel size are all interrelated as shown in Figure 24–24. Matrix size is the number of points in a picture matrix, 6400 (80 × 80) in Figure 24–24A and 25,600 (160 × 160) in both Figure 24–24B and C. The name **matrix size** is firmly entrenched in the CT literature, but it is a confusing name, because the "size" refers to the size of a unitless number and not to a physical size. **Field size** (x and 2x in Figure 24–24) refers to the outside dimensions of the CT slice (e.g., 27 × 27 cm in the original EMI scanner). Field size dictates the maximum size of anatomic part that can be examined. The smaller field size shown in Figure 24–24A and B might be used for head scans, while the larger size in Figure 24–24C could accommodate a larger part and might be used for body scans. Note that the matrix size is the same in Figure 24–24A and B and the pixel size is the same in Figure 24–24A and C.

Continuing with Figure 24–24, if exactly the same precision (counting statistics) were required for the pixel in all three blocks, the patient exposure would have to be increased four times in going from the 80 × 80 to either of the 160 × 160 matrices, because there are four times as many pixels in the larger matrix. As we shall discuss next, resolution is a function of pixel size. With equal exposures per voxel, resolution would be better in Figure 24–24B than in Figure 24–24A because the pixels are smaller in Figure 24–24B. Resolution would be equal in both Figure 24–24A and C, because both have the same sized pixels.

Resolution

Resolution, pixel size, quantum mottle, and subject contrast are so closely related

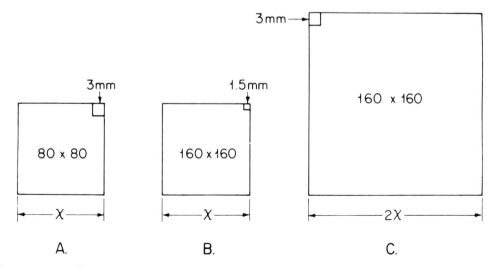

Figure 24–24 Comparison of field size (x, 2x), matrix size (80 × 80, 160 × 160), and pixel size (1.5 mm, 3 mm)

that it is difficult to talk about one without referring to the other three. **With high subject contrast and good precision, resolution is approximately 1½ times pixel size;**[12] that is, a 3- × 3-mm pixel should be capable of resolving objects with a diameter of 4.5 mm. Figure 24–25 demonstrates the effect of pixel size on resolution. The letters EMI are displayed on a 32 × 32 matrix (1024 pixels) (Fig. 24–25A). The large M is easily seen but the smaller E and I cannot be recognized. With the 80 × 80 matrix (6400 pixels), the quality of all the images improves, but the images of the smaller E and I improve more than the image of the large M (Fig. 24–25B). The unobtainable goal is in a matrix with an infinite (∞) number of points (Fig. 24–25C). Pixel size determines resolution for high-contrast objects so, theoretically, image quality improves with a large matrix (i.e., smaller pixels). CT scanners capable of resolving high-contrast structures less than 1 mm in diameter are now common.

Perhaps high contrast should be more accurately defined. In computed tomography the difference between Plexiglas and water is considered to be high contrast, and their linear attenuation coefficients differ by approximately 12% at an effective energy of 70 keV.[8] With this sort of contrast, resolution is pixel size-limited. The differences between air and water, or between water and bone are enormous by CT standards. For example, a tiny fleck of calcium in a pineal gland, a fleck too small to be seen on a radiograph, may be easily seen on a CT scan. **The calculated linear attenuation coefficient for a pixel is a weighted average of all materials in the pixel.** Photoelectric attenuation is so much greater for calcium than for water that a small amount of calcium weights the average towards the higher linear attenuation coefficient of calcium. With even a small amount of calcium, a whole picture element appears white. This effect is called **partial volume averaging.** The predominance of calcium over water has a deleterious effect on imaging in some circumstances. Figure 24–26 shows how the skull can obscure large areas of brain, especially in the more superficial cuts in which the tomographic slice traverses the calvarium obliquely. In slice A, five picture elements contain bone (shaded pixels) while only two contain bone in slice B. In the shaded area the brain is hidden from view by the calvarium.

Low-contrast resolution, or perhaps visibility is a better term, is more dependent on noise and object size than on pixel size. **The more homogeneous the background, the better the visibility of low-contrast images.** The noisier the background, the larger the low-contrast image must be before it can be detected. The only way that resolution can be improved for low-contrast objects is with better counting statistics, which produces a more homogeneous background. Low-contrast resolution is studied quantitatively by comparing two

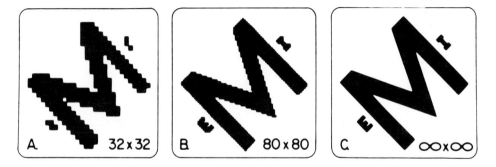

Figure 24–25   Resolution improves with a large matrix (smaller pixels)

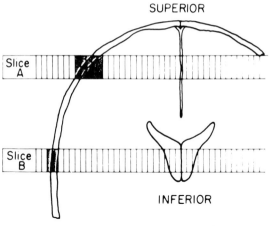

Figure 24–26   Apparent increase in skull thickness when the bone is cut obliquely, such as by slice A

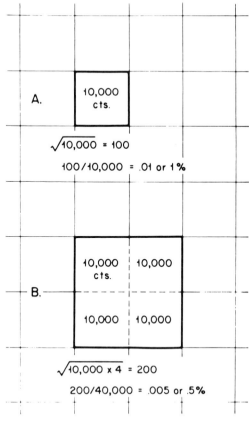

Figure 24–27   Statistical fluctuations are less with larger pixels

plastics, such as Lexan and Plexiglas, whose linear attenuation coefficients differ by approximately 1%.[12] At this level of subject contrast, resolution is limited to objects 6 to 10 mm in diameter. With a 1-cm object, a subject contrast of 1%, and a fixed patient exposure, visibility may be better with 3-mm pixels than it is with 1.5-mm pixels because the counting statistics are better with the large pixels (Fig. 24–27). The illustration represents a portion of a CT matrix, uniformly radiated to 10,000 counts per unit element (i.e., small squares). The number of counts in the smaller squares will vary statistically by 1%. This is the same percentage as the subject contrast, and the object will be obscured in this noisy background. With the larger pixels, the statistical fluctuation is only 0.5%, and the 1% subject contrast should be visible against this more uniform background.

Low-contrast resolution can be improved if subject contrast is enhanced. Some iodine-containing compounds are preferentially concentrated in certain tissues of the brain. Because iodine has a much higher atomic number than elements normally found in the brain, even small traces significantly enhance contrast in selected areas. It is now common practice to use iodinated compounds as part of many CT studies.

Spatial Uniformity

Spatial uniformity refers to the accuracy of readings over one area of the matrix relative to another area. The count rate for a perfectly uniform object (water phantom) should be the same over all areas of the matrix. Breaks in uniformity can be detected by plotting the counts for a single line as shown in Figure 24–28. The arrow in Figure 24–28A shows the matrix line plotted in Figure 24–28B. With good spatial uniformity, almost all the points fall within ±2 SD (Fig. 24–28B). The plot from a scanner with poor spatial uniformity is shown in Figure 24–28C. Counts fall below 2 SD at the margins of the field. Non-

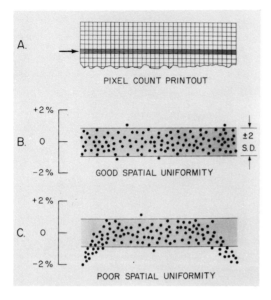

Figure 24–28   Spatial uniformity. (Modified from McCullough and Payne[12])

uniformity can be caused by beam hardening, detector flaws (nonlinearity or afterglow), or a poor mathematical reconstruction.

Size Adjustability

The original EMI scanner was designed specifically for head work, a wise decision, because the head can be easily immobilized, does not undergo any significant physiologic motion (such as breathing), and is reasonably small. The next step was to build a unit with a larger format, adaptable to any area of the body. Ideally, pixel size, field size, section thickness, matrix size, and speed (scanning times) should all be independently adjustable. Then a radiologist could select the precision (noise) and resolution (pixel size) needed to cope with a clinical situation.

PATIENT EXPOSURE

One of the more pleasant surprises with the original EMI scanner was the relatively small patient exposure. The radiation dose to the skin for a complete head examination (3 scans, or 6 slices at 4.5 minutes per scan) was 1.6 rad maximum and 1.0 rad mean.[4] Exposures were higher than this for a 3- or 4-film standard radiographic examination, in which the volume of irradiated tissue was also larger.

Theoretically, each small increment of tissue in a CT scan is exposed only during the time that the slice containing the increment is being tomogramed. At other times the increment is exposed only to scatter radiation, which is minimal because of the narrow beam. Because the scan fields do not overlap, the absorbed doses are not compounded. The theory is only partially true. Many CT units have relatively large focal spots and, as a result, prepatient collimation cannot delineate the margins of the beam sharply. Adjacent slices are partially exposed to stray radiation with each scan, and the cumulative dose is substantial. The exposure to the center of the head increases from 2.7 to 6.4 rad (2.4 times) in going from a one- to a five-slice study with an EMI-CT 5000 scanner set at 70 sec (slow speed).[12]

Doses are not uniform with CT scans, at least not when the gantry only rotates through 180°. The distribution from an

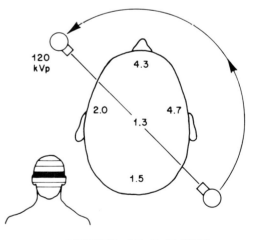

Figure 24–29   Radiation dose from CT. (Modified from McCullough and Payne[12])

EMI-CT 5000 is shown in Figure 24–29. The scanner is a body unit that was not designed specifically for head work. The doses are for a 10-inch field and a 20-sec (fast) scan time. The gantry in this unit only moves through a 180° arc, so the doses are much higher on the side of the head that is adjacent to the x-ray tube. The dose distribution is symmetric with a fan beam unit that rotates through a 360° arc.

ARTIFACTS

Under artifacts, we will discuss various technical problems that may arise during CT. The first is a major aberration that occurs at the interface between two objects with linear attenuation coefficients differing by greater than 60%. Iterative reconstructions "undershoot" the density of soft tissues (brain and cerebrospinal fluid) at junctions with bone, producing a lucent 2- to 6-mm ring adjacent to the bone. The same phenomenon occurs at air-soft tissue interfaces (pneumocephalus) but with "overshoot" (a ring of apparently greater density). The aberrations are less troublesome with a larger (160 × 160) matrix and with analytic rather than iterative reconstructions.[13]

Motion

Patient motion has a devastating effect on image quality. This was the primary reason for developing a body unit that could complete a scan during the time that a patient could hold his breath. Two types of patient motion produce artifacts. The first is a rotary and/or back-and-forth motion in which all elements in the CT slice remain in the beam throughout the exposure, but the elements change their orientation with respect to each other. The resulting scan contains black and white vertical bands for side-to-side motion and diagonal bands for rotary motion. This type of motion artifact is not as damaging to image quality as the second type, in which elements move completely out of the beam for a portion of the exposure. This type of motion is most dev-

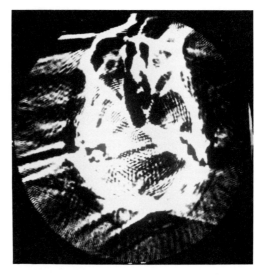

Figure 24–30   Motion artifacts. (Courtesy of Dr. Kenneth R. Maravilla, University of Texas Health Science Center at Dallas)

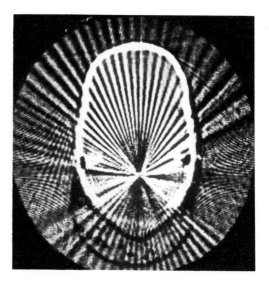

Figure 24–31   Star artifact from a metallic clip. (Courtesy of Dr. Kenneth R. Maravilla, University of Texas Health Science Center at Dallas)

astating when high-contrast objects such as bone or air move in and out of the beam (Fig. 24–30). They are especially likely to occur in the posterior fossa because of the close proximity of the petrous pyramids.

High-Density Foreign Material

The linear attenuation coefficients of metals (tantalum clips, missiles from penetrating injuries, droplets of Pantopaque) are much higher than those of any body tissue, including bone. A small metal fragment produces a star pattern, and the star effect is accentuated by any motion (Fig. 24–31). The only way to avoid the problem with current mathematical reconstructions is to change the angle of the slice to exclude the foreign body, which may also exclude a pathologic abnormality. A similar pattern is produced by gas, for example the residual of air from a ventriculogram, but the effect is less spectacular.

Detector

Artifacts from errors in detector calibrations and balance are common. The character of the artifact depends on the design of the particular scanner. Rotating fan beam scanners produce ring artifacts similar to those shown in Figure 24–32. The illustration greatly exaggerates the problem. At the time this image was made, we were calibrating our fan beam unit by scanning a water phantom. The detectors were badly out of balance and the multiple concentric rings are the consequence of this imbalance.

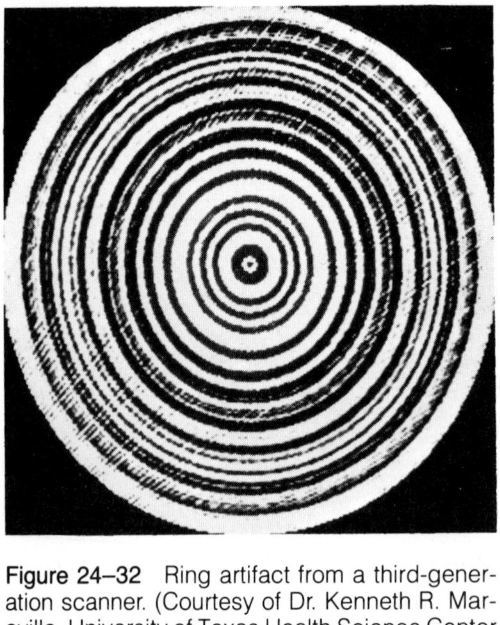

Geometric Oversights

The CT tomographic slice does not have parallel sides, as we have implied to this point.[5] Figure 24–33 shows the geometric configuration of an EMI slice with two detectors, each 13 mm in height and each recording a separate slice from a single focal spot (nominal 12 mm). The beginning of the scan (0°) is shown in Figure 24–33A, the end of the scan (180°) in Figure 24–33B, and the superimposition of the two in Figure 24–33C. The two scan slices partially overlap (shaded area in Figure 24–33C) and record some areas twice. The top surface of the upper slice and the bottom surface of the lower slice are concave in their centers and flared at their peripheries. This configuration does not lend

Figure 24–32 Ring artifact from a third-generation scanner. (Courtesy of Dr. Kenneth R. Maravilla, University of Texas Health Science Center at Dallas)

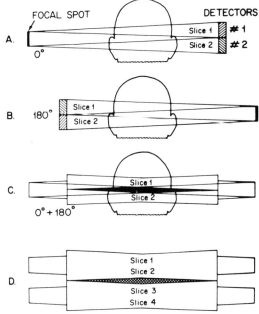

Figure 24–33 Configuration of the original EMI beam showing overlap (*shaded*) and skip areas (*cross-hatched*)

itself well to stacking. Consecutive slices are shown in Figure 24–33D. If scanned as drawn, the cross-hatched area would be completely excluded from both slices.

SUMMARY

CT is a radiographic technique for producing cross-sectional tomographic images by first scanning a slice of tissue from multiple angles with a narrow x-ray beam, then by calculating a relative linear attenuation coefficient for the various tissue elements in the section, and finally by displaying the reconstruction as a gray scale image on a television monitor. Two basic scan patterns are used: repetitive linear scanning through a 180° arc with one or several detectors, and fan beam scanning with a delta-shaped beam and a large array of either rotating detectors or a stationary ring of detectors. The fan beam offers the advantage of greater speed and more uniform patient exposures, and the disadvantages of greater cost, more scatter radiation, and a more complex mathematical reconstruction.

In the original EMI scanner, mathematical reconstructions were done with iterative methods, but now reconstructions are usually done with analytic techniques using either two-dimensional Fourier analysis, filtered back-projection, or a combination of the two. Analytic methods start computations as soon as the first ray projection is scanned, so they are fast and the reconstruction may be completed a few seconds after all the data are collected. The mathematical reconstruction is a display (on paper as numbers or on a cathode ray tube as a gray scale) of CT numbers, which are proportional to the linear attenuation coefficients of the tissues in the tomographic section. A relatively high-energy heavily filtered heterochromatic beam is used in all current commercial scanners, but a monochromatic beam would be superior, because the mean energy of a monochromatic beam is not affected by filtration and linear attenuation calculations would be more ac-

curate. Transmission counts are measured either by scintillation crystal detectors, which have a high counting efficiency but suffer from nonlinear response and afterglow, or by pressurized xenon detectors, which have a linear response and do not suffer from afterglow but are less efficient.

Contrast levels can be adjusted to augment specific areas in the image. All CT scanners have an arbitrarily expanded scale of relative linear attenuation coefficients, called CT numbers. Dense bone is assigned the highest value, air the lowest value (usually a negative number), and water a value of 0. In the original EMI scanner, dense bone was $+500$, water 0, and air -500. The difference in the linear attenuation coefficients of soft tissues, excluding fat, is about 4%, with fresh blood clots among the densest and cerebrospinal fluid the least dense. This 4% difference is easily demonstrated when a normal or pathologic anatomic structure is sufficiently large and appropriately located. The most serious factor limiting image quality is statistical noise. This problem can be partially solved by increasing scan times (more radiation) and picture element (pixel) size, but both of these alternatives are objectionable. Increasing scan times increases patient exposures and increasing pixel size decreases high-contrast resolution.

REFERENCES

1. Bracewell, R.N.: Strip integration in radioastronomy. Aust. J. Phys., 9:198, 1956.
2. Brooks, R.A., and DiChiro, G.: Theory of image reconstruction in computed tomography. Radiology, 117:561, 1975.
3. Cormack, A.M.: Representation of a function by its line integrals, with some radiological applications. J. Appl. Phys., 34:2722, 1963.
4. EMI Scanner: A New Perspective on Brain Tissues. Middlesex, England, EMI Limited, 1973.
5. Goodenough, D.J., Weaver, K.E., and Davis, D.O.: Potential artifacts associated with the scanning pattern of the EMI scanner. Radiology, 117:615, 1975.
6. Hounsfield, G.N.: Picture quality of computed tomography. Am. J. Roentgenol., 127:3, 1976.
7. Hounsfield, G.N.: Computerized transverse axial scanning (tomography). Br. J. Radiol., 46:1016, 1973.

8. Kuhl, D.E., and Edwards, R.Q.: Reorganizing data from transverse section scans of the brain using digital processing. Radiology, *91*:975, 1968.
9. McCullough, E.C., Payne, J.T., Baker, H.L., Hattery, R.R., Sheedy, P.F., Stephens, D.H., and Gedgaudus, E.: Performance evaluation and quality assurance of computed tomography scanners with illustrations from the EMI, ACTA, and Delta scanners. Radiology, *120*:173, 1976.
10. McCullough, E.C., Baker, H.L., Houser, O.W., and Reese, D.F.: An evaluation of the quantitative and radiation features of a scanning x-ray transverse axial tomography: The EMI scanner. Radiology, *111*:709, 1974.
11. McCullough, E.C., and Payne, J.T.: X-ray transmission computed tomography. Med. Phys., *4*:85, 1977.
12. McCullough, E.C., and Payne, J.T.: Performance evaluation: CT scanners. Presented at the International Symposium & Course on Computerized Tomography (CT). San Juan, Puerto Rico, 1976.
13. New, P.F.T., and Scott, W.R.: Computed Tomography of the Brain and Orbit. Baltimore, Williams & Wilkins, 1975.
14. Oldendorf, W.H.: Isolated flying spot detection of radiodensity discontinuities displaying the lateral structural pattern of a complex object. IRE Trans. Biomed. Electronics, *BMW 8*:1, 1961.
15. Phelps, M.E., Gado, M.H., and Hoffman, E.J.: Correlation of effective atomic number and electronic density with attenuation coefficients measured with polychromatic x-rays. Radiology, *117*:585, 1975.
16. Phelps, M.E., Hoffman, E.J., and Ter-Pogossian, M.M.: Attenuation coefficients of various body tissues, fluids, and lesions at photon energies of 18 to 136 keV. Radiology, *117*:573, 1975.
17. Radon, J.: Berichte über die Verhandlungen der koniglich Sashsischen Gesellschaft der Wissenschaften zu Leipzig. Mathematisch—Physische Klasse, *69*:262, 1917.

25

Ultrasound

X rays were put to practical use the moment they were discovered, and improvements in equipment and techniques progressed rapidly during the first few years. In contrast, ultrasound has been notoriously slow in its medical evolution. The technology for producing ultrasound and the characteristics of sonic waves have been known for many years. The first major attempt at a practical application was made in the unsuccessful search for the sunken Titanic in the North Atlantic in 1912. Other early attempts at applying ultrasound to medical diagnosis met with the same fate. Techniques were not sufficiently developed, especially imaging techniques, until the massive military research effort that accompanied World War II. Sonar (**SO**und **N**avigation **A**nd **R**anging) was the first important successful application. Successful medical applications began shortly after the war, in the late 1940s and early 1950s. Since then progress has been rapid, especially in the last decade with B-mode imaging, and even more recently with the addition of gray-scale presentations.

A simplified overview of a sonic imaging system is shown in Figure 25–1. The vital ingredients are (1) a transducer, (2) an ultrasonic beam, and (3) a display method, usually a cathode ray tube (CRT) or a television monitor. The transducer serves a dual function as both a transmitter and receiver. Sound is transmitted in approximately 1000 short bursts (pulses) each second. During the interval between pulses, the transducer functions as a detector, sensing the returning echoes from the previous pulse. An operator, frequently a physician, positions the transducer on the patient, moves it about to produce the appropriate echoes over the region of interest, and simultaneously manipulates the CRT controls for optimal image display. A permanent photographic record may be made of this image. In its current state of development, the interplay between the patient, operator, and instrument is much more complex than it is in diagnostic radiology, in which a technician can select a technique, push a button, and have a reasonably good chance of success. Ultrasonic imaging is more of an art than x-ray imaging. The operator must have a thorough enough knowledge of anatomy to interpret the images as they appear. The controls can then be adjusted and the transducer positioned to show subtle abnormalities that could not be demonstrated without this interplay.

CHARACTERISTICS OF SOUND

A sound beam is similar to an x-ray beam in that both are waves transmitting energy. A more important difference is that x rays pass readily through a vacuum while sound requires a medium for its transmission. The velocity of sound depends on the nature of the medium. A useful way to picture matter (the medium) is as a series of spherical particles, representing either atoms or molecules, separated by tiny springs (Fig. 25–2A). When the first particle is pushed, it moves and compresses the

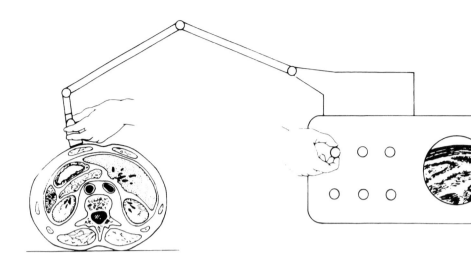

Figure 25–1   An ultrasonic imaging system

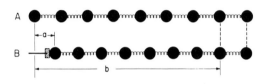

Figure 25–2   Propagation of a sound wave

attached spring, thus exerting a force on the adjacent particle (Fig. 25–2*B*). This sets up a chain reaction, but each subsequent particle moves a little less than its neighbor. The tension or pressure applied to the spring is greatest between the first two particles and less between any two down the line. If the driving force reverses its direction, the particles also reverse their direction. If the force vibrates to and fro like a cymbal that has been struck, the particles respond by oscillating back and forth. The particles in a sound beam behave in the same manner; that is, they oscillate back and forth, but over a short distance of only a few microns in liquids and even less in solids.

Although the individual particles move only a few microns, you can see from Figure 25–2 that the effect of their motion is transmitted through their neighbors over a much longer distance. During the same time, or almost the same, that the first par-

ticle moves through a distance a, the effect of the motion is transmitted over a distance b. The velocity of sound is determined by the rate at which the force is transmitted from one molecule to another.

Longitudinal Waves

Ultrasonic pulses are transmitted through liquids as longitudinal waves. The term "longitudinal wave" means that the motion of the particles in the medium is parallel to the direction of wave propagation. The molecules of the conducting liquid move back and forth, producing bands of compression and rarefaction (Fig. 25–3). The wave front starts at time 1 in Figure 25–3 when a vibrating drum compresses the adjacent material. A band of rarefaction is produced at time 2, when the drum reverses it direction. Each repetition of this back-and-forth motion is called a cycle, and each cycle produces a new wave. **The length of the wave is the distance between two bands of compression, or rarefaction,** and is represented by the symbol λ. Once the sound wave has been generated, it continues in its original direction until it is either reflected or absorbed. The motion of the vibrating drum, plotted against time, forms the sinusoidal curve shown along the left side of Figure 25–3.

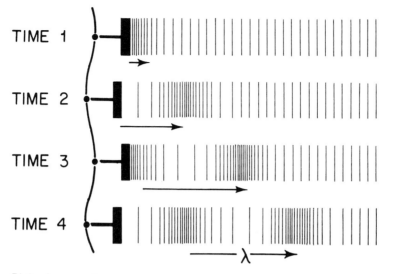

Figure 25–3 Birth of a sound wave

Ultrasound, by definition, has a frequency of greater than 20,000 cycles per second. Audible sound has a frequency between 15 and 20,000 cycles per second (the frequency of the average man's voice is about 100 cycles per second, and that of the average woman is about 200). The sonic beams used in diagnostic imaging have frequencies from 1,000,000 to 20,000,000 cycles per second. One cycle per second is called a Hertz; a million cycles per second is a megahertz (abbreviated MHz). The term "Hertz" honors the famous German physicist Heinrich R. Hertz, who died in 1894.

Velocity of Sound

For body tissues in the medical ultrasound range, **the velocity of transmission of sound is independent of frequency, and depends primarily on the physical makeup of the material through which the sound is being transmitted.** The important characteristics of the transmitting medium are (1) its compressibility and (2) density. Table 25–1 shows the velocity of sound in some common materials, including several types of body tissue. The materials are listed in order of increasing speed of transmission, and you can see that sound travels

Table 25–1. Velocity of Sound in Various Materials

MATERIAL	VELOCITY (m/sec)
Air	331
Fat	1450
Mercury	1450
Castor oil	1500
Water (50° C)	1540
"HUMAN SOFT TISSUE"	1540
Brain	1541
Liver	1549
Kidney	1561
Blood	1570
Muscle	1585
Lens of eye	1620
PZT-5A	3780
PZT-4	4000
Skull (bone)	4080
Brass	4490
Quartz	5740
Aluminum	6400

slowest in gases, at intermediate velocity in liquids, and most rapidly in solids. Note that all body tissues, except bone, behave like liquids, and therefore they all transmit sound at about the same velocity. A velocity of 1540 meters per second is used as an average for body tissue.

Compressibility

The velocity of sound is inversely related to the compressibility of the conducting material; that is, the less compressible a material, the more rapidly it transmits sound. Sound waves move slowly in gases because the molecules are far apart and are easily compressed. They behave as though they are held together by loose springs. A particle must move a relatively long distance before it can affect a neighbor. Liquids and solids are less compressible because their molecules are closer together. They only need to move a short distance to affect a neighbor, so liquids and solids propagate sound more rapidly than gases.

Density

Dense materials tend to be composed of massive molecules, and these molecules have a great deal of inertia. They are difficult to move or to stop once they are moving. Because the propagation of sound involves the rhythmic starting and stopping of particulate motion, we would not expect a material made up of large molecules (i.e., large in mass) such as mercury to transmit sound at as great a velocity as a material composed of smaller molecules, such as water. Mercury is 13.9 times denser than water, so we would expect water to conduct sound much more rapidly. Nevertheless, you can see from Table 25–1 that water and mercury transmit sound at fairly similar velocities. The apparent discrepancy is explained by the greater compressibility of water, which is 13.4 times as compressible as mercury.[3] The loss in mercury's ability to transmit sound rapidly because of its greater mass is almost exactly balanced by a gain because of its lesser compressibility. As a general rule, this same principle applies to all liquids, that is, density and compressibility are inversely proportional. Consequently, all liquids transmit sound within a narrow range of velocities.

The relationship between wavelength and wave velocity is as follows:

$v = \nu\lambda$
v = velocity of sound in conducting media (m/sec)
ν = frequency (Hz)
λ = wavelength (m)

In the ultrasonic frequency range, the velocity of sound is constant in any particular medium. When the frequency is increased, the wavelength must decrease. This is shown in Figure 25–4. In Figure 25–4A, the vibrator has a frequency of 1.5 MHz. Assuming the medium to be water, which propagates sound at a velocity of 1540 m/sec, the wavelength will be

$$1540 \text{ m/sec} = 1,500,000 \text{ (1/sec)}\lambda$$

and

$$\lambda = 0.001 \text{ m}$$

Therefore, 0.001 m (1.0 mm) is as far as the wave can propagate in the time available before a new wave starts. In Figure 25–4B, frequency is doubled to 3.0 MHz, but the waves move away at the same velocity, so their length is halved to 0.0005 m (0.5 mm).

Intensity

The intensity of sound, or loudness in the audible range, is determined by the length of oscillation of the particles conducting the waves. The greater the amplitude of oscillation, the more intense the sound. Figure 25–5 shows high- and low-intensity longitudinal waves of the same frequency, wavelength, and velocity. The compression bands are more compacted in the high-intensity beam. The harder the vibrator is struck, the more energy it receives and the wider its vibrations. These wider excursions are transmitted to the adjacent conducting media and produce a more intense beam. In time, the vibrations diminish in intensity, although not in frequency, and the sound intensity decreases, producing a lower intensity beam. Ultrasonic intensities are expressed in Watts (power) per square centimeter (note that

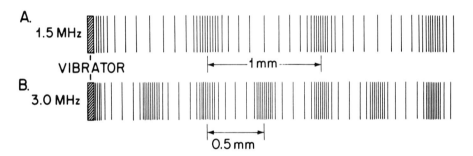

Figure 25–4 The wavelength of sound decreases as its frequency (MHz) increases

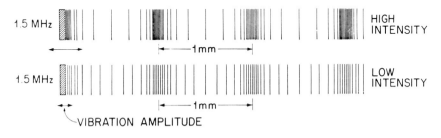

Figure 25–5 A larger amplitude of vibration produces denser compression bands and a higher intensity sound

these units are a mixture of SI and cgs units, but that's the way we do it). The mathematical expression that relates intensity to particle velocity, wave velocity, and medium density is rather complex and of no practical importance to radiologists, so we will not attempt to explain it here.

Relative Sound Intensity

Sound intensity is measured in **decibels.** A decibel is a relative unit, not an absolute one. Simply defined, a decibel (dB) is one tenth of a bel (B). A **bel** is a comparison of the relative power of two sound beams expressed logarithmically using the base 10. For those who may have forgotten, we will briefly review logarithms. Starting with the number 10 and raising it to various positive and negative powers, we get a series of numbers, as follows:

10 Raised to a Power	Corresponding Number	Log (base 10)
10^4	10,000	4
10^3	1,000	3
10^2	100	2
10^1	10	1
10^0	1	0
10^{-1}	0.1	-1
10^{-2}	0.01	-2
10^{-3}	0.001	-3

For example, 10 raised to the fourth power (10^4) is 10,000. The log of 10,000 is 4. Note that there is no zero in the center column. The log of zero is undefined. The number 10 raised to the 0 power is 1, and not 0 as might be expected at first glance.

Returning to our definition of a bel, it is a logarithmic comparison of the relative intensity of two sound beams. Table 25–2 summarizes the relationships between the bel, decibel, and intensity (or power) of an ultrasonic beam. Note that increasing intensity from 1 to 2 B increases relative intensity by a factor of 10. The number of

Table 25–2. Comparison of Relative Intensity, Bels, Positive and Negative Decibels, and Percentage of Sound Remaining in Ultrasonic Beam

BELS (B)	POSITIVE DECIBELS (dB)	INTENSITY (Watts/cm²)	NEGATIVE DECIBELS (−dB)	SOUND REMAINING IN BEAM (%)
0	0	1	0	100
1/10	1	1.26	−1	79
2/10	2	1.59	−2	63
3/10	3	2.00	−3	50
4/10	4	2.51	−4	40
5/10	5	3.16	−5	32
6/10	6	3.98	−6	25
7/10	7	5.01	−7	19
8/10	8	6.31	−8	16
9/10	9	7.94	−9	13
1	10	10	−10	10
2	20	100	−20	1
3	30	1,000	−30	0.1
4	40	10,000	−40	0.01
5	50	100,000	−50	0.001
6	60	1,000,000	−60	0.0001

decibels is obtained by multiplying the number of bels by 10. If an ultrasonic beam has an original intensity of 10 Watts/cm², and the returning echo is 0.001 Watts/cm², their relative intensity will be

$$\log \frac{0.001}{10} = \log 0.0001 = -4 \text{ B, or } -40 \text{ dB}$$

Decibels may have either a positive or negative sign. Positive decibels indicate a gain in power, while negative decibels express a power loss. Ultrasound loses power as it passes through tissue, so in the above example, the intensity of the returning echo relative to the original beam is −40 dB. Table 25–2 shows a column of negative decibels and the percentage of sound remaining in the beam at the new decibel level. In our example, the intensity of the returning echo (−40 dB) is only 0.01% that of the original intensity.

TRANSDUCERS

A transducer is a device that can convert one form of energy into another. Ultrasonic transducers are used to convert an electric signal into ultrasonic energy that can be transmitted into tissues, and to convert ultrasonic energy reflected back from the tissues into an electric signal.

The general composition of an ultrasonic transducer is shown in Figure 25–6. The most important component is a thin (approximately 0.5-mm) **piezoelectric crystal** element located near the face of the transducer. The front and back faces of the crystal are coated with a thin conducting film to ensure good contact with the two electrodes that will supply the electric field

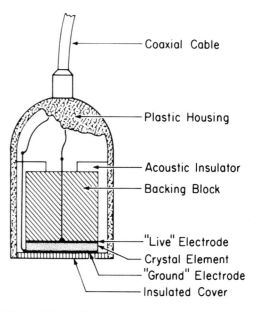

Figure 25–6 Ultrasound transducer

used to strain the crystal. The term "strain" refers to deformity of the crystal caused when a voltage is applied to the crystal. The surfaces of the crystal are plated with gold or silver electrodes. The outside electrode is grounded to protect the patient from electrical shock, and its outside surface is coated with a watertight electrical insulator. The inside electrode abuts against a thick backing block that absorbs sound waves transmitted back into the transducer. The housing is usually a strong plastic. An acoustic insulator of rubber or cork prevents the sound from passing into the housing. A large variety of sizes and shapes of transducers are available to perform specific functions, but they all have this general design.

The Characteristics of Piezoelectric Crystals

Certain materials are such that the application of an electric field causes a change in their physical dimensions, and vice versa. This is called the piezoelectric effect, first described by Pierre and Jacques Curie in 1880. Piezoelectric materials are made up of innumerable **dipoles** arranged in a geometric pattern (Fig. 25–7). An electric dipole is a distorted molecule that appears to have a positive charge on one end and a negative charge on the other (Fig. 25–7A). The positive and negative ends are arranged so that an electric field will cause them to realign, thus changing the dimensions of the crystal (Fig. 25–7B). The illustration shows a considerable change in thickness, but actually the change is only a few microns. Note that no current flows through the crystal. The plating electrodes behave as capacitors, and it is the voltage between them that produces the electric field, which in turn causes the crystal to change shape. If the voltage is applied in a sudden burst, or pulse, the crystal vibrates like a cymbal that has been struck a sharp blow and generates sound waves. The backing block quickly dampens the vibrations to prime the transducer for its sec-

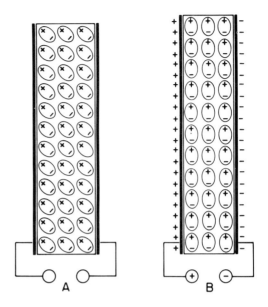

Figure 25–7 An electric field realigns the dipoles in a piezoelectric crystal

ond function, which is to detect returning echoes.

As the sound pulse passes through the body, echoes reflect back toward the transducer from each tissue interface. These echoes carry energy and they transmit their energy to the transducer, causing a physical compression of the crystal element. This compression forces the tiny dipoles to change their orientation, which induces a voltage between the electrodes. The voltage is amplified and serves as the ultrasonic signal for display on an oscilloscope or television monitor. Incidentally, the compression force and associated voltage are responsible for the name piezoelectricity, which means "pressure" electricity.

Some naturally occurring materials possess piezoelectric properties (e.g., quartz), but most crystals used in medical ultrasound are man-made. This group of artificial piezoelectric materials is known as **ferroelectrics,** of which a great variety exist. Barium titanate was the first of the ceramic ferroelectrics to be discovered. This has been largely replaced by lead zirconate titanate, commonly known as **PZT.*** Several types of PZT are available, with slight variations in chemical additions and thermal treatment producing different properties.

A great advantage of piezoelectric ceramics is that they can be formed into different shapes, depending on the application for which they are intended. Piezoelectric crystals can be designed to vibrate in either the thickness or radial mode (Fig. 25–8). Medical crystals are designed to vibrate in the thickness mode. They still vibrate to a lesser extent in the radial mode, however, so the receiving amplifier is gated to tune out all frequencies except those from the thickness mode. Results of current research suggest that certain plastic polymers, such as polyvinylidene fluoride, have favorable piezoelectric properties that will allow the future development of plastic transducers with characteristics superior to those of the synthetic ceramics now being used.

Curie Temperature

Ceramic crystals are made up of innumerable tiny dipoles but, to possess piezoelectric characteristics, the dipoles must be arranged in a specific geometric configuration. To produce this polarization, the ceramic is heated to a high temperature in a strong electric field. At a high temperature the dipoles are free to move, and the electric field brings them into the desired alignment. The crystal is then gradually cooled while subjected to a constant high voltage. As room temperature is reached, the dipoles become fixed, and the crystal then possesses piezoelectric properties. The Curie temperature is the temperature at which this polarization is lost. Heating a piezoelectric crystal above the Curie temperature reduces it to a useless piece of ceramic, so obviously transducers should never be autoclaved. The approximate Curie temperatures for several crystals are as follows:

Quartz	573° C
Barium titanate	100° C
PZT-4	328° C
PZT-5A	365° C

Resonant Frequency

An ultrasound transducer is designed to be maximally sensitive to a certain natural frequency. The thickness of a piezoelectric crystal determines its natural frequency, called its resonant frequency. Crystal thickness is analogous to the length of a pipe in a pipe organ. Just as a long pipe produces a low-pitched audible sound, a thick crystal produces a low-frequency ultrasound. The surfaces of a piezoelectric crystal behave like two identical cymbals, facing each other but separated in an open space. When one cymbal is struck, its vibrations set up sound waves that cause the other cymbal to vibrate. Vibrations are maximum in the second cymbal when the space sep-

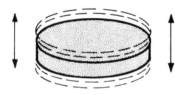

THICKNESS MODE

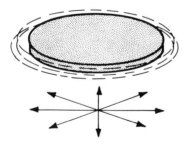

RADIAL MODE

Figure 25–8 Modes of vibration of a piezoelectric crystal

*PZT is a registered trade name of PZT materials from the Clevite Corporation.

arating the two is equal to one half of the wavelength of the sound. At this distance the sound waves from and vibrations of the two cymbals are exactly synchronized. The sound from one reinforces the vibrations of the other. A vibrating piezoelectric crystal transmits sound in both directions from each surface. The internally transmitted waves cross the transducer to synchronize with vibrations from the other side, just like the two cymbals in our example. When a crystal is struck with a single sharp voltage spike, it vibrates at its natural frequency, which is determined by its thickness. The natural frequency is the one that produces internal wavelengths that are twice the thickness of the crystal.

The crystal is designed so that its thickness is equal to exactly half the wavelength of the ultrasound to be produced by the transducer. The crystal is said to **resonate** (i.e., oscillate most efficiently) at the frequency determined by its thickness. The frequency that corresponds to half of the wavelength thickness is called the fundamental resonance frequency of the transducer. As an example, let us calculate the fundamental resonance frequency of a PZT-4 crystal that is 0.001 m (1 mm) thick. The velocity (v) of sound in PZT-4 is 4000 m/sec (Table 25–1), and we are told that the crystal will resonate at a frequency (v) equal to twice the crystal thickness (i.e., $\lambda = 2v = 0.002$ m). Substituting these values in the equation relating frequency, wavelength, and velocity of sound, we obtain

$$v = v\lambda$$
$$v = \frac{v}{\lambda}$$
$$v = \frac{4000 \text{ m/sec}}{0.002 \text{ m}}$$
$$v = 2{,}000{,}000/\text{sec} = 2 \text{ MHz}$$

Thus, a 2-MHz piezoelectric crystal made of PZT-4 will have a thickness of 0.001 m (1 mm). Similarly, a 1-MHz crystal will be 0.002 m thick. Note how crystals designed to resonate at high megahertz frequencies will be extremely thin.

A crystal can be forced to vibrate at the frequency of any alternating voltage, but the intensity of this sound is much less than it would be for a comparable voltage at the crystal's natural frequency. **In medical sonography, the crystal is usually subjected to a single voltage pulse and is allowed to vibrate at its natural frequency.** The fact that piezoelectric crystals have a natural frequency has considerable practical importance. With an x-ray machine the wavelength, or kilovoltage, can be adjusted by simply turning a few dials on a control panel. We do not have this freedom with ultrasound imaging. A frequency change requires another transducer, one designed for the desired frequency. Only a few different sizes and frequencies are needed to handle most clinical situations, which is fortunate because transducers are rather expensive.

Transducer Q Factor

The Q factor refers to two characteristics of piezoelectric crystals: the purity of their sound and the length of time that the sound persists. A high-Q transducer produces a nearly pure sound made up of a narrow range of frequencies, while a low-Q transducer produces a whole spectrum of sound covering a much wider range of frequencies. Almost all the internal sound waves of a high-Q transducer are of the appropriate wavelength to reinforce vibrations within the crystal. When an unsupported high-Q crystal (i.e., a crystal without a backing block) is struck by a short voltage pulse, it vibrates for a long time and produces a long continuous sound. The interval between initiation of the wave and complete cessation of vibrations is called the ring down-time. Figure 25–9 shows the ring down-time for high-Q and low-Q crystals.

The Q factor can also be defined mathematically in terms of the purity of the sound. As the result of the sudden application of an electrical pulse, a transducer will ring at its resonance frequency, but will

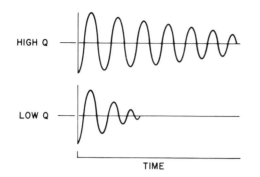

Figure 25–9 Ring down-time of a high Q and low Q transducer

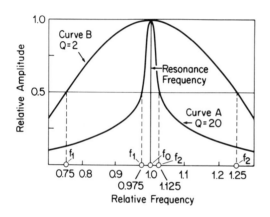

Figure 25–10 The Q factor related to frequency response for a high Q (curve A) and a low Q (curve B) transducer

the frequency response curve, and is defined as

$$Q = \frac{f_0}{f_2 - f_1}$$

Q = Q factor
f_0 = resonance frequency
f_2 = frequency above resonance at which intensity is reduced by half
f_1 = frequency below resonance at which intensity is reduced by half

In Figure 25–10, curve A illustrates a Q factor of 20. The transducer system generating curve A produces a narrow range of sound frequencies and has a long ring down-time. Such a system is useful for Doppler ultrasound transducers (we will discuss this in detail later). The transducer system producing curve B in Figure 25–10 has a Q factor of 2. This type of system will produce sound with a broad frequency range and will have a short ring down-time. Such a transducer (i.e., low Q) is needed for organ imaging (pulse-echo operation) because it can furnish short ultrasound pulses and will respond to a broad range of returning frequencies.

A long continuous sound is unsatisfactory for sonic imaging. **The transducer is both a transmitter and a receiver,** but it cannot send and receive at the same time. When continuous sound is being transmitted, the associated vibrations in the crystal produce continuously fluctuating voltages between the electrodes. If the internally generated sound waves are stronger than the returning echoes, as they may be, the returning signal is lost in the noise of the system. Another reason why continuous sound is undesirable for imaging is that depth resolution is generally determined by the length of the sonic pulse. (Depth resolution will be defined later in this chapter.) The length of the sonic pulse, called the **spatial pulse length,** is the number of waves multiplied by their wavelength. The sonic pulse from an unsupported high-Q crystal is long because the sound persists for a long time.

also produce sound waves at frequencies above and below the resonance frequency. The Q factor of a transducer system describes this frequency response. If the frequency response of a crystal is plotted, curves similar to those in Figure 25–10 are obtained. The points f_2 and f_1 represent the frequencies above and below the resonance frequency where the sound intensity has been reduced to half. The Q factor of a transducer system describes the shape of

The approximate Q factor of several piezoelectric materials is as follows:

Quartz	>25,000
PZT-4	>500
PZT-5A	75
Piezoelectric polymers	3

The Q factor of piezoelectric materials can be controlled by altering the characteristics of the backing block of the transducer. **A backing block is incorporated to quench the vibrations and to shorten the sonic pulse.** If the wavelength of sound from a transducer is 0.5 mm (0.0005 m), and the pulse is quenched after two wavelengths, the spatial pulse length is 1 mm (0.001 m). Ideally, the ultrasonic pulse should be a single wavelength. The ideal backing material should accept all sound waves that reach it (i.e., not reflect any back into the crystal) and should then completely absorb the energy from these waves. This means that the backing material must have a characteristic impedance similar to that of the transducer crystal (don't worry about characteristic impedance right now; we will discuss it shortly). Backing blocks are generally made of a combination of tungsten and rubber powder in an epoxy resin. The ratio of tungsten to resin is chosen to satisfy the impedance requirements, and the rubber powder is added to increase the attenuation of sound in the backing block. For example, addition of 5% by volume of rubber powder to a 10% by volume mixture of tungsten powder in epoxy increases the attenuation from 5.6 to 8.0 dB cm^{-1} at 1 MHz. As a general rule, high-Q crystals are more efficient transmitters and low-Q crystals are more efficient receivers.

Three other important topics concerning transducers are focused transducers, impedance matching, and quarter-wave length matching. These will be dealt with later in the chapter after the appropriate background material has been introduced.

CHARACTERISTICS OF AN ULTRASONIC BEAM

A single vibrating point sends out waves in all directions, much like those produced by a pebble thrown into a quiet pond; the waves move away from their point of origin as concentric circles. If two pebbles simultaneously land side by side, they each cause ringlike waves, and these waves may either reinforce or cancel each other, depending on their phase when they meet (Fig. 25–11). At time A, two waves are approaching each other from opposite directions. At time B, they are touching but not overlapping. One half-cycle later, at time C, the valley of one has reached the crest of the other and they cancel each other. Another half-cycle later, at time D, the crest and valleys are exactly superimposed, reinforcing themselves and doubling the

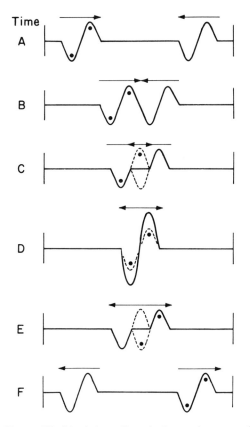

Figure 25–11   Interactions between two sound waves traveling in opposite directions

height and depth of the peaks and valleys. Another half-cycle later, at time E, the waves have separated, and finally go their own way, at time F, as two separate waves moving in the opposite direction.

Piezoelectric crystals behave as a series of vibrating points and not as the pistonlike surface that we have implied previously. The wave fronts are not uniform, at least not close to the crystal. In Figure 25–12 the crystal is depicted as five vibrating points, with each point producing multiple concentric rings or waves that eventually form a continuous front as they reinforce each other along a line parallel to the face of the crystal. The distance at which the waves become synchronous depends on their wavelengths. The shorter the wavelength, the closer the front forms to the surface of the transducer.

The intensity of ultrasound varies both from one side of the beam to the other and longitudinally along the length of the beam. Numerous ingenious methods have been employed to demonstrate these variations, with the more common summarized in Figure 25–13. The simplest way of depicting a beam is that shown in Figure 25–13A, in which the beam is drawn as a parallel bundle for a certain distance, beyond which it disperses. The parallel component is called the near or **Fresnel** (pronounced Fre-nel) **zone.** The diverging portion of the beam, that beyond **x′** is called the far or **Fraunhofer zone.** The no-

tation **x′** is used to identify the transition point between the Fresnel and Fraunhofer zones.

Figure 25–13B shows a schematic Schlieren photograph of a sonic beam, the same beam shown in Figure 25–13A. When sound passes through a transparent medium, such as water, it changes the refractive index of the medium. This change can be photographed with the proper lighting arrangement. The sound in the illustration originates from four point sources. The waves from these points reinforce and cancel each other in phase: the initial four beams become three, then two, and finally a single wave front at x′, the transition zone.

Figure 25–13C is produced by plotting the intensity of the beam along its central longitudinal axis. The plot shows the same variations in beam intensity that are shown photographically in Figure 25–13B. The black and white areas of Figure 25–13B appear as peaks and valleys in Figure 25–13C.

These illustrations all describe a continuously emitted sound beam, which is a little different than the pulsed beam used for imaging. The transition from continuous to pulsed beams is easy to picture with the aid of Figure 25–13D, which is a cross-sectional photographic display. The sonic pulse changes its character as it moves away from the transducer. It passes in rapid succession through each of the stages shown in the illustration. The pulse becomes homogeneous at the transition point. Beyond the transition point, the pulse remains homogeneous but increases in diameter and decreases in intensity.

The length of the Fresnel zone is determined by the diameter of the transducer and the wavelength of the ultrasound:

$$x' = \frac{r^2}{\lambda}$$

x′ = length of the Fresnel zone (cm)
r = radius of the transducer (cm)
λ = wavelength (cm)

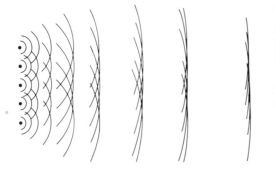

Figure 25–12 Superimposition of waves to form a wavefront

Note that we have left this illustration in

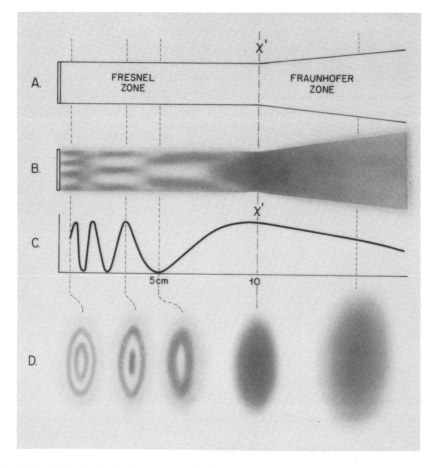

Figure 25–13 Methods of displaying a sonic beam

cgs units (cm), rather than switching to SI units (m). Table 25–3 shows the length of the Fresnel zone for various wavelengths and transducer diameters. The zone is longest with a large transducer and high-

Table 25–3. The Length of the Fresnel Zone for Various Sized Transducers and Frequencies*

FREQUENCY (MHz)	LENGTH OF FRESNEL ZONE (cm)				
	DIAMETER OF TRANSDUCER (cm)				
	0.5	1.0	1.5	2.0	2.5
1.0	0.37	1.6	3.4	6.5	10
1.5	0.58	2.4	5.1	9.7	15
2.0	0.79	3.2	6.8	13.0	20
2.5	1.01	4.0	8.5	16.0	25
5.0	2.01	8.1	17.0	32.0	50
7.5	2.97	11.9	25.0	48.0	75

*Based on a sound velocity of 1540 m/sec.

frequency sound, and shortest with a small transducer and low-frequency sound. For those who have difficulty interpreting tables, the same type of data are visually displayed in Figures 25–14 and 25–15. In Figure 25–14, the size of the transducer is constant at 1.5 cm, and the frequency of the sound is increased in stages from 1 to 3 MHz. The near zone increases in length with increasing frequency. In Figure 25–15, the frequency is fixed at 1 MHz and the size of the transducer is increased in stages from 1 to 2.5 cm. Again, the near zone increases in length with larger transducers.

High-frequency beams have two advantages over low-frequency beams: depth resolution is superior, and the Fresnel zone is

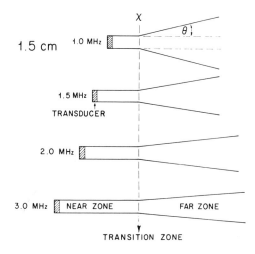

Figure 25–14 Elongation of the near zone with increasing frequencies

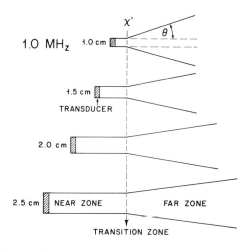

Figure 25–15 Elongation of the near zone with increasing transducer size

longer. It would seem logical to use high frequencies for all imaging. High frequencies, however, have a major drawback related to penetration. **Tissue absorption increases with increasing frequency,** so a relatively low-frequency beam is required to penetrate thick parts. It would also seem logical to increase the size of the transducer to keep the beam coherent for sufficient depth to reach the point of interest. Although larger transducers improve coherence, they deteriorate side-to-side resolu-

tion. This dilemma is at least partially resolved with the use of focused transducers (to be discussed later). The amount of dispersion in the far zone is shown in the uppermost illustration in Figure 25–15. The size of the angle is determined as follows:

$$\sin \theta = 1.22 \frac{\lambda}{D}$$

θ = dispersion angle of far zone
λ = wavelength (mm)
D = diameter of transducer (mm)

The equation is rather simple to use with mathematical tables or a calculator with trigonometric functions. For example, the dispersion angle for a 10-mm transducer and a wavelength of 1 mm (a frequency of 1.5 MHz) may be determined as follows:

$$\sin \theta = 1.22 \frac{1.0}{10} = 0.122$$

$$\theta = 7°$$

If the wavelength is shortened to 0.5 mm (a frequency of 3 MHz), and the transducer size is kept at 10 mm, the dispersion angle is 3.5°.

INTERACTIONS BETWEEN ULTRASOUND AND MATTER

The types of interactions between sound and matter are similar to those of light, and include the following: (1) reflection, (2) refraction, and (3) absorption.

Reflection

In x-ray imaging, the transmitted radiation blackens the film and creates the actual image. Attenuated radiation creates defects or holes in the transmitted beam, contributing to image formation in a passive way. Scattered radiation fogs the film and is detrimental to image quality. With ultrasound, however, the image is produced by the reflected portion of the beam. Transmitted sound contributes nothing to image formation, but transmission must be strong enough to produce echoes at deeper levels. The percentage of the beam reflected at tissue interfaces depends on (1) the tissue's acoustic impedance, and (2) the beam's angle of incidence. There is an ultrasound imaging mode called transmission mode imaging, but at this time technical problems remain to be solved before the information in the transmitted beam can be useful for routine clinical applications. We will not discuss transmission mode imaging.

Acoustic Impedance

Acoustic impedance is a fundamental property of matter. The impedance of a material is the product of its density and the velocity of sound in the material.

$$Z = \rho v$$

Z = acoustic impedance (Rayls)
ρ = density (g/cm³)
v = velocity of sound (cm/sec)

For example, the acoustic impedance of water is the velocity of sound in water (154,000 cm/sec) times the density of water (1 g/cm³), or

cm/sec × g/cm³ = g/cm² sec
154,000 × 1 = 154,000 g/cm² sec

This is an inconveniently large number, so it is divided by 100,000 (the same as multiplying by 10^{-5}) to reduce it to a more convenient size. Thus, the unit for acoustic impedance in the cgs system, the Rayl, is defined as g/cm² sec × 10^{-5}. **The velocity of sound in tissue is fairly constant over a wide range of frequencies, so a substance's acoustic impedance is a constant.** Table 25–4 lists the acoustic impedance, in Rayls, of various materials, including several body tissues and some piezoelectric materials used in ultrasound transducers. As sound waves pass from one tissue plane to another, the amount of reflection is determined by the difference in the impedances of the two tissues. The greater the difference, the greater the percentage reflected. Note that the difference between most body structures is fairly small, the two exceptions being air and bone. A soft tissue-air interface reflects almost the entire beam, and a soft tissue-bone interface reflects a major portion of it. The sum of the

Table 25–4. Approximate Acoustic Impedance of Various Materials

MATERIAL	ACOUSTIC IMPEDANCE (Rayls—g/cm² sec × 10⁻⁵)
Air	0.0004
Fat	1.38
Castor oil	1.4
Water (50° C)	1.54
Brain	1.58
Blood	1.61
Kidney	1.62
Liver	1.65
Muscle	1.70
Lens of eye	1.84
Piezoelectric polymers	4.0
Skull (bone)	7.8
Quartz	15.2
Mercury	19.7
PZT-5A	29.3
PZT-4	30.0
Brass	38.0

reflected and transmitted portions is 100%. For example, if 90% of a beam is reflected, 10% will be transmitted. At a tissue-air interface, more than 99.9% of the beam is reflected, so none is available for further imaging. Transducers, therefore, must be directly coupled to the patient's skin without an air gap. Coupling is accomplished by use of a slippery material such as mineral oil for contact scanning or by a water bath when the transducer cannot be placed directly on the patient.

Let us pause a moment and consider the unpleasant subject of the units used to express various quantities. In discussing acoustic impedance we have used the unit of the Rayl, which is a member of the cgs (centimeter-gram-second) system. In Chapter 1 we pointed out that it is now becoming more common to encounter units based on the SI system. In the SI system we must express the velocity of sound (v) in units of meters per second (m/s) and density (ρ) in units of kilograms per cubic meter (kg/m³), so acoustic impedance becomes

$$Z = \rho v = \frac{kg \cdot m}{m^3 s} = \frac{kg}{m^2 s} = kg\ m^{-2}s^{-1}$$

Table 25–5 lists acoustic impedance (Z)

Table 25–5. Acoustic Impedance as Written in the cgs and SI Systems

| MATERIAL | ACOUSTIC IMPEDANCE | |
	cgs System ($g\ cm^{-2}\ s^{-1}$)	SI System ($kg\ m^{-2}\ s^{-1}$)
Air	0.0004×10^{-5}	0.0004×10^{-6}
Water	1.54×10^{-5}	1.54×10^{-6}
Quartz	1.52×10^{-6}	1.52×10^{-7}
PZT-4	3.0×10^{-6}	3.0×10^{-7}

expressed in the cgs and SI systems for several materials. Note that SI units are only one tenth as large as cgs units. It may be useful to think of SI units as dimes, and cgs units as dollars, with ten dimes expressing the same quantity as one dollar.

Angle of Incidence

The amount of reflection is determined by the angle of incidence between the sound beam and the reflecting surface. The higher the angle of incidence (i.e., the closer it is to a right angle), the less the amount of reflected sound. Below a certain critical angle, the entire beam is reflected. The angles of incidence and reflection are equal, just as they are for visible light. In medical ultrasound, in which the same transducer both transmits and receives ultrasound, almost no reflected sound will be detected if the ultrasound strikes the patient's surface at an angle of more than 3° from perpendicular. When a sound beam strikes a smooth interface that is perpendicular to the beam, the amount of reflection is given by

$$R = \left(\frac{Z_2 - Z_1}{Z_2 + Z_1}\right)^2 \times 100$$

R = percentage of beam reflected
Z_1 = acoustic impedance of medium 1
Z_2 = acoustic impedance of medium 2

For example, to determine the percentage of a sonic beam reflected in going from the chest wall to the lung, substitute the acoustic impedance of lung and chest wall (muscle) from Table 25–4:

$$R = \left(\frac{1.70 - 0.0004}{1.70 + 0.0004}\right)^2 \times 100 = 99.9\%$$

As you can see, the number 0.0004 is so small that for practical purposes it can be ignored, and the beam is almost totally reflected, giving an intense echo but leaving no beam for further imaging. At a kidney-fat interface, the amount of reflection is

$$R = \left(\frac{1.62 - 1.38}{1.62 + 1.38}\right)^2 \times 100$$
$$R = \left(\frac{0.24}{3}\right)^2 \times 100 = 0.64\%$$

Approximately 0.64% of the beam is reflected at a kidney-fat interface. The brain is intermediate between the soft tissues and air. At a skull-brain interface, approximately 44% of the beam is reflected. The preceding equation applies only to perpendicular reflections.

It is also possible to calculate the amount of transmission of a sound beam that strikes a smooth interface perpendicular to the beam. The equation is

$$T = \frac{4Z_1 Z_2}{(Z_1 + Z_2)^2} \times 100$$

T = percentage of beam transmitted
Z_1 = acoustic impedance of medium 1
Z_2 = acoustic impedance of medium 2

Remembering that the sum of the reflected and transmitted portions of the sound beam must be 100%, let us calculate the percentage transmission at a kidney-fat interface and see if it balances the 0.64% reflection calculated in the preceding paragraph:

$$T = \frac{4\ (1.62)\ (1.38)}{(1.62 + 1.38)^2} \times 100$$
$$T = 99.36\%$$

Refraction

When sound passes from one medium to another its frequency remains constant but its wavelength changes to accommodate a new velocity in the second medium (Fig. 25–16). In the illustration, the velocity of sound is twice as fast in the first medium as in the second. Each wave is shown as a single horizontal line and reflection is ignored. When the waves reach the surface

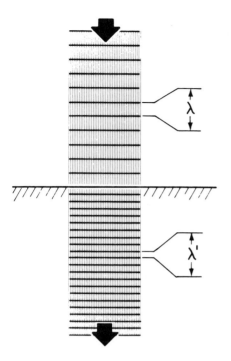

Figure 25–16 The wavelength of sound shortens when its velocity decreases

the arrows can be reversed in the illustrations to demonstrate the change that occurs when velocity increases in the second medium.

The angles of reflection (θ_x) and refraction (θ_t) are shown in Figure 25–18. The angle of refraction is governed by **Snell's law,** which is

$$\frac{\sin \theta_i}{\sin \theta_t} = \frac{V_1}{V_2}$$

θ_i = incidence angle (see Fig. 25–18)
θ_t = transmitted angle
V_1 = velocity of sound for incident medium
V_2 = velocity of sound for transmitting medium

Refraction can cause artifacts. Refraction artifacts cause spatial distortion (real structures are imaged in the wrong location) and loss of resolution in the image.

Absorption

Absorption of ultrasound in fluids is a result of frictional forces that oppose the motion of the particles in the medium. The energy removed from the ultrasound beam is converted into heat. To be precise, the term "absorption" refers to the conversion of ultrasonic to thermal energy, and "attenuation" refers to total propagation loss, including absorption, scattering, and reflection.

The mechanisms involved in absorption are rather complex, and our explanation will be greatly simplified. Three factors determine the amount of absorption: (1) the frequency of the sound, (2) the viscosity of the conducting medium, and (3) the "relaxation time" of the medium. We will discuss frequency last because it is affected by the other two factors.

If we picture sound as being composed of vibrating particles, the importance of viscosity is obvious. Particle freedom decreases and internal friction increases with increasing viscosity. This internal friction absorbs the beam, or decreases its intensity, by converting sound into heat. In liquids, which have low viscosity, very little absorp-

of the second medium they are slowed to half-speed, but they keep coming at the same frequency. Their spacing, or wavelength, must be reduced by half to accommodate the decrease in velocity ($\lambda' = \frac{1}{2}$).

Exactly the same thing happens when the sound beam strikes the second medium at an angle, but the change in wavelength necessitates a change in direction. The reason for the direction change is shown in Figure 25–17. At time 1, a wave front approaching from a 45° angle just barely makes contact with the second medium. As it progresses, straddling the two media, one edge is traveling at a different velocity than the other. The wave front remains continuous, but one edge lags behind the other until the beam finally emerges in the second medium with a different wavelength and a different direction. This bending of waves as they pass from one medium to another is called **refraction.** Exactly the same process occurs in optics. Because the beam could be traveling in either direction,

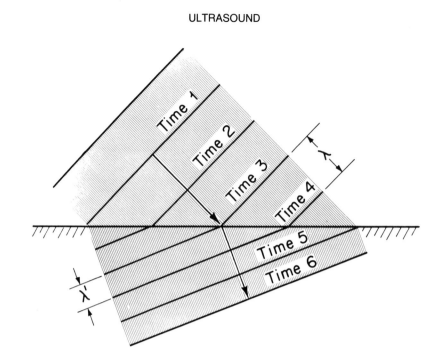

Figure 25–17   Refraction of sound waves

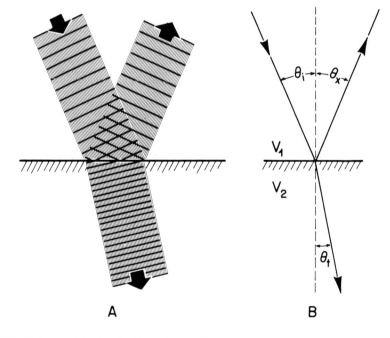

Figure 25–18   Refraction and reflection of sound waves

tion takes place. In soft tissues viscosity is higher and a medium amount of absorption occurs, while bone shows high absorption of ultrasound.

The relaxation time is the time that it takes for a molecule to return to its original position after it has been displaced. It refers to the resilience of a material. Two substances with the same viscosity may have different relaxation times. The relaxation time is a constant for any particular material. When a molecule with a short relaxation time is pushed by a longitudinal compression wave, the molecule has time to return to its resting state before the next compression wave arrives. A molecule with a longer relaxation time may not be able to return completely before a second compression wave arrives. When this happens, the compression wave is moving in one direction and the molecule in the opposite direction. More energy is required to reverse the direction of the molecule than was needed to move it originally. The additional energy is converted to heat.

In soft tissues there is a linear relationship between absorption of ultrasound and frequency. Doubling the frequency approximately doubles absorption and approximately halves the intensity of the transmitted beam. Knowledge of the absorption allows the correct transducer for a particular job to be selected. The common transducer frequencies available are 1, 2.25, 3.5, 5, 7, and 10 MHz. The proper frequency is a compromise between the best resolution (higher frequency) and the ability to propagate the energy into the tissues (lower frequency).

The attenuation of ultrasound also varies with the temperature of the tissues, but the relationship varies with different tissues. For example, at a temperature range of 7° to 35° C and a frequency range of 0.4 to 10 MHz, physiologic hemoglobin solutions show a decreasing attenuation with increasing temperature. By contrast, central nervous system tissues have been shown to exhibit increasing attenuation with increasing temperature.

The frequency of sound effects the amount of absorption produced by the viscosity of a material. The higher the frequency (i.e., the more often a particle moves back and forth in a given time), the more its motion is affected by the drag of a viscous material. Frequency also affects the amount of absorption produced by the relaxation time. At low frequencies, molecules have sufficient time to relax between cycles but, as frequencies increase, the relaxation time consumes a greater and greater proportion of the total cycle. These effects are already appreciable in the lower range of diagnostic frequencies (1 MHz), and they continue to increase at higher frequencies.

Only rather fragmentary data are available to quantitate the absorption of ultrasound. An absorption coefficient is usually employed. This coefficient is identical in concept to the linear attenuation coefficient described for x-rays in Chapter 5. The unit for the absorption coefficient is decibels/cm of thickness at a frequency of 1 MHz. The stipulation of 1 MHz is essential because absorption is frequency-dependent. At 2 MHz, the absorption coefficient is about twice as large. Table 25–6

Table 25–6. Absorption Coefficients for Various Materials at a Frequency of 1 MHz

MATERIAL	ABSORPTION COEFFICIENT (dB/cm)
Lung	41
Skull (bone)	20
Air	12
Muscle (across fiber)	3.3
Lens of eye	2.0
Kidney	1.0
Castor oil	0.95
Liver	0.94
Brain	0.85
Fat	0.63
Blood	0.18
Aluminum	0.018
Water	0.0022
Mercury	0.00048

lists absorption coefficients for various materials. A 1-cm thick slice of kidney, with an absorption coefficient of 1 dB/cm, reduces the sound intensity by 1 dB. Table 25–2 shows that -1 dB represents an absorption of 21% of the beam, and that 79% of the beam remains. A 1-cm thick slice of lung absorbs 41 dB, which reduces intensity by a factor of more than 10,000, leaving less than 0.01% of the beam remaining.

QUARTER-WAVE MATCHING

Now that we have (hopefully) developed a better understanding of absorption, reflection, and acoustic impedance, let us reconsider the ultrasound transducer. When a short electrical shock is applied to the piezoelectric crystal, four ultrasonic pulses are generated, two at each face of the crystal. Two pulses travel back into the transducer; one pulse from the back travels into the backing block, and one pulse from the front travels into the patient's tissues. We have discussed how the acoustic impedance (Z) of the backing block is matched to that of the crystal so that the sound directed away from the patient will be transmitted into, and absorbed by, the backing block. Another important consideration is the transmission of the ultrasound wave into the patient with a minimum loss of energy. The use of mineral oil between the transducer and the patient's skin is an effective means of transmitting energy from the transducer to the patient. Another method of improving energy transfer is that of mechanical impedance matching. If a layer of material (called the matching layer) of suitable thickness and characteristic impedance is placed on the front surface of the transducer, the energy is transmitted into the patient more efficiently (Fig. 25–19). The thickness of the matching layer must be equal to one fourth the wavelength of sound in the matching layer: hence the name quarter-wave matching. In addition, the characteristic impedance of the matching layer must be about the mean of the characteristic impedances on each side of the layer (this is probably not exactly true, but is close enough for our purposes).

$$Z_{matching\ layer} \cong \sqrt{Z_{transducer} \times Z_{soft\ tissue}}$$

For example, a characteristic impedance of about 6.8×10^6 kg m^{-2}s^{-1} is required for the matching layer between PZT-4 (Z = 3.0×10^7 kg m^{-2}s^{-1}) and water (Z = 1.54×10^6 kg m^{-2}s^{-1}). Such a layer could be manufactured using a mixture of aluminum powder and epoxy resin.

Use of quarter-wave matching will also improve the transmission of ultrasound pulses returning from tissues back into the transducer. The equations explaining the theory of quarter-wave matching have been described by Wells, and will not be discussed here.[16]

ULTRASONIC DISPLAY

The ultrasonic image is an electronic representation of data generated from returning echoes and displayed on a TV monitor, cathode ray tube, or storage cathode ray tube. The image is assembled, one bit at a time, much like a television image. Each returning echo generates one bit of data, and many bits together form the electronic image. The evolution of sonic imaging began slowly from a static one-dimensional base (A mode), improved somewhat when a component of motion was added (TM mode), made a giant leap forward with two-dimensional imaging (B mode), and reached its current zenith with gray-scale imaging. These advancements can all be attributed to refinements in electronic instrumentation. Further refinements are being made every year and, undoubtedly, other major improvements will occur before this book is published.

A Mode

In the A mode, echoes are displayed as spikes projecting from a baseline (Fig. 25–20A). The baseline identifies the central axis of the beam. Spike height is proportional to echo intensity, with strong echoes producing large spikes. A series of

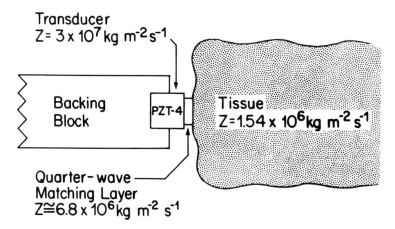

Figure 25–19 Quarter-wave matching

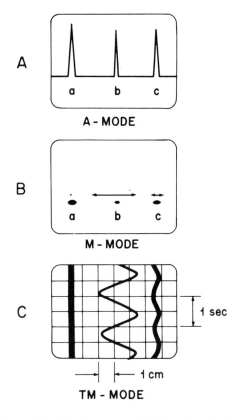

Figure 25–20 A mode and TM mode displays

sonic pulses is used for A-mode imaging but, for simplicity, we will begin with a single pulse. When a voltage pulse strikes a transducer, an echo spike is generated on the monitor to mark the beginning of the sonic pulse. As the pulse passes through the patient, sound is reflected to the transducer from each tissue interface. The depth of the interface recorded on the display is proportional to the time that it takes for the echo to return. Using a sound velocity of 1540 m/sec in average soft tissue, it is a simple mathematical task to convert time into distance. At a velocity of 154,000 cm/sec, sound travels 1 cm in 6.5 microseconds (μsec). An echo must make a round trip, however, so when the echo takes 13 μsec to return, it is displayed at a depth of 1 cm.

If the tissue planes are in a fixed position, and the transducer is held stationary between pulses, as is customary, then the echo spikes from subsequent pulses will fall in the same positions as those from the initial pulse. No memory is built into the display mechanism, so it discards previous pulses as it receives new ones. A permanent record is made by photographing the electronic display. In the A mode, or amplitude mode, the display on the cathode ray tube contains information about the depth of structures and the amplitude of the returning echo. Generally, little use is made of the amplitude of the echo spike. A mode is used in ophthalmology, echoencephalography, echocardiology, and as an adjunct to B-mode displays when accurate depth measurements are required. The A-mode cathode ray tube will display about 40 dB of amplitude information, corresponding to a variation in echo amplitude of about 100:1 (we will explain this shortly).

TM Mode

In the A mode, if the echoes are produced by moving structures, then the echo spikes will also move. If the echoes shown in Figure 25–20A had originated from the anterior chest wall (a), the posterior leaflet of the mitral valve (b), and the posterior heart wall (c), the echoes from the moving structures would move back and forth along the baseline. At any moment they might appear as shown in the illustration. A moment later, however, the mitral valve and heart wall would be in a different position, with the mitral valve moving more than the heart wall. For the TM mode, the spikes are converted into "dots" as shown in Figure 25–20B (M mode). The dots move back and forth, as indicated by the arrows. The M mode is an intermediate mode that cannot be meaningfully recorded. To make a permanent record, the motion must be recorded over a period of time. This is accomplished by moving the line of dots to the top of the scope and then gradually dropping them to the bottom. A record of the sweep is made with a camera using an exposure time longer than the sweep time. Such a record is shown in Figure 25–20C. Because this is a time-motion study, it is referred to as the TM mode. The sweep time in the illustration is 3 sec. If a longer sweep time is used, more beats are recorded and they are compacted from top to bottom, but their back-and-forth excursions remain unchanged. The obvious disadvantage of this method is the short time that can be recorded. A longer record can be made with an electronic strip chart recorder that can also simultaneously display several other parameters, such as the electrocardiogram. A strip chart record can be as long as the operator desires, and this method is increasing in popularity for echocardiography, in which the TM mode is most useful.

B Mode

Sonography came of age as an imaging technique with development of the B mode. The other modes produced valuable information, but they were only useful in limited areas. The B mode greatly expanded the role of ultrasound as a diagnostic tool, especially in abdominal diseases. **The B mode produces a picture of a slice of tissue.** Echoes are displayed as dots, similar to that in the TM mode but, in contrast to the TM mode, the transducer is moved so that the sound beam traverses a plane of the body. The transducer is like the handle of a saber, with the ultrasonic beam as the blade. The blade images a sagittal section when it cuts through the length of the body, and images a transverse or cross section when drawn from side to side. The images are similar to what we would see if the section could be exposed and viewed face-on.

In most B-mode scanning techniques the transducer is placed on the patient's skin, with mineral oil on the skin acting to exclude air and to ensure good acoustic coupling between transducer and skin. This is called contact scanning. The transducer may be left in one spot and rocked back and forth, producing a simple sector scan (Fig. 25–21A). More often, the transducer is moved across the body while it is being

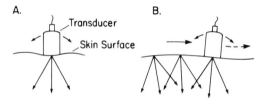

Figure 25–21 Simple sector B scan (A) and compound contact B scan (B)

rotated, producing a compound contact scan (Fig. 25–21*B*). This compound motion is required because anatomic structures in the body present various angles from which the ultrasound waves are reflected. If the angle between the perpendicular from the transducer surface and the interface to be imaged is greater than about 5°, the amount of reflected ultrasound returning to the transducer will be too little to produce an image. Thus, the compound scanning motion is required to present the surface of the transducer to the wide variety of interface angles requiring imaging. Assembling the echoes generated by compound scanning into a meaningful scan picture requires precise synchronization between the transducer motions and the cathode ray tube display.

In assembling the image, the localization of one echo relative to another is accomplished with a small computer that is fed information by an arm containing three joints (Fig. 25–22). The computer calculates the alignment of the baseline by the number of degrees in the three joints. Echo depth is determined by the time delay, as in the A mode. When the transducer moves from one position to another, from A to B in the illustration, the computer recalculates the angles and time delays to position returning signals in the display properly. Even though the echoes arise from two completely different transducer positions

(A and B), the computer correctly interprets them as originating from one point (P). Many thousands of these calculations and echoes produce an image that appears on the scope as a cut section. Various manufacturers employ different methods for measuring the three angles. The angles of the joints of the arm may be measured by potentiometers or by optical digital encoders that generate signals that change with transducer position and orientation.

To review, the scanning arm serves two functions: (1) it determines the spatial orientation of the sound beam; and (2) it constrains the motion of the transducer so that all components of a single image slice through the same plane in the patient.

The method used to display the image obtained by B-mode scanning must be different from the ordinary cathode ray tube used to display A-mode images. Two requirements must be met. First, the image must persist on the viewing screen long enough to allow it to be studied (the image on a routine cathode ray tube is only visible for a fraction of a second). Second, persistence of the image is required to allow a picture to be "built up" as a result of the compound scanning motion of the transducer. These requirements were initially met by displaying the B-mode scan on a modification of the cathode ray tube called a storage (or variable persistence) cathode ray tube. These tubes allowed the operator to view the B-mode scan as it was produced (an image could be viewed continuously for about 10 minutes). The design and function of a variable persistence cathode ray tube are not considered pertinent, so we will spare you (and ourselves) the agony of exploring the technical details. Also, this type of display is not used on current B-mode scanners. The overwhelming disadvantage of these direct viewing storage tubes is their limited ability to display shades of gray. In fact, some of them show no shades of gray, with the image being composed of only light or dark areas on the screen. This is termed a bistable image.

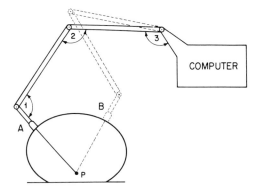

Figure 25–22 Computer localization of transducer alignment

Gray-Scale Imaging

B-mode scanning took a major step forward with the advent of gray-scale imaging in 1972. The purpose of gray-scale imaging is to display the great variation of the amplitudes of the echoes arising from tissues as varying shades of gray on a television monitor. This contrasts with the bistable or limited gray-scale image possible with direct viewing storage cathode ray tubes. Gray-scale imaging was made possible by the development of the scan conversion memory tube (usually called a scan converter). Unlike storage cathode ray tubes, the scan converter tube does not produce a visible image. Instead, the scan converter stores the information received from a transducer and then uses the stored information to generate a signal that is used to produce a visible image on a television monitor. A scan converter tube is similar to a cathode ray tube in that an electron beam is caused to scan a target capable of storing the information it receives. The electron beam is used alternately to "write" the information on the target, "read" the information to generate the signal sent to a television monitor, and "erase" the target in preparation for receiving a new set of information. The target of the scan converter tube is a complex affair made up of a silicon backplate about 25 mm in diameter on which more than a million tiny (about 10 μm) squares of silicon "wafers" are placed. It is reasonable to assume that, as a transducer is used to scan a patient in a compound contact scanning maneuver, several returning echoes from the same point will be received by the transducer. When the target of the scan converter receives multiple signals to the same area, it records only the strongest signal and discards all others. In this way the final "picture" is composed only of the strongest echo detected from each point of the scan, rather than of a random addition of numerous signals (called overwriting). This is why the operator is able to build up a more diagnostic picture by repeated movements of the transducer through the plane of each image. Once the image has been stored on the target of a scan converter tube, the electron beam can be made to scan the target and generate a signal suitable for display on an ordinary television monitor.

Two types of scan conversion memory tubes are in use. The analog scan converter was developed in 1972. More recently, the digital scan converter has replaced the analog unit. The terms "analog" and "digital" are rather vague to most physicians. Because of the explosion of "digital" components being introduced to diagnostic imaging procedures, we are making this topic the subject of an entire chapter (see Chapter 27). Briefly stated, a digital scan converter converts variations in amplitude of the echo signal received by the transducer into binary numbers. The information is sorted into 16 (4-bit) or 32 (5-bit) or more levels of gray that can be displayed on a television monitor.

The analog scan converters present some difficulty in clinical use because the gray-scale levels assigned to the echo amplitude tend to drift, causing deterioration of images and making comparison of scans obtained at different dates difficult. There is also an objectionable flicker of the image viewed on the television monitor. This flicker is related to the fact that a scan converter tube must simultaneously store (write) the image and transmit (read) the image to the television monitor. The tube must switch between writing and reading modes during the time an image is being received. An analog converter tube is able to do this switching at a rate of about ten times per television frame, producing visible on-off flicker. Once stored by an analog converter, an image can be viewed for about 10 min before image deterioration begins.

Digital scan converter tubes are free of gray-scale drift. They have a much faster writing speed than the analog unit, thereby eliminating the flicker on the television monitor. Once stored, the image on a digital storage tube can be viewed indefinitely. Digital scan converters are suitable for advanced computer processing and are adaptable to real-time imaging developments. Thus, the digital scan conversion memory tube promises to replace the analog systems.

Being able to read the information stored by a scan converter tube on a regular TV monitor offers several advantages. Such monitors are inexpensive, and accessories such as character generators (i.e., letters) can be easily employed to identify scans. The controls of the TV monitor can be used to adjust contrast and brightness. Other television accessories such as color, video tape, and video disc options can be adapted. A "zoom" display can also be employed by using only a portion of the stored image to generate the TV image. It is also possible to store several complete images on different parts of the scan converter target.

Let use briefly review the advantages of a digital scan conversion memory tube over direct view cathode ray storage tubes:

1. Reading the image on a routine TV monitor allows use of numerous accessories and additional image control.
2. Computer data processing options are available.
3. Gray-scale display is available.
4. Zoom display is available.
5. More than one image can be stored.
6. Resolution is better.
7. Prolonged viewing does not degrade the image.
8. There is negligible overwriting (only the strongest signal from each point in the scan is recorded).

Controls

The number and intensity of echoes from any particular area are extremely variable, and setting the scanner to demonstrate one area optimally frequently detracts from image quality in another area. Multiple controls are built into ultrasonic units, and all are designed to regulate the intensity of echoes from various depths. Usually several controls are manipulated simultaneously, so there is no logical sequence for discussion. The following controls may be available, although they may not all be provided by a single manufacturer:

1. Time gain compensator
2. Delay
3. Intensity
4. Coarse gain
5. Reject
6. Near gain
7. Far gain
8. Enhancement.

The echoes from deep structures are much weaker than those from closer structures. The two may differ by a factor of one million. If an echo from an object close to the surface produces a 10-cm spike, as displayed in the A mode, the echoes from deeper structures may be a mere 0.001 mm, less than the thickness of a hair. Obviously, something must be done to remedy this, and most controls are designed for just that purpose. The **time gain compensator (TGC)** is the most important control. Its function is shown in Figure 25–23. The echoes from deep structures are severely attenuated and produce small spikes (Fig. 25–23B). The TGC is depicted in Figure 25–23C as a sloping line, and the height of the slope is added to that of the pulses. The result, shown in Figure 25–23D, is a series of pulses of similar amplitude. The slope of the TGC adjusts the degree of amplification. The slope is shown as a straight line but it is actually exponential, because the deeper echoes require more of a boost than it would appear from the illustration. They may actually be amplified more than a thousand times. The delay control regulates the depth at which the TGC begins to augment weaker signals.

Three controls govern amplitude across the entire display without discrimination for or against a particular depth. The first is the **intensity control,** which determines the potential difference across the trans-

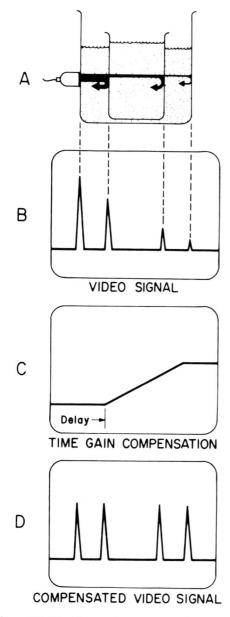

Figure 25–23   Time gain compensation

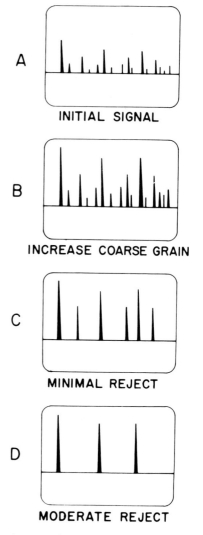

Figure 25–24   Coarse gain and reject controls

ducer (i.e., the strength of the voltage pulse). Increasing intensity produces a more energetic ultrasonic beam and thus stronger echoes at all levels. The second amplitude control is the **coarse gain,** which regulates the height of echoes from all depths. Increasing the coarse gain control enhances all echoes proportionately (Fig. 25–24). The initial echoes (Fig. 25–24*A*)

are all enhanced to nearly twice their amplitude by increasing coarse gain (Fig. 25–24*B*). The third amplitude regulator is the **reject control,** and it is slightly different from the other two. Although it does not discriminate against echoes from a particular depth, it does discriminate against those below a minimum amplitude (Fig. 25–24*C* and *D*). Reject cleans up the image by removing small useless signals. Selective rejection of weaker signals enhances the clarity of the stronger ones.

A **delay control** regulates the depth at which the TGC begins to augment the weaker signals (Fig. 25–25). Obviously the strong superficial echoes do not require amplification by the TGC; in fact, they may have to be dampened. This is accomplished with the **near gain control,** which is poorly named because it is used primarily to diminish and not to enhance near echoes. The distance over which near gain operates is controlled by the delay.

Two additional methods may be used to supplement distant echoes (i.e., those originating deep in the tissues): the **far gain** and the **enhancement controls.** Far gain is similar to near gain only at the opposite end of the TGC curve and is used to enhance all distant echoes. The enhancement controls augment a localized portion of the TGC curve (Fig. 25–25). It gates a specific depth and enhances echoes within the gate to any desired level. For example, the gate can be set to "frame" the near and far extremes of mitral valve motion; echoes from this specific region will then be amplified to delineate the valve more clearly.

The interplay between all these controls is extremely complex, and it is impossible to learn their effect on imaging from a book.

Pulse Rate

Pulse rate and frequency are different and unrelated. Frequency refers to a characteristic of the sound; that is, the number of times that conduction particles vibrate back and forth per second, usually between 1 and 20 MHz in medical sonography. **Pulse rate refers to the number of separate little packets of sound that are sent out each second** (Fig. 25–26). Each sonic pulse is short (only a few wavelengths), and its duration varies with the Q factor of the transducer. Between pulses, the transducer serves as a receiver. A commonly used rate is 1000 pulses/sec. At this rate, the total time available for each pulse is 0.001 sec. Approximately 0.001 of this time is devoted to transmission, so the transducer is a receiver almost 1000 times longer than it is a transmitter.

The pulse rate determines the total number of echoes returning to the transducer in a unit of time. Doubling the rate from 1000 to 2000 pulses/sec will double the number of echoes returning to the transducer each second.

Obviously, a high pulse rate is desirable, but too high a rate creates another problem. The transducer cannot send and receive at the same time. As the pulse rate increases, the receiving time decreases. If the receiving time is too short, echoes from distant parts may still be out, or on their way in, when the next pulse starts. The time between pulses, or the pulse rate, must be set to accommodate the thickest part that might be examined. This thickness is half the distance between pulses. Remember, the sound is making a round trip, so the maximum thickness that can be examined is only half of the distance that the sound can travel. Table 25–7 shows the maximum part thickness that can be imaged at various pulse rates. At the commonly used rate of 1000 pulses/sec, a 75-cm thick part can be examined. At a rate of 10,000, the thickest part is 7.5 cm, which is satisfactory for ophthalmology but not for abdominal imaging.

IMAGING PRINCIPLES

The sonographic image is influenced by the size and shape of both the object and

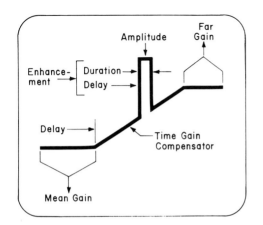

Figure 25–25 Various controls for the sonic display

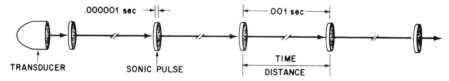

Figure 25–26 Multiple sonic pulses

Table 25–7. Maximum Part Thicknesses that can be Imaged at Various Pulse Rates

PULSE RATE (per second)	MAXIMUM PART THICKNESS (cm)*
1,000	75
3,000	25
6,000	12.5
10,000	7.5

*Based on a velocity of sound of 150,000 cm/sec; the sound must travel twice as far as the thickness to complete a round trip.

the transducer. The same principle applies to x-ray imaging. The effect of the x-ray focal spot size is made readily apparent if a pinhole is placed halfway between the target and film, with the resultant image being a picture of the focal spot, not the pinhole. At shorter object-film distances, or with larger objects, the effect is much less dramatic, and we call it penumbra or edge gradient, but the effect is there just the same. Transducers are much larger than focal spots, so transducer images are more evident. Figure 25–27 shows a B-mode scan of five equally spaced wire rods imaged with a focused transducer. (Focused transducers will be described later in this section.) The wires are small in diameter relative to the sound beam. As the beam moves from left to right, echoes begin when the leading edge of the beam reaches a wire and continue until the beam has passed beyond all the wires. The resulting images are pictures of the sound beam, not of the wire. Because beam width varies with depth, image width also varies with depth, being closest to the shape of the wire when the beam is narrowest. The wire is the sonographer's pinhole.

Resolution

When we talk about resolution with the A mode, we are only concerned with the ability of the beam to separate two objects at different depths. In the B mode, however, we must also be concerned with horizontal, or lateral, resolution: that is, the ability to separate two adjacent objects. We will refer to these as depth and lateral resolution. Neither is accurately defined, at least not by x-ray imaging standards, so our discussion will be in terms of general principles, and not of line pairs per mm.

Depth (Axial) Resolution

Depth resolution is the ability of the beam to separate two objects lying in tandem along the axis of the beam. Figure 25–28 shows a time sequence of an ultrasonic pulse resolving two surfaces, a and b, separated by x distance. At times 2 and 3, portions of the beam are reflected from surfaces a and b respectively. The reflected pulses are completely separated, and each produces its own signal. The separation of their leading edges is 2x, or twice the original separation, because the second echo had to travel back and forth across the distance x. The length of the sonic pulse, called the spatial pulse length, equals the wavelength of the sound multiplied by the number of wavelengths in the pulse. The number of wavelengths will depend on the Q factor of the transducer. For example, at a frequency of 1.5 MHz, the wavelength of the sound in water is 1 mm (λ = 1,500,000 cycles/sec ÷ 1,500,000 mm/ sec). If each sonic pulse consists of three wavelengths, the spatial pulse length will be 3 mm. Two objects will be resolved (recognized as being separate) if the spatial

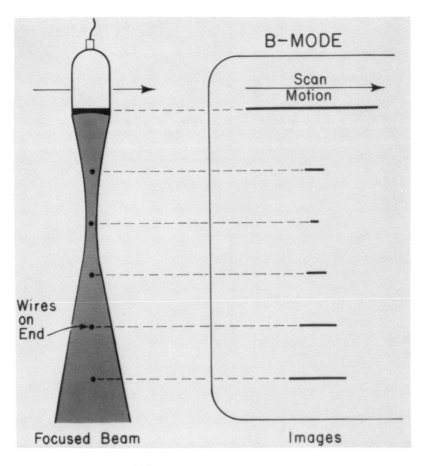

B—MODE

Scan
Motion

Wires
on
End

Focused Beam

Images

Figure 25–27 "Imaging" the sonic beam

pulse length is less than twice the separation. Figure 25–29 shows two objects separated by exactly half a spatial pulse length. At time 2 the pulse splits, but the first reflected pulse does not clear surface a before the second reflected pulse returns from surface b. The transducer only sees one pulse, so the two surfaces are not resolved.

Reverberation Echoes. When we discussed tomography we described phantom images as images that appear to the eye but have no physical existence. A similar image, called a **reverberation image,** occurs in sonography. Figure 25–30 shows how these spurious images are produced. The critical event occurs at time 4 when the returning echoes from b reflect off the back surface of a and initiate a third echo (time 5), which the transducer interprets as another object. Thus three surfaces are dis-

played, with the third being a reverberation image. Time 6 shows the beginning of a fourth image and, with a geometric configuration such as the one shown in the illustration, the number of reverberation images is limited only by the penetrating power of the beam and the sensitivity of the detector.

The transducer itself may act as a reflecting surface and produce a reverberation artifact, especially in ophthalmologic sonography. The artifact is recognized by manually changing the distance between the transducer and the globe of the eye. The factitious image moves in synchrony with the transducer.

Lateral (Horizontal) Resolution

Lateral resolution is the ability to separate two adjacent objects. Figure 25–31

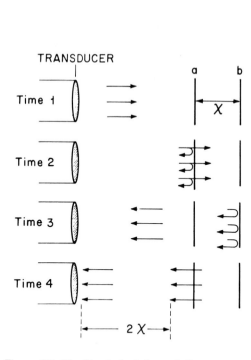

Figure 25–28   Depth (axial) resolution

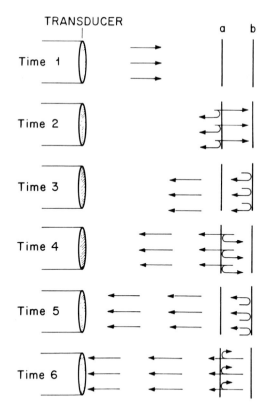

Figure 25–30   Reverberation images

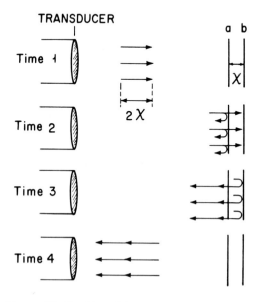

Figure 25–29 Unsatisfactory or unsuccessful depth resolution

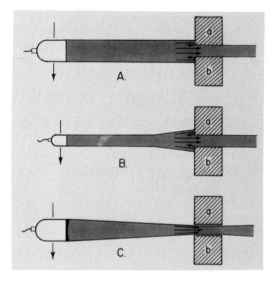

Figure 25–31 Lateral (horizontal) resolution

shows two objects separated by a narrow space. To recognize the objects as discrete entities, the beam must be narrower than the space separating the objects. In Figure 25–31A the beam is too wide, so that even when it straddles the space, echoes return from both objects, the display interprets an edge, and the space goes unrecognized. An obvious way to narrow the beam and to improve resolution is to use a smaller transducer. This works well in some clinical situations, for example in ophthalmology in which small diameter high-frequency transducers are used to produce superb resolution. The advantages of small transducers, however, are lost in the much thicker abdomen. The Fresnel zone is too short, even at high frequencies, to reach deep structures. Figure 25–31B illustrates the problem. The beam is well into the Fraunhofer zone at the object plane, and may actually be wider than the beam from a larger transducer.

Focused Transducers. The solution to the above imaging problem is use of a focused transducer, such as the one shown in Figure 25–31C. Focused transducers restrict beam width and improve lateral resolution but they are designed to focus at a specific depth or depth range, so they must be selected for optimal display of the depth of interest. In Figure 25–31C the beam is focused at the proper depth so that it can pass through the space between objects a and b, thus permitting them to appear as separate entities.

Sonic beams can be focused with either a curved piezoelectric crystal or with an acoustic lens. The lens material, usually polystyrene or an epoxy resin, propagates sound at a greater velocity than body tissues, so the sound is refracted, or bent, toward a point in space. Knowing the radius of curvature of the lens and the velocities of sound in the lens material and body tissues, the exact focal point can be calculated. **A close approximation of the focal length is the diameter of curvature of the lens** (Fig. 25–32). Focusing moves the transition point between the near and

far zones from its anticipated position at x' back toward the transducer to a new position at x'_f. The beam is maximally restricted and of greatest intensity at the focal point, but the point is not sharply defined. Like an optical lens, an acoustic lens has a focal zone, a distance over which the focal properties are fairly well maintained. The focal zone is shortest with a large diameter, short focal length lens. Focused transducers are classified as short, medium, or long, depending on the depth at which they focus, as follows:

Short	4–6 cm
Medium	6–8 cm
Long	8–11 cm

Tomographic Thickness. The expression "tomographic thickness" is only meaningful with B-mode scanning. It refers to the thickness of the slice in sharp focus or to the thickness that the sonic beam "sees." It is closely related to lateral resolution. We described a B-mode scanner as a saber cutting a gash through the body. Two sabers would be more accurate: two sabers side by side separated by the width of the beam and cutting out a slice of tissue. The thinner the slice, the more accurately the images will depict a plane. The final image is a composite of all objects in the slice. The thickness and shape of the tomographic slice are the same as those of the sonic beam. A cylindrical beam (unfocused) produces a pancakelike slice with parallel sides in the Fresnel zone and a flared-out bottom in the Fraunhofer zone. Slices from focused transducers flare out at both the top and bottom, and are narrowest in the center. The top flare is limited by the width of the transducer but the bottom flare increases with increasing depth.

Imaging Curved Surfaces

Curved surfaces are difficult to image with an echo system, and unfortunately most body surfaces are curved. In Figure 25–33 an attempt has been made to image the top of a sphere with a linear scan motion. As the probe moves across the sphere, beam alignment is optimum only at position 2. The reflected echoes from positions 1 and 3 never reach the transducer, so only

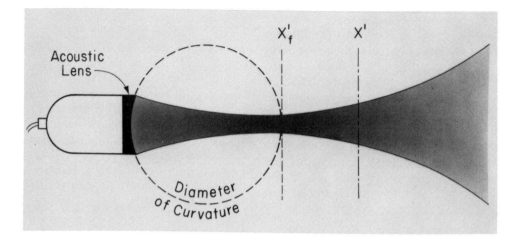

Figure 25–32 Focused transducer

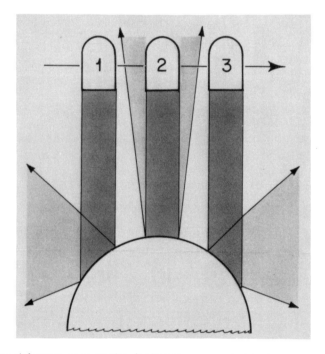

Figure 25–33 Unsatisfactory scan motion for imaging curved objects

the central portion of the sphere is imaged and the sides are left open.

The perfect imaging motion for a sphere, or any curved surface, is an arc whose center of curvature is located at the same point as that of the surface being imaged. Such an arrangement is shown in Figure 25–34. The transducer always remains perpendicular to the tangent of the sphere as it rotates through a 180° arc. The returning echoes all travel the same distance so they are equally attenuated, and the image is a perfect duplication of the object. Obviously, this ideal mode is impossible in clinical work, because there are no true spherical structures in the body, and even

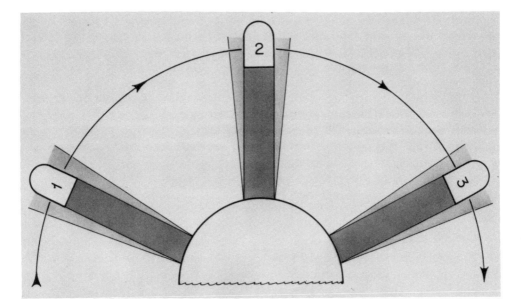

Figure 25–34 Optimum scan motion for imaging curved objects

if there were, we would not be able to locate their centers. A fair approximation of this system may be achieved, however, with cross-sectional scanning by sweeping the transducer around 180° of the body surface. Cross-sectional images, especially those obtained since the advent of the gray scale, are of excellent quality.

Figure 25–35 shows a third method for imaging curved surfaces, one using a compound scanning motion. The transducer moves slowly from left to right and at the same time oscillates back and forth through a 90° arc. During at least part of the scan the beam strikes a large portion of the curved surface at right angles. This method cannot be used for contact scanning, but it works well with the part immersed in a water bath.

Permanent Records of Sonic Images

After the desired image is displayed on the TV monitor or cathode ray tube, a permanent record is made for later review. The simplest method is probably a Polaroid picture of the display tube. Two other

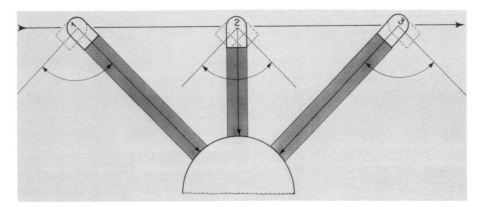

Figure 25–35 Alternative method for imaging curved objects

methods are gaining in popularity: transparencies, similar to x-ray film, and video tape or video disc recorders. The transparencies may be made with either roll film using a 70-mm or larger format camera, or with multiple exposures on a large cut film. Film for this use should be high-contrast, high-speed, orthochromatic, single-emulsion, 90-sec processable, on a clear or blue base. Such film is commercially available. Recently, video disc recorders have become more economical and are being used for ultrasonic display.

DOPPLER TECHNIQUES

The Doppler effect is a change in the perceived frequency of sound emitted by a moving source. The effect was first described by Christian Doppler in 1843. The cause of the frequency change is shown in Figure 25–36. In Figure 25–36A a vibrating source (p) produces a series of concentric waves, all moving out from the center, with the oldest in the most peripheral location (time 1) and the newest at the center (time 6). The velocity of sound in the particular medium and the frequency of the oscillator determine the wavelength (λ), or distance between crests. In Figure 25–36B the sound source is moving to the right as it vibrates. It sends out a wave crest and

then runs after the crest in one direction and away in the opposite direction. The sound usually moves faster than the source, so the source never catches the crest. Source motion does change the gap between crests, increasing the frequency and decreasing the wavelength to the right and decreasing the frequency and increasing the wavelength to the left. Sound velocity is not affected by source motion, so the sound moves at the same velocity in all directions. The wavelength change is caused by the source motion changing the spacing between crests.

The magnitude of the Doppler shift is shown in Figure 25–37. An ambulance moving 27 m/sec (60 miles/hr) is blowing its siren at a frequency of 1000 Hz. The frequency ahead of the siren is 1086 Hz, while the frequency behind it is 926 Hz. A pedestrian would hear a frequency shift of 160 Hz as the ambulance passed. The only persons hearing the true frequency of 1000 Hz would be the passengers in the vehicle.

In contrast to the other ultrasonic modes that we have discussed, all of which are visual, most current medical applications of the Doppler effect employ an audio mode. Doppler techniques are used to study motion, primarily that of the circulatory system. Two transducers are used in the audio

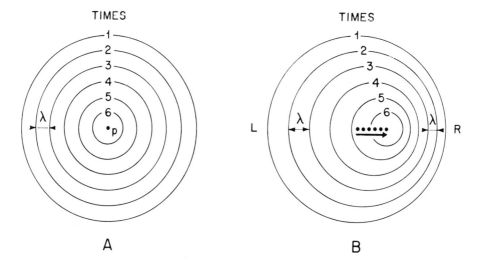

Figure 25–36 The Doppler shift

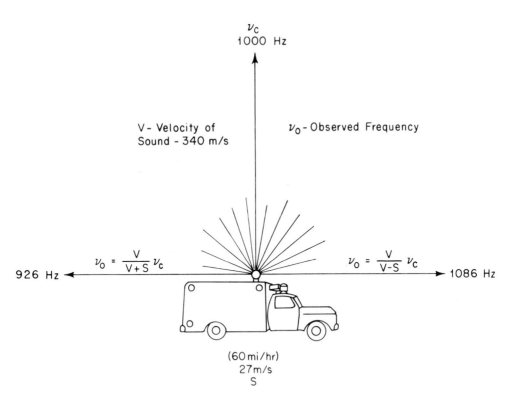

Figure 25–37 Magnitude of the Doppler shift

mode, one as a transmitter and the other as a receiver. Both operate continuously. Pulsed Doppler devices that allow discrimination of Doppler signals from different tissue depths are much different from continuous wave Doppler, and will be described separately.

Continuous Wave Doppler

The continuous wave Doppler mode employs two piezoelectric elements, both contained in a single head (Fig. 25–38). One crystal transmits a continuous sonic signal at a known frequency, usually between 3 and 8 MHz. The other crystal receives the returning echoes and records their frequency. The frequency of the initial signal is algebraically subtracted from that of the returning echoes. The difference, the **Doppler shift,** usually falls within the frequency range detectable by the human ear and, after amplification, this Doppler shift is the audio signal. Returning echoes orig-

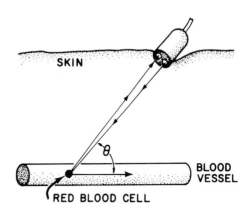

Figure 25–38 Audio mode Doppler transducer

inate from the cellular elements of the blood, particularly the red blood cell. The Doppler beam is used to detect the motion of the blood within the vessel rather than the motion of the vessel wall.

In contrast to pulsed sonography, in which the intensity of returning echoes is greatest when the beam is perpendicular to a reflecting surface, the Doppler shift is greatest when the beam strikes a vessel at a sharp angle. Figure 25–38 shows a vector of red blood cell motion toward the transducer even though the transducer is not in the direct path of flow. The smaller the angle between the sonic beam and the flow direction (θ), the greater the vector of motion toward the transducer, and the greater the Doppler shift. Theoretically, motion cannot be detected when the transducer is perpendicular to the direction of blood flow, but this theoretic situation does not actually occur because of divergence of the beam (i.e., some part of the beam is always off of the perpendicular). The frequency change of back-scattered echoes can be calculated with the Doppler shift equation:

$$\Delta v = \frac{2\ vs}{v} \cos \theta$$

Δv = frequency change (Doppler shift-Hz)
v = frequency of initial beam (Hz)
s = velocity of blood (m/s)
v = velocity of sound (1540 m/s)
θ = angle between sound beam and
    direction of blood flow (Fig. 25–38)

The vector of blood cell motion toward the transducer is represented by cos θ in the equation. If the angle is increased, there is a smaller vector of motion toward the transducer and consequently cos θ is smaller. If the number of degrees in the angle is decreased, the cos θ is larger, and it approaches 1 as the transducer looks directly into the blood stream.

At frequencies between 2 and 10 MHz, the Doppler shift falls in the audible range for most physiologic motions. An experienced listener can learn a great deal about the status of the circulatory system with a Doppler device. It can be used to detect blood flow or its absence in both arteries and veins, to identify vascular constrictions with their associated eddy currents and venturi jets, and to detect fetal heart motion earlier than any other method.

Let us calculate the Doppler shift that might be encountered in a typical exami-

nation of arterial blood flow. Assume blood flow to be at an average velocity of 20 cm/sec (s = 0.2 m/s), the operating frequency of the transducer to be 5 MHz (v = 5,000,000 Hz), and the angle θ that the sound beam makes with respect to the vessel lumen to be 60° (cos 60° = 0.5):

$$\Delta v = \frac{2(5,000,000)\ (0.2)}{1540}\ (0.5)$$
$$\Delta v \cong 650\ Hz$$

Thus, for relatively slow-moving structures, the Doppler shift signal falls within the audible range. Note that the Doppler shift equation tells us that the change in frequency of the ultrasound signal received by the transducer will be 650 Hz, but does not designate whether the change will be positive or negative (i.e., we may receive 5,000,650 Hz or 4,999,350 Hz). If the flow of blood is toward the transducer, the higher frequency is received; if blood flow is away from the transducer, the Doppler shift will be negative. Thus, the sign of the frequency change carries information about the direction of blood flow. Some Doppler systems are able to use this information to measure flow direction. Most simple Doppler systems only indicate that flow is present and do not indicate direction.

A review of the Doppler shift equation reveals that the magnitude of the shift (Δv) will vary with the velocity of blood flow and the frequency of the transmitted ultrasound beam. For ultrasound frequencies in the range of 2 to 10 MHz, Δv will range from 0 to about 10 KHz for velocities ranging from 0 to 100 cm/sec.

Transducers for Continuous Wave Doppler

The typical transducer used in continuous wave Doppler instruments contains two separate piezoelectric elements, one for transmitting and the other for receiving ultrasonic waves. The transmitted sound beam and the receiving pattern of the receiver are very directional. To obtain maximum sensitivity for detecting returning echo signals, the beam regions of the transmitter and receiver are caused to overlap. This overlap is achieved by inclining the transducer elements (Fig. 25–39) or by using focused elements. The region of beam overlap defines the most sensitive region of the transducer.

Several technical considerations apply to the design of a transducer for continuous Doppler operation. Because one is concerned with the Doppler frequency shift, it is important to produce a transmitted signal that has a minimum of frequencies outside the resonant frequency of the transmitting transducer. This is done by using a high-Q transducer material, which means that the transducer will produce a narrow range of sound frequencies. With continuous Doppler operation as much of the generated power must be transmitted into the patient as possible. There are two requirements for this: all the energy transmitted to the back face of the transducer must be reflected back to the front face; and all the power from the front face of the transducer must be transmitted to the patient. Reflection of energy from the back face of the transducer is accomplished by mismatching the acoustic impedance of the transducer material and the material behind it. This is usually done by backing the transducer with air, which has an impedance much lower than that of the piezoelectric transducer (usually PZT). Acoustic

transmission from the transducer face into the patient is now often accomplished with quarter-wave matching (previously discussed).

Doppler units designed to detect movement of the fetal heart must have as broad a beam as possible, so that small changes in the position of the fetus do not cause loss of the signal. Transducers for this purpose have several wide-angle transmitters surrounded by an array of similar receivers.

Choice of Operating Frequency

Remember that the transmitted Doppler frequency actually has a frequency spectrum rather than a single frequency spike, but we will continue to assume a single transmitted frequency signal to simplify our analysis.

The choice of the transmitted Doppler frequency is generally controlled by the need to obtain an adequate signal strength at the receiving transducer. As a general rule, the reduction in signal strength of a sound beam traveling through soft tissue is about 1 dB per cm per MHz. Thus, a 4-MHz wave traveling through 5 cm will have a loss of about 20 dB. Now, what does 20 dB mean? The answer is complicated, and we must be satisfied with only a partial answer. The definition of decibel given earlier

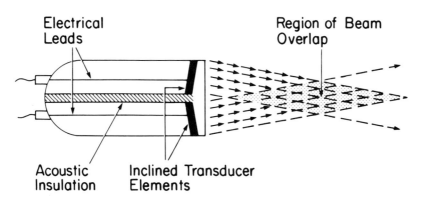

Figure 25–39 A typical Doppler ultrasound transducer with inclined transducer elements

in this chapter described a ratio between sound intensities:

$$\text{Intensity ratio in dB} = 10 \log_{10} \frac{\text{intensity}_1}{\text{intensity}_2}$$

A difference in the intensity ratio of 20 dB corresponds to a 100-fold difference in relative intensity between two sound beams:

$$20 \text{ dB} = 10 \log_{10} \frac{100}{1} = 10 \, (2) = 20$$

Here is the complication. The decibel system is also frequently used to express the relative amplitude of sound reflections. You may think of amplitude as the amount of displacement the sound beam causes on a certain area (such as the face of a piezoelectric crystal). Intensity and amplitude are related as

$$I = A^2$$
$$I = \text{intensity}$$
$$A = \text{amplitude}$$

Therefore, the equation expressing amplitude ratio in the decibel system becomes

$$\text{Amplitude ratio in dB} = 20 \log_{10} \frac{\text{Amplitude}_1}{\text{Amplitude}_2}$$

When discussing attenuation of a sound beam in soft tissue, we are using the amplitude ratio. Therefore, a 20-dB loss in amplitude ratio represents a loss by a factor of 10:

$$20 \text{ dB} = 20 \log_{10} \frac{10}{1} = 20 \, (1) = 20$$

Similarly, a 40-dB loss in amplitude corresponds to a factor of 100, and a 60-dB loss represents a factor of 1000. When discussing attenuation of sound traveling through body tissues, we are using the decibel system to relate a change in relative amplitude. The answer to the original question of what a 20-dB loss in relative amplitude means is this: loss in relative amplitude by a factor of 10:1.

Because higher frequency sound is more rapidly attenuated by soft tissue, why not use lower frequencies for Doppler examinations? Use of a higher frequency offers several advantages. When blood vessels are examined, the source of echo signals is the red blood cells flowing in the vessel. These very small objects cause scattering of the sound beam in all directions (as opposed to reflection, which occurs at large smooth interfaces). The intensity of this scattering increases with frequency, being proportional to the frequency raised to the fourth power. Thus, a higher frequency transducer will produce a stronger scattered signal. Higher frequency beams produce two other desirable effects: higher frequency sound beams can be more sharply defined, and higher frequency input also causes a larger Doppler shift, which increases the sensitivity of the unit.

For small superficial vessels Doppler probes operating at 8 to 10 MHz are commonly used. Applications in the carotid artery use a lower frequency to avoid excesssive attenuation by soft tissues, with 4 to 5 MHz being typical choices. For evaluation of even deeper arteries and veins, and in fetal monitoring, frequencies of about 2 MHz are common.

To review, choice of operating frequency of a continuous wave Doppler unit is a compromise between (1) high frequency, which gives a stronger returning signal, a larger Doppler shift, and a better defined beam, and (2) low frequency, which decreases amplitude attenuation of the beam in the body soft tissues.

Pulsed Doppler

With continuous wave Doppler instruments, reflectors and scatterers anywhere within the beam of the transducer contribute to the Doppler signal. Continuous wave Doppler lacks any form of depth resolution, and is thus not useful in the heart, in which everything is in constant motion. **Pulsed Doppler has provided the means of detecting the depth at which a returning signal has originated.** The depth can be positioned at any point along the axis of the pulsed Doppler ultrasound beam.

Pulsed Doppler is similar to a conventional pulse echo instrument in that bursts of ultrasound are emitted repetitively at a precisely controlled rate into the tissues. A new pulse is not transmitted until the echoes from the previous pulse have been detected. The depth at which a returning signal originated can be determined by knowing the time of transmission of the signal and the time of its return (i.e., the "time of flight" to an interface and the subsequent return). Short bursts of ultrasound, about 0.5 to 1.0 μsec, can yield good axial resolution with separation of interfaces to within about 1 mm.

To summarize, continuous wave Doppler instruments provide velocity information and pulsed Doppler instruments provide both velocity and position information simultaneously.

To determine the Doppler shift of an echo at a specific depth requires that the ultrasonic transducer produce very short duration (such as 1 μsec) bursts at a precise rate of repetition. After transmission of this short burst of ultrasound, the receiving transducer may be turned on (termed "gating on") for a short period at a specific time. Therefore, only signals arriving from a specific tissue depth are available for detection. The "gate" position may be adjusted by the operator to select Doppler signals from any volume along the axis of the transducer.

The basic facts of pulsed Doppler have now been presented. A very short burst of ultrasound traveling through soft tissues generates a Doppler shift signal from all moving structures along the beam's path. By gating on the receiving transducer for a short period at a specified time following transmission of the burst, only Doppler signals originating from a specified depth are recorded. As you have come to expect, certain technical considerations turn the simple into the complex.

Let us first calculate how much time "time of flight" is talking about. Remember the speed of sound in soft tissues is 154,000 cm per second. A simple calculation (e.g.,

$1 \div 154,000$) reveals that sound travels 1 cm in soft tissue in about 0.0000065 seconds, usually expressed as 6.5 μsec. So, a round trip of 1 cm requires 13 μsec. This sets a time limit on the repetition rate of the pulses: the required time between successive pulses is at least 13 μsec per cm of range in the sample volume. For example, a time of 80 μsec between ultrasound bursts would allow detection of flow from vessels as deep as 6 cm, because 6 cm × 13 μsec/cm = 78 μsec. A new pulse cannot be transmitted until the desired echoes from the previous pulse have been recorded.

To determine the Doppler shift originating at a particular depth requires that the transmitted bursts of sound be repeated at a precise rate. As an example, let us consider how a 1-μsec burst might be generated every 80 μsec. The "clock" used to time the events is a master oscillator, which operates in a continuous mode. The rate at which this master oscillator clock fires the repetitive bursts is expressed in terms of KHz, which can be confusing. As an example, consider a 1-MHz master oscillator used to generate a 12.5-KHz pulse repetition frequency. This means that the 1,000,000 cycle per second signal is divided into equal 12,500-cycle segments. If there are 1,000,000 pulses in one second, 12,500 pulses will occur every 0.0125 second (0.0125 second = 80 μsec). A pulse repetition rate of 12.5 KHz means that the pulses will be spaced precisely 80 μsec apart, and each pulse will be exactly in step with the master oscillator. It may be that a higher frequency master oscillator is used, such as 5 MHz, in which case a burst of 1-μsec duration would require the clock to fire 5-cycle bursts (5 cycles at 5 MHz = 0.000001 sec) at the 12.5-KHz rate. Because the time between pulses must be at least 13 μsec per cm of tissue being examined, the maximum allowable pulse repetition frequency of pulsed Doppler ultrasound is in the 8 to 15-KHz range.

There is a reason that the pulse repetition frequency of a pulsed Doppler ultrasound system must be variable. It can be shown mathematically (but not by one of us) that the maximum Doppler shift frequency that can be detected by a pulsed Doppler system is equal to half the pulse repetition frequency. With the 12.5-KHz pulse repetition frequency used in the previous example, the maximum Doppler shift frequency that could be detected would be 6.25 KHz. For practice you should now calculate the velocity corresponding to a 6.25-KHz Doppler shift assuming a 5-MHz transducer and an angle θ of 0° (the answer is about 96 cm per sec). The maximum depth at which this velocity could be detected is about 6 cm, as explained earlier. Detection of rapidly moving structures in the heart may require alterations of three parameters: (1) using a higher pulse repetition frequency; (2) using a lower ultrasound frequency; or (3) approaching the structure from a steeper angle (remember cos θ becomes smaller as the angle θ increases from 0° to 90°).

Let us briefly review pulsed Doppler ultrasound, which is a means of adding depth resolution to a Doppler system. Short bursts of ultrasound, lasting 0.5 to 1.0 μsec, are generated at a precise rate by a master oscillator "clock." The repetition frequency of about 8 to 15 KHz is limited by the "time of flight" of ultrasound in soft tissue. The repetition frequency will in turn limit the maximum Doppler shift frequency that can be detected.

Because pulsed Doppler alone does not provide information about the site of origin of an echo, it is usual to combine the pulsed Doppler instrument with a real-time imaging system or some other display mode. For example, cardiac evaluation might use an M-mode display to identify the left ventricular or left atrial outflow tract, and the "piggybacked" pulsed Doppler unit could then evaluate flow characteristics within the selected area. Similarly, a continuous wave Doppler instrument might be used to locate a blood vessel, and

a pulsed Doppler unit used simultaneously could image blood flow through various levels of the vessel. Such so-called "duplex" system combinations are currently being developed.

When a sound beam passes through a blood vessel, the back-scattered signal will consist of all the Doppler shifts produced by all the red cells moving through the sound beam. Because velocities of the red cells range from almost zero at the vessel wall to a peak velocity near the center of the vessel, a spectrum of Doppler shift frequencies will also be present. This spectrum may be quite complex with pulsating blood flow, especially when areas of vessel stenosis produce rapid and turbulent flow patterns. An experienced observer can hear the typical Doppler frequency shifts encountered with vessel stenosis. It is also possible to make a visible recording of the relative contribution of individual frequencies comprising the total Doppler signal. This technique is called spectral analysis of the Doppler signal.

REAL-TIME ULTRASOUND

Real-time imaging systems are those that have frame rates fast enough to allow movement to be followed. With a conventional B-mode system the operator produces a single image frame with the transducer. This single frame is viewed until it is erased and a new image is generated. A real-time ultrasound transducer can produce multiple frames in a very short time, typically at least 10 frames per second. This fast frame rate allows movement to be viewed in "real-time" as the images are generated. Because of the short persistence of vision, a flicker-free display requires at least 16 frames per second.

Line Density and Frame Rate

Line density refers to the number of vertical lines per field of view. The lines can be parallel to each other, as in a linear array, or can radiate from a point, as in sector scanners. The greater the number of lines per frame, the higher the resolution of the image (Fig. 25–40). Obviously, we assume that each line contains new information. In some early units the number of lines per frame was increased by duplicating lines, a maneuver that will produce a pleasant image but does not add any information.

The maximum pulse repetition rate, or frame rate, is limited by the speed of ultrasound in tissue. Consider a structure 15 cm deep in a patient. The time required for an ultrasound pulse originating at the skin to reach the structure and then return to the transducer (a round trip of 30 cm) will be about 200/1,000,000 of a second, usually expressed as 200 μsec. Because a new pulse cannot be generated until all echoes from the first pulse have returned, the maximum number of individual lines that can be generated in our example is 5000 per second (1,000,000 ÷ 200). If there were 61 lines per frame (this is a com-

mon situation), the circumstances in our example would allow a maximum of almost 82 frames per second. With 100 lines per frame, however, we are limited to 50 frames per second.

The purpose of the previous example is to illustrate the possible tradeoffs that must be considered with real-time imaging. Visualizing deep structures will require a slower frame rate (pulse repetition rate). High frame rates are desirable, however, when imaging fast-moving structures such as the heart. High line density is desirable to improve image quality, but more lines per frame requires a lower number of frames per second. As in film-screen radiography, some compromise is required.

Types of Real-Time Instruments

There are two basic techniques for producing real-time ultrasonic images. In one type a conventional single-element transducer, or group of single-element transducers, is mechanically moved to form images in real time. This is the group of **mechanical scanners.** The other technique uses an array of transducers. The transducers do not move, but are activated electronically so as to cause the ultrasonic beam to sweep across the patient. This is called **electronic array** real-time scanning.

Mechanical Scanning

Essentially there are three types of mechanical real-time scanning instruments. Two of these use a single transducer that is caused to oscillate, while the third uses two, three, or four transducers mounted on a rotating wheel. All produce an image with a sector format, usually encompassing an arc between 45° and 90°. This design produces a relatively rugged transducer that has a minimum of electronics and is of comparatively less complex design. The frame rate and sector angle can be varied in some instruments. Decreasing the sector angle will produce higher resolution, because the same number of vertical lines are compressed into a smaller area. Wide-

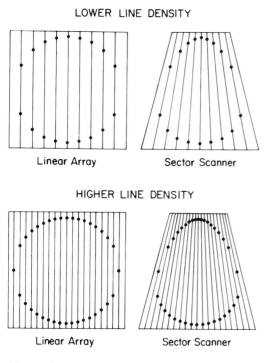

Figure 25–40 Image resolution improves in both linear array and sector real time images as the number of lines per frame increases

angle sectors give lower resolution but allow a larger field of view. One disadvantage of sector scanners is that the scan format is relatively fixed for any transducer, requiring a change of transducers if any special imaging is required (such as an M-mode recording of the heart). Let us look briefly at the three types of mechanical real-time transducers.

Oscillating Transducer: Unenclosed Crystal. A single transducer crystal is caused to oscillate through an angle. The frame rate depends on the rate of oscillation, and can be varied. The motor driving the transducer is connected to the transducer by gears or a lever (Fig. 25–41). Because the oscillating transducer touches the patient's skin (i.e., there is no interposed water bath), both the operator and patient can feel vibrations caused by the moving crystal. A sector-shaped image is produced. This oscillating transducer is often called a wobbler sector scanner. The angle of wobble can be varied from about 15° to 60°, and frame rates are generally about 15 to 30 per second.

With mechanical scanners the ultrasound beam may be reflected from a reflecting mirror, making it possible to move the mirror rather than the transducer crystal. We will not describe mirror systems in any more detail.

Oscillating Transducer: Enclosed Crystal. In this type of sector scanner the transducer is enclosed in an oil- or water-filled container. Castor oil is commonly used as

the fluid. The transducer may be driven by mechanical linkage to a motor. Another design attaches a permanent magnet to the back of the transducer and mounts the combination between the poles of an electromagnet. Changing the direction of current flow through the coils of the electromagnet causes the magnet and transducer to oscillate. The type of image produced by this system depends on the distance between the transducer and the front surface of the casing that is in contact with the patient's skin. If the transducer is near the surface, a sector image (similar to that in Fig. 25–41B) is produced. When the transducer is mounted several centimeters behind the front surface, a trapezoidal image is produced (Fig. 25–42). With this type of system the patient does not feel any vibration because the moving transducer does not touch the skin. The ultrasonic, or acoustic, window through which the ultrasound beam emerges is made of a flexible membrane, and it is this window that contacts the patient's skin.

Rotating Wheel Transducer. This type usually employs three or four transducers that are mounted 120° or 90° apart on a wheel (Fig. 25–43). The wheel diameter is usually between 2 and 5 cm. Several different methods are used to connect the wheel to a motor, which rotates the wheel at a constant rate in one direction only. The ultrasound beam emerges through an

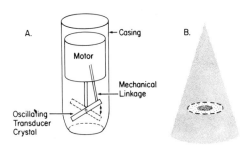

Figure 25–41 An oscillating transducer with an unenclosed crystal (A) produces a sector image (B)

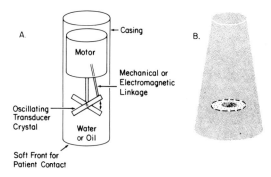

Figure 25–42 An oscillating transducer with an enclosed crystal (A) may produce a trapezoidal image (B)

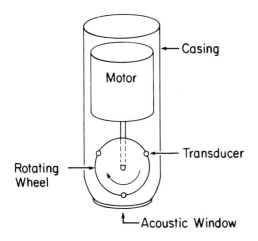

Figure 25–43 A rotating wheel transducer

acoustically transparent window. Only the transducer that is behind the acoustic window is allowed to transmit and receive ultrasound waves. Depending on design, either a sector- or trapezoid-shaped image may be produced.

Rotating transducer systems can also be designed to use a reflecting mirror. The sector or trapezoid field may be operated at an opening angle up to 90°. If only two transducers are used, it is possible to use a sector angle as large as 180°.

Electronic Array Scanning

There are basically two types of electronic real-time scanners. Both use arrays of transducers comprised of many small rectangular transducer elements (about 2 × 10 mm) arranged adjacent to each other. The two types are **linear array** (which produces a rectangular scan format) and **phased** or **steered array** (which produces sector scans). Unlike mechanical systems, the transducers in an electronic array real-time system do not move. The ultrasound beam is caused to move by electronic controls. We will attempt to describe the design of these transducers and to explain how electronics causes the ultrasound beam to move and become focused.

Linear Array. This consists of a number of small rectangular transducer elements (about 2 mm × 10 mm) arranged in a line, with their narrow dimensions touching. There could be 64 to 200 transducers forming an assembly from 4 to 10 cm long. In our examples we will assume an assembly of 64 transducers. From our earlier discussion you will recall that a good ultrasound image requires a satisfactory number of vertical lines per image. Early linear array instruments had 20 transducer elements, with each transducer being larger than those in more recent units. The resulting image had only 20 lines per frame, which did not produce a very satisfactory picture.

Increasing the number of lines per frame without increasing the total length of the transducer assembly would seem to have a simple solution: use more but smaller transducers. This is exactly how the problem has been solved, but a new problem is created. Please refer back to Figures 25–14 and 25–15 to remind yourself that the length of the Fresnel (near, or nondivergent) zone of an ultrasound beam is determined by the diameter of the transducer and the wavelength of the ultrasound:

$$x' = \frac{r^2}{\lambda}$$

x' = length of Fresnel zone
r = radius of the transducer
λ = wavelength

Thus, for a constant wavelength, decreasing transducer size will shorten the Fresnel zone and increase the angle of dispersion. If each transducer in a 64-unit assembly were fired separately, the resulting beam pattern would disperse rapidly and be of no diagnostic usefulness (Fig. 25–44A).

The problem of a sufficient number of lines per frame versus the need for satisfactory beam focusing (i.e., a long Fresnel zone) has been solved in two ways: first, by using an array with many narrow transducer elements to produce high line density; and second, by firing the transducers in groups, causing the group to act as a

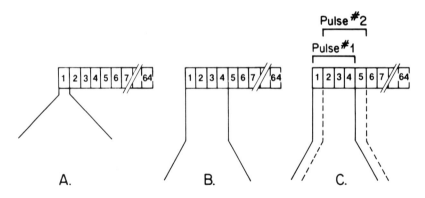

Figure 25–44 A linear transducer array

single larger transducer and thus provide better resolution (Fig. 25–44*B*).

The pulsed sequence of firing of groups of transducers in a linear array is illustrated in Figure 25–44*C*. We will assume that four transducer elements are operated as a group. In the illustration, pulse 1 is generated by simultaneously pulsing elements 1, 2, 3, and 4. After the echoes return to this first group, the next line in the frame is generated (pulse 2) by pulsing elements 2, 3, 4, and 5. This sequence continues until elements 61, 62, 63, and 64 form the final line in the frame. By this mechanism a linear array of 64 elements (individual transducers) pulsed in groups of four and stepped one element between lines will produce a frame with 61 lines. This is the origin of the 61-line frame we mentioned in the introduction to this section. The entire array will be pulsed in approximately 1/20 to 1/50 sec, producing 20 to 50 frames per second. The number of lines per frame will depend on the number of transducers in the array, the number of transducers pulsed at one time, and the sequence of pulsing.

We must now turn to the question of how the ultrasound beam originating from a linear array is focused. This is done electronically in one dimension, and with a plastic lens in another dimension.

You will recall that an ultrasound beam can be focused in a manner similar to the effect of lenses and mirrors on visible light.

Focusing can increase the intensity of an ultrasound beam by factors greater than 100. Plastics are used as the lens material. Because the speed of sound in plastic is greater than that in water and soft tissue, a concave lens is necessary for focusing an ultrasonic beam (note that this is the opposite of the effect of optical lenses on visible light). For our example, we will consider that the linear array is made up of a series of 2-mm × 10-mm transducers (elements). Focusing along the 10-mm dimension is accomplished by placing a long concave lens in front of the elements (Fig. 25–45). Remember, the concave lens will

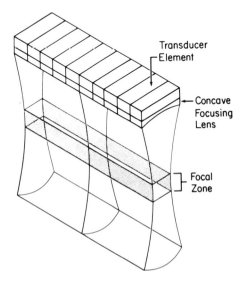

Figure 25–45 A concave lens used to focus a linear array

not bring the beam to a focus at a single point, but will create a focal zone (i.e., a distance over which the focal properties are fairly well maintained). This focusing lens determines the width of the ultrasound beam in the plane perpendicular to the image plane, and determines the thickness of the image slice.

A fixed lens cannot be used to focus the beam in the plane parallel to the image because the location of the beam is constantly moving along the array as the elements are switched on and off. Focusing to improve resolution in this plane is termed "improved azimuthal resolution," and is accomplished electronically (Fig. 25–46). How can an ultrasonic beam generated by a group of transducers be focused electronically? We will discuss this in some detail because the same principle applies to steered array real-time scanners. The student interested in details about electronic focusing should consult the elegant article and illustrations of Wells.[15]

To improve azimuthal resolution, the method of pulsing each individual transducer element within each group is changed. Figure 25–47 shows how a group of four transducer elements can be focused electronically. First, refer back to Figure 25–12, which shows that the concentric rings of sound originating from different

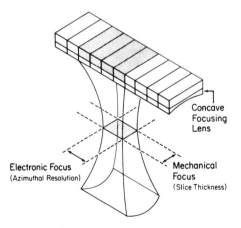

Figure 25–46 Focusing a linear array transducer

points within a single piezoelectric crystal reinforce each other to form a wave front in front of the crystal. Similarly, each element in a group can be considered to emit a circular wavelet when stimulated. When each transducer element in the group is stimulated at the same time, the wavelets will reinforce each other to form a wave front that travels normal to the surface of the array (Fig. 25–47A). When all elements in a group are pulsed at the same time, the resultant wave front behaves like a nonfocused single-element transducer equal in diameter to the width of all the elements in the group.

Producing a focused beam using a group of transducer elements can be accomplished by stimulating the individual elements at slightly different times (Fig. 25–47B). If the two central elements are pulsed several nanoseconds (1 nanosecond = 10^{-9} sec) after the outer two elements, the wavelets from the individual elements combine to form a focused beam. When speaking of ultrasound propagation in tissue, a nanosecond is a very short time. You will recall that ultrasound travels one centimeter in soft tissue in about 6.5 μseconds (microsecond = 10^{-6} second), and the timing between pulses is usually slower than one pulse every 80 μsec (the time required for a round trip of 6 cm). It is possible to vary the sharpness of the focus (length of the focal zone) and the depth of focus by varying the time delay between the pulsing of the central and outer elements of the group. In some systems the operator has some control of sharpness of focus and depth of focus. As the operating group of elements is switched along the entire array, the associated delay (i.e., focusing) signals must be appropriately switched along the array to maintain the focusing action.

The typical linear array real-time scanning transducer used in adult abdominal examinations employs a transducer array about 120 mm long by 10 mm wide, and a frequency of between 2 and 3 MHz. The basic principles of the instrumentation are

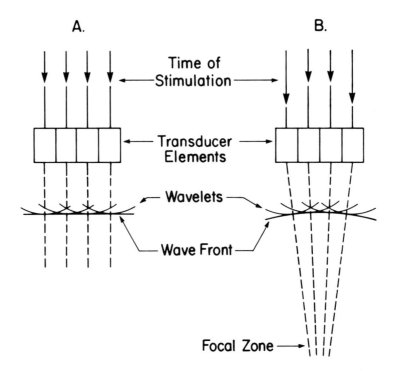

Figure 25–47 Electronic focusing of the ultrasonic beam produced by a transducer array

said to be relatively simple, allowing portable battery-operated units to be designed.

Steered or Phased Array. The term "steered array" or "phased array" may be used for this type of real-time scanning.

With a steered array transducer a sector scan is obtained, but the transducer is not moved while the scan is being generated. Rather, the ultrasound beam is caused to sweep back and forth across the patient by using electronically controlled steering and focusing.

For linear array scanning we discussed how an ultrasound beam produced by a group of transducers could be focused by the appropriate choice of time delays. Similarly, the beam may be directed, or steered, to a desired angle by a similar mechanism of time delays. By choosing the appropriate delay between stimulation of the individual elements of the transducer, it is possible to steer the beam, or to steer and focus the beam simultaneously. This concept is illustrated with simple block diagrams in Figure 25–48. Note that it is necessary to change the pulsing sequence constantly for each element in the array.

A steered array transducer is similar in size to a single-element transducer used for conventional B-mode scanning. A typical transducer contains 32 elements and operates at a frequency of 2 to 3 MHz. With a steered array transducer all the elements are pulsed to form each line of the image, as opposed to the linear array in which only a few (typically four) elements produce each line in the image. The scan format is a sector with its apex at the center of the array. The ultrasound beam is caused to sweep through the sector angle at a rate fast enough to form a real-time image. A similar delay pattern is introduced into the received signals, which causes the transducer to be sensitive only to echoes returning along the same path as the transmitted beam.

The steered array system can be used to produce a time-motion tracing from a single line, while simultaneously displaying the entire sector image. It has found its

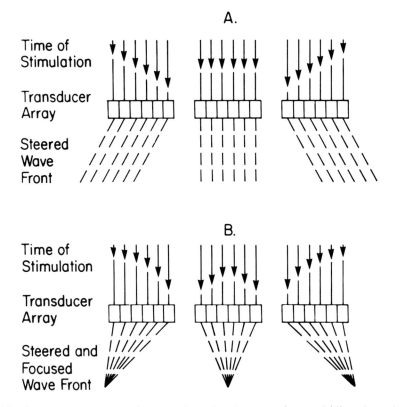

Figure 25–48 A steered array transducer system showing a nonfocused (*A*) and an electronically focused (*B*) beam

major application in cardiac imaging and in evaluation of vessel pulsation in abdominal imaging. Two problems presently limit more general use of this technique. First, image quality is not uniform across the entire beam pattern, and resolution may not be as good at the edges of the sector as in the center. Second, this instrument is very expensive because of the complex computer-controlled electronics necessary to steer and focus the beam.

SUMMARY

Ultrasound is sound with a frequency greater than 20,000 cycles/sec (Hertz, Hz). Medical sonography employs frequencies between 1 megahertz (MHz) and 20 MHz. These high frequencies are produced by subjecting a special ceramic material, a piezoelectric crystal, to a short-voltage spike. A group of synthetic piezoelectric materials

called ceramic ferroelectrics have replaced the piezoelectric crystal materials that were used earlier. Although PZT is currently the most widely used material, research suggests that certain plastic polymers may soon replace these synthetic ceramics in the construction of ultrasound transducers. The electric field created by the voltage spike realigns crystalline elements (dipoles) in the ceramic, thereby suddenly changing the crystal's thickness. This sudden change in thickness starts a series of vibrations that produces sound waves.

The piezoelectric crystal is housed in the front of a transducer, a plastic box that protects the crystal from mechanical trauma and provides sonic and electrical insulation. Electrodes are plated onto the surface of the crystal, and the outside electrode is grounded to protect the patient from electrical shock. A backing block dampens vibrations between voltage spikes, so the transducer can be used to generate multiple short pulses of sound. Each transducer vibrates at its own natural frequency, called the resonant frequency, when struck with a short-voltage spike. If a clinical situation dictates a different frequency, another transducer must be selected, one designed with the appropriate frequency. Piezoelectric crystals can be damaged by heat. Above a critical temperature, called the Curie temperature, a crystal loses its piezoelectric properties and becomes a worthless piece of ceramic. The Q factor is a measure of the purity of tone (narrowness of frequency range). The ring down-time is the time that it takes a transducer to stop vibrating.

An ultrasonic beam is a series of longitudinal waves that transmit energy. These waves travel through average body tissue at a velocity of 1540 m/sec. Their velocity is independent of frequency. The velocity of sound depends on the density and compressibility of the conducting medium, and is equal to the frequency multiplied by the wavelength. As a sound beam passes through the body, the beam is attenuated, or reduced in intensity, by a combination of diffusion, reflection, refraction, and absorption. The sonic beam is fairly coherent with parallel sides in the near, or Fresnel, zone. Beyond a certain critical distance, the transition point, the beam reaches the far, or Fraunhofer zone, and begins to flare out and disperse. The length of the near zone is proportional to the square of the diameter of the transducer and inversely proportional to the wavelength of the sound. The beam is rapidly attenuated by dispersion in the far zone. Reflection occurs at tissue interfaces. The incident and reflected angles are equal. The amount of reflection depends on the difference in the acoustic impedance of the two surfaces and on the angle of incidence of the beam. Acoustic impedance is the product of the density and velocity of sound in the conducting medium. Reflection is greatest with a large difference between the acoustic impedance of the two media and with a small incident angle. Reflection is least, and transmission greatest, at an incident angle of 90°.

When the velocity of sound changes as it passes from one medium to another, the frequency remains constant but the wavelength changes. If the wave front strikes the second medium at an angle, the sound is refracted, or bent. The degree of refraction depends on the angle of incidence and on the difference in the velocity of sound in the two media. Absorption, which is the conversion of sound into heat, depends on the frequency of the sound and on both the viscosity and relaxation time of the conducting medium. Absorption in tissue is proportional to frequency; that is, increasing from 1 to 2 MHz doubles absorption and halves the penetrating power of the beam. Therefore, high-frequency sound cannot be used to examine thick body parts.

A longitudinal wave is propagated by multiple particles (molecules) oscillating in the direction of propagation to produce bands of compression and rarefaction in the conducting medium. When these bands are back-scattered to the piezoelectric crystal as echoes they change the crystal's thickness, which produces an electrical signal. This signal forms the basis of the ultrasonic image. The sound is transmitted in short bursts, or pulses, usually 1000/sec. The pulses are short, about 0.000001 sec in duration. Between pulses the transducer acts as a receiver, recording returning echoes. The time delay between the initiation of a pulse and the return of an echo is converted into depth in all imaging modes. The images can be displayed in several modes. The A mode displays a one-dimensional static image showing echoes as spikes projecting from a baseline. The baseline identifies the central axis of the beam. The TM mode is similar to the A mode, except that the echoes are recorded as dots instead of spikes, and the TM mode is used to study moving parts. Motion is recorded on a strip chart recorder or by sweeping the dots across an oscilloscope during a timed exposure.

The B mode is a two-dimensional display of the image produced by moving a transducer either longitudinally or in cross section. The transducer is similar to the handle of a saber with the sound beam as the blade. Multiple controls are provided to augment weaker echoes. The most important control is the time gain compensator, which logarithmically enhances echoes from selected depths after an adjustable delay.

Depth resolution, the ability to separate two objects in tandem, depends on the spatial pulse length, which is the number of waves in a pulse multiplied by the wavelength. Depth resolution is best with transducers that have a short spatial pulse length. Lateral resolution, the ability to separate two adjacent objects, depends on the width of the sonic beam. The beam can be narrowed with an acoustic lens, which bends the sound toward a focal point.

The Doppler effect is a change in the perceived frequency of a sound emitted by a moving source. Doppler devices are used to detect motion. They accomplish this by continuously transmitting a sound beam through one transducer while a second transducer records returning echoes. The difference between the two frequencies usually falls in the audible range for most physiologic motions. After amplification the difference becomes an audio signal. Continuous wave Doppler instruments can provide velocity information, but lack any form of depth resolution. Pulsed Doppler instruments provide both depth and velocity information simultaneously. A pulsed Doppler instrument is usually combined with some other form of ultrasound imaging system in a "piggybacked" system. Spectral analysis of a Doppler signal, by allowing evaluation of the spectrum of frequencies making up a Doppler signal, allow evaluation of the nature of blood flow in normal and stenotic blood vessels.

Real-time imaging systems produce image frames fast enough to allow motion to be followed. A compromise between line density per frame and frame rate is required. Frame rates are usually at least 16 frames per second. The real-time image may be generated by a mechanical scanner or by an electronic array arrangement. Mechanical scanners generate a sector format image with either an oscillating transducer or a rotating wheel transducer. Electronic array real-time scanners may use a linear array transducer, which produces a rectangular scan format, or a steered array transducer, which produces a sector format image. Focusing the electronic array ultrasound beam requires both a concave plastic lens and electronic focusing. Satisfactory beam geometry requires that the individual elements in a linear array transducer be pulsed in groups, commonly four elements at a time, with each group producing one line in the resulting image. With a steered array transducer, all elements of the transducer are pulsed to form each line of the image.

REFERENCES

1. Baker, D.W.: Applications of pulsed Doppler techniques. Radiol. Clin. North Am., 18:79, 1980.
2. Barnes, R.W.: Ultrasound techniques for evaluation of lower extremity venous disease. Semin. Ultrasound, 11:276, 1981.
3. Carpenter, D.A.: Ultrasonic transducers. Clin. Diagn. Ultrasound, 5:31, 1980.
4. Cooperberg, P.L., David, K.B., Sauerbrei, E.C.: Abdominal and peripheral applications of real-time ultrasound. Radiol. Clin. North Am., 18:59, 1980.
5. Hendee, W.R.: Medical Radiation Physics. Chicago, Year Book Medical Publishers, 1979.
6. James, A.E., Fleischer, A.C., et al.: Ultrasound: Certain considerations of equipment usage. In The Physical Basis of Medical Imaging. Edited by G.M. Coulam, et al. New York, Appleton-Century-Crofts, 1981, p. 169.
7. James, A.E., Goddard, J., et al.: Advances in instrument design and image recording. Radiol. Clin. North Am., 18:3, 1980.
8. Knox, R.A., and Strandness, D.E.: Ultrasound techniques for evaluation of lower extremity arterial occlusion. Semin. Ultrasound, 11:264, 1981.

9. Price, R.R., Jones, T., Fleischer, A.C., and James, A.E.: Ultrasound: Basic principles. *In* The Physical Basis of Medical Imaging. Edited by G.M. Coulam, et al. New York, Appleton-Century-Crofts, 1981, p. 155.

10. Rose, J.L., and Goldberg, B.B.: Basic Physics in Diagnostic Ultrasound. New York, John Wiley and Sons, 1979.

11. Sanders, R.C., and James, A.E.: The Principles and Practice of Ultrasonography in Obstetrics and Gynecology. New York, Appleton-Century-Crofts, 1980.

12. Sarti, D.A., and Sample, W.F.: Diagnostic Ultrasound Text and Cases. Boston, G.K. Hall and Company, 1980.

13. Skolnick, M.L.: Real-Time Ultrasound Imaging in the Abdomen. New York, Springer-Verlag, 1981.

14. Souquet, J., Defranould, P., and Desbois, J.: Design of low-loss wide-band ultrasonic transducers for noninvasive medical application. IEEE Trans. Sonics Ultrasonics, *Su-26*:75, 1979.

15. Wells, P.N.T.: Real-time scanning systems. Clin. Diagn. Ultrasound, *5*:69, 1980.

16. Wells, P.N.T.: Biomedical Ultrasonics. London, Academic Press, 1977.

17. Woodcock, J.P., and Skidmore, R.: Principles and applications of Doppler ultrasound. Clin. Diagn. Ultrasound, *5*:166, 1980.

18. Zagzebski, J.A.: Physics and instrumentation of Doppler ultrasonography. Semin. Ultrasound, *11*:246, 1981.

19. Zwiebel, W.J.: Doppler cerebrovascular examination. Semin. Ultrasound, *11*:293, 1981.

26

Protection

HISTORICAL REVIEW

Many somatic dangers of radiation became evident a few months after x rays were discovered. Roentgen announced his discovery in December of 1895. In 1896, 23 cases of radiodermatitis were reported in the world literature.[1] Between 1911 and 1914, three review articles identified 54 cancer deaths and 198 cases of radiation-induced malignancy. The first American radiation fatality occurred in 1904 when Thomas Edison's assistant, Clarence M. Dally, died of cancer. A few farsighted individuals cried out for radiation controls, but their pleas were largely ignored. Catastrophes continued until the whole medical community became alarmed. Finally, in 1921, the first official action was taken when the British X-Ray and Radium Protection Committee was founded to investigate methods for reducing exposures. Their efforts were severely hampered, however, because they did not have a satisfactory unit of radiation measurement. The crude units of the time, the erythema dose and "slight film fogging," proved completely inadequate. In 1928, the Second International Congress of Radiology (ICR) appointed a committee to define the Roentgen (R) as a unit of exposure. The committee did not finish its assignment until 1937, but the Roentgen became the accepted unit of measurement even though it was not accurately defined.

The first dose-limiting recommendation was made by a group of American scientists, the Advisory Committee on X-Ray and Radium Protection, in 1931, 46 years after Roentgen's discovery. The recommendation was 0.2 R per day. The name of the committee has been changed several times, and it is now called the National Council on Radiation Protection and Measurements (NCRP). It is a private organization of scientists, experts in various aspects of radiation, who operate under a congressional charter but without legal status. The NCRP publishes its recommendations periodically in handbooks. These are purely advisory, but most state and federal laws are based on NCRP recommendations. Since the first recommendation of 50 R per year (0.2 R per workday), made in 1931, the maximum permissible dose (MPD) has been lowered on three separate occasions (Table 26–1). The MPD is now only one tenth of its initial level. Recommended exposures have been lowered because of growing concern over the increasing use of diagnostic radiation, and apprehension about the mounting evidence that small doses can cause leukemia and carcinoma.

Table 26–1. Historical Review of Maximum Permissible Dose (MPD) Recommendations of the National Council on Radiation Protection and Measurements

DATE	ANNUAL MPD (rem)
1931	50
1936	30
1948	15
1958	5

BIOLOGICAL EFFECTS OF RADIATION

All ionizing radiation is harmful! This is the premise that mandates a radiation protection policy. The harmful effects fall into two broad categories: somatic, those effects harmful to the person being irradiated; and genetic, those effects harmful to future generations. We are not qualified to discuss the biologic effects of radiation in any detail, so our description will be quite superficial. The interested reader should read one of the texts listed at the end of this chapter.[2,3,6] **One important point must be emphasized: the data are not available to indicate if there is a threshold below which no harmful effect will occur.** Without this knowledge, we cannot say that there is a safe dose. Therefore, a recommendation that 5 rem per year is the maximum permissible dose really means "that, in light of present knowledge, this dose is not expected to cause appreciable bodily injury to a person at any time during his lifetime."[5] **In actual practice, radiation levels should be kept at the lowest practicable level, and we should not think of permissible doses as being perfectly safe.**

The most important somatic effect of radiation is carcinogenesis, and leukemia is the most common neoplasia. The exact risk is unknown. Hall made the statement that "the 20-year risk from leukemia plus all other radiation-induced neoplastic diseases is 6 cases per 100,000 individuals exposed per rem."[2] He admitted that this estimate was made on limited data and involved many tenuous assumptions. Nevertheless, most experts agree that low doses of radiation can cause neoplasms. Usually there is a long latent period, ranging from 5 to 20 years for leukemia and from 10 to 30 years for other tumors.

The genetic effects of radiation are more frightening than the somatic ones, because they may not manifest themselves for several generations. Each new mutant constitutes a potential burden to society, and the burden must be kept at the lowest level consistent with good medical practice. Because of the fear of these genetic effects, dose limits are placed on exposures to large segments of the population, as opposed to maximum permissible doses. This emphasizes the need to restrict exposures. The **genetically significant dose (GSD)** is defined as the dose that, if received by every member of the population, would be expected to produce the same total genetic injury as the actual doses received by the various individuals. For example, if the world population consisted of 1000 individuals and each received a radiation dose of 0.1 rem, the genetic effect would be the same as if 10 individuals received 10 rem and the other 990 received nothing:

$$1000 \times 0.1 = (10 \times 10) + (990 \times 0)$$

The concept implies that the effect of large exposures to a few individuals is greatly diluted by the total population and thus has little overall genetic impact. Radiation workers may receive relatively large exposures without significantly changing the population's genetically significant dose.

RADIATION UNITS

Before discussing maximum permissible dose (MPD) recommendations, we are going to digress and define three units of radiation measurement: the Roentgen, the rad, and the rem.

The Roentgen (R) is defined as a unit of **radiation exposure** that will liberate a charge of 2.58×10^{-4} Coulombs per kilogram of air.[4] This definition is relatively meaningless to most radiologists, because the Coulomb is not part of our daily vocabulary. In more familiar terms, a Roentgen is the approximate exposure to the body surface for an AP film of the abdomen for a patient of average thickness. As a measure of exposure, the Roentgen is independent of area, or field size (Fig. 26–1). When a large square (A) is exposed to 1 R, each increment of the square receives 1 R. If the square is divided into multiple

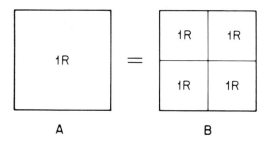

Figure 26–1 The exposures in A and B are identical

Table 26–2. Approximate Absorbed Dose (Rad) per Roentgen of Exposure

TYPE OF TISSUE	RAD PER ROENTGEN OF EXPOSURE	
	50 kVp	1 MeV
Soft tissue	0.95	0.95
Bone	5.0	0.90

smaller squares (B), each of these squares receives 1 R of exposure. It would be improper to add the exposures of the smaller squares and say the total was 4 R, because no area has received that much exposure. This is a familiar concept in other areas of our daily lives. For example, rainfall is measured in inches without regard to area. A 1-in. rain produces a 1-in. deep layer of water in a drinking glass or a washtub, provided they both have flat bottoms and perpendicular sides. Roentgen exposures are exactly the same.

The **rad** is the unit of **absorbed dose.** One rad is equal to the radiation necessary to deposit energy of 100 ergs in 1 gram of irradiated material (100 erg/g). It is independent of the composition of the radiated material and energy of the beam. The number of rads deposited per Roentgen of exposure, however, varies both with energy of the beam and with the composition of the absorber (Table 26–2). The energy deposited in soft tissue per Roentgen is approximately 95 erg/g in the diagnostic energy range. It may be five times as much in bone at low energies and actually a little less than 95 erg/g at 1 MeV. As a general rule, the absorbed dose is proportional to the degree of attenuation.

The **rem** is a unit of **dose equivalent.** It is equal to the absorbed dose multiplied by a **quality factor (QF):**

$$\text{Rem} = \text{rads} \times \text{quality factor}$$

The rem is a measure of the biologic effectiveness of irradiation. Some practical quality factors are shown in Table 26–3.[7] These are only approximations; the actual numbers depend on the energy of the beam. Because the quality factor for x rays is 1, the rad and rem are equal. In fact, at diagnostic energy levels the rad, rem, and Roentgen may all be considered to be equal, because the energy deposited in soft tissues by 1 R of exposure is only 5% more than a rad:

$$1\ R \simeq 1\ \text{rad} = 1\ \text{rem}$$

X rays and beta particles have the same quality factor. This is logical, because the beta particle is a moving electron and the end product of x-ray attenuation is also a moving electron. They are used as the standard, and assigned a quality factor of 1. Larger particles deposit more energy per unit length of travel. The amount of energy deposited per unit length of travel, expressed in keV per micron, is called the **linear energy transfer (LET).** If an electron and proton start with the same energy, the proton will be attenuated more quickly. Because of the proton's large size, it encounters more "friction" as it passes between atoms. Having started with the same

Table 26–3. Quality Factors for Various Types of Radiation

TYPE OF RADIATION	QUALITY FACTORS
X rays	1
Gamma rays	1
Beta particles	1
Protons	5
Neutrons:	
Slow	3
Fast	10
Alpha particles	20

amount of energy as the electron, the proton deposits more energy per unit length of travel, so it is a higher LET radiation. The amount of biologic damage is determined by the linear energy transfer of the radiation. A tissue absorbing 100 rads of proton radiation sustains five times as much biologic damage as a tissue absorbing the same quantity of x rays. Thus, protons have a quality factor of 5. For radiation protection purposes the quality factor is multiplied by the absorbed dose in rads to determine the dose equivalent in rems.

The **relative biologic effectiveness (RBE)** is another expression used to compare the effectiveness of several types of radiation. It must be determined for each type of radiation and biologic system and, by convention, is reserved for laboratory investigation.

CURRENT POPULATION EXPOSURES

Mankind has been exposed to radiation since the beginning of time. Initially the exposure all came from natural sources but, over the past few decades, exposures from man-made sources have gradually increased. Annual exposures in the United States from the various types of radiation are summarized in Table 26–4.[5] These are approximations, and serve only as a general guide. They may vary by a factor of 10 under some circumstances.

Table 26–4. Current Radiation Exposure in the United States from Various Sources

SOURCE OF RADIATION	ANNUAL DOSE (mrem)
Natural Radiation (average 125)	
External (average 100)	
Cosmic	30–70
Gamma	30–130
Internal	25
Medical procedures	50–70
Applied in human research	—
Occupational	1
Man-made environmental	4
Total	140–300

Natural Radiation

Natural radiation exposure arises from external and internal sources. The external sources are cosmic and gamma radiation. Exposure from cosmic radiation varies slightly with latitude and considerably with altitude. It ranges at sea level from 30 mrem/year in Florida to 35 mrem/year in Alaska, and up to 70 mrem/year at an altitude of 1 mile. Gamma-ray exposures are a little lower inside buildings than on the outside. The exposure comes primarily from radionuclides in the rock and building materials. In the United States, gamma-ray exposures average about 60 mrem outside and 55 mrem inside of a building. The total exposure from external sources averages about 100 mrem/year.

Internal exposure comes from radionuclides in food, water, and air, and is estimated at about 25 mrem/year. The principal contributors are radium and thorium (and their decay products), radiopotassium (^{40}K), and radiocarbon (^{14}C).

The total natural radiation dose in the United States is estimated at 125 mrem, and may range up to 400 mrem/year. No deleterious effect has been validated in persons receiving the higher exposure, but we cannot derive great consolation from this fact since no satisfactory epidemiologic study has ever been undertaken.

Man-Made Radiation

Exposure to man-made radiation sources contributes less to population exposure than natural sources, but the man-made contribution is constantly rising and is cause for concern. At present, the major contributor to the genetically significant dose (GSD) is medical radiation for diagnostic and therapeutic procedures, estimated at between 50 and 75 mrem/year. Other man-made sources (e.g., radiation used in research, occupational exposure, and man-made environmental radiation) make only a minor contribution. Occupational exposures may be as high as 5000 mrem/year (although they are usually much less), but the total number of exposed persons is relatively small, and the contribution to the GSD is estimated at only 1%.

Man-made environmental radiation includes effluents from atomic facilities and fallout from nuclear explosions. The radionuclides of principal concern are iodine (^{131}I), strontium (^{89,90}Sr), cesium (^{137}Cs), and cerium (^{144}Ce). Consumer products contribute little because of tight controls. Exposure comes primarily from some television receivers and from luminous watches, clocks, and signs. Fortunately, shoe-fitting fluoroscopes are gone. The average national increment from man-made environmental radiation is estimated to be about 4% of the exposure from natural radiation.

DOSE-LIMITING RECOMMENDATIONS

The principal objective of radiation protection is to ensure that the dose received by an individual (other than the patient) does not exceed the applicable maximum permissible value. A secondary objective is to prevent damage or impairment of function of radiation-sensitive film or equipment.[4]

To accomplish the principal objective, we must know maximum permissible values and understand the tools that we have available to reduce exposures to these levels. We will discuss permissible exposures and dose limits next, and deal with methods later.

For the purpose of regulating radiation exposures, individuals are divided into two categories: the occupationally exposed and the occasionally exposed. The recommendations affecting radiation protection policy deal only with these two categories. A third category, or group, is the population at large. Different exposure recommendations are made for each of these three groups (Table 26–5).[5] Briefly summarized, **the maximum permissible dose for an occupationally exposed individual is 5 rem/year; the dose limit for the occasionally exposed is one tenth as much, or 0.5 rem/year; and the dose limit for the population is one third of the occasional level, or 0.17 rem/year.** These recommendations apply to radiation incurred under occupational conditions, and exclude exposure from the following:

1. Background radiation
2. Medical-dental procedures (diagnostic x rays)
3. Man-made devices outside the occupational environment (TV sets, luminous dial watches, etc.)

Occupational Exposure

The occupationally exposed individual accepts some risk. He takes this slight risk for some tangible benefit, usually gainful employment. As a general rule, he is somewhat knowledgeable of the risks involved, and his numbers are relatively small so his exposure does not contribute appreciably to the genetically significant dose. For this reason, his maximal permissible dose is larger than that of the other groups. By law, no one under 18 years of age may be employed in an occupationally exposed position.

The MPD for the whole body and other critical organs (the gonads, red bone marrow, and lens) shall not exceed 5 rem in any 1 year, or 3 rems in one quarter, or a cumulative dose of 5 rem, multiplied by the age in years minus 18:

Maximum permissible cumulative dose
$$= (N - 18) \times 5 \text{ rem}$$

For example, if a technologist is 30 years of age, his permissible cumulative dose would be $(30 - 18) \times 5 = 60$ rem. This is the maximum permissible accumulation that he is allowed to receive up to the age of 30 years. If a radiation worker accidentally receives a dose exceeding his maximum permissible cumulative dose, he must avoid any further exposure until his cumulative dose falls below that recommended by the formula. The MPD for the skin, hands, forearms, and other organs is higher, as shown in Table 26–5. Fetal ex-

Table 26–5. Dose-Limiting Recommendations

CATEGORY OF INDIVIDUAL	MAXIMUM PERMISSIBLE DOSE (rem)	
	Annual	Quarterly
Occupationally exposed		
Whole body (gonads, lens, and bone marrow)	5	3
Hands	75	25
Forearms	30	10
Other organs	15	5
Fetus (entire gestation)	0.5	

	DOSE LIMITS (rem)
Occasionally exposed	0.5
General population	
Genetic	0.17
Somatic	0.17

posures are restricted to only one tenth of the whole body dose, or 0.5 rem during the entire 9 months of gestation.

Occupationally exposed individuals work in a controlled area, which is an area under the supervision of an individual responsible for radiation protection. Exposures in controlled areas must be kept at a level that would allow a radiation worker to stay in the area during his entire working day without exceeding his MPD. The customary time interval used to calculate exposures for controlled areas is 1 week. Dividing the 5 rem maximum permissible annual dose by a 50-week work year gives a maximum permissible weekly exposure of 0.1 Roentgen. Note that we have changed units from rems to Roentgens, but this is permissible because the two are almost equal in the diagnostic energy range. If exposures in the entire controlled area are kept below 0.1 R/week, then a radiation worker is free to move about the area in safety.

Occasional (Nonoccupational) Exposure

The nonoccupationally exposed individual is in a different situation than the radiation worker. Usually the occasionally exposed individual has no knowledge of the risk involved, receives no compensation for taking a risk and, most important, has no freedom to decide if he will accept the risk.

When a member of the general population, for example a visitor, enters a radiation area, he becomes an occasionally exposed individual. The radiation is thrust on him, frequently without his knowledge. Also, the population size of the occasionally exposed is not controlled, so large numbers of individuals could be involved, which would have a greater impact on the genetically significant dose. For all these reasons, the dose limits for the occasionally exposed is 0.5 rem/year, or one tenth of the MPD for the occupationally exposed.

Areas occupied by occasionally exposed persons are designated as uncontrolled areas. The area may be a corridor, waiting room, elevator, parking lot, and so forth. If the area is exposed to radiation, and nonradiation workers have access to it, its radiation restrictions are more stringent than controlled areas. Exposures must be kept at a level consistent with the continuous occupancy by an occasionally exposed individual without exceeding his dose limit of 0.5 rem/year, or 0.01 R/wk.

In summary, the occupationally exposed individual has a maximum permissible dose of 5 rem/year and occupies a controlled area with a permissible weekly exposure of 0.1 R. The occasionally exposed individual has a dose limit of 0.5 rem/year and occupies an uncontrolled area with a permissible weekly exposure of 0.01 R.

PROTECTIVE BARRIERS

Three methods can be used to control radiation exposure levels: distance, time, and barriers. Distance is obviously an effective method, because beam intensity is governed by the inverse square law. Exposures can be controlled with time in various ways: by limiting the time that the generator is turned on; by limiting the time that the beam is directed at a certain area; or by limiting the time that the area is occupied. All these factors are taken into consideration in planning a new installation. When they prove inadequate, however, the only alternative is a protective barrier, usually lead or concrete. Barriers are designated as either primary or secondary depending on whether they protect from primary radiation (the useful beam) or stray radiation (a combination of leakage and scatter radiation).

Primary Barriers

Figure 26–2 summarizes the factors that must be considered in determining primary barrier requirements for a radiographic installation. The number of factors seems imposing, but the total concept is quite simple.

Our first task is to evaluate the exposure to the area in question. Once we know the exposure, we can use either half-value layers or tables to determine barrier requirements. Five factors must be evaluated in exposure calculations. These are shown along the central axis of the illustration and include the following:

1. Workload (W) in mA · min/wk
2. R per mA · min at 1 m ($\overline{E}$)
3. Use factor (U)
4. Occupancy factor (T)
5. Distance (d) in meters

We will go through the list one step at a time, but first note that no mention is made of attenuation by the patient. Even though patient attenuation may be 90%, it is completely ignored in calculating barrier re-

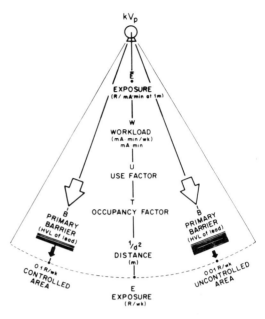

Figure 26–2 Summary of factors involved in primary barrier determinations

quirements. The x-ray energy used for protection calculations is the maximum voltage (kVp) of the generator, even though the machine will frequently be operated at lower potentials. No distinction is made between single- and three-phase generators.

Step 1. The **workload (W)** is the quantity of x rays generated per week. It is the product of tube current in mA and time in minutes of exposure per week (mA · min/wk). For example, if a 125-kVp chest room is being designed to handle 12 patients/hour, the workload is calculated by multiplying the mAs per exposure times the number of exposures per week and then dividing by 60 to convert seconds into minutes. At 125 kVp, we will estimate 2 mAs for a PA and 8 mAs for a lateral film (i.e., 10 mAs/patient):

$$\frac{mAs}{pt} \times \frac{pts}{hr} \times \frac{hr}{wk} = mAs/wk$$
$$10 \times 12 \times 40 = 4800 \text{ mAs/wk}$$

To convert mAs to mA · min, we simply divide by 60:

$$4800 \div 60 = 80 \text{ mA} \cdot \text{min/wk}$$

The workload recommended by the NCRP can be used when more specific information is not available. Their recommendations are given in Table 26–6.[4] The recommendations for our 125-kVp chest room is 400 mA · min/wk, which is five times the 80 mA · min/wk that we calculated. The NCRP recommendations provide a generous margin for error, which is the goal of radiation protection policies. Note in the table that the workload diminishes as energy increases. The workload for a radiographic room is 1000 mA · min/wk at 100 kVp and only 200 mA · min/wk at 150 kVp. The recommended workload is diminished because fewer mAs are required to expose a film at the higher kVp. Patient handling limits the number of procedures that can be accomplished in a day. Therefore, the recommended workloads in Table 26–6 are all considered equal. This may not seem logical, but it makes good sense. A room can only handle a certain number of patients a day. It takes approximately the same number of milliroentgens to expose a film at 100 kVp as it does at 150 kVp. When the kVp is raised, the mAs can be lowered and the net mR output stays about the same.

Step 2. Because the recommendations regarding maximal permissible dose are all given in Roentgens, we must have a way of converting workload into Roentgens. The customary way of expressing exposures is in terms of **Roentgens/mA · min at a distance of 1 m** from the x-ray source. Table

26–7 shows the x-ray output for various x-ray energies.[7] This exposure is multiplied by the workload to determine the total Roentgen output per week. For example, at a maximum energy of 100 kVp with a workload of 1000 mA · min/wk, Table 26–7 shows an exposure of 0.9 R/mA · min at 1 m. This is a weekly exposure of (1000 mA · min/wk × 0.9 R/mA · min) 900 R/wk at 1 m. The inverse square law is used to determine the exposure at other distances. Note that the exposure per mA · min increases with increasing kVp, and this compensates for the lower workload recommendation described in the previous section.

Step 3. The **use factor (U),** which should really be called the **beam direction factor,** is the fraction of time that the beam is directed at a particular barrier. If it is anticipated that the beam will only be directed at a wall 10% of the time, then U is 0.1. If a wall holds a fixed film changer for chest radiography, where the direction of the beam cannot be changed, then U for that particular wall is 1.0; all other walls are secondary barriers. When specific information is not available, recommended use factors can be obtained from Table 26–8.[4] U for ceilings is always zero, because the

Table 26–7. X-Ray Output in R per mA·min at 1 m ($\bar{E}$) for Various Energies

PEAK KILOVOLTAGE (kVp)	$\bar{E}$ (R/mA · min at 1 m)
50	0.15
70	0.40
100	0.90
125	1.4
150	2.0

Table 26–6. Recommended Workloads for Radiographic and Fluoroscopic Installations

MAXIMUM ENERGY (kVp)	WORKLOAD (mA · min/wk)	
	RADIOGRAPHIC ROOM	FLUOROSCOPIC ROOM
100	1000	1500
125	400	600
150	200	300

Table 26–8. Use Factors for Diagnostic Exposure Rooms

	USEFUL BEAM (Primary Barrier)	STRAY RADIATION* (Secondary Barrier)
Floor	1	1
Walls	1/16	1
Ceiling	0	1

*Stray radiation is the sum of leakage and scatter radiation

beam is rarely directed at the ceiling. **U for secondary barriers is always 1,** because the entire room is exposed to stray radiation whenever the x-ray beam is turned on.

Step 4. The **occupancy factor (T)** is the fraction that the workload should be decreased to correct for the degree of occupancy of the area in question. It has the same basis as U, and is expressed as a fraction that represents the amount of time that the area will be occupied. If the floor of an exposure room is in the basement of a hospital, and no subbasement will ever be constructed, then the floor's T is 0, and it is neither a primary nor a secondary barrier. The following list shows recommended occupancy factors for various areas for nonoccupationally exposed persons when more specific information is not available:[4]

Full occupancy (T = 1): Areas that will be occupied by the same individuals for their full work day, such as offices, laboratories, and nurses stations.

Partial occupancy (T = 1/4): includes corridors, restrooms, and elevators using operators.

Occasional occupancy (T = 1/16): includes waiting rooms, stairways, unattended elevators, janitor closets, and outside areas used for pedestrian and vehicular traffic.

If the area in question is **a controlled area** (i.e., within the x-ray department), it **is assigned an occupancy factor of one.** A radiation worker may spend only a small amount of time in any particular area, but wherever he goes in the department, he will be in a position of potential exposure, so all areas are assumed to be continuously occupied. Therefore, the occupancy factors listed above are only for areas occupied by nonoccupationally exposed individuals.

Step 5. Distance (d) is one of the most effective means of radiation protection, because exposures change inversely with the square of the distance (the inverse square law). Distances are measured in meters to

be consistent with the units used in Table 26–7. If an exposure is 2 R at 1 m, then at 4 m it will be

$$2R \times \frac{1}{4^2} = 0.13R$$

It is usually assumed that an individual will be at least 1 ft from a barrier for distance measurements. Some radiation is absorbed in air, but with energies over 50 kVp and distances less than 100 ft, the amount is negligible, and it is ignored.

The product of the factors described in steps 1 through 5 gives the "effective" weekly exposure to any particular point. The term "effective" is used here to emphasize that the actual exposure may be different, depending on the occupancy factor:

$$E = \bar{E}WUT \times \frac{1}{d^2}$$

E = weekly exposure reaching the point in question (R/wk)
$\bar{E}$ = R/mA · min at 1 m
W = workload (mA · min/wk)
U = use factor (no units)
T = occupancy factor (no units)
d = distance in meters from the x-ray tube to the point in question

The categories of protected areas were discussed earlier ("Dose-Limiting Recommendations"). Two types of areas require protection, those occupied by occupationally exposed individuals and those occupied by persons only occasionally exposed. The recommendations are 5 rem/year for the occupationally exposed and 0.5 rem/year for the occasionally exposed. Dividing by a 50-wk work year, the weekly maximum permissible exposures are 0.1 R for occupationally occupied and only 0.01 R for occasionally occupied areas. After an area has been assigned to a category, its weekly exposure must be kept below recommended levels. If the total exposure (E) at the point in question is less than 0.1 R/wk for a controlled area, or 0.01 R/wk for an uncontrolled area, no barrier is required. If E is greater than these maximal permissible exposures, then a protective barrier is required. Calculation of its thickness is discussed next.

Methods for Calculating Primary Barrier Thickness

Having determined the amount of radiation reaching the area in question, we must reduce this exposure to an acceptable level that depends on the category of the area. This is accomplished by interposing a barrier of either lead or concrete. Two methods are commonly used to calculate barrier requirements for diagnostic installations: (1) half-value layers (HVL), and (2) precalculated shielding requirement tables. A third method, employing attenuation curves, is commonly used for therapy installations. The attenuation curves are difficult to read at diagnostic exposure levels and are rarely used by physicists, so we will not bother describing the method.

Half-Value Layers (HVL)

The first method for calculating barrier requirements, and the simplest to understand, is with half-value layers (HVL). The concept of HVL was first used in radiation therapy to express the quality of an x-ray beam. **The half-value layer is the thickness of a specific substance that, when introduced into the path of a beam of radiation, reduces the exposure rate by one half.** A beam with a HVL of 0.2 mm of lead is more penetrating than a beam with a HVL of 0.1 mm of lead. HVLs in millimeters of lead and inches of concrete are given in Table 26–9.[4] Barrier thickness is calculated by repetitively halving the exposure until it reaches a permissible level, and then multiplying the number of halves times the HVL of the beam. For example, if the actual exposure at some point is 3.2 R/wk, and the permissible exposure 0.1

Table 26–9. Half-Value Layer (HVL) Thicknesses of Lead and Concrete for Various X-Ray Energies[4]

PEAK KILOVOLTAGE (kVp)	LEAD (mm)	CONCRETE (in.)
50	0.05	0.17
70	0.15	0.33
100	0.24	0.6
125	0.27	0.8
150	0.29	0.88

R/wk, the required number of HVLs is determined as follows:

$$3.2 \div 2 = 1.6$$
$$1.6 \div 2 = 0.8$$
$$0.8 \div 2 = 0.4$$
$$0.4 \div 2 = 0.2$$
$$0.2 \div 2 = 0.1$$

Five HVLs reduces 3.2 R/wk down to 0.1 R/wk. If the HVL of the beam were 0.25 mm of lead, the barrier would be

$$0.25 \times 5 = 1.25 \text{ mm of lead}$$

A problem arises in using half value layers with heterochromatic radiation. Remember, filtration changes the quality of a diagnostic beam as it passes through a barrier. The beam increases in mean energy, or is hardened, so if we use its initial HVL we could underestimate barrier requirements.

Table 26–10 explains how this problem arises. We start with a 150-kVp heterochromatic beam with a mean energy of 50 keV, a HVL of 0.29 mm of lead, and a hypothetical 100 R/wk from the beam. These are the characteristics of the beam as it emerges from the x-ray tube. It has already been filtered by both inherent and added filtration. To reduce the intensity to 50 R, we place 0.29 mm (1 HVL) of lead at point A. The 0.29 mm of lead further filters the radiation, increases its mean energy from 50 to 57 keV, and therefore increases its HVL. Now we must place 0.32 mm of lead at point B to reduce intensity by one half. In the example given, it is as-

Table 26–10. Filtration Changes the Quality of a Diagnostic X-Ray Beam

		0.29 mm Pb	+	0.32 mm Pb	+	0.34 mm Pb	=	0.95 mm Pb
		A		B		C		P
Peak Energy (kVp)	150		150		150			150
Mean Energy (keV)	50		57		63			66
HVL (mm lead)	0.29		0.32		0.34			0.35
R in beam*	100		50		25			12.5

*Assumes no reduction in intensity from the inverse square law; that is, the distance between points A, B, and C is zero.

sumed that there is no intensity loss from inverse square. As we continue adding newly determined HVLs to reduce intensity to 12.5 R at point P in the table, we change the mean energy from 50 to 66 keV and the HVL of the beam from 0.29 to 0.35 mm of lead, 0.06 mm more than its initial thickness. Summing the three HVLs placed at points A, B, and C shows that 0.95 mm of lead is required to reduce the intensity at point P to 12.5 R. If we had assumed that three of the original HVLs would have accomplished this objective, we would have underestimated the barrier, because 0.29 × 3 is only 0.87, which is 0.08 mm less than that actually required. The error is not significant, however, if the original HVL is for an already hardened beam. The numbers given in Table 26–10 are for such a beam. In other words, the radiation has been passed through numerous HVLs, and the last one is used to express beam quality.

Precalculated Shielding Requirement Tables

Most physicists use precalculated tables such as Table 26–11 to determine barrier requirements for diagnostic installations.[4] The tables are easy to use because the inverse square effect and barrier thicknesses are precalculated. All that needs to be done is to determine the effective workload by multiplying the actual workload (W) by the use factor (U) and occupancy factor (T).

The effective workload is still in mA · min/wk, because the use and occupancy factors have no units. Knowing the kVp and distance, the table indicates primary and secondary barrier requirements in both lead and concrete. For example, to determine the barrier requirements at 10 feet for a busy 100-kVp radiographic room with a workload of 1000 mA · min/wk with the use and occupancy factors both 0.25, we would multiply the workload by the use and occupancy factors:

$$W \cdot U \cdot T = mA \cdot min/wk$$
$$1000 \cdot 0.25 \cdot 0.25 = 62.5$$

We then go to Table 26–11 and find 62.5 mA · min/wk in the 100-kVp column. Moving to the right to a distance of 10 ft, we find primary barrier requirements of 0.5 mm of lead for a controlled and 1.25 mm for an uncontrolled area. In the same column we can find barrier requirements in concrete and also secondary barrier thicknesses. All this is accomplished with little mathematical manipulation, which explains the popularity of the tables.

Secondary Barriers

Secondary barriers provide protection from scatter and leakage radiation, which we will lump together and call stray radiation. As a general rule, **no secondary barrier is required for areas protected by a primary barrier;** that is, the primary serves as both a primary and secondary barrier.

Table 26–11. Shielding Requirements for Radiographic Installations[4]

WUT* in mA·min/week			DISTANCE IN FEET FROM SOURCE (X-RAY TUBE TARGET) TO OCCUPIED AREA									
100 kVp	125 kVp	150 kVp										
1000	400	200	5	7	10	14	20	28	40			
500	200	100		5	7	10	14	20	28	40		
250	100	50			5	7	10	14	20	28	40	
125	50	25				5	7	10	14	20	28	40
62.5	25	12.5					5	7	10	14	20	28
TYPE OF AREA	**MATERIAL**		**PRIMARY PROTECTIVE BARRIER THICKNESS**									
Controlled	Lead, mm		1.9	1.65	1.4	1.2	1.0	0.75	0.5	0.3	0	0
Noncontrolled	Lead, mm		2.65	2.4	2.2	1.95	1.7	1.5	1.25	1.0	0.8	0.5
Controlled	Concrete, inch		5.9	5.2	4.6	4.0	3.3	2.7	2.1	1.6	1.0	0.4
Noncontrolled	Concrete, inch		8.0	7.3	6.7	6.0	5.4	4.8	4.1	3.5	2.9	2.2
			SECONDARY PROTECTIVE BARRIER THICKNESS									
Controlled	Lead, mm		0.55	0.4	0.2	0.1	0	0	0	0	0	0
Noncontrolled	Lead, mm		1.2	1.0	0.8	0.6	0.45	0.25	0.1	0	0	0
Controlled	Concrete, inch		1.9	1.4	0.8	0.2	0	0	0	0	0	0
Noncontrolled	Concrete, inch		3.8	3.2	2.6	2.1	1.5	1.0	0.4	0	0	0

*W—workload in mA· min/week, U—use factor, T—occupancy factor.

All the factors that played a role in calculating barriers for the useful beam will have to be reconsidered in determining secondary barriers, except for U. U is really a beam direction factor and, because stray radiation goes in all directions, U is always 1.

Protection From Scatter Radiation

To determine primary barrier thickness, we make numerous estimates and allow a generous margin for error. Secondary barrier calculations are even less precise. The two most important factors, the intensity and energy of the scatter radiation, are both unknown. Therefore, before we can go any further, we must make two assumptions.

First, the energy of the scatter radiation is assumed to be equal to that of the primary radiation (provided the primary is less than 500 kVp). This assumption is reasonably accurate, especially below 100 kVp, where little energy is lost in Compton scattering, and where the secondary beam is hardened (its mean energy increased) by passing through the patient. If the assumption errs, it errs on the side of conservatism.

Second, the intensity of 90° scatter radiation, relative to the primary beam, is reduced by a factor of 1000 at a distance of 1 m for a field size of 400 cm². The 1-m distance is measured from the center of the beam on the patient's surface. When radiation can be forced to scatter more than once, for example with a maze, its intensity is reduced to inconsequential levels, well below permissible exposures, so we will not concern ourselves with multiple scatterings.

Field size is one factor that controls scatter radiation, so it is not surprising that it plays a role in determining secondary barrier requirements. The other two factors that control scattering, peak kilovoltage and patient thickness, are ignored. Field size is measured at the patient's surface. A correction factor is used for fields other than 400 cm².

$$\text{Correction factor} = \frac{F}{400}$$

$$F = \text{actual field size (cm}^2\text{)}$$
$$400 = \text{control field size (cm}^2\text{)}$$

The correction factor has no units, because both F and 400 are in square centimeters, and they cancel each other. For fields smaller than 400 cm², the correction factor is less than 1; for larger fields, it is greater than 1. For example, with 200 cm², the correction factor is

$$\text{Correction factor} = \frac{200}{400} = 0.5$$

The Roentgen output of the x-ray tube (exposure in R/mA · min at 1 m; i.e., $\bar{E}$), workload (W), and occupancy factor (T), are the same as they were for the primary barrier calculations. Inverse square attenuation is also the same except that the distance is measured from the center of the patient rather than from the center of the x-ray tube. The use factor is dropped because it is always 1. A correction factor is added for field size, and the total exposure is divided by 1000 for right angle scattering:

$$E_s = \bar{E}WT \times \frac{1}{d^2} \times \frac{1}{1000} \times \frac{F}{400}$$

E_s = weekly exposure from scatter radiation (R/wk)
$\bar{E}$ = R/mA · min at 1 m
W = workload (mA · min/wk)
T = occupancy factor (no units)
d = distance (in meters from the center of the beam on the patient's surface)
F = actual field size (cm²)

The weekly exposure is then handled in the same manner as for primary barrier calculations. Exposures are reduced to permissible levels by one of the two previously described methods (i.e., HVLs or precalculated tables).

Protection From Leakage Radiation

Leakage radiation is radiation that passes through the lead shielding in the tube housing when the beam is turned on. By law, the **maximum permissible leakage exposure 1 meter from a diagnostic x-ray tube is 0.1 R/hour** with the tube operating continuously at its maximum kVp and mA. This does not mean the maximum mA that the tube is capable of generating, but rather the maximum mA at which the tube can be run continuously without overheating. The tube may be rated at 150 kVp and

1000 mA, but it cannot be operated continuously at this level. At 150 kVp, its maximum mA will probably be around 500 mA, and it will only tolerate that for a few milliseconds. The maximum mA at which the tube can be run continuously must be determined from anode heat cooling charts. Figure 26–3 shows a cooling chart for a Dynamax "69" tube. The maximum continuous mA is the maximum amount of heat per second (1400 heat units in this case), divided by the peak voltage, which may be from 100 to 150 kVp. At 150 kVp, the maximum continuous mA would be

$$1400 \div 150 = 9.3 \text{ mA}$$

The Dynamax "69" is a large tube. Smaller tubes have maximum continuous loads of 3 to 5 mA. The manufacturer must build the housing to limit exposure to 0.1 R/hour at 1 meter with the tube operating at peak potential, and the highest mA that does not exceed the housing's ability to dissipate heat.

In calculating exposures from primary and scatter radiation, we could look up the Roentgen output at 1 meter ($\bar{E}$) for each mA of workload. Both the exposure and workload involve the primary beam. For leakage radiation, we need a comparable unit of exposure (i.e., R/mA · min at 1 m), but the "mA · min" refers to the useful beam and the "R at 1 meter" to the leakage radiation. Leakage occurs whenever the x-ray beam is "on." It is completely independent of the useful beam itself, and will occur even if the collimator shutter is completely closed. As long as x rays are being generated within the tube housing, leakage radiation occurs.

Figure 26–4 shows the relationship between the workload of the primary beam and the permissible leakage level of 0.1 R/hour. In the illustration, 5 mA is given as the maximum continuous current that the tube can tolerate. If the tube runs at this level for only 1 sec, the exposure is 5 mAs, which is the unit technicians use to describe radiographic techniques. To be consistent

ANODE THERMAL CHARACTERISTICS

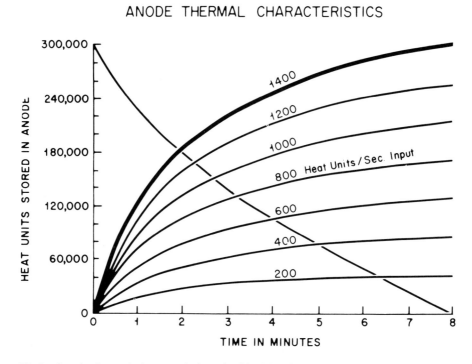

Figure 26–3 Anode thermal characteristics of a Machlett Dynamax "69" x-ray tube

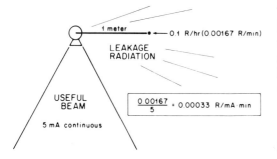

Figure 26–4 Maximum permissible leakage exposure at 1 m in R/mA · min with a maximum continuous exposure of 5 mA

with our previous methods, however, we will continue using the unit mA · min, which is the number of mA multiplied by the "on" time in minutes. Thus, in 1 minute of continuous operation, the output will be 5 mA · min. The leakage exposure is 0.1 R/hour at a distance of 1 meter from the x-ray tube. To convert to R/min, we simply divide by 60:

$$0.1 \text{ R/hr} \div 60 \text{ min/hr} = 0.00167 \text{ R/min}$$

This is the leakage exposure that results from the tube being "on" for 1 minute. The workload of the primary beam for the same minute was 5 mA · min. To determine the leakage exposure at 1 meter for each 1 mA · min of workload, we must divide by 5:

$$\frac{0.00167 \text{ R/min}}{5 \text{ mA} \cdot \text{min/min}} = 0.00033 \text{ R/mA} \cdot \text{min at 1 m } (\overline{E}_L)$$

Now that we have determined the exposure in R/mA · min at 1 m ($\overline{E}_L$), it is easy to calculate the exposure at some other point. We multiply the number of R/mA · min by the workload, occupancy factor, and inverse square of distance, as we did for primary and scatter exposure calculations:

$$E_L = \overline{E}_L WT \times \frac{1}{d^2}$$

E_L = weekly exposure from leakage radiation (R/wk)

$\overline{E}_L$ = leakage exposure at 1 m per mA · min of workload (R/mA · min)

W = workload (mA · min/wk)

T = occupancy factor (no units)

d = distance from x-ray tube in meters

The customary method for reducing leakage exposures to permissible levels is with HVLs of barrier. Leakage radiation is already heavily filtered by the lead in the tube housing, so the half-value method is quite accurate.

There is one last "rule of thumb" regarding radiation protection. If the difference between the barrier requirements for scatter and leakage radiation is greater than three half-value layers, use the large one and ignore the smaller one; if less than three half-value layers, add one half-value layer to the larger and ignore the smaller. For diagnostic installations, however, this rule is relatively meaningless. Leakage exposures are almost always within the permissible range without any barrier. Even more important, the walls of diagnostic rooms are almost always planned as primary barriers, and they provide ample protection from stray radiation.

Example

Figure 26–5 shows a general radiographic room with an upright Bucky mounted on the wall protecting area C. The generator, a three-phase unit, is rated at 125 kVp and 600 mA. We will calculate barrier requirements for areas A, B, and C, where A is a radiologist's office, B is the floor above a basement pathology laboratory, and C is a restroom. The distances from the points in question to the x-ray tube are given in the illustration, and note that the points are 1 foot from the wall, which is the NCRP recommendation.[4] We will assume that the x-ray tube is never directed at area A.

Because we do not know how many patients will be done in an 8-hour shift, we will accept the NCRP recommendation for a busy general radiographic room of 400 mA · min/wk for a 125-kVp installation. Then we need not concern ourselves with the generator's mA capacity, and, of course, single- and three-phase units are treated in the same way. We can look up the occupancy factors, use factors, and Roentgen output at 1 m in the appropriate tables. Because the beam is never directed at area A, its use factor as a primary barrier is 0, and it will only require a secondary barrier. In actual practice, it would be better to provide a primary barrier for area A so that the room's function could be changed at a later date without the need for additional protection. We will return to area A when we discuss secondary barriers. The use factor for point B, the pathology

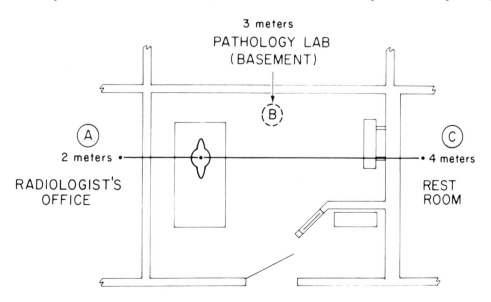

Figure 26–5 Floor plan of the general radiographic room described in the example

laboratory, is 1 because it is a floor, and the use factor for a floor is always 1 (Table 26–8). The table shows a use factor of 1/16 for walls, but a large number of upright chest examinations are anticipated, so we will use a use factor of 1/4 and not follow the NCRP recommendations. The occupancy factors are 1/4 for the restroom and 1 for the pathology laboratory. We will calculate primary barriers first, and in this example we will use both methods to determine barrier thickness.

Primary Barriers

Precalculated Tables. We will start with the table method, because it requires the least mathematics. To use the method, we must find the product of the workload (W), use factor (U), and occupancy factor (T):

$$
\begin{array}{cccccc}
 & W & \cdot & U & \cdot & T & = mA \cdot min/wk \\
\text{Point B:} & 400 & \cdot & 1 & \cdot & 1 & = 400 \\
\text{Point C:} & 400 & \cdot & \frac{1}{4} & \cdot & \frac{1}{4} & = 25 \\
\end{array}
$$

We can look up barrier requirements for points B and C in Table 26–11, but we have a bit of a problem, because the distances in the table are given in feet and our distances are in meters. One meter equals 39.37 inches, or approximately 3.25 feet. Converting from meters to feet, we get

Point B: 3 × 3.25 = 10 ft
Point C: 4 × 3.25 = 13 ft

To look up the barrier thickness for point B in Table 26–11, we find 125 kVp and 400 mA · min/wk at a distance of 10 ft. Both the pathology laboratory and restroom are uncontrolled areas. The primary barrier thickness is 2.2 mm of sheet lead, or 6.7 inches of concrete, for an uncontrolled area. Because B is in a basement, we would simply make sure that the concrete floor is at least 6.7 inches thick. Point C is done similarly, but 13 feet is not shown in the table so we have to extrapolate between 10 and 14 feet. At 25 mA · min/wk, a lead thickness between 1.25 and 1.0 mm, say 1.20 mm, would be needed for an uncontrolled area. No secondary barrier

would be required for these walls, because the primary barrier would provide ample protection from stray radiation.

Half-Value Layers. To use HVLs, we must calculate the potential exposure at the points in question. The Roentgen output at 1 m ($\overline{E}$) is 1.4 R/mA · min (Table 26–7):

$$
\begin{array}{ccccccccc}
 & E = & \overline{E} & \cdot & W & \cdot & U & \cdot & T & \cdot & 1/d^2 \\
\text{Point B:} & E = & 1.4 & \cdot & 400 & \cdot & 1 & \cdot & 1 & \cdot & \frac{1}{3^2} & = 62 \\
\text{Point C:} & E = & 1.4 & \cdot & 400 & \cdot & \frac{1}{4} & \cdot & \frac{1}{4} & \cdot & \frac{1}{4^2} & = 0.154 \\
\end{array}
$$

The pathology laboratory and restroom are both uncontrolled areas with maximum permissible exposure levels of 0.01 R/wk. The exposures to both points are excessive (i.e., above permissible levels), so our next step is to determine the number of HVLs required to reduce them to permissible levels.

Point B:	Exposure	— HVLs
	62 R/wk	— 0
	31	— 1
	15.5	— 2
	7.75	— 3
	3.88	— 4
	1.94	— 5
	0.97	— 6
	0.48	— 7
	0.24	— 8
	0.12	— 9
	0.06	— 10
	0.03	— 11
	0.015	— 12
	0.01	— approx. 12.6 HVLs
	0.007	— 13

If the number of half-value layers does not come out evenly, we can extrapolate as we did above, but it is simpler to use the whole number that reduces exposures below the permissible level (13 in this case), a practice that errs on the side of conservatism. Table 26–9 shows the HVL for 125 kVp to be 0.27 mm for lead and 0.8 inches for concrete. We multiply these values by the 12.6 HVLs required to attenuate the beam to permissible levels:

Lead:	0.27 × 12.6 = 3.4 mm
Concrete:	0.8 × 12.6 = 10 in.

Because B is the floor, we would probably use the 10 inches of concrete. Following the same procedure for point C:

Point C: Exposure — HVLs
               0.14 R/wk — 0
               0.07   — 1
               0.35   — 2
               0.17   — 3
               0.10   — approx. 3.3 HVLs
               0.085   — 4

Lead: 0.27 × 3.3 = 0.89 mm
Concrete: 0.8 × 3.3 = 2.6 in.

The barrier thicknesses are different for the two methods (tables and HVLs), but this is not important because our purpose here is to explain principles. Also, the differences emphasize the fact that radiation protection is not a precise science.

Secondary Barriers

Wall A protects a radiologist's office and will require a secondary barrier. It is a controlled area with a maximum permissible exposure of 0.1 R/wk, and because it is a controlled area, its occupancy factor is 1. For convenience, we will calculate the exposures for both leakage and scatter radiation at a distance of 2 meters as shown in Figure 26–5.

Precalculated Tables. Table 26–11 gives both primary and secondary barrier requirements. We simply multiply the workload (W), use (U), and occupancy (T) factors (WUT), and find the barrier thickness for the appropriate distance:

W   · U · T   = mA · min/wk
400 · 1 · 1   = 400 mA · min/wk

Converting the distance of 2 meters into feet, we get a little over 6 feet. At 125 kVp, the secondary barrier thickness for a controlled area (Table 26–11) is 0.55 mm of lead for 5 feet and 0.40 mm for 7 feet. We will need a thickness between these two, say 0.5 mm, and this would handle both the leakage and scatter radiation. In other words, we would be finished. But we will go on to make the calculations for scatter and leakage radiation separately using half-value layers.

Half-Value Layer Method for Scatter Radiation. The workload will be the same as it was for the primary barrier: 400 mA

· min/wk at 125 kVp. The occupancy factor is 1 because it is a controlled area. The exposure is 1.4 R/mA · min (Table 26–7). This exposure is at 1 meter, which we will assume is the patient's surface. This is a reasonably accurate assumption because most films are taken from a distance of 40 inches. We will estimate an average field size of 14 × 14 in. (196 in.^{2}). There are approximately 6.5 cm^2/in.^{2} (2.54 × 2.54 cm), so our field will be 1270 cm^2 (6.5 cm^2/in.^{2} × 196 in.^{2}). We will also assume one right angle scattering:

$$E_s = \overline{E} \cdot W \cdot T \cdot 1/d^2 \cdot 1/1000 \cdot F/400$$
$$E_s = 1.4 \cdot 400 \cdot 1 \cdot 1/2^2 \cdot 1/1000 \cdot 1270/400$$

$$E_s = 0.45 \text{ R/wk}$$

Using the HVL method to reduce this exposure to the permissible level of 0.1 R/wk:

The HVL at 125 kVp (Table 26–9) is 0.27 mm
of lead and 0.8 inch of concrete.

Point A: Exposure — HVLs
               0.45 R/wk — 0
               0.225   — 1
               0.113   — 2
               0.10   — 2.3 HVLs
               0.056   — 3

Lead: 0.27 × 2.3 = 0.62 mm
Concrete: 0.8 × 2.3 = 1.8 in.

Half-Value Layer Method for Leakage Radiation. We will assume that 6 mA is the maximum continuous exposure the tube will tolerate without overheating. To determine the R/mA · min ($\overline{E}_L$), we divide the 0.1 R/hour permissible leakage exposure by 60 min/hour and 6 mA · min/min:

$$(0.1 \div 60) \div 6 = 0.00028 \text{ R/mA} \cdot \text{min}$$

The weekly leakage exposure at point A will be

$$E_L = \overline{E}_L \cdot W \cdot T \cdot 1/d^2$$
$$E_L = 0.00028 \cdot 400 \cdot 1 \cdot \tfrac{1}{2}^2 = 0.028 \text{ R/wk}$$

An exposure of 0.028 R/wk is less than the permissible level for a controlled area, so no barrier is required for leakage radiation. The total secondary barrier would be the 0.62 mm of lead required for scatter radiation.

SHIELDING REQUIREMENTS FOR RADIOGRAPHIC FILM

A secondary objective of radiation protection is "to prevent damage or impairment of function of radio-sensitive film or equipment."[4] We will limit our discussion to x-ray film. "An exposure of 1 milliroentgen (mR) over a portion of a film may produce undesirable shadows."[4] For protection purposes, an exposure of 0.2 mR is considered safe. This is the maximum permissible exposure that the film should receive during its entire storage life. We (radiologists) think more of our films than we do of ourselves. The maximum permissible exposure for film is only 0.2 mR as compared to 100 mR/week for ourselves, 500 times as much, and this assumes that the film will only be stored for one week.

Protective barrier calculations for film are exactly the same as those for controlled and uncontrolled areas, with one exception. The permissible exposure for the film varies with storage life. For one week of storage, the customary time interval for protection calculations, the permissible level is 0.2 mR. For monthly storage (4 weeks), the film is only permitted a weekly exposure of 0.05 mR (0.2 mR ÷ 4 weeks). The number of HVLs of lead and concrete must be sufficient to bring exposures to the appropriate level. Barrier thicknesses can also be determined from a table similar to Table 26–11.[4]

SUMMARY

Man has lived with, and tolerated, natural radiation since the beginning of time. Evidence is accumulating, however, that small doses of radiation can cause both mutations and neoplasms. No one knows just how much radiation is tolerable, but it is clear that the genetically significant dose has been increasing from man-made sources. The National Council on Radiation Protection's recommendations are designed to protect both the general public and radiation worker. Many of the recommendations have been turned into laws.

The most important recommendations are those involving maximum permissible doses, which are currently 5 rem/year for a radiation worker and 0.5 rem/year for the occasionally exposed individual. These levels are broken down into weekly permissible exposures of 0.1 R/wk for controlled areas occupied by radiation workers and 0.01 R/wk for uncontrolled areas occupied by the occasionally exposed individuals. Three modalities are available to reduce radiation exposures: time, distance, and barriers. Time plays its role in three ways: in the amount of time that the machine is turned "on" at a particular current, expressed as mA · min/wk, and called the workload; in the amount of time that the beam is directed at a particular area, called the use factor; and in the amount of time that an area is occupied, the occupancy factor. Distance attenuates the beam by the familiar inverse square law. If time and distance fail to bring exposures to permissible levels, then the third method, a barrier, is required. Barriers are usually constructed of either sheet lead or concrete, depending on which is cheaper.

Protection must be provided against three types of radiation: the primary, or useful beam; scatter radiation; and leakage radiation. The latter two together are called stray radiation. If the useful beam can be directed at a wall, the wall must be a primary barrier. If the useful beam cannot be directed at a wall, it is a secondary barrier and need only protect from stray radiation. Primary barriers serve a dual function as both primary and secondary barriers.

The exposure from the primary beam can be calculated by multiplying the workload, use factor, occupancy factor, and inverse square of the distance by an R output at 1 meter for each mA of workload. If this exposure, expressed in R/wk, exceeds permissible levels, then a barrier is required. Barrier thicknesses can be calculated in two ways: 1) with precalculated tables or 2) with HVLs of lead or concrete. A secondary barrier protects against stray radiation and is only required when the useful beam cannot be directed at a particular wall. Secondary barriers protect against scatter and leakage radiation. For scatter radiation, the exposure is assumed to be attenuated by a factor of 1000 (i.e., reduced to 0.001 at a distance of 1 m for each right angle scattering), and it is also assumed that its quality does not change. A correction factor is added for field size and the use factor is always 1, because scatter and leakage radiation go in all directions. Otherwise, the calculation is the same as for the primary beam. The R output at 1 meter for each mA · min of workload is multiplied by the workload, occupancy factor, and inverse square of the distance, a conversion factor for field size, and 0.001 for a right angle scattering.

The exposure from leakage is based on the law that the maximum radiation level at 1 meter is 0.1 R/hour, or 0.00167 R/min. This exposure must be converted to R/mA · min. The maximum operating mA for continuous exposure at maximum kVp is determined from anode heat rating charts, and it is usually about 5 mA. The conversion to R/mA · min is accomplished by dividing the 0.00167 R/min by the maximum continuous mA. This exposure at 1 meter is multiplied by the occupancy factor and inverse square of distance to determine the leakage exposure at the point in question. If the barrier requirements for scatter and leakage differ by more than 3 HVLs, the larger suffices; if less than 3 HVLs, add 1 HVL to the larger.

REFERENCES

1. Buschong, S.C.: The Development of Radiation Protection in Diagnostic Radiology. Cleveland, CRC Press, 1973.
2. Dalrymple, G.V., Gaulden, M.E., Kollmorgen, G.M., and Vogel, H.G., Jr.: Medical Radiation Biology. Philadelphia, W.B. Saunders, 1973.
3. Hall, E.J.: Radiobiology for the Radiologist. Hagerstown, MD, Harper & Row, 1973.
4. Medical X-Ray and Gamma-Ray Protection for Energies up to 10 MeV—Structural Shielding Design and Evaluation. Washington, D.C., National Council on Radiation Protection and Measurements, NCRP Report No. 49, 1976.
5. Basic Radiation Protection Criteria. Washington, D.C., National Council on Radiation Protection and Measurements: NCRP Report No. 39, 1971.
6. Pizzarello, D.J., and Witcofski, R.L.: Basic Radiation Biology. 2nd Ed. Philadelphia, Lea & Febiger, 1975.
7. Schultz, R.J.: Primer of Radiation Protection. 2nd Ed. New York, GAF Corporation. X-Ray Products Division, 1969.

27

Digital Radiography

The field of digital radiography has developed to its present state by the implementation of largely conventional radiographic techniques using digital electronic apparatus. No unfamiliar basic physics principles need to be introduced in describing the operation of digital radiographic systems currently in use. Most techniques (including intravenous injection for arteriography) have already been used with film-screen systems, so there is considerable common ground between digital radiography and the more familiar film-screen techniques. We will emphasize these sometimes striking similarities between digital radiography and more conventional radiography. In addition, the discussion of digital techniques offers an opportunity to demonstrate clearly some fundamental limits on radiographic imaging systems. The main topic remaining is an extension of the understanding of computer image manipulations as discussed for computed tomography (CT), without having to consider the complicated reconstruction mathematics. Finally, because there are so many promising areas for development in this field, we will take a brief look at some current research.

A DIGITAL FLUOROSCOPY SYSTEM

The most common type of digital radiography system at present is digital fluoroscopy (DF). Such a system can be used to demonstrate most digital radiography principles, so we will begin with a general

system description that will be of subsequent use. At the block diagram level, the design of a DF system can be considered to be a fairly conventional fluoroscopic unit, with an added digital image processing unit.

Fluoroscopy Unit

Figure 27–1 shows a fluoroscopic unit suitable for digital applications, and obviously it is only the block diagram of a conventional unit with several minor ad-

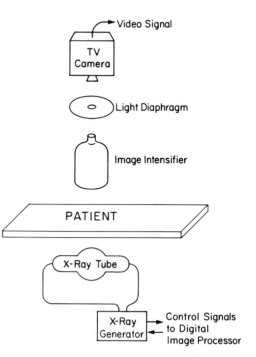

Figure 27–1 Block diagram of a fluoroscopic unit

ditions. Digital applications, however, place some special demands on a fluoroscopy unit.

Mask Subtraction Application

For instance, consider intravenous injection angiography, in which subtracted images are displayed on a 512 × 512 pixel matrix. We will call this technique mask subtraction. Currently it is the most commonly used technique in digital radiography, and it is one of the methods of performing digital subtraction angiography. **Digital subtraction angiography (DSA) is the generic term for any digital radiographic method of implementing subtraction angiography.** We will discuss several other methods later.

Mask subtraction is the DSA technique that most closely resembles film-screen angiography. The patient is prepared and a catheter is placed under fluoroscopic control. The patient is then injected, either intravenously or intra-arterially, with an x-ray contrast material that contains a high atomic number element such as iodine. Individual x-ray exposures are made at a typical rate of one exposure/sec or more. The exposure series begins before the contrast material is expected to arrive in the vessels of interest, and extends past the time when the contrast material is expected to have cleared the vessels. Each individual pulsed exposure forms a single image within the series. A precontrast mask and a contrast-containing image are roughly equivalent to an angiographic film pair. The subtraction of the mask image from the contrast-containing image is the basis of this mask subtraction technique. If a peripheral venous injection is used, the contrast material reaching the arteries is so diluted that only small attenuation differences exist between contrast- and non-contrast-filled arteries. The x-ray exposures needed for producing acceptable images in this situation are similar to those used for serial photospot camera images, or perhaps even higher.

A good x-ray generator and x-ray tube of conventional design are probably adequate for the mask subtraction procedure, but an excellent image intensifier is required, and the television system must be of higher quality than normally needed for routine fluoroscopy.

X-Ray Generator and X-Ray Tube

The principal function of the generator is to provide very repeatable exposures. **A small difference in the x-ray tube current or kilovoltage** supplied by the generator for two exposures in a series **will result in an improper mask subtraction** of the images of unchanged areas of the body. This improper subtraction may obscure the visualization of the actual structures of interest (such as opacified vessels), which have very small subject contrast differences on the two images. The digital image processing unit generally has some control over the generator. In the case of mask subtraction, this control can be limited to the initiation and termination of the individual exposures in a series. The generator connections required for this type of control are usually rather simple, and are similar to those needed for rapid film changers.

An x-ray tube similar in design to one that might be used in film angiography is appropriate for most DF applications. The primary beam magnification and x-ray tube loading parameters in typical digital angiographic procedures are quite similar to those encountered in film angiographic procedures, so specially designed x-ray tubes have not been found to be necessary as yet. In the specific application of the mask subtraction example, a 512- × 512-pixel image matrix was specified. This places resolution limitations on the final image that make the use of very small focal spots (such as those used in magnification radiography) unnecessary. We will discuss these resolution limitations shortly. In fact, very small focal spots are undesirable for this application because of the x-ray tube heat loading requirements.

Image Intensifier

A high quality image intensifier is needed for digital applications, but all the necessary image intensifier (II) characteristics are also desirable for some more conventional applications. **A very high contrast ratio is needed,** which mandates use of a recently designed II. In the case of our 512- × 512-pixel matrix, however, high spatial resolution is not needed for the II, so a thick input phosphor can be used for high x-ray detection efficiency. The power supply for the II must be quite stable, because small changes in accelerating potential for the electrons can produce changes in the brightness gain of the II. The power supply fluctuations are more likely to occur at radiographic tube current levels than at fluoroscopic tube current levels because of loading of the generator. The resulting change in II intensity might not be detectable in photospot or cine images, but two images from a digital series may not subtract properly.

Light Diaphragm

To this point, all components have been of a type that might be found in routine use for fluoroscopy or photospot imaging. For instance, we might have chosen a modern three-phase twelve-pulse generator, angiographic x-ray tube, and high-contrast II from those available for other uses. The selection of components that would not be part of the system were it not for our mask subtraction application begins with the light diaphragm.

The light diaphragm is used to control the amount of light from the II that reaches the TV camera tube, exactly as in the case of changing photographic f stops. In a typical procedure, the patient first undergoes some fluoroscopy with an x-ray tube current of about 2 mA at some given kVp. Subsequently, the patient undergoes a serial digital procedure in which 200 mA may be used to reduce quantum mottle. Let us choose light diaphragm sizes so that the amount of light reaching the TV camera

tube for a single television frame will be approximately the same in either the fluoroscopic or the serial portion of the study. If we do not make the right choice, we will either saturate the TV camera tube with light during our high mA serial exposures, or we will use only a small portion of the TV camera tube's range for display of fluoroscopic images. In this example we will collect a large fraction of the light from the II output phosphor for fluoroscopic images, and about 1% of that fraction for the serial images. In actuality, a combination of different sizes of light diaphragms and different electronic video gains may be employed. There is also some advantage in using a light diaphragm that is adjustable over a range for serial exposures, because this increases the flexibility of the system.

Television Image Chain

The second component which is of a type not normally found in fluoroscopic systems for nondigital use is **a special TV chain, one of the most critical components in the entire DF system.** The II tube absorbs a certain fraction of the incident x-ray photons and produces a quantity of light proportional to the number of incident x-ray photons. The basic function of the TV chain is to produce an electronic video signal from this light. The size of this signal should be directly proportional to the number of x-ray photons that exit the patient. Eventually this video signal will be fed to the digital image processing unit, where it will be digitized. At present, **a TV camera tube with a lead oxide vidicon target (plumbicon) is favored.** A plumbicon tube of this type has low lag and has a video output that is directly proportional to light input.

As noted in Chapter 17, a TV camera with high lag will produce a smeared ghost that follows a rapidly moving object on the TV image. A ghost is objectionable in any procedure. The most desirable type of TV camera tube (all other factors being equal) would be one in which the image on the input phosphor is completely erased during the readout of each frame. In the case of images for digital subtraction, a tube with excessive lag can cause a situation in which the "current" frame actually has residual information that properly belongs in the past. **A TV camera tube with low lag is desirable,** especially in dynamic studies in which rapid image changes are encountered.

Perhaps the most important property that **the TV chain must possess** is **extremely low electronic noise.** In fluoroscopy at 2 to 3 mA, there is so much quantum mottle in the image that relatively high electronic noise can be tolerated. As we shall see later, however, the combination of a much larger number of x-ray photons and working with subtracted images requires use of a different (and expensive) TV camera tube to avoid having electronic noise obscure low-contrast structures.

Television Scan Modes

Another feature that is sometimes desirable for digital fluoroscopy is a choice of television scan modes. Most television systems operate in an **interlaced mode.** In the United States, each 262.5-line field is scanned in 1/60 second, so that the entire 525-line frame is scanned in 1/30 second. This scan choice is adequate to avoid the perception of flicker, but it does have drawbacks for some digital applications. As normally employed, the TV tube scans continuously. When an x-ray exposure begins, first the generator and all other components must become stable, during which time the TV system continues to scan. In digital mask subtraction these stabilization frames must be discarded for several reasons. For instance, during the time the exposure is increasing, there would be no brightness in the first portion of the TV frame and considerable brightness in the last portion of the frame. This would produce objectionable flicker between the two fields of the frame and, for most of the frame, the TV camera tube would not be operating in its optimum brightness region. Another reason for discarding the early frames is the very severe demands that would be placed on all components. Each component would have to reach exactly the same operating point in the same amount of time for each exposure to ensure good subtraction. The net result of throwing away some TV frames is that the patient may be given some unnecessary x-ray exposure. There are a number of solutions to this particular problem, one of which is to change to a different x-ray exposure and TV scanning mode.

The pulsed progressive readout method involves two steps for obtaining a single TV frame image. First, TV camera scanning is halted and an exposure is made. Second, the TV camera target is operated in a **progressive scan mode,** which means that every line is read out in order, rather than in a field-interlaced fashion. Now we only need to ensure that each exposure in a series is reproducible. The exposure may be of any duration up to several seconds, and all the dose is used to form the image. Because this mode must allow time between frames for the exposures (and perhaps also for "scrubbing" any residual image off the camera target), framing rates are somewhat slower than in the interlaced mode. There is no reason why continuous progressive framing cannot be employed, but the same stabilization time penalty described for interlaced scanning will be applicable.

Another method of scanning the television target that would be unsatisfactory for real-time visual presentation is a **slow scan mode.** This method is currently being used for implementing fairly large (1024- × 1024-pixel) digital fluoroscopic matrices. Implementing a 1024 × 1024 matrix on a 1050-line television system running in interlaced mode at 30 frames per second would require an increase in the band width of the television system to four times that for a 525-line system (see Chap. 17 for an explanation of television band width).

If we do not insist on 30 frames per second, each TV line can be scanned twice as long as in the 525-line system (thus doubling horizontal resolution), and twice as many lines can be scanned (doubling vertical resolution) without increasing the video band width. This limits the framing rate (7.5 frames per second) to one fourth of "real time" (30 frames per second). There are two advantages over the 30-frame per second approach. First, the television chain electronics and the digitizer section can have the same band width as a 525-line system, which significantly simplifies system design. Second, **at high band width, electronic noise is significantly increased,** which is avoided by slow scan. Naturally, the television camera tube must be inherently capable of higher spatial resolution than that needed for a 525-line system. Also, there are some sources of electronic noise that are worse at the higher resolution and that are not helped by the use of slow scan techniques.

Digital Image Processor

A typical digital image processor for DF is shown in Figure 27–2. This block diagram is a functional one, because different image processor units may have different physical configurations. Therefore, unlike the fluoroscopic unit, we may not be able to indicate a particular component and say that it corresponds to a particular block of our diagram. Nevertheless, all DF image processors are intended to have the same basic functions, and the same basic principles apply. Their major functions are 1) digitizing TV frames and processing them into digital images, 2) storing the digital images for later recall, 3) displaying digital images on a TV monitor and photographing these images, and 4) manipulating digital images (e.g., averaging, subtracting, changing contrast scales).

Basic Operation

A rough description of the functions of the individual blocks in Figure 27–2 seems to be in order before discussing them individually in more detail. The central control computer is in charge of all the other components of the image processor (and, we hope, is absolutely subservient to us). Suppose we tell the computer to run a series of a certain number of exposures and

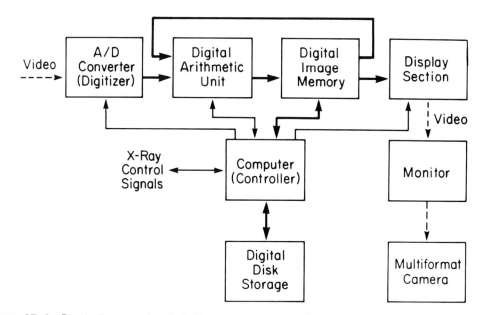

Figure 27–2 Block diagram of a digital image processor unit

to store each image of the series in digital form for later use. During the run the computer is to use the first image as a mask and is to display each subsequent image in subtracted form. We set exposure techniques on the generator and instruct the computer to begin. The computer informs the generator when to start and to stop each exposure. It sets up the digitizer (analog-to-digital converter) to convert an entire TV frame into a digital image, and starts the digitizer at the appropriate time. Meanwhile, the computer has instructed the arithmetic unit on what to do with the first digitized image, which is simply to place the image in appropriate form and to store it in a particular block of image memory. The computer tells the digital disc where that particular block is located in image memory, how big the image is, and when to start storing the image. Similar instructions are given to the display section.

To handle the second exposure, the control computer issues the same commands as before to all components except the arithmetic unit and display section. The arithmetic unit must handle the incoming digitized data, and stores this "raw" data in a block of image memory that the digital disk will access. Simultaneously, the arithmetic unit must access the previously stored first image (the mask), subtract the mask from the incoming second image, and store the result in a third block of image memory that the display section can access. The computer has already set the display section for contrast levels appropriate for subtracted images and has told the display section which block of image memory to show. For the third and subsequent exposures, the computer has no new tasks to perform. It only has to pay attention to coordinating the subordinate activities until the run is complete or until we abort the run from the generator.

Note that in our system the control computer only tells its subordinates what to do and coordinates their actions, a strictly managerial task. As previously indicated, the block diagram is functional rather than physical. The actual computer that is incorporated may be very primitive and without much control, so that the subordinates operate very much in a preset fashion. Conversely, the computer may be quite complex and take over most of the menial tasks from the subordinates. Both approaches have some merit. A complex general purpose computer can be very flexible and perform virtually any current or future task that may be required for digital fluoroscopy. Of course, an ingenious programmer may be required to implement the task. On the other hand, we shall see that high calculation speeds are required for even routine operations. A general purpose computer capable of such speeds can be very large and expensive. It makes sense to have less expensive specialized machine cretins that do very simply routine tasks at the required speeds, provided that the system as a whole is able to do the entire job. New applications may not be easily implemented, however, if the system is too inflexible. The present trend seems to be use of a flexible but not extremely fast general purpose computer for control and complex tasks, and use of a set of fairly flexible subordinate units for fast or more mundane work.

Analog-to-Digital Conversion

The analog-to-digital converter (ADC) converts the video images from the TV chain into digital form. Figure 27–3A is a photograph of a displayed video image of a skull. The format is a frame consisting of 525 TV lines from two interlaced fields. If we consider only one of the horizontal TV lines through the center of the image from the II, the electronic video signal that defines the line for the monitor will resemble that shown in Figure 27–3B. The video signal has a voltage that varies during the scan from left to right along the line. The voltage is initially low, indicating a dark region on the camera input face. The voltage then rises sharply in a brighter region, drops

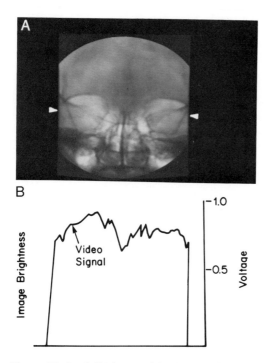

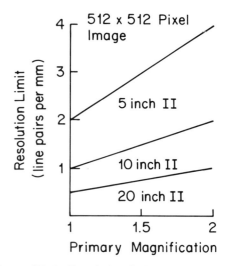

Figure 27–3 A TV frame of the image of a skull phantom (*A*) and the video signal from one line of the frame (*B*)

again in a darker region, and so forth. The size of the voltage at any point along the scan should directly represent the number of x-ray photons that struck the corresponding point on the II input phosphor. The time required to scan along the line from left to right is a little over 60 μsec for standard TV in this country.

The only portion of the video frame that needs to be digitized is the portion that contains the II image. To digitize the central TV line, the digitizer notes the start of the line, waits an appropriate amount of time until the first point on the edge of the II is expected, and then measures the voltage. The measurement is simply a number that the digitizer sends along to the waiting arithmetic unit. The digitizer immediately grabs the next point along the line, measures its voltage, and passes this second number to the arithmetic unit. After all 512 points along this line have been digitized, the digitizer sits back and waits for the next

line to come along. When the digitizer has performed the same operation on 512 appropriate lines of the 525 available, the entire frame has been digitized. The video image has been converted into digital form, and the digitizer can wait for the next TV frame. Digitizers are seldom given awards for high intelligence.

Matrix Size. In the above example, each television frame has the image from the II digitized into a 512- × 512-pixel matrix. It is important to note that the choice of **matrix size limits the spatial resolution** that can be achieved by the system. This is analogous to matrix size in CT. Consider the number of line pairs that can be displayed on a 512- × 512-pixel matrix. To define a single pair of lines aligned along the vertical dimension, at least two pixels in the horizontal dimension are required, one for the bright line and one for the dark line of the pair. Thus, the 512 horizontal pixels can define (at most) 256 line pairs. This limitation can be applied to the size of the image represented by the matrix, which is roughly the II input mode size (Fig. 27–4). If the II image represents about 12.5 cm (about 5 inches) in diameter, then 125 mm into 250 line pairs gives us a limit on system resolution of 2 line pairs per mm, assuming

Figure 27–4 Resolution limits imposed by a 512 × 512 pixel matrix

no primary beam magnification. So, even with a small field of view, a 512- × 512-pixel matrix will be expected to be the most important limiting factor on resolution, given reasonable focal spot sizes and primary beam magnifications. **The limitation becomes more severe for larger II input sizes.** With an II operating in a 25-cm (about 10 in.) mode under the same conditions, resolution would be limited to about 1 line pair per mm at the II input face. Similarly, displaying a 50-cm diameter image of a chest would result in maximum resolution of only 0.5 line pair per mm. Naturally, if the matrix size is increased to 1024 × 1024, the limitations imposed by matrix size will not be as great, and system resolution will be potentially double.

Binary Number System. We need to digress for a moment to review the binary number system. Those who speculate on such things suggest that the decimal number system is one inevitable counting method for beings with ten fingers, that a being with eight fingers (or their equivalents) would probably have an octal number system, and perhaps the argument is valid. But humans are beginning to use a binary as well as a decimal system because of computers. The validity of this statement can be checked easily by asking a bright 10-year-old.

Table 27–1 compares the binary and decimal number systems. A binary (base 2) "digit" can assume only one of two values, rather than one of ten as for a decimal (base 10) digit. So, binary counting (with the decimal counterpart in parentheses) is in the following sequence: 0 (0), 1 (1), 10 (2), 11 (3), 100 (4), 101 (5), 110 (6), 111 (7), 1000 (8), 1001 (9), 1010 (10), 1011 (11), 1100 (12), and so forth. With one **binary digit, or bit,** any whole number from 0 through 1 may be counted only two discrete values. Two bits allow the representation of 00 (0), 01 (1), 10 (pronounced one-oh, not ten; decimal 2), and 11 (pronounced one-one; decimal 3), a total of four discrete values.

We note that 2^2 is 4. Three binary digits allow eight discrete values, or 2^3. We would correctly expect that with n binary bits, some 2^n discrete values could be counted. Most DF display units handle individual pixels with eight-bit accuracy for displayed brightness (we will discuss the brightness scale later). An individual pixel can therefore have any brightness value from 0 through 255 decimal, a total of 2^8 (decimal 256) possible brightness values. The bottom of Table 27–1 provides an example of how to calculate the decimal value of a binary number. The decimal representation of the number 26 can be interpreted to mean that the value of the least significant digit (6) is multiplied by 10^0 (note that 10^0 = 1). The second significant digit (2) is multiplied by 10^1 (10). The third significant digit (not stated, but actually 0) is multiplied by 10^2 (100), and so forth. The actual number is the sum of the values represented by each digit (0 + 0 + 20 + 6 = 26). The decimal representation of a binary number may be calculated in the same fashion, except that the digits are multiplied by powers of 2 rather than by powers of 10. For the binary number 011010 (pronounced oh-one-one-oh-one-oh), the value of the least significant digit is 0×2^0. The value of the second digit is 1×2^1, and so forth. The result is 0 + 16 + 8 + 2 + 0 = 26.

Digital information is any information that is represented in discrete units. Analog information is any information that is represented in continuous, rather than discrete, fashion. The common meaning of the term "digital" is beginning to drift toward a usage associated only with electronics, computers, and the binary number system. We wish to use the perhaps outmoded meaning, however, to indicate the difference between analog and digital information. A video signal is an analog voltage representation of the quantity of light that strikes the input face of a TV camera tube. If this voltage analog of light intensity has a total range between 0 and 1 V, then

Table 27–1. Comparison of Number Systems

	DECIMAL	BINARY
Allowed values of a single digit counting sequence	0, 1, 2, 3, 4, 5, 6, 7, 8, 9	0, 1
	0	0
	1	1
	2	10
	3	11
	4	100
	.	.
	.	.
	.	.
	255	11111111
	256	100000000
	.	.
	.	.
	.	.
	1023	1111111111

Calculation of decimal values

10³	10²	10¹	10⁰		2⁵	2⁴	2³	2²	2¹	2⁰
··· 0	0	2	6	···	0	1	1	0	1	0

$$(0 \times 10^3) + (0 \times 10^2) +$$
$$(2 \times 10^1) + (6 \times 10^0)$$
$$= 0 + 0 + 20 + 6$$
$$= 26$$

$$(0 \times 2^5) + (1 \times 2^4) + (1 \times 2^3) +$$
$$(0 \times 2^2) + (1 \times 2^1) + (0 \times 2^0)$$
$$= (\text{decimal } 16 + 8 + 0 + 2 + 0)$$
$$= (\text{decimal } 26)$$

any quantity of light from zero intensity to some maximum intensity can be represented exactly (ignoring such things as electronic noise for illustration purposes). On the other hand, if a decimal digital system with two digits is chosen to represent the amount of light, only discrete values between .00 and .99 (a total of 100 values) are possible. The error caused by using digital representation can be as great as 0.005. The 0.005 is 0.5% of the maximum value. The error as a percentage of the true value can be greater than this. For instance, a value of 0.0151 would be represented as .02, an error of more than 30% of the true value.

Digitization Accuracy. There are many different types of digitizers. The actual principles of operation of each type are rather simple, but it does not seem worthwhile describing the operation of any of them. What counts in this case is the result. A comparison of analog video voltage and digitized values is shown in Figure 27–5. The analog video indicates that a smooth

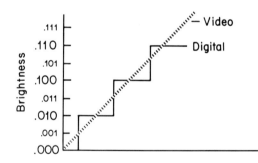

Figure 27–5 Comparison of analog video voltage and digitized values

variation in brightness occurs from completely dark at left to maximum brightness at right. (There would actually be some irregularities caused by noise.) The digitized values of brightness represent the output of a two-bit digitizer, so there are only two binary digits of precision. The values that the digitizer will obtain are .00 (at the left), then .01, .10, and finally .11 (at the right). Three-bit digitization would provide a stairway with smaller steps and less error, and four bits would be still better. As more bits of digitization are added, eventually the steps become so small that the changes between steps are almost completely hidden in the electronic noise from the video chain.

The statistical fluctuations in the number of x-rays that strike a small area of the II input screen can also be considered to be a source of noise, as will be discussed a little later. **Noise limits the accuracy of the image, and an appropriate digitizer will add very little to the inaccuracy.** An appropriate digitizer will have enough bits so that noise hides the steps (typically about ten bits). A very large number of bits, however, will add essentially nothing to the overall accuracy. It is easier and frequently much cheaper to build digitizers, arithmetic processors, and other system components if they only have to manipulate a small number of bits at a time. The argument extends to image memory and to digital disc storage, because useless bits are as expensive to store as significant ones.

DIGITIZED IMAGE

There are many tradeoffs that must be made in the formation of any radiographic image, and this is particularly apparent in a digital fluoroscopic image. X-ray and video chain equipment must be chosen with the digital application in mind, and all the conventional tradeoffs regarding such factors as patient dose and spatial resolution are still present. The equipment chosen and the image manipulations employed will have great influence on the diagnostic usefulness of the final image, but there is very little that is fundamentally different between a digital radiographic image and a film radiographic image. In general, the choices made in conventional film radiography and in digital radiography will have similar consequences.

Brightness Versus Log Relative Exposure Scale

We have been careful so far to maintain a linear relationship between the number of x-rays exiting the patient and the magnitude of the digital value that is measured. If the image is displayed on a monitor, as illustrated in Figure 27–6A, adding a given number of x-rays adds a constant amount of brightness to the image. At present, almost all digital fluoroscopic images are changed from this linear relationship to a logarithmic one. In the logarithmic relationship, increasing log relative exposure by a given amount will increase brightness by a constant amount (Fig. 27–6B). This type of relationship is a familiar one. Specifically, the H & D curves of film-screen systems are plotted as density versus log relative exposure. The brightness scale under discussion is quite similar to the density scale of film-screen systems. In fact, we will use brightness as being almost synonymous with film density. (Many authors speak of a "gray scale," which is the same as our "brightness scale.") This is one of many instances in which there is a striking parallel between digital and film-screen images.

In the film H & D curves of Figure 27–7 (same as Fig. 11–14), the relationship is density versus log relative exposure. A long contrast scale is achieved in the broad latitude film B, while A has a much smaller latitude in its exposure range. Of course, the short latitude film will result in higher contrast within the exposure range in which its H & D curve is steepest. A given change in log relative exposure anywhere within this more or less straight line portion of the curve will give about the same change in density. The size of the change will be small for film B, indicating low contrast, and will be large for film A, indicating high contrast. An increase in speed would be seen over film A if an H & D curve of similar shape were drawn to the left of the H & D curve for film A.

Windowing

The analogy becomes more exact if we digress for a moment to discuss windowing. The selection of window widths and levels

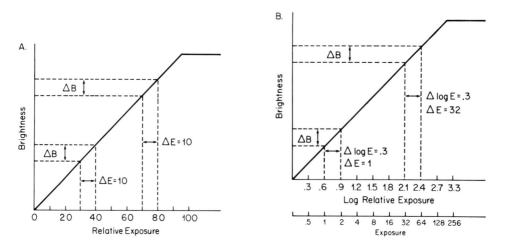

Figure 27–6   Comparison of a linear brightness scale (*A*) with a logarithmic brightness scale (*B*)

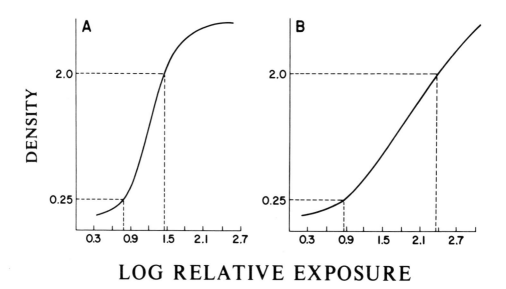

LOG RELATIVE EXPOSURE

Figure 27–7   Film H & D curves

is familiar from the discussion of CT displays, and serves the same fundamental purpose in digital radiography. As shown in Figure 27–8, if the original digitized image were displayed following logarithmic conversion, a broad latitude of log relative exposure values could be seen (*solid line*). The windowing operation selects only a certain range of log relative exposure values to display, and uses the full brightness scale of the TV monitor to display only that selected range of log relative exposures

(*dashed line*). A narrow log relative exposure range, or window, is roughly analogous to use of a high-contrast film. Moving the window to the left has the same general effect as choosing a faster film. In principle, **it is possible for the digital system to** produce almost any shape of response curve, or to **mimic the shape of an H & D curve almost exactly** if that seems desirable. The implication is that we are making a single exposure and then changing the brightness of each point in the image to

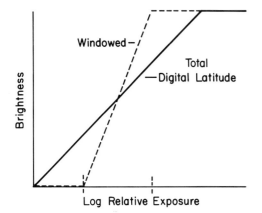

Figure 27–8 The selection of a window to display a smaller exposure latitude

make the image appear different. The fact that it is possible to make images with film-screen systems with different H & D curves causes no conceptual difficulty, so we will not allow a change in the brightness curve to cause us difficulty.

A brightness scale is analogous to the density scale for a film H & D curve. Stating that a point on a TV monitor has a certain brightness level is akin to stating that a particular point on a film has a certain density. The brightness scale is not defined as rigidly as the density scale for a particular film, of course. The brightness scale may be changed according to the DF user's preference. Conceptually, we might speak of a given structure as having a density of 2 on radiographic film. Equivalently, the same structure might have a brightness of 200, for example, on a DF image.

The importance of this analogy is that most manipulations being performed in DF have the same basic effect as those done with film. Thus, knowledge of film-screen radiographic imaging can be used directly, rather than considering a digital system as performing some new magic. Now we can return to a discussion of why the transformation to a logarithmic scale is useful.

Logarithmic Transformation

On a film radiograph a vessel of a given size will appear at about the same contrast with its background, regardless of where on the image the vessel appears. Without worrying about whether this is the most satisfactory situation, we can note that most DF images are displayed with similar characteristics. **Logarithmic transformation ensures that equal absorber thickness changes will result in approximately equal brightness changes, whether in thin or thick body parts.** The consequence of linear and logarithmic brightness relationships will be illustrated with the aid of subtracted DF images from a phantom, and an example will be offered to explain the relationships.

Figure 27–9A is a photograph of a phantom that will help to illustrate several points in the following discussion. The phantom consists of a step wedge of tissue-equivalent material, with crossing bars of bonelike material in its base. A shelf on top of the phantom makes it easy to add small structures for later subtraction. Figure 27–9B is an image of this phantom made on a DF system. Figure 27–9C is an image of only a small region of the phantom from the upper right quadrant made with the fluoro collimator jaws closed down to define only a small area. The image of this region will be used frequently, generally in conjunction with subtraction, and with photographic enlargement to show detail.

Figure 27–10 presents two subtracted digital fluoroscopic images for comparison of linear and logarithmic conversions. The subtracted image of Figure 27–10A was formed by a three-step process: (1) a mask image was obtained using logarithmic conversion; (2) a second image with some added "vessels" was obtained in an identical fashion; and (3) a subtraction of the two images was performed. This is the actual method used to implement the mask subtraction technique described previously. The subtracted image is displayed using a rather narrow window (read "high-contrast film" if you wish) to enhance contrast. There is no apparent difference in the vessel brightness (read "film density differ-

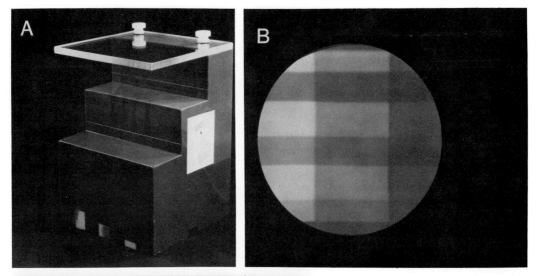

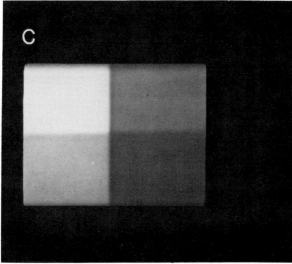

Figure 27–9   A phantom for tests of a DF unit

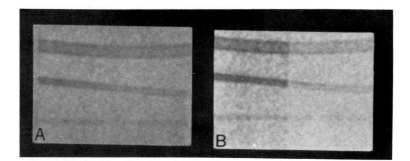

Figure 27–10   Subtracted images using logarithmic conversion *(A)* and no logarithmic conversion *(B)*

ence") between thin and thick phantom regions. (The differences in quantum mottle will be discussed later.) The image of Figure 27–10*B* was made in the same way, except that no logarithmic conversion was performed on the mask or second original image. The difference in vessel brightness between thick and thin body regions is obvious.

Figure 27–11 offers a numerical illustration for the difference in appearances of the images in Figure 27–10. A phantom with two different thickness parts has two vessels of equal size that can be filled with radiographic contrast material (Fig. 27–11*A*). Either vessel will absorb about the same fraction of the x-ray beam that strikes it. But, as seen in Figure 27–11*B* (a linear relationship), the difference in the absolute number of photons transmitted by the contrast-filled vessels is greater for the thin than for the thick part. The result of the linear relationship, after subtraction, is that the vessel within the thin part appears to have been denser than the vessel in the thick part. The logarithmic relationship of Figure 27–11*C* makes equal fractional changes in the number of x-ray photons result in equal brightness changes. The same percentage change, therefore, whether for a large number of photons (the thin phantom region) or for a small number of photons (the thick region), will provide the same apparent vessel density after subtraction.

Subsequently, we will see that some other sources of image degradation may make some modification of the strictly logarithmic shape advisable, but the assumption of a logarithmic conversion will be adequate for our present purpose.

There are many ways in which the individual pixel brightness values can be converted from a linear exposure relationship to a logarithmic exposure relationship. The exact method, provided that the end result is obtained in a reliable manner, does not really matter. There is one interesting method that illustrates a common type of

computer data manipulation. Before the advent of the hand calculator, we used tabulated values instead of calculating trigonometric and logarithmic functions. Of course, there is a way to calculate the value of a logarithm from scratch, but none of us could remember many details beyond the fact that it was not too much fun. A logarithmic table for looking up two decimal digits of precision would only need 100 entries ($10^2 = 100$). A typical DF system might digitize to ten bits (binary digits) of precision, and thus would need a table with only a little over 1000 entries ($2^{10} = 1024$). The advantages are the same for the machine as for a human, simplicity and speed. Computers take advantage of tables quite a bit in the "calculation" of values from data with limited precision. All that is necessary is for the arithmetic processor to look up the logarithmic value of pixel brightness furnished by the digitizer, and to store that value in its image memory. If we do not like a logarithmic transformation, we can put anything we want into the table and the machine will never know the difference. Note that when it is time to convert from digital pixel values back into analog video levels, an appropriate table can tell what analog level to assign to what digital value. Thus, it is easy to change window levels and widths, or to make other changes in the shape of the display response curve (nominally brightness versus log exposure) without altering the values stored in memory.

Image Noise

Our ability to measure any quantity in the real world is ultimately limited by noise. The statement sounds something like, "If nothing else kills you, a meteor will." Unfortunately, noise is an important problem throughout imaging. This is especially true in the case of radiographic imaging, in which x-ray photon statistics are always a problem. The addition of electronic image chain noise further complicates matters for digital radiography. The quantum noise in

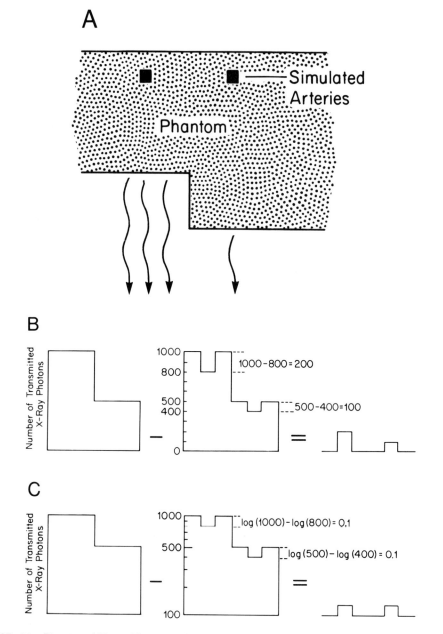

Figure 27–11   Phantom (A) used for numerical illustration of linear subtraction (B) versus logarithmic subtraction (C)

digital subtraction angiographic images is particularly prominent, as is true for images from CT and nuclear medicine.

Most important sources of noise in radiographic imaging are random in nature. By comparison, an image basically consists of a distribution of densities or brightness variations arranged in some set spatial pattern. Random noise, as the name implies, does not have a set spatial pattern. Mathematically, random noise and all that it produces can be described statistically. An expanded discussion of some statistics of random noise seems to be in order here.

(The authors reluctantly concede that a love of statistics is not necessarily prima facie evidence of mental instability.) Our emphasis is practical, and the discussion is mandated by recent developments in medical imaging. We will present an example of DF images degraded by different amounts of noise, followed by several examples explaining different aspects of noise degradation effects.

The major sources of random noise in a digital fluoroscopic image are electronic noise from the television chain and quantum noise from statistical fluctuations in x-ray photon density. The digital portion of the system should not further degrade the image by the addition of still more noise. A well-designed digital system can meet this responsibility, so there is nothing inherent in digital radiography that necessarily leads to more noisy images.

Quantum Mottle

Quantum mottle, caused by the statistical fluctuations in the number of photons that exit the patient, is ultimately a limiting factor for all x-ray imaging. If quantum mottle is regarded as fluctuations in the brightness or density of the image, the effects of the mottle become a bit easier to describe. The concept is illustrated in Figure 27–12. Figure 27–12A, B, and C are the mask-subtracted images of simulated blood vessels superimposed on the region of the phantom shown in Figure 27–9C. Each image is heavily dominated by quantum mottle, and electronic noise is negligible. Subtracted images shown in Figure 27–12A, B, and C are displayed using the same window width and level. The image in Figure 27–12A was made with each individual unsubtracted frame taken at fluoroscopic dose levels (about 0.1 mAs at 80 kVp). The image in Figure 27–12B represents about four times that dose, and the image in Figure 27–12C has 16 times the dose of Figure 27–12A. Note how smaller detail becomes visible on the subtracted images as dose is increased. Figure 27–12D is the same as

Figure 27–12C, except that the window has been narrowed to increase contrast and to show more clearly that even the smallest vessel is now visible. **The visual prominence of noise increases as the display window is narrowed.**

Standard Deviation

One x-ray exposure is not identical to a second x-ray exposure, even though the same x-ray tube, generator, kVp, mA, and time are used. Also, the number of photons incident on different areas of the patient is not identical for a single exposure, simply because the production of x-rays is a random statistical process. The concept of standard deviation (SD) was introduced in Chapter 13. The standard deviation (SD) for x-ray photon statistics can be calculated by

$$SD = \sqrt{N}$$

where N is the number of photons involved. For instance, suppose that an average of 10,000 photons per mm^2 exit a phantom and are incident on the face of an II during the time of one TV frame. (An actual pulsed DF image might contain 100,000 photons/mm^2 or more. We are using 10,000 photons/mm^2 to simplify arithmetic.) The standard deviation in 10,000 photons is SD = $\sqrt{10,000}$ = 100. The calculation is simple, but the practical meaning of standard deviation requires more explanation.

The statistics of random processes allows us to calculate the probability of occurrence of certain situations. Table 27–2 presents some probabilities based on standard deviations. The first line of Table 27–2 indicates that, about two out of three times, a particular value will be within 1 SD of the average value. For the case in point, a particular 1-mm^2 area on the face of the II will be expected to have between 9,900 and 10,100 photons incident on it about two out of every three TV frames, if there is no change in the phantom or x-ray beam parameters. Another valid interpretation is

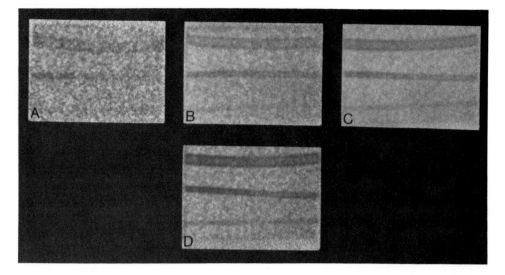

Figure 27–12 The effect of quantum mottle on mask-subtracted images. Images have relative exposures of 1 (*A*), 4 (*B*), and 16 (*C*). The image in *D* is the same as in *C*, but is windowed to enhance contrast

Table 27–2. Some Probabilities Based on Standard Deviations

NUMBER OF STANDARD DEVIATIONS	AVERAGE FRACTION OF READINGS		
	WITHIN	OUTSIDE	BELOW
1	2/3	1/3	1/6
2	19/20	1/20	1/40
3	997/1,000	3/1,000	3/2,000
4	99,994/100,000	6/100,000	3/100,000

that, for a phantom of uniform thickness, about two out of every three randomly chosen 1-mm² areas of the II will have between 9,900 and 10,100 incident photons.

Suppose that a nodule with a 1-mm² cross-sectional area absorbs about 1% of the photons that strike it (Fig. 27–13*A*). This is the same as saying that the average subject contrast between this nodule and its surroundings is 1%. The addition of the nodule to the phantom will result in the absorption of 100 of the 10,000 photons that would otherwise strike the II face, on the average (Fig. 27–13*B*). Our chances of examining one TV frame and detecting that the nodule has been added are very poor. According to Table 27–2 (column 3), statistical fluctuation causes 1/3 of all the 1-mm² areas of the TV screen to have more than 10,100 or less than 9,900 incident

photons. About 1/6 of the areas that are the same size as the added nodule will actually be darker than the area beneath the nodule (column 4). We must also keep in mind that, for a given TV frame, the added object may produce more or less actual subject contrast with its surroundings. The average fraction of the photons absorbed is equal to the average subject contrast (1%), because 100/10000 = 0.01, or 1%. In fact, the number of photons beneath the object (average of 10,000 − 100 = 9,900) will be between 9,800 and 10,000 photons only about 2/3 of the time. The situation improves rapidly with increasing x-ray absorption.

Subject Contrast

Higher subject contrast lessens the importance of noise. A 1-mm² nodule that

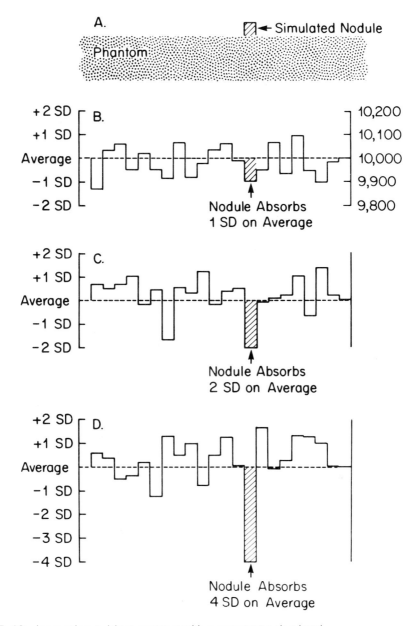

Figure 27–13 Increasing subject contrast with a constant noise level

absorbs 2% of the photons incident on it (2% average subject contrast) will exhibit an average of two standard deviations difference (200 photons, or 2% of 10,000) with its surroundings (Fig. 27–13C). About 19 out of 20 1-mm² areas will be within two standard deviations of the average of 10,000 photons. Only one area in 40 will be less than 9,800 photons (i.e., 2 SD below

the average, line 2 of Table 27–2). There are so many 1-mm² areas on the II face that the addition of a 1-mm² nodule with 2% subject contrast still cannot be reliably detected, using our 10,000 photons per mm² example.

A nodule that has an average subject contrast of 4% has a very good statistical chance of being detected reliably in this situation (Fig. 27–13D). A 4% contrast level represents 400 photons, or 4 SD. Only three 1-mm² areas of 100,000 such areas will have less than 9,600 photons. Therefore, the chance that statistical fluctuations will mimic a 4% contrast 1-mm² nodule is only three per 100,000 in our example using 10,000 photons per mm².

Increasing Exposure

Increasing exposure reduces quantum mottle. Figure 27–14 illustrates quantum mottle at different exposure levels. Figure 27–14A corresponds to the situation in Figure 27–13B. Suppose that exposure (in milliampere seconds) is increased fourfold. In the example just discussed, with 1% subject contrast for a nodule of 1-mm² area, quadrupling the exposure increases the number of photons per square millimeter from 10,000 (where the SD was 100) to 40,000/mm². Figure 27–14B shows this increased number of photons. The standard deviation of 40,000 photons is SD = $\sqrt{40,000} = 200$. Another way to calculate this is to note that the new SD = $\sqrt{4 \times 10,000} = \sqrt{4} \times \sqrt{10,000} = \sqrt{4} \times 100 = 2 \times 100$. The obvious extension of this is to increase mAs by 16 times (Fig. 27–14C). Thus, the SD = $\sqrt{16} \times \sqrt{10,000} = 4 \times 100 = 400$.

There appears to be a problem here. We know that increased dose means less quantum mottle, yet the number of photons in one standard deviation is larger for larger doses. The solution to the quandary is to consider the average number of photons removed by the nodule. Because 1% of 40,000 photons is 400 photons, a 1% contrast level represents 400 photons when there are 40,000 photons in the region of interest. The standard deviation of 40,000 is only 200, which means that the number of standard deviations represented by the

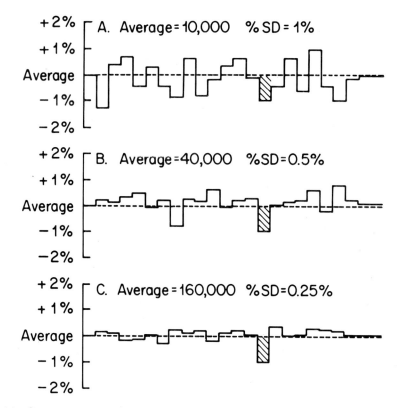

Figure 27–14   Constant subject contrast with a decreasing noise level (increasing dose)

1% contrast level is 400/200 = 2 (Fig. 27–14*B*). Increasing the mAs fourfold increases the number of photons by four (from 10,000/mm² to 40,000/mm²), which increases the number of photons absorbed by four times (from 100 to 400) but only increases the standard deviation by $\sqrt{4}$ = 2 times. Statistical fluctuations (quantum mottle) now represent a smaller percentage of the total number of photons (200/40,000, or 0.5%), and are therefore less likely to be confused with the nodule (1% average subject contrast). For simplicity, we will regard this as being equivalent to reducing quantum mottle to half of its previous level. Figure 27–14*C* represents 16 times the dose of Figure 27–14*A*. The quantum mottle is reduced to one fourth (i.e., $1/\sqrt{16}$) of the original value. **Increasing the dose M times reduces quantum mottle by $\sqrt{M}$ times.**

Noise and Observer Performance

In practice the relationship of image statistics to the performance of an observer is qualitative rather than quantitative. Improving statistics in a particular imaging situation does improve visibility to the point where other imaging limitations such as resolution become more important. It may be possible to state that increasing dose will improve the visibility of small low-contrast objects in DSA images of a particular body region. It would not be valid to declare that mammograms are "better" than chest radiographs because the former has more photons. Direct comparisons are valid only when such parameters as background structures, size of image features, and contrasts are reasonably similar. For instance, we can legitimately compare the effects of increasing contrast with the effects of increasing dose in DSA images. Reducing noise (quantum mottle, in this case) by half (by increasing dose by four times) has the same effect on detection probabilities as doubling subject contrast. In fact, a subtracted image of the high-dose example using a narrow window would be virtually indistinguishable from a subtracted image of the high subject contrast example using a broader window.

Noise and Subtracted Images

At first glance the quantification of the effects of noise on subtracted images seems to be a more difficult concept. One simple consideration, however, allows us to describe noise in subtracted images in a very straightforward way. The key is to consider the total number of photons within the region of interest for both the mask and the contrast-containing frame. Again, using 10,000 photons per mm² within a single frame for an example, a subtracted image requires at least two frames, one for the mask and one for the contrast-containing image. The final subtracted image is formed by using about 20,000 photons per mm² in the regions that contain no contrast material, and SD = $\sqrt{20,000} = \sqrt{2} \times 100$. Only one of the original images contains contrast material. If the contrast-containing object absorbs 1% of the incident x-ray photons (in compliance with our first example), an average of 100 photons will represent the subject contrast in the final image. The statistical fluctuations are higher ($\sqrt{2} \times 100 = 141$) than for a single frame, yet the contrast-containing structure is represented by the same number of photons as in a single frame. **The noise in subtracted images is worse than in either the mask or in the contrast-containing image.**

Noise and Object Size

The importance of quantum mottle tends to be much greater for small objects than for large ones. In the example of a 1-mm² lesion, which absorbs 1% of the 10,000 incident photons, we noted that there is about one chance in six that any randomly chosen 1-mm² area of the image could be mistaken for the lesion itself. The situation with a 4-mm² lesion is much better. **Quantum mottle is much less significant for detecting large structures than for** detecting small ones because the larger structures have both higher inherent subject contrasts and cover larger areas. The diameter is doubled, so the area is four times that of the 1-mm² lesion and attenuation in twice as great. The x-ray attenuation of the 4-mm² lesion is 2%, and there are about 40,000 photons within the area; thus, an average of 800 photons is absorbed. The SD of 40,000 is only 200, so the lesion should produce an average difference with its surroundings of about four standard deviations (800/200 = 4). The probability of occurrence of statistical fluctuations with four standard deviations is much less than for one standard deviation, as previously noted. Table 27–2 indicates that only about three lesion-sized areas out of 100,000 will be expected to have statistical fluctuations that could cause an incorrect identification of quantum mottle as being the 4-mm² lesion in this case. In a clinical situation observer performance would be improved, but not nearly as much as these simple statistics would suggest.

Independent Noise Sources

Every source of image noise contributes to image degradation to some extent. For the most common types of random noise, the total degradation can be calculated by using the percentage standard deviations of the individual noise sources. For our purposes, the percentage standard deviation (% SD) can be defined as the percentage fluctuation in the brightness (or density) of an image. For instance, the percentage standard deviation caused by x-ray photon statistics with 10,000 photons is 1% (100 is 1% of 10,000). In the case of DF, the major noise sources are random electronic noise from the TV system (% SD_{TV}) and quantum statistical fluctuations in the number of detected x-rays (% SD_Q). An equation for calculating the composite percentage standard deviation (% SD_C) for this situation is

$$\%SD_C = \sqrt{(\%SD_{TV})^2 + (\% SD_Q)^2}$$

The result is that the % SD (the magnitude of image fluctuations) is greater than would be seen as a result of either of the two noise sources operating alone. This is consistent with our overall convention of considering noise as fluctuations in the final image.

A poor TV system for DF use might have random noise at a midbrightness level with a % SD_{TV} of 1%. This is the percentage fluctuation in the image that would be produced by electronic noise alone. If the quantum noise at some x-ray exposure level has a % SD_Q of around 0.4%, then % $SD_C = \sqrt{(1)^2 + (0.4)^2} = 1.077\%$. The composite image noise in this case is only a little worse than that of the TV chain alone. One common method of reducing the noise in DF images is to increase the exposure per frame. That clearly will do no significant good here, because even reducing the quantum noise to a small fraction of the 0.4% level will produce little improvement in image quality.

A better TV chain might have random noise at a midbrightness level with a % SD_{TV} of around 0.2%. Under the same exposure conditions, % $SD_C = \sqrt{(0.2)^2 + (0.4)^2} = 0.45\%$. The image is dominated by quantum noise, and the system is good enough to make efficient use of patient dose. Note that for very low exposures per frame such as are typically seen in routine fluoroscopy (about 0.1 mAs per frame), the quantum noise will be much worse than for pulsed DF exposures (perhaps 10 mAs per frame), and even the "poor" TV system might be perfectly adequate.

Frame Integration

Another common method of reducing the noise in DF images is to average or to add together several frames, sometimes called frame integration. Frame integration reduces the effect of all types of random noise. The composite % SD_C is reduced by $\left(\dfrac{1}{\sqrt{M}}\right)$ where M is the number of frames averaged together. The specific equation is not of much interest to us. Whether M frames are averaged together or the dose per frame is increased by M, the final image represents the same number of x-ray photons. The difference is that **increasing the dose per frame reduces only the x-ray quantum noise effects, but integrating frames reduces both electronic and quantum noise effects.** Exposure levels and TV chain quality determine whether this distinction is important. On the practical side, averaging also has the advantage of reducing the importance of the x-ray exposure used during the stabilization time (if any). Of course, frame integration has the disadvantage of longer exposure times.

X-Ray Scatter

X-ray scatter produces the same fundamental types of degradation in digital radiographic applications as in any other radiographic applications. Some potentially valuable techniques in digital radiography, however, impose severe demands on an imaging system. Therefore, effects that were not especially significant in past applications now become more limiting. **Scatter has three major effects that degrade images:**

1. Scatter reduces radiographic contrast.
2. Scatter causes small structures with equal attenuation to appear to have different contrasts with their surroundings, depending on whether the structures are in thin or thick body regions, even after logarithmic conversion.
3. Scatter raises the patient dose required to obtain a given x-ray photon statistical confidence level.

The action of scattered x-ray photons in reducing subject contrast has been discussed in Chapters 8 and 13, so we will concentrate on the second and third effects.

Figure 27–15 illustrates the effect of scatter on contrast in different thickness body regions for subtracted images. The region of the phantom in Figure 27–15A has tight collimation to define a very small x-ray field and thereby to reduce scatter. Figure 27–15B was made with a wider collimator opening and was then photographically cropped to show the same region. The unsubtracted image in Figure 27–15C is darkest in regions of greatest thickness, as has been our custom to this point. The simulated vessels produce less contrast in thick body part areas than vessels in the thin region. The effect occurs because scatter tends to appear as the addition of a uniform x-ray background all across the image. The explanation of the effect requires an examination of the logarithmic conversion that was performed during the collection of these images.

Scatter was not discussed in the section on logarithmic conversion. We implicitly assumed that a structure that attenuated some fixed fraction of the number of incident photons would remove that fixed fraction of the number of photons from the final image. Unfortunately, that assumption is not valid. Figure 27–16 shows the situation when a uniform background of scattered x-ray photons is added to Figure 27–11B. Recall that the transformation of Figure 27–11B to a logarithmic scale produced Figure 27–11C, in which each opacified vessel caused a change of 0.1 with respect to local background. The familiar effect of the addition of scatter is that contrast is reduced. This can be seen by using a calculator, and noting that in the thick body region of Figure 27–16, log 2000 − log 1800 = 0.046 instead of 0.1 Another effect of scatter is that the vessels in thin and thick regions no longer produce the same contrast change. Note that log 1500 − log 1400 = 0.03, which is less than the change produced by the vessel in the thin region (0.046). In other words, when equal amounts of scatter are added to all parts of an image, the removal of a small number

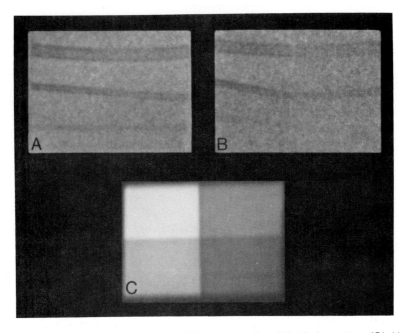

Figure 27–15 Effect of scatter on contrast. *(A)*, Low scatter. *(B)*, High scatter. *(C)*, Unsubtracted image is shown for comparison

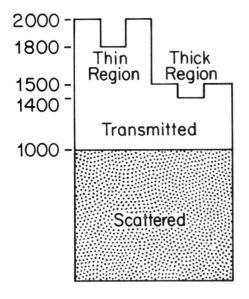

Figure 27–16 Effect of a constant scatter background on thin and thick body regions

of photons from the thick area will not produce as large a percentage difference as the removal of a larger number of photons from the thinner area.

The most obvious potential solution to force thin and thick body parts to display true attenuation is to subtract out the scatter. Unfortunately, the amount of scatter depends on such x-ray beam parameters as kVp and field size. Scatter also depends on the composition, thickness, and location of the structure being imaged. Finally, scatter is not really uniform across the entire image. It is not feasible, therefore, to correct an image completely for scatter by simply subtracting the same fixed fraction of photons from every image. In practice, an attempt to correct for scatter partially is often employed with DSA images. A modification to the "logarithmic table" (or an equivalent method) is commonly employed.

Scatter also makes quantum noise worse, which leads to the discussion of the third major effect. Our well-worn example of 10,000 photons per mm^2 (primary) will serve one last time. If 30,000 photons per mm² of scatter are added (not unreasonable), the quantum noise in the image is caused by 40,000 photons per mm² (i.e., primary plus scatter), but the useful image is still formed by using only 10,000 photons per mm² (primary only). Small low-contrast objects still attenuate the same number of primary x-ray photons. The vessel that attenuates 1% still removes about 100 photons. The standard deviation with scatter is 200, and without scatter it is only 100. Thus, quantum noise is worse by a factor of two in this case with scatter present. Even if it were feasible simply to subtract scatter after it was detected, the discussion of subtracted images suggests that the worsening of quantum noise by scatter would still persist.

Other solutions are feasible. Increasing dose by four times will reduce quantum noise by $\sqrt{4}$, or twice. This means that 160,000 photons per mm² (scatter plus primary) will give the same statistical confidence level in the final image as for 10,000 photons per mm² without scatter. Increasing dose is not only bad for the patient, but the II-TV chain would have to handle 16 times as many x rays. The TV chain would also need better noise characteristics to handle the smaller percentage contrast differences without degradation of the image.

Note the implication that less dose is required for images with an x-ray grid as opposed to images without a grid for the same low-contrast detectability. This option is not easily implemented with film-screen radiography because enough x-rays must be absorbed to expose the film to useable densities.

The best solution to all problems caused by scatter is to eliminate all scatter completely, if possible. X-ray grids and primary beam magnification help to some extent. Another particularly effective method of eliminating scatter will be discussed in a later section.

Veiling Glare

There are other effects that also contribute to a reduction in image contrast. For instance, image intensifiers reduce image contrast because of light scatter and other phenomena within the II (see Chap. 15). Veiling glare is a term used in optics to describe the light that is scattered and reflected within a lens system. For convenience, consider image veiling glare to consist of all those processes except x-ray scatter that produce a similar result in a DF system. The II contributes most of this veiling glare, and the remainder is contributed by the optical coupling to the TV chain and even the TV chain itself. Veiling glare becomes worse at larger field sizes. The effects of veiling glare on the image are similar in some respects to those of x-ray scatter. The addition of a background brightness to the image provides the same problem of thickness-dependent contrast levels following simple logarithmic conversion. The correction of an image for veiling glare is similarly difficult, and of course image contrast is somewhat reduced. Veiling glare, however, does not significantly affect x-ray photon statistics. Thus, images with and without veiling glare will need about the same patient dose for equivalent confidence levels, based on x-ray photon statistics alone.

DIGITAL SUBTRACTION TECHNIQUES

We have defined digital subtraction angiography (DSA) as the generic term for any digital radiographic method of implementing subtraction angiography. There are many techniques that may be applied to DSA, and we will discuss four. These are (1) mask subtraction (previously described), (2) dual energy subtraction, (3) time interval differencing, and (4) temporal filtering. Each technique is mentioned under several names in the current literature, so our choice of terminology is somewhat arbitrary. Mask subtraction is by far the most common at present, but each of the other three techniques is beginning to see clinical use. The field of digital radiography is advancing rapidly, and any or all of these specific techniques may be supplanted before they are widely used.

Mask Subtraction

The general method by which mask subtraction is implemented was described at the beginning of this chapter. We have since noted a number of limits on radiographic imaging systems in general, and a few that apply specifically to digital radiographic systems.

The image spatial resolution at present tends to be limited by the digital matrix sizes used. The ability to resolve low subject contrast objects is limited by the number of x-ray photons used (quantum mottle) and by the electronic noise of the video chain. Quantum mottle may be reduced by increasing the x-ray tube mA, thereby increasing the number of x-ray photons in each frame. Frame averaging is often employed to reduce the effects of video chain noise (as well as quantum noise) in forming a single image in the series. Scattered x rays and image veiling glare also reduce contrast and cause other problems. Patient motion between the time the mask is taken and the time the contrast-containing image is taken is a severe problem that does not have any optimal solution at present. The discussion of partial solutions to this motion artifact problem will be deferred for now.

Dual Energy Subtraction

Another technique for performing DSA is dual energy subtraction, a method that does not require the acquisition of images before and after the arrival of contrast material. In dual energy subtraction, two images are taken within a very short period, during which time there is no change in the patient. These two images are obtained by making exposures with different x-ray energy spectra as would be obtained, for instance, from a high-kVp exposure and a low-kVp exposure.

Film-Screen Method

We will first offer an idealized example of dual energy subtraction using a film-screen system. This example will illustrate the basic principle of how to eliminate soft tissue, leaving only bone. Figure 27–17A shows the exposures transmitted through different thickness of soft tissue at high kVp, and the resulting densities recorded on a high-contrast film-screen system. The x-ray attenuation is low at high kVp, and the difference in log relative exposure values between the thinnest body part and the thickest body part is 0.5 (log relative exposures of $1.7 - 1.5 = 0.5$). The high-contrast film records soft tissue over a density range of 1.5 (densities of $2.5 - 1.0 = 1.5$). Figure 27–17B shows the exposures transmitted through the same soft tissue thicknesses at low kVp (and higher mAs). Low kVp inherently provides higher subject contrast than high kVp, so a low-contrast film was chosen to record the low-kVp image. The low kVp and mAs would have to be adjusted experimentally to give the desired density range for a particular patient, so our example is not very practical. In principle, though, this could be done. The difference in log relative exposures between thin and thick body parts is 0.8 for the low kVp, but, as a result of the choice of a low-contrast film for low kVp (and our judicious tinkering with x-ray technique factors), the thinnest soft tissue part is displayed at the same density (2.5) as on the high-contrast film used in the high-kVp image. The thickest part is also displayed at the same density (1.0) on both images.

Recall that successively adding equal thicknesses of tissue will cause equal changes in density within the straight line portion of the H & D curve. This means that an intermediate soft tissue thickness will also give the same film density (1.75) on either the high- or low-kVp image. The net result is that the high-kVp image (recorded on high-contrast film) may be subtracted from the low-kVp image (recorded

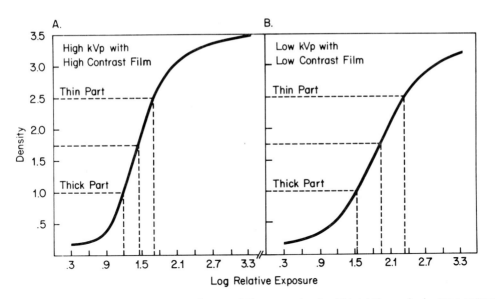

Figure 27–17 Film in *A* was selected to have soft tissue contrasts at high kVp equivalent to contrasts of film in *B* at low kVp

on low-contrast film), and soft tissue structures will cancel. What about bone?

It is no surprise that the differential attenuation between bone and soft tissue at low kVp is much greater than their differential attenuation at high kVp, a point made in Chapter 5. Perhaps the best practical example is high-kVp versus low-kVp chest films. The bone contrast in the high-kVp films is reduced much more than is the soft tissue contrast. For review, bone has the higher atomic number, and thus has a lot more attenuation because of the photoelectric effect. Because the photoelectric attenuation drops off very rapidly as kVp is increased, bone attenuation changes much more than soft tissue attenuation. Figure 27–18 has the same soft tissue thicknesses as the previous figure, but a small bone has been added to the object. In the regions that do not contain bone, soft tissues still cancel, but bone attenuation has changed more than has soft tissue attenuation. Regions that contain bone will not cancel completely. Thus, the final image consists of only bone plus the inevitable noise. If soft tissue film contrasts are made equivalent between low- and high-

kVp images, bone contrasts will not be equivalent.

Digital Method

The dual energy subtraction operation can be implemented in practice using digital image processing. The basic principle is the same, so consider the example just presented using film-screen subtraction. Figure 27–19A corresponds closely to Figure 27–18A. The same three thicknesses of soft tissue and the same added bone, kVp, and so forth are illustrated. The digital brightness scale has been modified so that the windowed digital line and straight line portion of the film H & D curve would superimpose. Similarly, the low-kVp digital window depicted in Figure 27–19B and the film H & D curve in Figure 27–18B are essentially identical. The brightness levels of thick (50), thin (250), and intermediate (175) soft tissue regions that contain no bone are the same either on the narrow window (high display contrast), high-kVp image, or on the broad window (low display contrast), low-kVp image. Soft tissues will cancel except for noise. As before, the final image will consist of bone only. The small

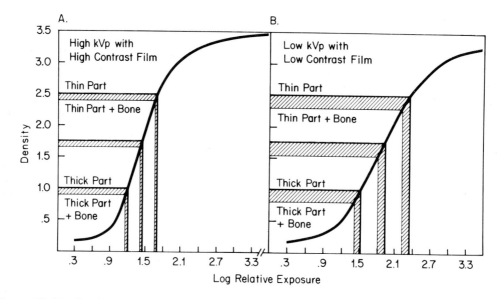

Figure 27–18 Dual energy subtraction principle. Bone contrasts change more with kVp than do soft tissue contrasts

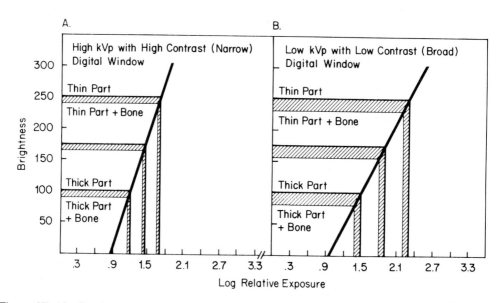

Figure 27–19 Dual energy subtraction by setting appropriate windows on a digital radiographic system

bone reduces brightness by 20 whether in thick $(100 - 80 = 20)$ thin, or intermediate regions of the low-kVp image. But the same bone only reduces the brightness by 10 in the high-kVp image.

Implementing dual energy subtraction by film-screen systems is very difficult. The advantage of the digital approach is flexibility. The beam energies and x-ray doses can be chosen with comparatively little concern for whether a good subtraction will result. The "windows" are chosen after the images are acquired (conceptually equivalent to choosing film types before exposure), and can be readily modified for the patient's requirements. A set of windows appropriate for the subtraction of bone rather than soft tissue can obviously be used if desirable for a particular problem. A single high-kVp and low-kVp image pair can yield chest images of either bone only, soft tissue only, or both. It should be noted that our use of display windows is for explanation, and that the technique is implemented by hardware performing functionally equivalent operations internally.

Problems of Dual Energy Subtraction

There are inevitably some disadvantages attached to this approach to imaging. All the problems associated with radiographic imaging in general and with DSA in particular are still present, except perhaps for anatomic motion. There are also some special problems unique to the use of dual energy subtraction.

First, the high-kVp image still has some bone within it. When the soft tissue densities are eliminated by subtracting windowed high- and low-kVp images, some of the bone density is also reduced. This implies that to obtain the same contrast differences as with a mask subtraction technique, more display contrast enhancement would be necessary with the dual energy scheme. As always, enhancing display contrast also increases the visibility of noise. More patient dose is required to suppress the visibility of this quantum mottle for dual energy subtraction.

Second, a more complex x-ray machine is indicated. An x-ray generator capable of switching kVp and mAs rapidly is needed to overcome problems with anatomic motion. Also, bone contrast in the subtracted image is greatest with two x-ray beams of greatly different energy spectra. The energy spectra can be varied even more by several methods. For instance, very different peak voltages can be employed, and extra filtration can be added to the higher kVp beam. The additional filtration adds some load to the x-ray tube that would not otherwise be necessary. Some mechanism for rapidly changing filters between exposures is also necessary.

Third, we actually made an invalid assumption in our example. A polychromatic x-ray beam is in fact hardened as it traverses the body. Beam hardening is the term used to describe the preferential removal of the lower energy x-rays as the beam traverses a thick body structure (see Chap. 5). The main cause of beam hardening is the photoelectric effect, which drops off rapidly at higher photon energies. The net effect is that the effective energy of the beam increases as it passes through thick body parts. Note that the photoelectric effect is greater in higher atomic number materials, so higher atomic number materials have a greater beam hardening effect. Also, higher kVp x-ray beams will have different beam hardening as compared to lower kVp beams. Beam hardening does not cause much of a problem in the simple mask subtraction technique, because only one x-ray beam energy is employed. The amount of beam hardening caused by bone and soft tissue is the same for each image, and small quantities of contrast material have only a small additional beam hardening effect. Unchanging structures still cancel without leaving residual images. The situation with dual energy subtraction is more complex because of the two beam energies employed. If each beam exhibited exactly the same amount of beam hardening in each region of the body, proper subtraction of bone and soft tissue would not be significantly affected. The broad range of thicknesses of soft tissue and bone, however, affect the two beams differently. A final image that should contain soft tissue structures only may in fact have significant amounts of residual bony structures that were improperly subtracted.

Finally, three different beam spectra are required to handle three substances with greatly differing atomic numbers. This might be termed three-energy subtraction.

The reason that three images at different beam energies are necessary can be understood by some simple algebra. Each pixel in a single image has information about unknown thicknesses of soft tissue, bone, and contrast material. Each of the three energies gives up independent (i.e., different) information about the thickness within that pixel. So, we have three unknown thicknesses and three equations that can be used to solve for the unknowns. For most angiography work using energy subtraction techniques alone, three exposures would be necessary to yield a subtracted image of iodine only. The iodine contrast would be even lower than for a dual energy subtraction, and the third image would contribute still more quantum noise. The display window would need to be narrowed even more than for the dual energy subtraction technique. The increased quantum mottle in the contrast-enhanced final images would become more prominent. Three exposures per image implies an increase in dose over the two exposures per image used for dual energy subtraction.

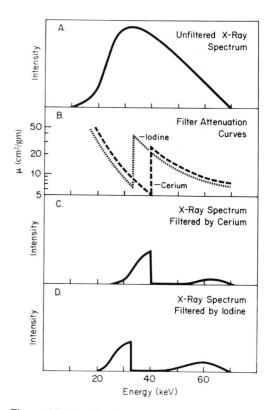

Figure 27–20   K-edge filtration

Other Dual Energy Subtraction Methods

K-Edge Subtraction

A technique called K-edge subtraction using film-screen systems received considerable research interest several years ago. Interest waned partly because of the difficulty of using film as the recording medium. The technique was named because of the K-shell absorption edge seen on a photoelectric attenuation curve. Figure 27–20 summarizes a method of using K-edge absorption x-ray filters to improve dual energy subtraction for contrast materials such as iodine. One of the two images should have the highest possible iodine x-ray contrast, and the other image should have little or no iodine x-ray contrast.

Iodine attenuates diagnostic x-rays almost entirely by the photoelectric effect.

One method for achieving high iodine subject contrast is removal of all x-rays from the beam except those that lie just above the K-shell binding energy of iodine (about 33 keV). An x-ray filter made of the rare earth named cerium can do this quite well. Figure 27–20A shows the x-ray tube bremsstrahlung spectrum to be filtered. As can be seen from Figure 27–20B, the K-edge photoelectric absorption of cerium begins at about 40 keV (binding energy of cerium's K-shell electrons). A thick filter of cerium inserted into the beam will remove most of the x rays above 40 keV by the K-shell photoelectric effect. Many x rays in the range of 30 to 40 keV will get through the filter. The x-ray spectrum through this filter will have its highest intensity just above the K-shell binding energy of iodine (Fig. 27–20C). This spectrum is nearly ideal for providing the highest possible x-ray subject contrast for iodine. This is the advantage of K-edge filtration, whether or not the technique is to be used with dual energy subtraction.

The image to be subtracted (roughly equivalent to a mask) should have little or no iodine subject contrast. The appropriate x-ray spectrum should contain few x rays that could be absorbed by iodine (Fig. 27–20D). If a thick iodine filter is placed in the beam, then almost all the x rays that could be absorbed by iodine have been absorbed before reaching the iodine within the patient. The resulting image will have very low iodine subject contrast.

The K-edge subtraction to form the final image is still a type of dual energy subtraction, and is accomplished by a method similar to that previously described. The problems with dual energy subtraction images, including incomplete bone-soft tissue cancellation with only two beam spectra, are still present, but the very high and very low subject contrast iodine images make most of those problems somewhat less important. The exception is that the technique is most effective with thick filters that remove most of the original beam intensity, and the high mAs required as a result makes x-ray tube load problems much worse. There are other problems, including those regarding patient dose and choice of materials for the most efficient filters, which we will not discuss.

Hybrid Subtraction

Another promising use for dual energy subtraction techniques is hybrid subtraction. A simple mask subtraction technique is combined with dual energy subtraction (thus "hybrid"). The technique is designed for the situation in which anatomic motion is expected to be a problem. The data are collected much as in simple mask subtraction, with images being collected at about 1-sec intervals over the course of the passage of contrast material through the vessels. The difference is that where each single image of the series is collected for mask subtraction, a high kVp-low kVp image pair is collected for hybrid subtraction. If there is no patient motion, the low-kVp image series can be used as if a simple mask subtraction had actually occurred.

Very little patient motion can be tolerated in simple mask subtraction between the time the mask is taken and the time the contrast material arrives in the vessels of interest. The soft tissues (large structures without sharp edges) cancel properly if patient motion is not too great, but bone edges cause severe artifact problems. Consider the subtracted images to consist of only two atomic number materials, iodine and bone. The hybrid subtraction technique produces two sets of subtracted images, one from the low-kVp and the other from the high-kVp series that were collected simultaneously. The same bone and iodine structures are present on both sets. Dual energy subtraction can now be used to eliminate bone, leaving only iodine. The final image will have lower contrast and more noise than if the dual energy operation had proved unnecessary, but the critical diagnostic information may be saved.

Dual energy and three-energy subtraction techniques have so much promise that they may be successful in spite of their obvious problems. First, the elimination of either bone or soft tissue by dual energy subtraction may be worthwhile, especially in chest radiography. Second, hybrid subtraction may be helpful in imaging situations in which normal anatomic motion is expected, as well as in the case of the uncooperative patient. Third, it may be possible in some instances to obtain the same diagnostic information in three exposures with a three-energy technique that would require about 20 exposures in temporal mask subtraction. Finally, there is the promise of obtaining subtraction images of contrast material for such procedures as laminography and cholecystography where the time span between pre-contrast and post-contrast images is long.

Time Interval Differencing

Time interval differencing (TID) is another digital subtraction technique, and it has seen some application in cardiology. The technique is closely related to simple mask subtraction. In simple mask subtraction an early image is chosen as the mask, and this single mask is subtracted from each succeeding image of the series to form the series of subtracted images. In the TID technique, a new mask is chosen for each subtraction.

For simplicity, assume that images are collected and stored at the rate of 30 images per sec for several seconds. Choose image 1 as the first mask, and subtract the mask from image 7 (0.2 sec later in time) to form the first subtracted image. Next, choose image 2 as the second mask, and subtract from image 8 (again, 0.2 sec time interval) to form the second subtracted image. The third subtracted image is a subtraction of image 3 from image 9, and so on. **Each subtracted image is the difference between images separated by some fixed interval of time.** The successive subtracted images are frequently displayed in a rapid sequence that is repeated to show dynamic function.

Each individual image of the series might have rather poor statistics that can be improved by frame integration at the expense of increased blurring caused by anatomic motion. For four-frame integration, images 1, 2, 3, and 4 are added together to form the first mask. Frames 7, 8, 9, and 10 are added together, and the first mask is subtracted from the result to form the first subtracted image. The second subtracted image uses frames 2, 3, 4, and 5 as the mask, subtracted from the sum of frames 8, 9, 10, and 11. This particular TID technique involves adding a number of images to form a mask that represents information about one time period, and subtracting the mask from the sum of another group of images that represents information about another time period. In principle this is very similar to another digital subtraction technique called temporal filtering.

Temporal Filtering

Time interval differencing can actually be considered to be a temporal filtering technique. The word temporal means of or limited by time, and clearly applies. We will not attempt a mathematical description of filtering either here or later in the examples of spatial filters. The description of the TID filtering operation is sufficient to explain the principle for present purposes. A set of final data (images) was formed from a set of original data (also images) by applying a consistent set of rules. Each successive final image was formed in exactly the same fashion, except for a shift along the time axis of the data. This operation of adding and subtracting part of a set of data together according to a set of rules to get one answer, and then shifting and repeating to get the next answer, is a filtering operation.

Time interval differencing is not usually regarded as a filtering technique, but of course it is actually a valid example. Temporal filtering is very general, and there are temporal filters that can be used to perform DSA (sometimes the awesome term "temporal filter" is even used). A simple example will show the general operation.

The passage of contrast material through an artery following intravenous injection will result in a contrast dilution curve with the general shape shown in Figure 27–21. Suppose that we wish to use our knowledge regarding the curve to perform DSA. The first step is to inject a bolus of contrast material intravenously. A second step might be to operate the x-ray tube in a continuous fashion at 10 to 20 mA, during which time individual frames are collected and stored at 30 frames per second. Now for the final step. One obvious approach is to choose either an early or a late frame with no contrast material present as a mask, and to subtract later frames from the mask as was done for simple mask subtraction. Unfortunately, the low mA leads to very high quantum noise in single frames. Another almost equally obvious approach is to add together several of the early frames and several of the late frames to form the mask. An equal number of

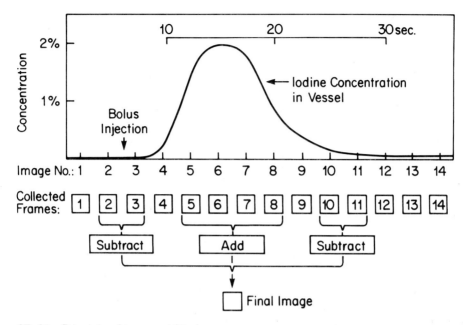

Figure 27–21 Principle of temporal filtering

frames that contain contrast can be added together to form a contrast-containing image. DSA is now accomplished by subtraction of the low-noise mask from the low-noise contrast-containing image.

In other words, individual images (single TV frames) are added together or subtracted from each other to form a composite image. The exact time of arrival of the contrast material is sometimes difficult to predict in reality, so the manual selection of the most appropriate frames to use for the individual steps could be quite time-consuming. Perhaps it would be better to allow the computer to do the selection using some consistent set of rules, and then to generate a large number of individual composite DSA images so that the best may be chosen. We now have a filter for doing DSA. Again, this filter generates one final image by adding and subtracting some of the original images together, and then shifting and repeating to form the next image. Obviously a temporal filter of almost any shape can be selected. The one used in this example was chosen for sim-

plicity of didactic explanation, and is not the optimal shape for the application.

One advantage of the temporal filtering approach is that less severe demands are placed on the video image chain than for simple mask subtraction, because the x-ray tube can be operated at much lower tube current values. Typically, mask subtraction requires around ten times the tube current needed by temporal filtering for comparable contrast detectability. An obvious disadvantage is that a large number of individual frames must be handled for temporal filtering.

Comparisons of patient dose and the sensitivity of the system to artifacts caused by patient motion are difficult to make at the present stage of development. Both patient dose and anatomic motion sensitivity are highly dependent on the way in which the techniques are implemented.

DIGITAL IMAGE PROCESSING

The field of image processing has received much attention since about the mid-1970s. Much of the impetus for this attention has come from the space program.

The startling images from satellites are typically manipulated by digital image processing techniques prior to being photographed for presentation to the public. Clearly, it is possible to manipulate medical images by computer in a manner analogous to the way in which these satellite images are manipulated. Nuclear medicine images in particular have had increasingly sophisticated digital processing techniques applied to them for years. At this point, digital x-ray image processing must be regarded as being in its infancy. No attempt will be made here to survey the rapidly growing field of digital x-ray image processing, but some discussion of present techniques and areas receiving attention is appropriate. Our examples will be linked to simple illustrations of a few general types of manipulations, rather than to specific complex (and changeable) processing operations now in use.

There are many ways to classify types of image manipulations (image processing operations). Engineers tend to classify on the basis of the type of mathematical operation that is implemented. We will classify them on the basis of the fundamental purpose of the manipulation.

First, there are manipulations that are intended to correct a deficiency in the imaging system or to place the information in a form more suitable for later processing. This might be termed "preprocessing," and it is usually performed during or immediately after data collection. Second, preprocessed images may be further manipulated by such methods as subtraction to form viewable images of the type desired for a particular application. Enough examples of these manipulations have been given in the discussion of DSA methods to illustrate this point. Third, there are manipulations employed to enhance the visibility of certain types of structures or certain features of images. Finally, certain manipulations are not intended to result in an improved visible image at all, but rather are aimed at allowing the computer to extract information such as projected crop yields in Canada, volcanic activity on Jupiter's moons, or the probability that a patient has cardiac insufficiency. A single type of mathematical operation may find application in all four of these types of image manipulations. Similarly, a single application may require all four general types of image processing.

For instance, several processing steps are applied in the mask subtraction technique of DSA. The individual images are first preprocessed by a logarithmic or similar conversion. Next, individual images are subtracted from each other to remove structures that are not of interest. A narrow display window is then selected to increase displayed vessel contrast. The first of these manipulations falls most conveniently into the preprocessing category. Subtraction provides a viewable image suitable for the application (DSA), our second category. The increase of displayed contrast by windowing is an example of image enhancement. Numerous researchers are working on methods for extracting numerical information regarding blood flow from DSA images, which would fall into our fourth general category. Obviously, categorization of image processing operations by intended purpose of the operation is somewhat arbitrary, because an argumentative person could successfully place a given manipulation into some category other than the one which we have chosen.

Image Correction and Preprocessing

In general, preprocessing of images is done to increase the value or accuracy of the data for later processing steps. The utility of a preprocessing step is very dependent on the later use to be made of the images. For instance, one of the most useful features of logarithmic conversion is that equal-sized vessels appear equally dense after the later subtraction.

An operation that would be immediately useful is the correction of images for x-ray scatter and image system veiling glare.

Such corrections are needed to increase the utility of numerical densitometry techniques (to be mentioned shortly). In another area, the II-TV system introduces geometric distortion in the image. This geometric distortion causes few problems in simple image viewing, but makes exact evaluation of spatial relationships somewhat difficult. Generally, the specific operations employed for preprocessing are not intended to compensate for all problems in the original data exactly. The common approach is to use approximate methods to attack only those problems most important to the application. Something similar to logarithmic conversion is very important for DSA, and scatter and veiling glare corrections would be helpful, but geometric corrections would be superfluous for most DSA applications.

Image Enhancement

For our purposes, image enhancement operations are performed at the viewer's option after the basic image of a particular type has been formed. This might be termed postprocessing of images. There are so many image enhancement methods available that books on the subject survey only a small fraction of the available techniques, and are obsolete before they are published. Three postprocessing operations that are common in digital radiography are mask reregistration, noise smoothing, and edge enhancement. A common feature of these three operations (and enhancement operations in general) is that "enhancement" is actually the suppression of information that the viewer deems to be unnecessary for a particular problem.

Mask Reregistration

Mask reregistration is sometimes useful when there is patient motion between the time the mask is taken and the time that contrast material arrives in the vessel of interest. The problem is illustrated in Figure 27–22, in which portions of the two digital images are shown. Each pixel is represented by a number (brightness level) in a digital matrix. Bony structures within the patient that should subtract on the two images are not recorded in the same position on the mask frame as the same structure on the contrast-containing frame. The subtracted image of Figure 27–22A shows the misregistered bony edges that produce motion artifacts whose magnitudes are greater than the magnitudes of the contrast-containing vessels of interest. The same problem occurs in film-screen subtraction angiography, in which the mask and contrast-containing image are aligned by eye until the "best" subtraction is obtained. This may be considered to be a form of manual reregistration, and is successful when patient motion is moderate. A similar approach will work for DSA. When the reregistered mask is subtracted from the contrast-containing image, Figure 27–22B does not contain the motion artifact. The aim is to throw away the information represented by the motion artifact.

The reregistration of the mask may be accomplished either manually (viewer-controlled) or automatically (computer-controlled). Manual reregistration is similar to alignment of the films. The viewer rotates the mask and translates it vertically or horizontally while viewing the subtracted image until a satisfactory subtraction is obtained. Automatic reregistration depends on computer calculations, and may be done in several ways. One method is first to calculate the sum of the "absolute values" of all pixels in a subtracted image. The absolute value of a negative number (− 5, for instance) is just the number without the negative sign (5), and is the same as the absolute value of the same positive number. The sum of the absolute values of − 5 and + 5 is 10.

Now an observation can be made. The contrast material is present on a subtracted image whether the mask is properly registered or not. In the case in which the image is properly registered, the only

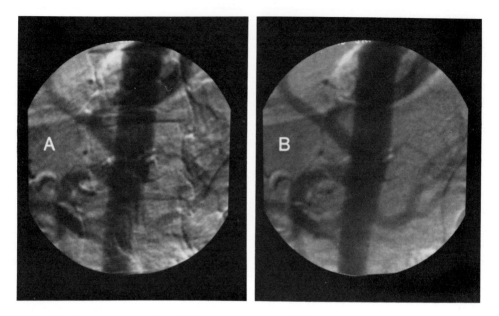

Figure 27–22   Mask reregistration. *(A)* Poor registration. *(B)* Good registration of mask and contrast-containing image

image features present are contrast and noise. Misregistration adds such factors as bony edges to the subtracted images, and the sum mentioned above should be higher than for a properly registered mask. The computer can therefore try numerous positions for reregistration, calculate the sum of absolute pixel values for each, and pick the reregistration position for which the sum is a minimum. Under good conditions, this minimum sum position will produce acceptable subtracted images.

There are numerous situations in which mask reregistration will be of limited value. The patient is three-dimensional, and mask reregistration operations are effective only for motions confined to a plane. Upper structures project onto different lower structures when the patient rolls onto one side as compared to being flat on his back. Reregistration cannot exactly compensate for this type of motion. The motion of structures within the patient (especially bowel gas and larynx) also changes the relative positions of prominent structures, and again reregistration cannot compensate exactly. In the case of automatic reregistration, there are numerous situations in which the minimum sum position of the mask (or some other calculation criterion) is not the position that even the most forgiving viewer would judge to be optimum for subtraction.

Noise Smoothing

Noise smoothing is an attempt to decrease the visual prominence of noise so that low-contrast objects of moderate to large size may be better appreciated. All method of smoothing x-ray quantum noise sacrifice some resolution in the process of smoothing the image. One method is illustrated in Figure 27–23. The technique operates by reducing the statistical fluctuations in each pixel by averaging the pixel with its closest neighbors. The first pixel in the smoothed image is formed by averaging the nine nearest neighbors in the upper left corner of the original image (rows 1, 2, and 3). The second pixel in the smoothed image is formed by shifting one column to the right in the original image and averaging, and the process continues until the entire first row has been formed.

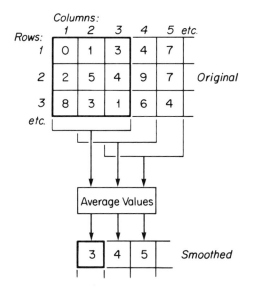

Figure 27–23 Smoothing noise by blurring an image

The second and subsequent rows are formed similarly. One shifts down a row in the original image and averages the nine adjacent pixels (rows 2, 3, and 4 of the original) to form the first pixel in the second row. The final image is a blurred version of the original. The visual prominence of noise has been suppressed through the process of averaging noise within small areas, but the disadvantage is that resolution is decreased.

The operation just described is a filtration operation. A final image was generated by applying a consistent mathematical operation to the original image to form the first pixel, and then shifting and repeating to form subsequent pixels. The operation of the filter suppressed small structures (high spatial frequencies) and had little effect on large structures (low spatial frequencies). This type of operation is sometimes called low-pass spatial filtering, indicating that low spatial frequencies are passed and high spatial frequencies are filtered out. For general information, the specific mathematical operation described in the preceding paragraph is a convolution. We note in passing that the literature contains references to "spatial domain" filtering (of which the above is an example) and "frequency domain" or "Fourier" filtering as mathematical approaches. The specific mathematical approach is largely a matter of computational convenience, because a given filter can generally be implemented either by Fourier methods or by spatial domain methods. With that, we put the mathematics of filters to rest.

Edge Enhancement

Edge enhancement is intended to increase the visibility of small structures with moderate to high contrast. The basic goal is to discard most of the information about the large structures and keep the information that relates to small structures. The appearance of a xeroradiograph is very familiar to most radiologists. The principal features of the xeroradiograph that distinguish it from film radiographs and DF images are that the xeroradiograph has a very broad latitude but still shows edges at high contrast. Problems with the xeroradiograph are that the necessary patient exposure becomes significantly higher as the kVp is increased. Also, once xeroradiography is chosen, it becomes difficult to display these images as the more conventional film radiographs. For these and other reasons, xeroradiography is not widely used for general radiographic applications.

If a conventional radiograph could be processed into an image that resembled a xeroradiograph in appearance, then it might be possible to have the advantages of both methods readily available. The combination of the blurred (low-pass filtered) image just described and the original image contain everything necessary to implement edge enhancement and mimic a xeroradiograph. The low-pass filter contains only the information about large structures and has low noise, while the original image contains additional information about the edges plus noise. The subtraction of the low-pass filtered image from the original yields an image in which edges and small structures remain. Edge enhancement is accomplished by suppressing information regarding large structures. Unfortunately, noise is also prominent in this edge-enhanced image. The final image has effectively been high-pass filtered, and the operation is sometimes referred to as a blurred mask subtraction. Many other specific mathematical operations could be used to perform exactly the same overall operation.

Information Extraction

A most promising area in digital radiography is the extraction of numerical or graphic information from images. The extraction of such information from nuclear medicine images is now routine in some applications. Many nuclear medicine blood flow measurements and similar dynamic techniques can be implemented using DF images. The development of useful methods for extracting information from DF images is still in its infancy at present.

It might be useful to have a technique that could accurately measure both the quantity of contrast material contained within some organ and the way in which the quantity of contrast changes with time. A DSA series of images contains the needed information. A somewhat trivial technique (not workable as described here) begins when a viewer circles the region of interest on one of the images. The brightness level in any given pixel in the subtracted image is directly proportional to the quantity of contrast material in the patient volume imaged onto the pixel for the idealized case (ignore scatter, veiling glare, geometric image distortion, and magnification). The total quantity of contrast within the region of interest could be calculated by simply adding together the contributions from all the individual pixels. Successive images of the same region of interest could be processed in the same way to produce the information needed for a graph of time versus total contrast material. Unfortunately, all the factors that were ignored are important to the accuracy of the results. The person charged with the resolution of these technical problems may have an easy task as compared to the person who is responsible for evaluating the technique for efficacy.

FUTURE EQUIPMENT DEVELOPMENTS

Alternate Image Receptor Systems

At present, digital radiography is almost synonymous with digital fluoroscopy in clinical use. A large fraction of DF systems are installed on C-arm units, and almost all are limited to use in one room or in two closely adjacent rooms. The average DF unit utilizes a 9-inch II and is capable of generating digital images on a 512- $\times$ 512-pixel matrix. Most manufacturers now offer 1024×1024 matrices as options, and 12- to 14-inch IIs are available for C-arm use. Both the large matrices and the large IIs are expensive. In addition to limitations on field of view and matrix-imposed resolution, we have discussed sources of image degradation inherent in conventional x-ray IIs and in TV video cameras and chains.

There are many alternatives to the conventional II-TV-based imaging chain. These have been investigated for many years, but digital x ray imaging lends new urgency to the search for new imaging systems. Image receptor systems for three areas of application are receiving most of the research attention. The first is slit radiography using linear detector systems. The second is two-dimensional detectors for replacement of film-screen cassettes. The third area now uses automatic film changers. We are short on crystal balls, so each example offered has been chosen to illustrate a diversity of approaches rather than to predict an ultimate winner of the technologic sweepstakes for that area.

One-Dimensional Image Receptors

Most radiographic imaging utilizes two-dimensional image receptor systems. An entire volume of the patient is projected onto the two-dimensional receptor (typically a film-screen cassette or II) during a single exposure to form the final image. In a technique called slit radiography, the x-ray beam is collimated into a fan-shaped beam so that a thin line is defined on the final image. Postpatient collimation is used to define further the line of the final image that is being formed, and to reject scatter that would strike other regions of the image receptor. A long x-ray exposure is used, during which the beam-defining collimator slit and the scatter rejection postpatient slit are swept in synchrony from the head to the foot of the patient.

The single most important reason for the development of slit radiography is the very high scatter rejection characteristics of the technique. Figure 27–24 compares scatter rejection for a slit radiography system and a two-dimensional film-screen imaging system with a grid. The only radiation reaching the image receptor during the exposure for slit radiography is that portion of the primary radiation that does not undergo any interactions within the patient, and radiation that is scattered over very small angles. Radiation scattered over wide enough angles to miss the postpatient slit and almost all multiple scattered radiation are absorbed before reaching the image receptor. The gridded system also rejects singly scattered photons, although perhaps somewhat less efficiently than for slit radiography. Also, multiple scattered photons may reach the image receptor. The importance of scatter for radiographic imaging in general, and digital radiography in particular, has been discussed in detail. Scatter rejection increases contrast, increases dose efficiency by reducing x-ray quantum requirements, and provides a final image that reflects true attenuation in thin or thick regions more accurately.

Detector systems commonly in use for x-ray CT may be considered to be one-dimensional. Experiments with slit radiographic techniques were done with some of the earliest CT scanners. Many modern CT scanners have some type of scout image capability (such as the GE Scoutview), which is in fact slit radiography. GE calls the technique "scanned projection radiography." The biggest problem is that, because of the size of individual detector elements, spatial resolution is poor for general radiographic work. A typical scanning slit imaging system with a single-line image receptor currently being applied to chest radiography digitizes the line into 1024 separate pixels. There is controversy over whether 1024 elements in one dimension is adequate for chest radiography, and image matrix sizes of greater than 1024 × 1024 may be necessary.

The slit radiography approach that depends on a single-line image receptor does have some significant drawbacks. Each individual line of the image requires that enough x-rays be detected to define that line. It is true that fewer x rays (and less patient exposure) are required to arrive at the same contrast detectability in the absence of scatter, and it is also true that the detector system might be more efficient in stopping x rays. The slit radiography system, however, still requires that a certain minimum number of x rays be delivered to each line of the system. For a 1024-line image, this essentially amounts to making 1024 separate exposures. Each exposure

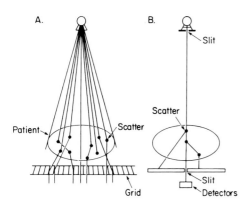

Figure 27–24 Comparison of scatter rejection for a grid (*A*) and for slit radiography (*B*)

will be considerably less than required for a single film-screen radiograph, but the sum of all individual exposures will still be quite large.

The net result is that the x-ray tube must deliver about 100 times the radiation for the single-line slit radiography system as would be required for a film-screen exposure with similar photon statistical contrast detectability characteristics. These exposure requirements can be met in a dedicated chest imaging system. The problem becomes more acute when higher exposures are needed, as in abdominal imaging. Also, much more time is required to obtain an image. Inaccuracy in collimating the beam and in moving the beam-defining slit increases patient dose. Some of the most valuable types of dynamic digital subtraction angiographic procedures, therefore, are clearly impossible. The extension to a larger image matrix would make the x-ray tube load and exposure time drawbacks even more significant.

There are some extensions to the technique that might help to solve some of these problems. For instance, the slit might be made larger, and several lines of detectors might be used to increase the number of lines defined per exposure. Unfortunately, this tends to increase the complexity and consequently the cost of the system. Slit radiography was originally developed on a film-screen system, which is a two-dimensional image receptor. There may be little net advantage for digital radiography in using a receptor system that is inherently one-dimensional versus using one that is inherently two-dimensional.

Fixed Two-Dimensional Image Receptors

For fixed systems there are alternatives to IIs and TV cameras. An old idea for replacement of conventional x-ray IIs was to use optical coupling of the light image formed on an x-ray screen, followed by light amplification. Each absorbed x ray produces so much light than an efficient lens system can guarantee that each x ray will be detected in the light amplifier. It is easy to amplify the light enough so that the presence of the x ray is detected in the final image. Compared to a small x-ray II, the solution is both bulky and expensive. For larger field sizes, however, the approach does have some merit. The input x-ray screen can be flat if that is desirable. Good optical systems with low veiling glare characteristics can be designed.

There are also alternatives to conventional TV cameras that are under development. One of the most promising, which has a light-sensitive region about the size of the input phosphor on a conventional TV camera tube, is similar in appearance to a large semiconductor electronic chip. A two-dimensional array of light detectors is embedded in this light-sensitive area. Each element of the array defines a single pixel of the image, and is essentially independent of all other pixels. The advantages, in addition to size, are that the system is more light-sensitive than most types of conventional TV tubes, and has much lower electronic noise.

Film-Screen Cassette Replacement

The benefits of having an image receptor that can be carried to remote locations and used with virtually any existing radiographic x-ray machine are obvious. An image receptor similar to a film-screen cassette in portability, resolution, and x-ray detection efficiency will eventually be developed for use in digital radiography. There are many possibilities. For instance, xeroradiographic plates initially accumulate an image in the form of a charge distribution that has been altered by the absorption of x rays. Several methods have been proposed and tried for scanning this charge distribution to convert the charge image into an electronic video image directly. Cassettes similar to xeroradiographic cassettes could be used at any convenient location and then brought to a central facility for "processing" and storage as digital images.

Archiving and Display of Large Image Matrices

At present, almost all DF display matrices are 512 × 512 pixels. Archiving is usually accomplished by recording the video display of the DF images onto film.

The development of a digital radiography apparatus that uses larger image matrices will require better display systems than those presently in use. Some expensive display systems are available with resolution of 2048 × 2048 pixels or better, but currently these are expensive and not very reliable. Presumably a radiology department that handles all images in digital format will require a large number of such display consoles, each with a moderate amount of image postprocessing and enhancement capability. Each console will probably need some rapid method of transferring images from a central area for display of recently acquired radiographs, and a somewhat slower method for transferring images from archival storage.

The digital archive storage problem appears to be intractable with currently available technology. Given 2048 × 2048 images, each image would require the storage of about 4,000,000 pieces of data. Digital discs capable of storing 250 such images are becoming more economical (larger and more expensive discs are also available), but storage of even 1 week's radiographs for a sizable radiology department would be prohibitively expensive. Other digital disc technology (such as the much publicized optical or laser discs) is under development. Archiving large numbers of images in digital form presents a formidable challenge.

Fortunately, medical imaging is not the only area with the need for better digital displays and storage retrieval methods. Applications as diverse as robotics, earth resources satellites, and computer games are adding impetus to development of the necessary technology. There no longer seems to be a question about whether an all-digital radiology departmnent will be possible. The question now is how long it will be before such a department actually comes into being.

SUMMARY

The most common type of digital radiography system is digital fluoroscopy (DF). A DF system requires an image intensifer (II) with a high contrast ratio and a TV chain with low lag and low electronic noise. The TV system may be operated in an interlaced, progressive, or slow scan mode.

The digital image processor performs four basic functions: forming the image, storing the image, displaying the image, and manipulating the image.

An analog-to-digital converter converts the analog video image into digital form. The computer handles numbers in binary form. Digital information is any information represented by discrete units. Analog information is any information represented in continuous, rather than discrete, fashion.

Manipulating the window width of the digitized image changes image contrast in a manner analogous to changing film gamma in routine radiography. Changing the digital window level is analogous to changing film-screen speed. Logarithmic transformation of the digitized image ensures that equal absorber thickness changes will result in approximately equal brightness changes, whether in thin or thick body regions. Film-screen radiographs inherently contain an analogous transformation.

The major sources of noise in a digitial fluoroscopic system are electronic noise and quantum noise. Higher subject contrast, increased patient exposure, large object size, and frame averaging all reduce the prominence of noise.

X-ray scatter rejection increases contrast and dose efficiency by reducing x-ray quantum requirements, and provides a final image that reflects true attenuation in thin or thick body regions more accurately. Veiling glare reduces contrast.

We have described four techniques for digital subtraction angiography:

1. Mask subtraction (most common)
2. Dual energy subtraction
3. Time interval differencing
4. Temporal filtering.

Digital image processing is intended to accomplish one or more of four basic functions:

1. Image correction and preprocessing
2. Formation of viewable images appropriate to the application
3. Image enhancement
4. Image information extraction.

Exciting new types of hardware are being developed. Many technical problems must be overcome before all medical images are routinely acquired and manipulated by digital computers.

REFERENCES

1. Brody, W.R., and Macovski, A.: Dual-energy digital radiography. Diagnost. Imag., *18*: 1981.
2. Foley, W.D., Lawson, T.L., Scanlon, G.T., Heeschen, R.C., and Bianca, F.: Digital radiography using a computed tomography instrument. Radiology, *133*:83, 1979.
3. Frost, M.M., Fischer, H.P., Nudelman, S., and Rohrig, H.: Digital video acquisition system for extraction of subvisual information in diagnostic medical imaging. SPIE *127*:208, 1977.
4. Kruger, R.A., Mistretta, C.A., Crummy, A.B., Sackett, J.F., Riederer, S.J., Houk, T.L., Goodsit, M.M., Shaw, C.G., and Flemming, D.: Digital K-edge subtraction radiology. Radiology, *125*:243, 1977.
5. Mistretta, C.A., and Crummy, A.B.: Digital fluoroscopy. *In* The Physical Basis of Medical Imaging. Edited by G.M. Coulam, J.J. Erickson, F.D. Rollo, and A.E. James. New York, Appleton-Century-Crofts, 1981, p. 107.
6. Mistretta, C.A., Crummy, A.B., Strother, C.M., and Sackett, J.F.: Digital Subtraction Arteriography: An Application of Computerized Fluoroscopy. Chicago, Year Book Medical Publishers, 1982.
7. Ovitt, T.: Noninvasive contrast angiography. Proceedings of a Conference on Noninvasive Cardiovascular Measurements. Palo Alto, CA, Stanford University Press, 1978.

28

Nuclear Magnetic Resonance

Nuclear magnetic resonance (NMR) is a powerful technique for the investigation of chemical and physical properties at the molecular level. Since its inception in the mid-1940s, it has been used extensively as an analytical tool for biologic studies as well as for physical and chemical investigations. The first imaging technique is attributable to Lauterbur.[4] In 1972, at Stony Brook, New York, he was able to generate the first two-dimensional NMR image of proton density and spin lattice relaxation time. Lauterbur coined the term "zeugmatography" (from the Greek *zeugma,* meaning that which joins together) for his technique. Joined together are a radio frequency magnetic field and spatially defining magnetic field gradients that produce the NMR image. (If you try to pronounce the word, or even spell it, it is easy to see why "NMR imaging" is used more extensively.) We will discuss Lauterbur's method later in the chapter.

Over the past decade, many different imaging techniques have been proposed and shown to be capable of producing NMR images. Bottomley has given an excellent review of imaging, with many references.[1] At the present time, we doubt that there is a consensus concerning which method might be the best for the clinical environment. What we are sure of is that NMR imaging has brought excitement to radiologists and physicists (medical, at least) rivaling that formerly produced by the introduction of CT imaging. We should not forget the important information that can be obtained by the use of NMR non-imaging techniques. It certainly is not clear where NMR imaging will stand in the radiological scheme, but there is little doubt that it will be somewhere among the imaging modalities in the future. In addition, there is no doubt that NMR investigations will produce a better understanding of the chemistry of physiology.

Perspective

We are going to look in detail at the physics (without the mathematics) of NMR, and then we will briefly discuss NMR imaging, because the physics is fairly well established while the NMR imaging is still in a state of flux. Note that the physics of NMR is completely different from anything that has been introduced and used in the radiological sciences. This very fact is going to make NMR more difficult to understand than was, for example, CT. For CT scanning we already understood the principles of x rays, detectors, and attenuation; all we needed to learn were image reconstruction, computer capabilities, and how to read the cross-sectional images. For NMR we need to start with the very basic concepts of the nucleus and proceed from there.

So the road is clear, if somewhat rocky. We must describe nuclear structure (some of which we learned in nuclear medicine) and nuclear angular momentum, and then discuss gyroscopic behavior (beautifully illustrated by the toy top). The combination of angular momentum and gyroscopic effects will lead us to the resonance (R) part of NMR. Resonance here refers merely to the change in energy states of the nuclei caused by absorption of a specific radio frequency (RF) radiation (but not of RF radiation at any other frequency). The resonance concept is one that we have already seen in x-ray production. Finally, we will find that resonance can occur in an external magnetic field, which of course is the magnetic (M) part of NMR.

We will present a brief discussion of nuclear physics, quantum mechanics, some electromagnetic theory, and even a bit of classical mechanics. (Normally six graduate physics courses cover this material.) One of the biggest problems we will find as we go along is to represent three-dimensional entities with two-dimensional drawings; some of the drawings are more successful than others, but we have tried our best.

NUCLEAR STRUCTURE AND ANGULAR MOMENTUM

The description of NMR must be made in terms of the **angular momentum of the nucleus,** so let us introduce the concept of angular momentum now. Angular momentum is one of the sacred cows of physics because, like energy, it is a constant of motion. **Angular momentum describes the rotational motion of a body.** Unlike energy, **angular momentum has direction (it is a vector) as well as magnitude.**

The angular momentum of a body may be changed by applying a torque on the body. Torque is a force that tends to rotate the body, rather than moving it in a straight line. Sometimes the change in angular momentum increases or decreases the rotational motion of the body. Sometimes the change in angular momentum merely changes the direction of the axis about which the body is moving. Later we will see these statements illustrated by the spinning top.

There are two types of rotational motion, **orbital** and **spinning.** As you might guess, there is an angular momentum associated with each of these motions. The earth and sun are good examples. The earth is orbiting the sun in a stable (unchanging) orbit and completes an orbit in 1 year. The angular momentum caused by orbiting, the **orbital angular momentum,** depends on the earth's mass and velocity and on the radius of the orbit. In addition, the earth is rotating (spinning) about its own axis. This rotation, or spin, produces the day-night period; there is one complete rotation about its axis in 1 day. In nuclear physics we call the day-night rotation "**spin,**" which has a **spin angular momentum** associated with it. The spin motion is an intrinsic property of the earth and does not depend on its interaction with the sun. If the sun were to disappear, the earth's orbital motion would cease; it would move off in a straight line but would continue to rotate on its axis. Of course, that would matter little to us since we would all be frozen very quickly.

Electron Angular Momentum

We will briefly discuss electron angular momentum even though electrons are not involved in NMR. The electrons in atoms have both orbital and spin rotation. The electron's orbital angular momentum depends on its relative motion to the nucleus (i.e., which shell it is in), but the electron's **spin angular momentum is an intrinsic property** that it has by existing. The total electron angular momentum is some combination of the spin and orbital angular momenta. The value of the spin angular momentum of every electron in the cosmos is the same. The detectable spin angular momentum of an electron equals the spin quantum number multiplied by a constant. The spin quantum number (usually more simply called electron spin) is given the symbol s, and s always equals $\frac{1}{2}$. The constant is given the symbol $\hbar$ and equals $h/2\pi$ (h = Planck's constant = 6.6×10^{-34} Joule seconds). The symbol $\hbar$ is pronounced "h-cross."

In Chapter 1, the value of h was given

as 4.13×10^{-18} keV sec. Both keV and Joules are energy units, so that the difference in the value of h is just a matter of the size of the energy unit we are using. In Chapter 1, h was introduced in its relation to the energy of a photon. In this chapter, h is introduced as the fundamental unit of angular momentum. It is the same constant in both of these applications. (Isn't it astounding that the same constant can be used to express both the energy of a photon and the angular momentum of a particle?)

Two interacting electrons always exist in the lowest possible energy state unless they are disturbed from the outside world. **The lowest energy state for the interaction is when the spin angular momenta are in antiparallel directions.** The direction of the spin is along the axis of rotation. Imagine a ball with a sharpened pencil through it (Fig. 28–1A). Now rotate the ball about the pencil so that the fingers of your right hand curl in the same direction the ball is rotating and your thumb points to the sharp end of the pencil. In this simple model, the pencil represents the spin angular momentum of the electron (represented by the ball. Physicists really don't like to think of

electrons as spherical particles, but for this text the picture is acceptable). The point of the pencil is aimed in the direction of the spin angular momentum of the electron. With two balls representing two electrons (Fig. 28–1B), the lowest energy state exists when the pencils are parallel but pointing in opposite directions (i.e., the spin angular momenta are in antiparallel directions). This configuration of the lowest energy state between electrons is usually called **spin-pairing,** a term we will use frequently in this chapter. In the helium atom, there are two K-electrons. These two electrons are spinning in opposite directions, called by physicists **"spin-up"** and **"spin-down."** We suspect that if there were two earths in the earth's orbit, the sun would rise in the west and set in the east on the other earth. This certainly represents the concept of spin-up and spin-down. In atomic structure, electrons will nearly always pair up with one spin-up and one spin-down. **The net spin angular momentum for a spin-up and spin-down pair is zero.**

There are a few exceptions in which the lowest energy state of a group of electrons is not produced by spin pairing. Nonspin pairing results in ferromagnetic materials,

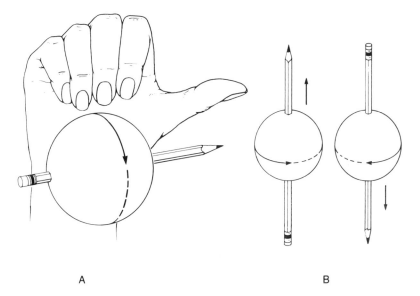

A   B

Figure 28–1 Spin angular momentum direction (A) and spin pairing (B)

of which iron is the best-known example. The very strong magnetic properties of iron are caused by nonpairing electrons.

Nuclear Angular Momentum

The nucleus is composed of neutrons and protons. Recall from Chapter 2 that protons have one unit of positive charge (equal to the unit of negative charge on the electron) while the neutron has none. Their mass is about the same, about 1836 times larger than the electron's mass. The collection of protons and neutrons, called collectively nucleons, is confined to a very small volume called the nucleus.

It should be obvious that the nucleus is not held together by an electrostatic force (i.e., Coulomb force, which is the force between charged particles), because the like charges of the protons would be expected to repel each other. There is a nuclear force, much larger in magnitude but shorter in range than the Coulomb force, that holds the nucleus together. (The origin of the nuclear force will not be discussed here.) The concept of the protons and neutrons maintaining their identity while in the nucleus is acceptable although not entirely correct. This concept most readily allows discussion of nuclear magnetism, and is the picture that we will use. Therefore, we have the nucleus with protons and neutrons being contained in a small volume by large nuclear forces.

One further step is required. The nucleons (both protons and neutrons) do, in some fashion, orbit about the center of the nucleus and have **orbital angular momentum.** The orbital motion of the nucleons is actually caused by the spinning motion of the entire nucleus rather than by independent orbital motion of the individual particles within the nucleus. An analogy is Mount Everest orbiting about the earth's axis of rotation. **In addition, both protons and neutrons have the same spin and therefore the same spin angular momentum as does the electron.**

Furthermore, there are energy levels for the nucleons very similar to the electronic levels (shells) in atomic structure. By now it comes as no surprise that the protons will fill these energy states by pairing themselves with spin-up and spin-down, or that the neutrons do the same. A proton will not pair with a neutron. This pairing of protons or neutrons produces cancellation of their spin angular momentum. The nucleus, however, does have angular momentum. **The angular momentum of the nucleus is determined by the spin of unpaired particles and by the orbital angular momentum of the neutrons and protons.** Something very interesting happens here. The combination of all these functions produces a very simple number for the value of the nuclear spin, designated by the letter I. The maximum detectable nuclear angular momentum is $I\hbar$. The letter I is called the nuclear spin (analogous to s, the electron spin).

Maximum detectable nuclear angular momentum = $I\hbar$

I = nuclear spin

$\hbar = h/2\pi$ (h is Planck's constant)

The nuclear spin, I, is always either zero, multiples of $\frac{1}{2}$, or whole numbers. (Note that this is a bit more complicated than with electrons, for which s is always $\frac{1}{2}$.) **Thus there arc only three kinds of nuclei as far as the spin is concerned:**

1. If the mass number A (protons plus neutrons) is odd, the nuclear spin, I, is a multiple of $\frac{1}{2}$ ($\frac{1}{2}$, $\frac{3}{2}$, $\frac{5}{2}$, $\frac{7}{2}$) (one unpaired nucleon).
2. If the mass number A and the atomic number Z (protons) are both even, I is 0 (no unpaired nucleons).
3. If the mass number A is even but the atomic number Z is odd, I is a whole number (1, 2, 3, 4, or 5) (two or more unpaired nucleons).

There are no other possibilities. Although the concepts concerning the nuclear angular momentum are difficult, the nuclear spin I that gives the value of the nuclear angular momentum is rather an uncomplicated number.

Why do we include angular momentum? Angular momentum is a physical quantity that describes the rotational motion of a body (i.e., a spinning nucleus has angular momentum). Why is angular momentum of the nucleus important to NMR? Without angular momentum, a nucleus would not precess when placed in a magnetic field. Without precession there would be no resonance, and the R part of NMR would not exist. We hope this introduction to angular momentum will help you develop a better understanding of nuclear resonance.

Up to this point we have discussed the fact that the charged nucleus is spinning and has angular momentum. Now we must investigate the magnetic effects caused by this spin. We will introduce the subject by using illustrations involving electrons flowing in a wire.

MAGNETISM AND THE MAGNETIC DIPOLE MOMENT

Magnetic Field Due To Electron Flow

To see how magnetism occurs in the nucleus, and also in the orbiting electrons, we need to retreat from the world of tiny particles to the more conventional world. Consider electrons flowing through a wire. The electron flow will produce a magnetic field (H) surrounding the wire. The direction of the magnetic field can be determined by a left-hand rule (Fig. 28–2A). With the thumb of the left hand pointing in the direction of electron flow, the fingers will curl in the direction of the magnetic field. (Note that most physics tests define current in terms of positive charge motion. For such a definition, all the left-hand rules become right-hand rules.) When the wire is formed into a circle, the same electron flow will produce a magnetic field upward inside the circle and a field downward outside the circle (Fig. 28–2B). The magnetic field about the loop of wire looks very much like the field surrounding the short bar magnet of Figure 28–3A. Note that Figure 28–3B is the same as Figure 28–2B.

Of more immediate interest is what happens if both the bar magnet and the wire loop with electrons flowing through it are placed in another (or external) uniform magnetic field. In Figure 28–4A, the bar magnet will have equal but opposite forces on the ends (actually, nearly the ends where the magnetic poles are located), and therefore will have no net force (a net force would cause the bar to move up or down). Each pole has a torque, however, that will cause a rotation about the center of the bar. The rotation will be such that the arrow from the S pole to the N pole will align with the arrows representing the magnetic field. We say that the magnet aligns itself along the field. As the magnet moves to align along the field, the torque decreases to zero when the bar is parallel to the field. We have just described a magnetic compass.

A.

B.

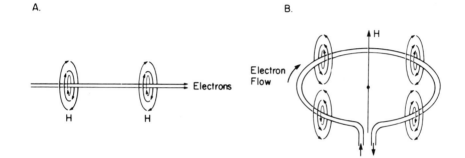

Figure 28–2   Magnetic field (H) caused by electron flow

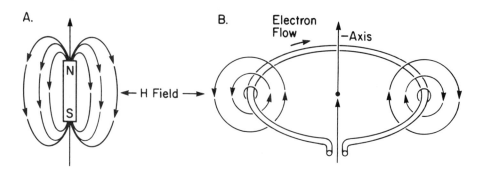

Figure 28–3 Magnetic field (H) comparison between bar magnet (*A*) and loop of electron flow (*B*)

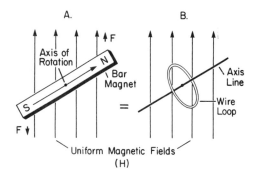

Figure 28–4 Effect of external field on bar magnet (*A*) and wire loop (*B*)

The loop with electrons flowing in it will also have a net torque and will rotate to align the loop itself perpendicular to the field. The axis line is defined as a line that is perpendicular to the plane of the loop and that passes through the center of the loop (Fig. 28–4*B*). This axis is analogous to the axle of the wheel. When the loop is aligned perpendicular to the magnetic field, the axis line is along the field, just like the bar magnet in Figure 28–4*A*. The loop alignment in a field is the principle on which voltmeters and ammeters operate.

Magnetic Dipole Moment

The **magnetic dipole moment (MDM)** is a property of a magnet or of a loop of wire with electrons flowing through it. **The reason for introducing the MDM is that the nuclei we use in NMR also have a magnetic dipole moment.** If we understand the effects of the MDM for these large bar magnets, we can more easily understand the effects for the smaller, invisible nuclei.

Perhaps the best way to describe the MDM is to say that **it is that property or characteristic of a magnet (or wire loop) that indicates how quickly the magnet will align itself along a magnetic field.** For a bar magnet, the stronger the magnet, the more quickly it will align with the field. In addition, the length of the magnet is significant: long magnets will align faster than short ones, all else being equal. For the loop of wire, the larger the electron flow, the more quickly the loop will align itself. In addition, larger area loops will align faster than smaller loops for a given electron flow.

If we were clever, we would define the MDM so that the direction or orientation of the MDM would give us the orientation of the object possessing the MDM. It seems obvious that the MDM for a bar magnet would give the orientation of the bar magnet if the MDM were along the length of the magnet. For the loop, however, we cannot draw a single line along the entire loop, but we can draw a line through the center of the loop. If that line were perpendicular to the loop, that line would give the orientation of the loop. In Figure 28–4*A* the MDM for the bar is a line going through the S and N poles and pointing out the N end. For the loop the axis line becomes the line of the MDM. The MDM, however, can be along the axis in one of two directions. The proper direction is obtained by another left-hand rule: curl the fingers of your left hand in the directions of electron flow, and your thumb will give the direction of the MDM. Test yourself on Figure 28–3*B*.

Magnetic Dipole Moments for Rotating Charges

Please note that a single electron orbiting about the nucleus constitutes an electron flowing in a circle (loop); it has a MDM. If the electron orbit is the smallest possible orbit (K shell), the MDM is called a **Bohr magneton.** For an electron in a higher shell (e.g., L, M), the MDM is the orbit number (L = 2, M = 3, etc.) multiplied by the Bohr magneton.

In addition to its orbital rotation, the electron has intrinsic spin. This spin rotation also represents a rotating charge. **The electron has a MDM of one Bohr magneton associated with the spin (this is in addition to the Bohr magneton associated with orbital motion).** We will give the value of the Bohr magneton (μ_B) in two systems of units:

$$\mu_B = 9.27 \times 10^{-24} \text{ J/Tesla (SI units)}$$
$$\mu_B = 9.27 \times 10^{-21} \text{ erg/Gauss (cgs units)}$$

We include cgs units because NMR magnets are sometimes described in terms of Gauss rather than Tesla. Remember that a Joule or an erg is a unit of energy, and Tesla and Gauss are units of magnetic field strength (really units of magnetic induction; see "Addendum" for a discussion of H and B at the end of this chapter.) One Tesla = 10^4 Gauss, and 1 J = 10^7 erg. Refer to Chapter 1 for a brief description of SI units.

If spinning electrons represent a rotating charge, a nucleus must also be a rotating charge. The differences between a proton and electron are the sign of their charge and their mass. In deriving the Bohr magneton, the electron mass shows up in the equation (not shown here). If we merely replace that electron mass by the proton mass, we have the nuclear magne-

ton. The nuclear magneton is designated by the symbol μ_N.

Let us consider the meaning of this term "magneton." **A magneton is a unit used to express the value of the magnetic dipole moment.** There are two units (these units are related in a manner analogous to inches and feet):

1. The Bohr magneton is used to express the MDM of electrons.
2. The nuclear magneton is used to express the MDM of nuclei.

The MDM of nuclei are not calculated, but instead are measured for each individual nucleus. These values are then expressed as a certain number of nuclear magnetons. Similarly, the MDM of the proton or neutron is measured in the laboratory and found to be different from the nuclear magneton. Even more strange, the MDM of the nuclei cannot be calculated by adding up the MDM of all the protons and neutrons in the nucleus. What all this teaches us is that nuclei, protons, and neutrons are not the simple structures we once thought them to be. To be complete, we will list the values of the nuclear magneton (μ_N), the MDM for the proton (μ_p), and the MDM for the neutron (μ_n):

$$\mu_N = 5.05 \times 10^{-27} \text{ J/Tesla}$$
$$\mu_p = 2.7928\mu_N$$
$$\mu_n = -1.9128\mu_N$$

where μ_N is the nuclear magneton, μ_p is the proton MDM, and μ_n is the neutron MDM.

For spinning particles, the MDM is always along the spin axis. (We described the spin axis as the pencil passing through the center of a ball, Figure 28–1.) A positive value indicates that the MDM and the angular momentum (remember the ball, pencil, and right-hand rule) are in the same direction. A negative value indicates that the MDM points in the opposite direction from the angular momentum.

Magnetic Dipole Moments of Nuclei

The MDM of nuclei depend on the number and arrangement of the protons and neutrons. We have already seen, though, that the protons and neutrons produce spin-up-spin-down pairs in the nucleus. The nuclear MDM is not just a simple addition of the MDM of the nucleons. In fact, the MDM of nuclei have been measured. We can note that if the nucleus has no spin (I = 0; i.e., it has no angular momentum), it will have no MDM. **Nuclei with no MDM will not be detectable by NMR.** Therefore, all nuclei whose mass number A (protons plus neutrons) and atomic number Z (protons) are both even cannot be used in NMR studies. Table 28–1 presents a number of elements that are of interest in medical NMR.

Alignment of Nuclear MDM in a Magnetic Field

We have tried to show you and to explain why some nuclei have spin angular momentum and a magnetic dipole moment. **The term MDM can be translated,** if you are so inclined, **to "tiny magnet."** MDM might be considered as that property of a nucleus that causes it to behave like a tiny magnet (if the tiny magnet is spinning around its north pole-south pole axis, it will possess spin angular momentum). When placed in a magnetic field, the tiny magnets will try to align along the field. Unfortunately, things in the tiny world don't always behave as we anticipate. In the present example, **the tiny magnet is allowed only a limited amount of alignment in the field.** Here we have a quantum rule very similar

to the electronic condition in atomic structure that electrons can only be in certain energy shells.

We must digress a moment and mention quantum physics. Quantum physics dictates certain rules that govern the behavior of objects the size of electrons and nuclei. Large objects, such as our examples of balls, bar magnets, and wire loops, are not limited by these quantum rules, which is why the analogy between magnets and spinning nuclei is not always precise. For example, magnets are able to align themselves exactly with a magnetic field, but spinning nuclei are limited in their alignment (Fig. 28–5). The possible alignments (orientations) are shown for nuclei with positive MDM and I = ½ (Fig. 28–5A) and I = 1 (Fig. 28–5B). (We really don't think that medical NMR will be applicable to nuclei with higher values of I, with the possible exception of Na.) Refer to Table 28–1 for some nuclei that might have medical applications.

The nucleus with I = ½ can spin in either of the two orientations shown in Figure 28–5A, but no others. The nucleus cannot come into exact alignment with the magnetic field. The bar magnet and wire loop would sooner or later come into exact alignment, because they are too large to be dominated by the quantum rules. Figure 28–5B shows that there are three orientations for the I = 1 nuclei.

Suppose we have a large number of nuclei of spin I = ½. With no applied mag-

Table 28–1.   Table of Nuclear Properties

ISOTOPE	MDM × NUCLEAR MAGNETON	SPIN, I	GYROMAGNETIC RATIO ($\times 10^7$ 1/T·sec)	LARMOR FREQUENCY FOR H = 1 T MHz/T
n	−1.91	½	−18.3	29.16
^{1}H(p)	2.79	½	26.8	42.58
^{2}H	0.85	1	4.1	6.53
^{13}C	0.70	½	6.7	10.70
^{14}N	0.40	1	1.9	3.08
^{19}F	2.63	½	25.3	40.05
^{23}Na	2.21	3⁄2	7.1	11.26
^{27}Al	3.64	5⁄2	7.0	11.09
^{31}P	1.13	½	10.8	17.24

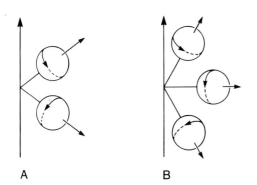

Figure 28–5 Nuclear alignment in a magnetic field

netic field H, the nuclei (and MDM) would be in random orientation in all directions. By applying a magnetic field, all the MDM would move into the two orientations, with some in one and some in the other (Fig. 28–5A). As might be expected, the two orientations have two different energy values. The up orientation has the lower energy, and the down orientation a slightly higher one. The number of nuclei that move into the lower energy state (up orientation) is only a little greater than those that move into the higher energy state (down orientation). The ratio of the numbers is determined by the difference in energy between the two states, the magnetic field, and the temperature. For instance, in a population of 2,000,000 nuclei, 1,000,000 + 1 might go to the lower energy state, while 1,000,000 − 1 might go to the higher state. This isn't very much difference. For a sample with about 10^{23} nuclei, the difference in the population of the two states would be about 10^{17} nuclei. The NMR signal is produced only by the 10^{17} excess nuclei. Therefore, of all the nuclei, very few participate in the NMR signal.

When the little magnets reach the orientation allowed by the quantum rule, the magnetic field is still trying to move them into exact alignment. This means that there is still some torque on each of the little magnets. In the next section, we will see that

this remaining torque is responsible for the MDMs precessing about the magnetic field.

Why do we include a discussion of magnetic dipole moment? First, it gets us thinking of certain nuclei as tiny (nuclear-sized) magnets. Second, we can see how these tiny magnets align themselves in an external magnetic field. Now that we understand this, we have the M part of NMR.

Angular Momentum and Precession

We have just described a nucleus with spin angular momentum and a MDM in a magnetic field. The nucleus still has some torque on it. In this section we need to describe the effect of this torque on the motion of the nucleus. We feel, and most other experts agree, that the best way to visualize the motion of the nucleus is to describe the motion of a spinning top in a gravitational field. Once again we are trying to use a large object to illustrate a quantum-sized object. Fortunately, in this example, we will not find a discrepancy in the analogy because of the size of the two objects. One of the most interesting motions in the world is the motion of a tilted spinning top. (We should really be talking about spinning jacks because one of us (JED) could never wrap a string around a top, throw it down, and get it to spin. His always just bounced off the floor. But he could really spin those jacks with his thumb and finger.) A top that is spinning at some tilted angle (we normally define tilted as being at some angle to up and down that we automatically define as the direction of gravity) will continue to spin with its axis at the tilted angle, but the axis of rotation will move in a circular path about the direction of gravity. The motion of the axis about the direction of gravity is called **precession.**

The precessional path of the center of the top is shown in Figure 28–6A as the circle at the apex of the top. Of course, this point (apex) is just exactly where the spin axis (L) emerges from the spinning top. (In physics texts the letter L is used to represent angular momentum, so we use it here.)

A.

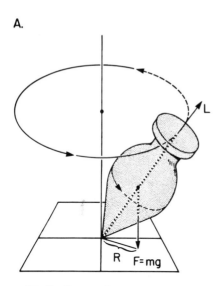

B.

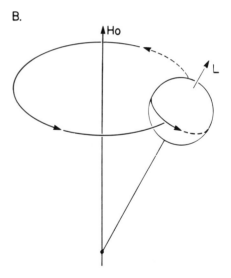

Figure 28–6   Precession

Remember, the spin angular momentum is also along the spin axis and, in this case, will point up from the top (along L). We know that a toy top will slow down and that the precessional circle will get larger until the side of the top touches the floor. (That's when it goes rolling across the floor.) The slowing down is a result of frictional forces at the point of rotation (and even frictional forces between the top and air molecules). Two assumptions have been made that are rather subtle: 1) there is sufficient frictional force to hold the tip of the top in place; and 2) the top is symmetric about the spin axis. If the first were not true, we would see something other than a top spinning on a fixed tip. More than likely, the tip would be moving in a circle on the floor. If the second assumption were not true, there would at least be wobble in the precessional motion and, very likely, no spinning about a single axis. We would really hate to try to spin a top with chewing gum on its side.

We are tempted to explain why a spinning top precesses but a nonspinning top falls off its tip. As a matter of fact we tried, but got bogged down in such matters as perpendicular vectors called torque, weight, angular momentum, and the change in angular momentum. Therefore,

we are going to assume that you believe that a spinning top will precess when in a gravitational field, and that a nonspinning top will fall over onto its side.

Larmor Frequency

All we need for precessional motion is a **symmetric body with spin angular momentum and some torque that is perpendicular to the angular momentum.** We have just that situation with a spinning nucleus in a magnetic field (Fig. 28–6B). Furthermore, there is no frictional force, so the nucleus will not slow down and fall sideways. The frequency of precession, called the **Larmor frequency,** is of fundamental importance in NMR. You will recall from Chapter 1 that the Greek letter ν (nu) was used as the symbol for frequency. Similarly, ν_L is the symbol for the Larmor frequency (sometimes the letter f is used for frequency). The Larmor frequency depends on the magnetic field and the gyromagnetic ratio, γ (gamma). This relationship is expressed by

$$\nu_L = \gamma H/2\pi$$
ν_L = Larmor frequency
γ = gyromagnetic ratio
H = magnetic field

(We sometimes see the Larmor frequency written as $\omega = \gamma H$. Here omega, ω, is really the angular velocity, and $\omega = 2\pi\nu$.)

The gyromagnetic ratio (also called the magnetogyric ratio) is the ratio of the MDM to $I\hbar$. Therefore,

$$\gamma = \frac{\mu}{I\hbar}$$

γ = gyromagnetic ratio
μ = MDM
I = nuclear spin
$\hbar$ = h/2π, h is Planck's constant
h = 6.6 $\times$ 10^{-34} Joules sec

The values of γ are included in Table 28–1. The gyromagnetic ratio is a unique value for each type of nucleus. For example, the γ values of the hydrogen isotopes (^{1}H, ^{2}H, ^{3}H) are all different from each other, and also different from the γ values of helium isotopes.

The defining equation for the Larmor frequency shows that **each type of nucleus will precess at a unique frequency in a given magnetic field.** Two different nuclei will precess at two different frequencies in a given field. Therefore, **the Larmor precession is a process that, for a given field, can distinguish between nuclear types.** We also need to note that a given type of nucleus will precess at different frequencies when in different magnetic fields.

For example, a hydrogen nucleus (proton) has a gyromagnetic ratio of 26.8×10^7 1/Tesla-sec (Hz/Tesla). In a magnetic field of strength 0.2 Tesla, the proton will precess at a frequency of about 8.5 MHz (8,500,000 cycles/sec). Calculate this yourself using the equation $\nu_L = \gamma H/2\pi$, being careful to keep track of units and powers of 10. Similar calculations show that the Larmor frequency for the proton in a 1-Tesla field is about 42.58 MHz, as listed in Table 28–1. We can find the resonance (Larmor) frequency of any of the nuclei listed in Table 28–1 in any magnetic field strength simply by multiplying the field strength (in Tesla) by the listed value of the Larmor frequency in a 1-Tesla field (last column of Table 28–1). Remember the

conversion from Gauss to Tesla: 1 Tesla = 10^4 Gauss.

Of course, the magnetic field need not vary much over a group of identical nuclei for those nuclei to precess at detectably different frequencies. This concept of identical nuclei in slightly different magnetic fields is the concept on which a great deal of NMR work is based. The chemical shifts, measured so extensively in chemistry laboratories, are just instances of identical nuclei finding themselves in slightly different fields because of local environmental perturbations on the applied magnetic field. Of more interest in NMR imaging is the purposely varied field to help establish different Larmor frequencies for a given nuclear type (usually hydrogen) across the object to be imaged. We will return to this imaging method later in the chapter.

Figure 28–6B shows a nucleus ($I = \frac{1}{2}$) spinning in the spin-up orientation. Note that in the spin-down orientation (not shown), the nucleus, as far as the magnetic field is concerned, has reversed its direction of spin. (Note the direction of the arrows in Figure 28–5A and B). The torque on both spin-up and spin-down nuclei, however, is the same. Therefore, both spin-up and spin-down nuclei precess in the same direction.

Energy States for Nuclear Spin Systems

We feel compelled to return to a discussion of the energy states associated with the spinning nucleus in a magnetic field. We have already mentioned that there are two energy states for an $I = \frac{1}{2}$ nucleus that finds itself in a magnetic field. Remember that the spin-up orientation has the lower energy.

When this chapter was originally written, we included a calculation for the energy of a bar magnet when placed in a magnetic field. That calculation is not really difficult, but we feel it would be sufficient for our purpose to give the results. When a bar magnet is aligned with a field, as in Figure

28–4A, its energy (potential energy) is just E = −μH (μ = MDM), while in the reversed orientation its energy is E = μH. The difference in energy between these two orientations is 2μH. This is also true for the loop.

The energy of a nucleus may also be written in exactly the same way. Figure 28–7A shows the two energy states for the $I = \frac{1}{2}$ nucleus. Remember that spin angular momentum has direction as well as magnitude. We use the direction of spin to indicate whether a nucleus is in the spin-up or spin-down state. In this example, $I = \frac{1}{2}$ indicates spin-up and $I = -\frac{1}{2}$ indicates spin-down. Note that the spin-up ($I = \frac{1}{2}$) state is lower in energy than the spin-down ($I = -\frac{1}{2}$) state. The energy (E) of these states ($E_1 = \mu H$ and $E_2 = -\mu H$) may be expressed in terms of the gyromagnetic ratio (γ). Because the equation defining the gyromagnetic ratio contains the terms I and μ (MDM), such an expression can be obtained with a little simple algebra (i.e., $E_1 = \mu H = \gamma I \hbar H$). With this substitution, the difference in the spin-up and spin-down energy states, as illustrated in Figure 28–7A, may be expressed as $\Delta E = \gamma h H$. $E_1 - E_2 = \gamma I_1 \hbar H - \gamma I_2 \hbar H$. For E_1, $I_1 = +\frac{1}{2}$; for E_2, $I_2 = -\frac{1}{2}$. Substituting these

values for I, we obtain $E_1 - E_2 = \frac{1}{2}\gamma\hbar H - (-\frac{1}{2})\gamma\hbar H = \gamma\hbar H$.

Now let us use this expression to describe how Larmor frequency relates to the frequency of the transition radiation between these two spin states. Transition radiation refers to the energy absorbed by the nucleus when it flips from the lower energy state to the higher energy state. This is analogous to the photoelectric effect when electrons absorb energy and go from a lower energy level to a higher energy level (e.g., from the K shell to the L shell).

There is a reason for all this. If the nucleus flips from the lower energy state to the higher, it must absorb an amount of energy equal to the energy difference. We have certainly seen this concept before. Remember that the production of characteristic x rays looks like this. Consequently, if a nucleus flips from the lower to the higher energy state, it must absorb this amount of energy from somewhere. When it returns to the lower energy state, it must give up this amount of energy. (We will see later that the emission of a photon is not the principal means of energy transfer when the nucleus returns from the higher to the lower energy state.) For x rays the emission was electromagnetic radiation that we called a photon. For nuclear transitions the energy is transformed to the lattice (the material structure surrounding the nucleus). This type of transition is called a radiationless transition, and usually heats the surrounding material (lattice).

In Chapter 1, we showed that the energy of a photon was given by E = hν (Planck's constant multiplied by frequency). Because we have the energy difference between the two nuclear spin states (E = γℏH), we can find the frequency of the photon absorbed to produce a spin state transition. That is, the energy (hν) of the photon producing the spin state transition must be exactly equal to the difference in energy (γℏH) between the two spin states. Let us write this statement in the form of an equation, and

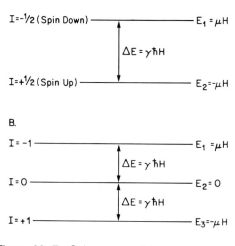

A.

$I = -\frac{1}{2}$ (Spin Down) ———————— $E_1 = \mu H$

$\Delta E = \gamma \hbar H$

$I = +\frac{1}{2}$ (Spin Up) ———————— $E_2 = -\mu H$

B.

$I = -1$ ———————— $E_1 = \mu H$

$\Delta E = \gamma \hbar H$

$I = 0$ ———————— $E_2 = 0$

$\Delta E = \gamma \hbar H$

$I = +1$ ———————— $E_3 = -\mu H$

Figure 28–7 Spin energy states

then solve the equation for the frequency (ν) of the photon producing the transition:

$$E = h\nu = \gamma\hbar H$$
$$\nu = \gamma H/2\pi$$

E = energy of photon absorbed
ν = frequency of the photon
γ = gyromagnetic ratio
H = magnetic field
h = Planck's constant ($\hbar = h/2\pi$)

This equation for the frequency of the photon producing the transition should look familiar. It is exactly the same as the Larmor frequency of precession of nuclei about a magnetic field. **The Larmor frequency of precession is exactly equal to the frequency of radiation absorbed in a transition from one spin state to another.** In the literature, statements about the radiation of transition are referred to as radiation at the Larmor frequency. Now we know why that is acceptable.

As an example, the Larmor frequency of a hydrogen nucleus (proton) in a 1-Tesla (10^4-Gauss) magnetic field is about 42 MHz (42,000,000 Hz). Let us compare this to more familiar electromagnetic radiation: the frequency of 300-nm (3000 A) visible light is about 10^9 MHz, and a 124-keV x-ray photon has about 10^{13} MHz. Inspection of the electromagnetic radiation frequency spectrum reveals that 42 MHz falls within the radio frequency range. All NMR studies are performed in the radio frequency range (about 1 KHz to 100 MHz).

For interest, the energy states of an I = 1 nucleus are shown in Figure 28–7B. But be careful; there are three, one of which is zero. Only the two transitions shown are possible. The transition from the upper state (I = −1) to the lower state (I = 1) is impossible; it is one of those "forbidden" transitions from quantum physics. Note that the allowed transitions give an energy difference just like the I = ½ nucleus. Thus, we are back to Larmor frequency for the absorbed radiation.

The basis of NMR is to induce transitions between these energy states by the absorption and transfer of energy. What-ever description is used to picture NMR, here or elsewhere, the whole concept basically deals with the transitions between these spin states. NMR is nothing more than the flooding of a sample with radiation at the Larmor frequency, and then measuring the Larmor frequency signal coming from the sample.

Earlier we said that for a sample with some 10^{23} nuclei, only about 10^{17} nuclei would be involved in the NMR process (these are the excess nuclei). Only 10^{17} nuclei! We cannot even image 10^7, let alone 10^{17}, nuclei. It is impossible to visualize what these nuclei are doing. Normally, then, we replace all these individual nuclei having individual MDMs by a single vector termed the **"magnetization,"** and give it the symbol M. We will discuss magnetization in the next section.

NMR PARAMETERS

Magnetization Vector

Recall that, in a normal-sized sample, there is an extremely large number of nuclei and, in a magnetic field, only a little more than half are in the spin-up state precessing at the Larmor frequency. A little less than half are in the spin-down state, also precessing at the Larmor frequency. Remember that each nucleus has a MDM and an angular momentum that are parallel, and that each nucleus looks like a tiny magnet. If we add up the MDM of all these tiny magnets, the resulting sum is the magnetization, M, of the sample. Because the nuclei have a spin angular momentum parallel to the MDM, there will also be a net angular momentum parallel to M.

In Figure 28–8A, we attempt to show several of the large number of nuclei (these are identical nuclei), some spin-up, some spin-down. Each MDM can be considered to have one part along the field and one part perpendicular to the field. (Because the MDM is a vector, it has components parallel and perpendicular to the field.) This is illustrated in Figure 28–8B, in

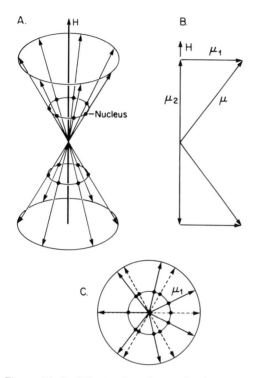

Figure 28–8 Effects of nuclear spins in an external field, H

which μ_1 is the component of the MDM perpendicular to the magnetic field, H, and μ_2 is the component of the MDM parallel to the magnetic field. There are similar components of the spin angular momentum. All the MDM components along the field for the spin-up nuclei add together and give a net result that is pointing up. The sum of components along the field for the spin-down nuclei also add together, but give a net result that is pointing down. When these two results are added together, there is a net result that points in the direction of the field because there are more nuclei in the spin-up than in the spin-down state. Effectively, then, **the excess nuclei in the lower energy state give a net MDM component along the field.**

Figure 28–8C attempts to show the top view of Figure 28–8A. What we see are the components (the μ_1 components of Fig. 28–8B) of the MDMs that are perpendicular to the field. Even with this small sample of nuclei, the tendency for these components to add up to zero (or to average to zero) may be seen. **For all nuclei, the perpendicular components of the MDM for both spin-up and spin-down add up to zero.**

We can replace all the nuclei in the sample by the single vector that is the sum of the components of the MDM for the excess nuclei. This vector is called the magnetization, M, for the sample. **The magnetization behaves like a magnet that has a spin angular momentum.** That is, the magnetization can precess about a magnetic field if the magnetization and the magnetic field are not parallel.

Precession requires spin angular momentum and a torque perpendicular to the angular momentum. Because the magnetization, M, as shown in Figure 28–8B, is exactly parallel to the magnetic field, H, no torque will be acting on M. This means that M cannot precess about H (a difficult concept, because the individual nuclei that make up M continue to precess). Without precession we are unable to detect any spin angular momentum of the magnetization vector, even though such spin angular momentum is present. If M were to be displaced from H, M would precess about H because there would now be a torque on M. In the next sections we will see 1) how to displace M from H and 2) how to observe and measure the resulting precessional motion of M.

RF Magnetic Field (Radio Frequency)

We would like to displace M from its direction along H and watch M as it tries to go back to its alignment along H. In the next few paragraphs we will discuss the method by which M can be displaced. It is not as easy as it sounds to make M move away from H because, as soon as M is displaced, it starts precessing about whatever magnetic field is present. If, by some means, M were displaced a bit from the H direction, M would precess about the H field with the Larmor frequency (Fig. 28–9A).

One way to displace M would be to apply a second magnetic field, H_1, but this second field H_1 would have to have a particular characteristic. Suppose H_1 were a constant (static) field. All we would see is the little dipole magnets realigning themselves and beginning to precess about the net magnetic field, which would become the vector sum of H and H_1. Of course, H_1 could be turned on and off quickly, in which case we would get a small displacement of M and it would then precess about H and gradually realign itself along H (Fig. 28–9A).

Or, we could have H_1 rotating about H at the Larmor frequency. In this case H_1 would follow M in the precessional motion about H. At this point most authors introduce a rotating coordinate system to discuss the motion of M and H_1. We can illustrate a rotating coordinate system by using mathematics, a merry-go-round, or a record player. We feel a record player would be best to use (because we can't draw horses).

Suppose we draw two perpendicular lines on a record and set the record on the turntable. Now our coordinate system would be the two perpendicular lines (x^1 and y^1) on the record, and the vertical line through the spindle (z^1) of the turntable (Fig. 28–9B). When the record player is turned on, x^1 and y^1 will rotate with the turntable at the angular velocity ω (instead of the familiar rate of $33\frac{1}{3}$ rpm, we are talking about a few million revolutions per second). Note that z^1 is not rotating. Compare that to the fixed coordinate system (x, y, z) of Figure 28–9B. Of course, z and z^1 do not change relative to each other, but x^1 and y^1 move relative to x and y. If we were to place z^1 along the H field and rotate the player at the Larmor frequency, we would have a system that would rotate with the same frequency as M, if M were slightly displaced from H so that it could precess. **Therefore, M would not seem to be moving in the $x^1y^1z^1$ system while it precessed about H.**

The situation with the merry-go-round analogy would be the same. A person standing on the ground (a fixed coordinate system such as xyz in Figure 28–9B) would see the little horses moving around and around. When he stepped onto the merry-go-round (a rotating coordinate system such as $x^1y^1x^1$ in Fig. 28–9B), the little horses wouldn't seem to be moving (of course, the rest of the world would be whizzing by).

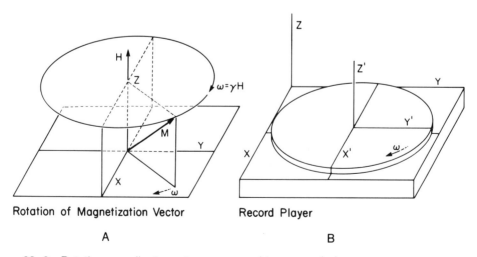

Rotation of Magnetization Vector

A

Record Player

B

Figure 28–9 Rotating coordinate system compared to a record player

In NMR studies, H is normally much larger than H_1, so the precession of M about H is much faster than M about H_1. Remember that the Larmor frequency will be greater in a larger magnetic field for identical nuclei: $\nu_L = \gamma H/2\pi$. Figure 28–10A attempts to show the spiral path that the tip of M will follow when both H and the rotating H_1 are present. This drawing represents the path seen from a fixed coordinate system, which represents the laboratory and the observer. The number of spiral loops is determined by the sizes of H and H_1.

The reason for choosing this particular rotating coordinate system (rotating at the Larmor frequency) is that the effective magnetic field appears to be zero (H appears to disappear) prior to applying the H_1 field. When we apply the H_1 field, it is the only magnetic field that the magnetization vector sees. This is why the magnetization vector, M, will leave its original direction (along H) and precess about the applied H_1 field. In any other rotating coordinate system (with H_1 rotating with it), part of the original field H would still be affecting M. At most, what we would see would be a perturbation of the magnetization precession about the H field. More than likely, M would continue to be along H and we would see nothing new because of the H_1 field.

We had better reconsider the last paragraph. We said that if we rotate around a magnetic field, H, at the Larmor frequency of a precessing nucleus, the magnetic field will disappear as far as the precessing nucleus is concerned. That sounds like magic and, indeed, physicists use the term "fictitious forces" when discussing rotating coordinates (and you thought we weren't going to get into science fiction).

Consider the analogy of a boy whirling a ball on a string. If you are standing near the boy, you will see the ball going around and around, faster if the boy applies more force on the string (this force is normally called tension) and slower with less tension. The tension in the string is analogous to the magnetic field, H. Now suppose you can make yourself very small and that you jump onto the ball (and have enough frictional, not fictitious, force so that you will stick to the ball). An amazing thing happens; from your new vantage point (your coordinate system) the ball is no longer moving. Because it was the force that the boy applied to the string that caused the ball to move in a circle as you looked at it from the ground, your new assumption must be that the boy is no longer applying any force to the string. Of course, your friends on the ground still see the ball whirling around (and you now see them whirling around while you stand still). By whirling around at the same speed as the ball, therefore, you no longer detect a force that makes the ball whirl. You really detect no net force, but because the boy is still

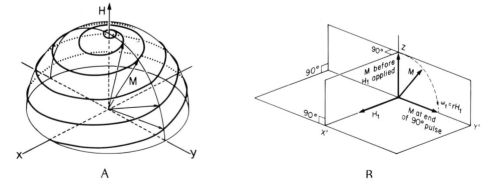

Figure 28–10 Beehive path of the magnetization vector, M, during a 90° pulse (A) and path of M during a 90° pulse as seen from a rotating coordinate system (B)

applying tension by the string, some new force must have arisen to counteract that tension. That new force is the fictitious force, and appears only because you are on a rotating coordinate system. We may use the term "fictitious," but you can certainly feel these forces. Jump on a merry-go-round and right away you are trying to slide away from the center; if you don't hold on you will indeed fall off.

We do the same sort of thing by standing on the earth. The earth is moving rapidly, but we have the sensation of standing still. This allows us to extend the analogy a bit further. Standing on the moving and rotating earth, we do not detect the force causing the motion. If another force comes along (such as a strong wind), however, we respond to the new force. Similarly, in our coordinate system rotating at the Larmor frequency, the nuclear magnets no longer detect the H field, so they are able to respond to the new H_1 field as if it were the only one present. Note that if the speed of rotation is not at the exact Larmor frequency of the nucleus in question, some of the H field will still be detected by its interaction with the magnetization vector, M.

You might think of this detectable part of H in terms of chasing the whirling ball in a tiny airplane. If your speed is exactly the same as that of the ball (i.e., if your airplane is moving in a circle with the ball), the ball will appear stationary relative to you. If your circular speed is a little slower or faster than the ball, however, the ball will appear to move ahead or behind you. This motion of the ball would be your detection of a portion of the original tension (force) applied to the string. Now back to the magnetization vector.

Because M cannot detect H in a coordinate system rotating at the Larmor frequency, M is free to interact with H_1 as if H_1 were the only magnetic field present. If H_1 is also rotating at the Larmor frequency, H_1 will appear to be a constant (unchanging) magnetic field. If H_1 is applied so that it is perpendicular to H, then Figure

$28-10B$ represents the precession motion of M about H_1. This precession motion is much easier to see than is the spiral motion of M as seen in the fixed laboratory system. We must remember, though, that the coordinate system $x^1y^1z^1$ and the entire Figure $28-10B$ is rotating about z^1 at the Larmor frequency $\nu_L = \gamma H/2\pi$. All that said and done, it is still within the fixed coordinate system that we actually observe the motion of M. Indeed, we will see M move in the "beehive" motion shown in Figure $28-10A$.

The spiral path concept of M moving from being parallel to H to being perpendicular to H is hard to visualize, so we would like to give an analogy before continuing. Consider a jeep perched on top of a steep mountain. Obviously, you cannot drive the jeep straight down the side of the mountain. Rather, the jeep must circle down and around and around the mountain in a gradual descent. Similarly, M leaves H and moves along a spiral path until it reaches the plane perpendicular to H and parallel to H_1 (for 90° motion, at least). A little later we will allow M to return parallel to H; it will move "up the mountain" in a spiral path, but the path will be a different spiral from that used on the downhill trip (see Fig. 28-11A).

When M finally reaches the xy plane, we have an interesting condition. There is no magnetization component along the z axis, which means that the spin-up-spin-down states are equally populated. The entire M vector is a result of the little magnets (nuclear magnetic dipole moments) grouping together as they precess about H. In Figure 28-8C, this would be seen as an excess number of nuclei on one side of the circle. We might call this grouping together as being "in phase." Note that the transverse component of M (that component perpendicular to H) is produced by the in-phase grouping of the dipoles. The parallel component of M (that component parallel to H) is produced by the population ratio of the two spin states. (We will return to a more complete discussion of in phase later.)

We need to determine how to produce H_1 so that it will rotate at the Larmor frequency about H and be perpendicular to H. Fortunately, a sinusoidally varying magnetic field that is perpendicular to H will look exactly like a constant field in the rotating coordinate system, and this is what we want. We can then produce the H_1 field by a conductor with electrons flowing through it if we design the conductor configuration in such a way that H_1 is perpendicular to H. (We will present more on this structure later; see "Radio Frequency Coils.") Remember that H_1 must rotate at the Larmor frequency, which is in the radio frequency range. Therefore, the electron flow in the RF coil must vary at the Larmor frequency (thus the term RF [radio frequency] magnetic field).

If this discussion of the precession of M about H_1 is sufficient, we can define two more terms before describing NMR parameters. If H_1 is on long enough to rotate M by 90°, we have what is called a **90° pulse.** If H_1 stays on twice as long, so that the precession of M carries M all the way to the $-z$ axis, we have rotated M by 180°. The RF pulse necessary to produce the 180° rotation is called a **180° pulse.**

Free Induction Decay

We are now ready to discuss NMR parameters, which are those quantities that are measurable with the NMR technique. It is important here to state that the NMR signal cannot be described in terms of photon emission alone, as we do with x-rays. Rather, we must move M away from the H direction and observe M moving back along H. We are going to describe the parameters first and then discuss some possible reasons for observing what we do.

Recall that we can rotate M away from H by applying an RF field at the Larmor frequency. If M precesses about the varying RF field by 90°, we have applied a 90° pulse (see Fig. 28–10B). Suppose we apply a 90°

pulse; the RF field is on until M is entirely in the plane perpendicular to H, and then H_1 is turned off. Thus, we see that a 90° pulse is simply the length of time that H_1 is turned on (the time will be different for different values of H_1). When H_1 is turned off, M will continue precessing about H. At the same time, the dipole magnets (spinning nuclei) will start returning to the equilibrium distribution (i.e., the distribution that existed before H_1 was turned on). In other literature you may encounter the term **thermal equilibrium;** this is exactly the same thing that we have called equilibrium distribution.

So, we have M precessing about H and moving back toward the direction of H. Figure 28–11A shows the path along which M returns to H. The coil shown in Figure 28–11B is an RF coil (more than likely the one used to produce the field H_1). Remember that M can be considered to be a magnet. When the end of the M magnet sweeps past the windings of the RF coil, a current (electron flow) is induced in the coil. For all jeep drivers, you may visualize Figure 28–11A as though you were in a helicopter hovering exactly over the top of a mountain while watching the jeep make its spiral climb back up the mountain. In Figure 28–11B, M at 1 is not inducing a current; at 2 the induced current has a maximum value; it is zero at 3; and at 4 the induced current is again a maximum but in the opposite direction from that at 2. It is the opposite direction because M is sweeping the loops in opposite directions at 2 and 4. Remember that M is getting closer to H between 1 and 4 (the jeep is getting closer to the top of the mountain, so it will appear to be closer to the center top of the mountain), so the current at 4 has a smaller maximum than at 2. For each trip of M around H we have the same shape of induced current, with the maximum values getting smaller. This decreasing induction continues until M is along the H direction.

The total signal induced in the coil is shown in Figure 28–12A. What we see is

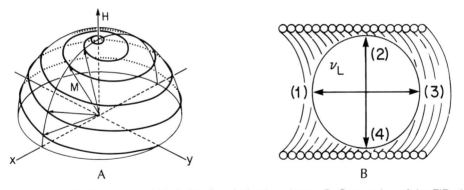

Figure 28–11   *A.* Beehive path of M during free induction decay. *B.* Generation of the FID signal

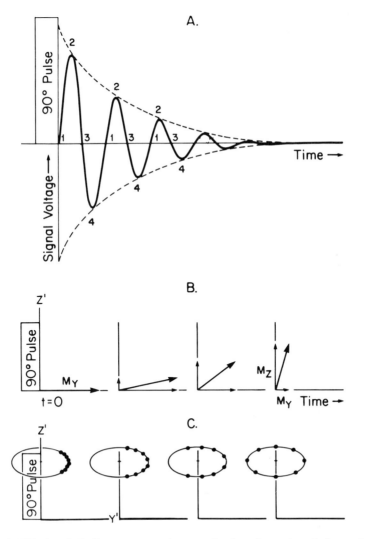

Figure 28–12   *A.* FID signal. *B.* Components of magnetization along y′ and z′ axes following a 90°
pulse. *C.* M_y decreases with increasing dephasing

an alternating voltage (produced by the induced current) that has the Larmor frequency. It also decays to zero (at least, to background noise) exponentially. (X-ray beams decay exponentially. At least, a monochromatic beam would be attenuated exponentially by some attenuating material.) This signal produced by the free return of M to the H direction is called the **free induction decay (FID).**

The return of M to the H direction is accomplished by two different mechanisms. Note that as M returns to the H direction, the component of M along y^1 (called M_y in Figure 28–12B) decreases to zero. The M_z component (the component of M along H), however, increases from zero during the FID. **We will need to discuss these two components as separate topics. They produce two other parameters of NMR, namely T_1 and T_2, the relaxation times.**

Spin-Spin Relaxation Time (T_2)

Having mentioned the FID, it would be appropriate here to introduce the concept of spin-spin relaxation time, T_2, **because T_2 is closely related to the FID.** Before explaining what T_2 represents, we need to discuss what happens after a 90° pulse to get M pointing back along H.

Refer back to Figure 28–8C, which showed that the little magnets (the nuclear MDM) were precessing about H so that their components perpendicular to the H field added up to zero. Obviously, this is not the case after a 90° pulse. We can visualize the little magnets as being placed in phase by the 90° pulse.

Figure 28–12B and C attempt to show how the nuclei are in phase at the end of a 90° pulse when M_y is greatest. As M_y decreases with time, the nuclei are resuming the random distribution that existed before the 90° pulse (H_1) was applied. The drawing represents an extreme case in which all the nuclei group together in phase, which is hardly to be expected in actuality. (The next paragraph will explain why the nuclei

(dipoles) return to a random distribution after the 90° pulse.) Going in phase may be compared to closing one of those old-fashioned folding fans that high-society matrons used to carry to the opera, and going out of phase is analogous to opening the fan. In fact, some authors use the term "fanning out" instead of going out of phase.

When the 90° pulse is ended, the little dipole magnets start precessing about H, each with a Larmor frequency. The Larmor frequency for each little magnet is not necessarily the same because of local magnetic fields that are produced by the environment (the material structure surrounding the dipole) and by poor H-field uniformity. Remember, the Larmor frequency will vary if the magnetic field varies. The in-phase dipole magnets start to separate, because some precess faster than others (we will later call these fast and slow dipoles). When the M vector is back along H, we again have a random distribution of the dipoles about H. The return to random distribution from the in-phase distribution is an exponential function of time. T_2 is the time constant for this exponential function when only the interaction between the dipoles is considered. The exponential function is presented in Figure 28–12A as the dashed line connecting to the tops of the peaks. We would like to draw that function again in Figure 28–13.

Note that T_2^* is introduced in Figure

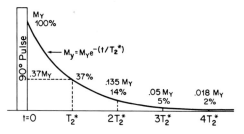

Figure 28–13 Graphic representation of the decay constant T_2^*

28–13 as a constant in the exponential portion of the equation

$M_y = M_Y e^{-t/T_2^*}$

M_y = component of M along the y axis

M_Y = component of M along y at the end of the 90° pulse

t = time following the 90° pulse

T_2^* = decay constant for randomization of the in-phase dipoles

We do exactly the same thing in x-ray attenuation where we introduced the attenuation coefficient, and we do the same thing in radioactive decay by introducing the disintegration constant. With these two constants we then proceeded to find the half-value layer and the half-life. We would like to do something slightly different here. Consider the exponential expression from Figure 28–13, e^{-t/T_2^*}. If time (t) is made equal to T_2^*, then $t/T_2^* = 1$ and the exponential becomes e^{-1} (remember that $e^{-1} = 1/e$). Therefore, at $t = T_2^*$, the value of the magnetization in the y^1 direction has decreased to $1/e$ of its maximum value at $t = 0$. (In this paragraph, e is the base of the natural log; it is not the electronic charge. $1/e$ has the value of 0.37.) In Figure 28–13, **T_2^* is the time required to reduce the value of magnetization along the y^1 axis (the transverse magnetization) to $1/e$ of its value following the 90° pulse.**

Therefore, T_2^* is the decay constant for randomization of the in-phase dipoles. T_2^* relates to randomization analogous to the way in which an isotope's half-life relates to the decay of the radioactive sample. It takes several T_2^* periods for the in-phase dipoles to approach randomization. The dispersion of the dipoles is determined by the local Larmor frequency, which is determined by the local magnetic field. The local magnetic field depends on, first of all, the applied field, H. The variations in the local field, however, depend on the fluctuating fields produced by neighboring charged particles and on permanent inhomogeneity in the applied field, H. The permanent inhomogeneity in the H field

simply means that it is impossible to make a perfect magnet. If the applied field, H, were perfectly uniform (no inhomogeneity), the T_2^* would be exactly equal to the spin-spin relaxation time, T_2. Because this is never the case, we will see later (see "Spin-Echo Technique") that T_2 is measured experimentally by procedures designed to eliminate the effects of the field inhomogeneity.

During the dephasing of the dipoles, energy may be transferred from one dipole to another, but no energy is transferred to the surrounding material. The transfer of energy to the surrounding environment brings about the return of the nuclear dipole to the lower energy spin state. There is another time constant for the return of the dipoles to the lower energy spin state.

Spin-Lattice Relaxation Time (T_1)

Recall that at equilibrium in a magnetic field, the spin-up (lower energy) population of nuclei contain about 1 in 1,000,000 more nuclei than are contained in the spin-down (higher energy) population. The excess nuclei in the spin-up state are responsible for producing the component of the magnetization vector, M, that is parallel to the magnetic field, H.

At the end of a 90° pulse, the two spin states of the nuclei are equally populated, and there is no component of the magnetization vector (M_z) in the H direction. This means that some (half) of the excess nuclei in the lower energy state have absorbed energy and have flipped to the higher energy state. At the end of the 90° pulse, those nuclei (or their relatives) transfer energy to the structure (called the lattice) that surrounds them, and return to the lower energy state. As they return to the lower state, the component of M along H is reestablished as the equilibrium distribution of the nuclei is reestablished. Here again, we find that the number of excess nuclei remaining in the higher energy state as time passes is an exponential function of time. (Remember that the number of x-ray photons remaining in a beam is an exponential function of absorber thickness.) Therefore, the number of nuclei that have returned to the lower state is obtained by subtracting those remaining in the higher energy state from the total number of excess nuclei that were in the higher state at the end of the 90° pulse. (This is exactly analogous to the number of x-ray photons removed from the x-ray beam.)

As always, we have a constant for this exponential function (like the attenuation coefficient for x rays) that we call **T₁, the spin-lattice relaxation time.** T_1 is the time for 63% of the nuclei to return to the lower energy state following a 90° pulse. The equation for the return to equilibrium following a 90° pulse is

$M_z = M_z (1 - e^{-t/T_1})$
M_z = component of M along H at time t
M_z = component of M along H at equilibrium
 t = time following a 90° pulse
T_1 = spin-lattice relaxation time.

When t is equal to T_1, we have $e^{-t/T_1} = e^{-1} = 0.37$.

One more interpretation of T_1 might be in order. **T₁ is a rate constant.** The rate (the number of nuclei per unit of time) at which the nuclei are flipping from the higher to lower energy state depends on the number of nuclei available for the transition and on some constant, T_1, that is a function of the environment in which the nuclei find themselves. Thus, the number of nuclei per unit of time that undergo a transition approaches zero because fewer nuclei are available to make the transition. (This again is completely analogous to x-ray attenuation or radioactive decay.)

Figure 28–14 shows the return to equilibrium population following a 90° pulse in terms of the component of M along H, M_z. Note that we are close to the equilibrium population after a time of 4 to 5 T_1 has passed. (For this reason, in pulsed NMR, in which repetitive pulses are used, the pulses should be separated in time by more than 4 to 5 T_1.)

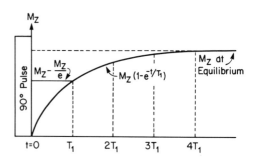

Figure 28–14 Graphic representation of the time constant T_1

Things have been going too well in the discussion of T_1 and T_2. So it's time for a small problem. **The return of the nuclei to equilibrium distribution does not give an NMR signal** (Remember that T_2^* could be measured by the FID signal produced by the transverse M_y.) This means that T_1 cannot be measured directly by NMR techniques. But, more importantly, **it means that at the end of the FID signal, there may still be some excess nuclei in the higher energy state.** In general, the nuclei will dephase (remember the T_2 discussion) before all the nuclei return to the equilibrium distribution following a 90° pulse, or **time T_1 will be longer than time T_2.** Sometimes T_1 and T_2 are nearly the same, as in liquids, and sometimes T_1 is much longer than T_2, as in solids.

There are several ways to measure T_1. Probably the simplest is to use an RF pulse sequence of a 90° pulse followed by a short latent period, followed by another 90° pulse (Fig. 28–15A). Pulse sequences are used extensively in NMR, with each designed to provide some particular bit of information. The sequence given above may be written as $90° - \tau - 90°$. (A sequence is normally notated by some shorthand notation such as this.) In the $90° - \tau - 90°$ sequence, the first 90° pulse rotates the M vector. During the time, τ, relaxation occurs as some of the nuclei flip from the higher to the lower energy state. Another 90° pulse is used to produce an FID that is made by fewer nuclei (because we are not

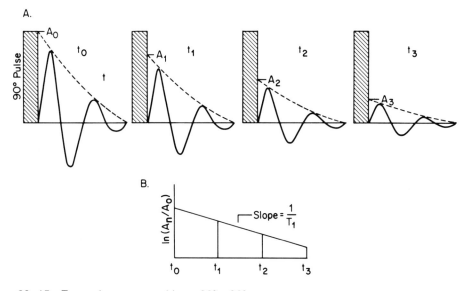

Figure 28–15 T_1 can be measured by a 90°-τ-90° sequence

at thermal equilibrium at the start of this pulse). The ratio of the FID amplitudes immediately after the two 90° pulses is a measure of how many nuclei flipped from the higher to lower state during the time, τ, between the pulses. This procedure is repeated for various values of τ, and T_1 can then be calculated from the data (Fig. 28–15B). Many people may prefer using a 180° pulse sequence: $180° - τ - 90°$.

Spin Density

The density of the spinning nuclei is proportional to the amplitude of the FID. Density here means the number of identical nuclei per unit volume that are found in an identical environment or, if you prefer, the number of nuclei per unit volume that have the same Larmor frequency. We would expect the magnetization to increase with an increased number of nuclei simply because there would be more dipoles to help form the magnetization. As the magnetization vector sweeps past the RF coil to produce the FID, we have already seen that the induced signal size depends on the size of the transverse component of the magnetization. Therefore, we would expect

larger values of magnetization to produce larger FID amplitudes.

Because the number of nuclei at the Larmor frequency determines the size of the FID signal, we need only measure the FID amplitude to obtain the spin density. We must ensure that no other effect is changing the amplitude of the FID. For example, the nuclei must be in the equilibrium distribution before applying the 90° pulse to evoke the FID. Usually, for NMR measurements, we use more than one pulse to help improve the signal-to-noise ratio (S:N). That means that a repetitive pulse sequence is normally used to form the final NMR signal. We must wait for a period equivalent to 4 to 5 T_1 between pulses to ensure that the nuclei are close to equilibrium.

MECHANISMS FOR RELAXATION

We have said that photon emission alone cannot explain the spin-lattice relaxation time, T_1. (This is different from the production of characteristic x rays, which we described entirely as photon emission.) Consequently, we must discuss what methods can be used by the nuclei to get rid of energy so that they can flip from the higher to the lower energy state.

For a proton in a 1-Tesla magnetic field, the energy separation between the two spin states is only 1.759×10^{-7} eV. We generally think in terms of kiloelectron volts when dealing with x rays which means that the energy state separation here is some 10^{-10} smaller than the energy separation of the inner atomic electrons. (You can try this calculation if you use 1 Tesla $= 1$ kg/C · sec, 1 MHz/Tesla $= 1$ C/kg, 1 eV $= 1/6 \times 10^{-19}$ J, and h $= 6.6 \times 10^{-34}$ J · sec). Look up the gyromagnetic ratio of a proton in Table 28–1, and remember the formula $\Delta E = \gamma \hbar H$.

When there are two quantum energy states (either spin states or electron energy shells), there is competition between photon emission and radiationless transfer of energy to the environment (sometimes called the lattice). For the nuclear spin flips, most transitions occur by radiationless transfer of energy to the lattice.

There are several ways, depending on the lattice structure in which the nuclei find themselves, by which the nuclei may transfer their energy to the lattice. The main requirement is that the nuclei be in the presence of locally fluctuating magnetic fields produced by the environment. Therefore, any means by which varying magnetic fields can be produced can be a means to transfer energy. The larger the field, the more quickly the energy can be transferred. In gases (and liquids), rotating molecules produce large local fields, and T_1 (rate of nuclear flips) is short, about a few milliseconds. In solids, on the other hand, the lattice is firmly fixed, which means no molecular rotation. In solids the energy is mainly transferred by dipole-dipole interactions. The magnetic field of the dipoles (those tiny magnets) interact with electronic dipole moments, which in turn interact with other nuclear dipoles. These interactions transfer energy from the nuclear dipole to the lattice as heat energy.

In no way do we intend to leave the impression that the T_1 interactions are simple and easy to catalog. Much of the work in NMR is in the area of trying to understand the interactions that produce the T_1 time. **We should note that the time T_1 is an indication of the environment in which the dipole is located.** This may be useful in NMR imaging. For example, gray and white nervous tissue differ in water content only by about 10%, but their T_1 values differ by a factor of 1.5

Spin-Echo Technique

We have seen that the dephasing (T_2^*) of the nuclear dipoles following a 90° pulse is determined by two quantities, 1) the spin-spin relaxation time and 2) the H-field inhomogeneity. We should keep in mind that the H-field inhomogeneity is built into the magnet and is undesirable but unfortunately quite permanent. Furthermore, the field inhomogeneity varies from point to point within the H field. **The spin-echo technique was developed to remove the effect of the H-field inhomogeneity.**

The spin-echo process starts with a 90° pulse along the x^1 axis (Fig. 28–16A). Of course, at the end of the pulse, dephasing starts among the spin dipoles. Some dipoles will be in a field larger than the H field because of local fields adding to the H field. They will precess faster than the M vector, which is precessing at the Larmor frequency. Some will be slower than M because they are in a smaller field than H. Remember, the frequency of precession is related to the strength of H:

$$\nu = \frac{\gamma H}{2\pi}$$

We can refer to these dipoles as fast and slow dipoles. In Figure 28–16B, the x^1y^1 coordinate is rotating at the Larmor frequency and, therefore, M appears not to be rotating. Those slow dipoles will then appear to be rotating in the $-y^1$ direction (i.e., they appear to be falling behind M) while the fast dipoles appear to be rotating in the $+y^1$ direction (they appear to be

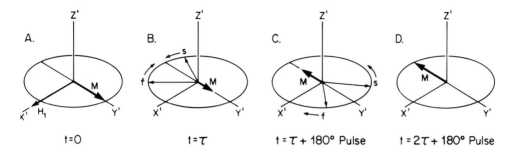

Figure 28–16 Spin-echo sequence

pulling away from M). That is, the fast and slow dipoles are rotating in opposite directions relative to M.

So, we have the 90° pulse. After a time, τ, a 180° pulse is applied along the x^1 axis. (Remember again that x^1y^1 are rotating at the Larmor frequency. Our electronics must keep track of how far the x^1 axis has rotated during the time, τ, so the 180° pulse can be applied along the x^1 axis.) The 180° pulse simply inverts the magnetization components. For the spin-echo technique, the component along H (M_z) is of no consequence. The spin grouping, however, is inverted about the x^1 axis for the transverse components.

It is noteworthy that, after the 180° pulse, the fast dipoles are behind M and the slow ones are ahead of M (Fig. 27–16C). After a time, τ (the same as before), the fast dipoles will catch up with M at the same time that M catches up with the slow dipoles. Everything will again be in phase, and the magnetization, M, along the y^1 axis will be maximal (Fig. 28–16D).

The effect is similar to that of a group of runners starting a mile run. Because they run at different speeds, the runners spread out as they get farther from the starting line. If, at an arbitrary time, τ, they are suddenly told that they are going the wrong way, they will turn around and head back for the starting line. The fast runners will be farther from the starting line than the slow runners. Because the runners who are the farthest away are the fastest, all will arrive back at the starting line together at

a time equal to 2τ (assuming that everyone runs back at a constant speed). This analogy would be more accurate if we kept the runners going in the same direction all the time. By magic, at time t we would interchange the fast and slow runners. Then, at time 2τ, the fast runners would exactly catch up with their slower companions. Of course, the dipoles (as would the runners) immediately start dephasing again as the fast dipoles pass the slow ones. As the dipoles come together (we get a reverse FID) and separate (another FID), we get a pulse that looks like 2 FIDs back to back (Fig. 28–17). **This back-to-back FID is the spin-echo.** Because we have used a 180° pulse, we effectively remove the H-field inhomogeneity from the dephasing.

The dephasing caused by spin-spin relaxation, however, would continue. The amplitude of the echo is smaller than the initial FID. The decrease in amplitude is an exponential function of T_2, the spin-spin relaxation time. T_2 can be measured by repeating the 180° pulse every 2τ and by measuring the time constant of the decrease of the amplitude of the echoes. This

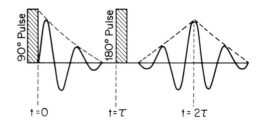

Figure 28–17 Spin-echo signal

type of pulse sequence has the name Carr-Purcell echo sequence, and it (or some modification) is usually used to measure T_2.

Fourier Transforms

We have previously mentioned Fourier transforms (FT) in connection with the modulation transfer function (see Chap. 13) and computed tomography reconstruction methods (see Chap. 24). The application of the FT to magnetic resonance is very straightforward, perhaps somewhat easier to understand than our previous examples. The signal received from NMR (the FID, for instance) is in the form of amplitude versus time. The FT of a signal of this type is in the form of signal strength (corresponding to spin density) versus frequency.

For instance, consider a simple sine wave, which has a time for one complete cycle period of T (Fig. 28–18A). This sine wave has only one frequency (f), so the FT of the sine wave is only a single line in the plot with a height that is proportional to the total strength of the sine wave (Fig. 28–18B). (Of course, in any practical situation, we cannot obtain a true single-frequency sine wave because additional frequencies result from starting and stopping the wave form.) It is interesting to note that both curves of Figure 28–18 contain the same information and that, given one, we

can get the other by means of the FT. Note that two sine waves with different frequencies would add together to give a complicated-looking signal in the "time domain" (before the FT of the signal), but would simply be two lines in the "frequency domain" (after the FT of the signal) whose heights would represent the relative strengths of the sine waves.

The sine curve looks something like an FID, except that the FID decays to zero. Thus, we might expect the FT of the FID to be something like the FT for the sine curve. If the FID is composed of dephasing nuclei in similar environments, the Larmor frequency of the FID is essentially a single-frequency decaying sine curve. We might expect the local environmental magnetic fields to cause the dipoles to precess at slightly different frequencies. Furthermore, we might expect that those slightly different frequencies would show up in the FT of the FID.

Figure 28–19 gives an FID and its FT. There are some points to note about the FT curve. First, it is a Lorentzian shape. (We make this observation only because you may have read this elsewhere.) The term "Lorentzian" is used to provide information (to mathematicians) about the symmetry of the line about the Larmor frequency. The second point is that the line width at half its maximum value (called the FWHM, the full width at half-maximum) is $2/T_2^*$. This result is verifiable by mathematics but is a terrible task involving integral calculus. Remember that $2/T_2^*$ has the unit of 1/time, which is the same unit that the frequency has.

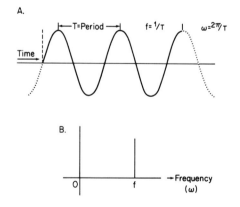

A.

B.

Figure 28–18 Fourier transform of a single-frequency sine wave

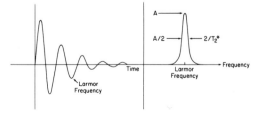

Figure 28–19 Fourier transform of a single FID

Suppose we have a sample with two groups of nonidentical nuclei. If their gyromagnetic ratios were different, there would be two Larmor frequencies. (Remember, $\nu_L = \gamma H/2\pi$, where ν_L = Larmor frequency, γ = gyromagnetic ratio, and H = applied magnetic field.) In such a case, the FID would be the sum of the two exponentially decaying sine waves, one at each of the Larmor frequencies. If, by chance, **we had two groups of identical nuclei in different magnetic fields, we would also see the composite FID of the two Larmor frequencies.** We will depict the two Larmor frequencies (Fig. 28–20A), the composite FID (Fig. 28–20B), and the FT of the FID in Figure 28–20. Note that Figure 28–20B shows a time function and, by use of the FT, this has been converted in Figure 28–20C to a frequency function.

We can see from these examples that the **FT of the FID can reduce a rather complicated signal to relatively simple frequency lines that indicate the spin density**

at each frequency. This is an important concept for NMR imaging. In some NMR imaging, we purposely vary the field across the subject so that the resonance Larmor frequency will be different for points across the subject. Figure 28–21 diagrams the effects of varying the field for three samples of identical nuclei. The single received signal (composite FID), when the FT is taken, shows us that there are three groups of nuclei. Furthermore, we are told that the three groups have equal spin density (i.e., the same number of nuclei per unit volume in all three samples).

Now, if we relate the Larmor frequency back to the magnetic field, we know that group 1 is where H_1 exists, and so forth. If we happen to make the change in the magnetic field a linear change, then we know the value of the field everywhere along the sample. This allows us to transform the information given in terms of frequency to sample location in spatial coordinates, and that is exactly what we need

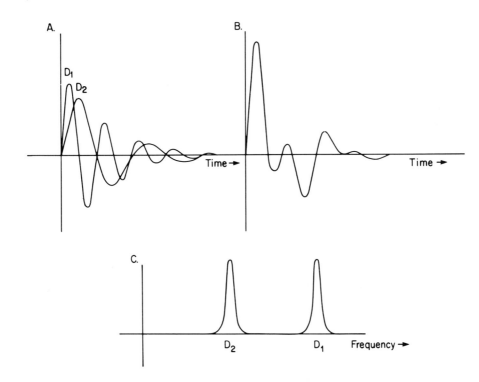

Figure 28–20 Fourier transform of a composite FID

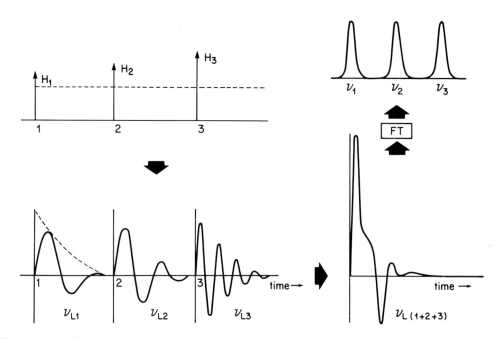

Figure 28–21 Fourier transform of three groups of identical nuclei in different magnetic fields

to do for spatially imaging a sample. If we could do all these simple steps, we could image, at least, a one-dimensional spatially varying sample.

INSTRUMENTATION

Magnets

It would seem from the foregoing discussion that there are several pieces of apparatus that are essential for the production, detection, and display of an NMR signal These include a magnet to produce the H field, some equipment to produce the varying H_1 field, a device to detect the FID of M, and the electronics to assimilate and display the NMR signal.

In NMR, producing and holding H constant is one of the most difficult jobs. Generally, the H-field value should be as large as possible because the signal-to-noise ratio (S:N) of the output information depends on H. The higher the value of H, the larger the S:N ratio. We must be aware that NMR requires an RF magnetic field that must penetrate tissue to image a body in cross section. A higher H value requires an in-

crease in the RF frequency, which does not penetrate the body as well as low-frequency RF. A higher H-field value may present problems with skin penetration by the RF field. In addition, H must be uniform (i.e., have the same strength and direction) over the entire volume of sample under investigation. Of course, when we make statements like the last two, we have to amend them immediately. We will probably find that stronger fields can improve the S:N ratio just so much, and then we see no further improvement with larger and more costly magnets. There will always be a tradeoff between field strength, uniformity, and magnet cost. We have always been in that position, however, when considering new imaging equipment.

Bar Magnets and Electromagnets

When discussing magnets we feel that it would be instructive to start with an iron bar magnet and to work forward and upward from there. In Figure 28–22A, the lines labeled "H" represent the magnetic field. The lines are usually called the "magnetic lines of force," and indicate the di-

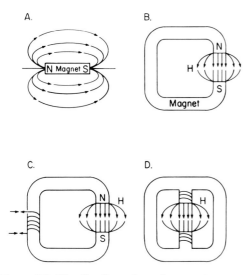

Figure 28–22 Configuration of magnets

rection of the magnetic field at each point along the line. If we are careful, but not too rigid, the lines may also indicate the field strength: the closer the lines are together, the larger the field strength. (More formally, the field strength at a point is the number of lines passing through a unit area centered at this point.) With this notation, a uniform field would be represented by straight lines evenly spaced. Obviously, if our drawing is any good at all, there is no uniform field area around the bar magnet.

Note the space called the "gap" of the C magnet in Figure 28–22B. There the lines are fairly straight and evenly spaced in the middle region. Toward the outer regions of the gap the lines become curved, which would indicate that the field is no longer uniform. The gap region of the C magnet could be used as the H field for NMR studies, but the sample to be investigated should be entirely within the uniform field area. Of course, bar magnets could be bent into a horseshoe shape to give a uniform field in the gap. Permanent magnets can be used for NMR imaging if they are big enough.

Figure 28–22C and D indicate the fields produced by two configurations of electro-

magnets. The field strength depends on the current; larger currents produce larger fields. Physics and chemistry laboratories worldwide use magnets based on the "yoke"-type construction for NMR studies (Fig. 28–22D). The magnets vary in size and construction, but all have one common property: the space between the pole faces is small, being at most a few inches wide. The restricted space between the pole faces restricts the size of the sample that may be investigated. (People will certainly not fit within the pole gap of commercially available electromagnets that have iron cores.)

Resistive Coil Air Core Magnets

Magnetic fields can be produced by current-carrying conductors. (This concept was discussed earlier in this chapter.) Suppose we have a coil of wire with current (electron flow) passing through it. In Figure 28–23A we have current (I) passing through a coil of wire (more than one loop), which produces the magnetic field (H) indicated. In Figure 28–23B the coil of wire is pulled out to form a solenoid (resembles a wire spring). The field inside the solenoid is fairly uniform, while outside the solenoid the field looks like the field around a bar magnet.

Further investigation would reveal that the field uniformity could be improved by a pair of Helmholtz coils, although the field strength might be somewhat lower than for a comparable solenoid. Figure 28–24A represents a pair of Helmholtz coils. A Helmholtz pair of coils consists of two parallel coils in which the current is flowing in the same direction.

The coil arrangement in Figure 28–24B consists of two sets of Helmholtz coils that can be used to produce sufficiently uniform fields with ample room for NMR imaging. A person could be placed in this field by sliding him in the direction of H through the opening in the coils. With the four coil arrangement (two sets of Helmholtz coils), field uniformities of one part per thousand over about a 50-cm diameter

A.

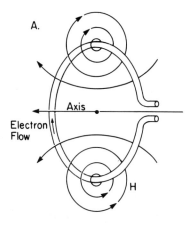

B.

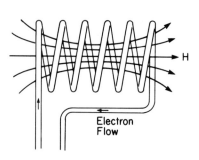

Figure 28–23   Magnetic field in a solenoid

A.

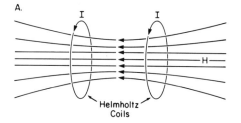

B.

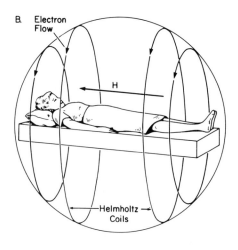

Figure 28–24   Magnetic field of a Helmholtz pair (A) and a resistive coil air core magnet (B)

can be achieved. Field strength, H, is somewhere in the half-Tesla region. **This type of magnet is called a resistive coil air core magnet.** The resistive coil part of the name implies that current must be supplied during the entire time that the magnet is activated. Therefore, electrical power is consumed during the entire time that the magnet is producing the magnetic field. Resistive coil magnets that are commercially available have rather low field strength, some instabilities because of power supply regulation, and high power consumption.

Superconducting Magnets

An alternative to the resistive coil magnet is the superconducting magnet. **"Supercons,"** as they are called, **take advantage of the zero resistance that certain materials have at very low temperatures.** At zero resistance a current, once started, will continue to flow without further power input. That means that supercons are initially connected to a power supply, brought up to the design field strength, and then disconnected from the electrical power source. The current continues and the magnetic field remains constant. There is just one little problem! **The entire magnetic system must be maintained at about 4° K,** which makes the North Pole look like Palm Springs. This low temperature can be maintained if the magnetic coils are submerged in liquid helium.

The supercon contains a solenoid of superconducting material, perhaps NbTi, in the form of filaments embedded in a copper matrix. The solenoid is surrounded by liquid helium; around the liquid helium is a vacuum (a very poor heat conductor). The helium must be in a container (stainless steel) surrounded by another container. A vacuum is hopefully maintained between these two containers. A double-walled container designed to hold low-temperature material is called a Dewar. Next to the vacuum region is a layer of liquid nitrogen, then another vacuum, perhaps some insulation, and an outside polished container.

Note that the entire structure outlined above is designed to keep heat energy from being transferred from the room temperature around the magnet to the liquid helium inside the magnet. Such structures are not perfect, and some heat will get to the liquid helium. The heat energy will convert some liquid helium to helium gas (liquefied gases have very low boiling points). If all the liquid helium is "boiled away," the temperature of the superconducting material will start to increase. If the temperature increases above that temperature at which superconductivity starts, the magnet will lose its field. **It is most important to keep liquid helium in the magnet.** Therefore, about once a week, the magnet must be filled with liquid helium (and nitrogen, too).

We are not good enough artists to draw the inside of a supercon, but we can present some photographs. Figure 28–25 shows a 5-in. bore supercon. The bore is the diameter of the center area into which the sample to be investigated is inserted (with all the RF coils necessary to make the measurements). The bore of the 5-in. magnet is vertical, and the samples must be inserted from the top or bottom. The small cylinders on top are tubes with which to fill the magnet with liquid nitrogen and helium

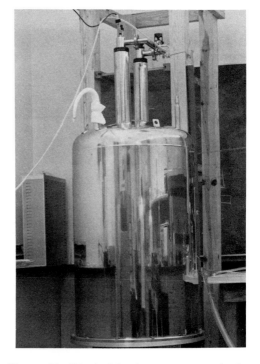

Figure 28–25 A 5-in. bore superconducting magnet

and to monitor the temperatures and liquid levels inside the magnet. The field strength, H, is 5 Tesla at the center of the bore (along the center line halfway from top to bottom), and the field homogeneity is one part in 10^7 over a 2-cm^3 volume.

Figure 28–26 shows a horizontal 12-in. bore magnet. In this picture you can see the bore area. As yet there are no RF coils in the bore of this magnet. Note the filling tubes on top. The field strength is 1.9 Tesla at the center, with one part in 10^6 homogeneity over a 2-cm^3 volume.

Some cautionary measures are in order. If the temperature of any segment of the solenoid goes above the temperature for superconduction, that segment will then have some resistance. Power loss in this resistance ($P = I^2R$) would be converted to heat, and the adjoining segments would be raised to nonsuperconducting status. This would continue until the entire solenoid would no longer be superconducting and

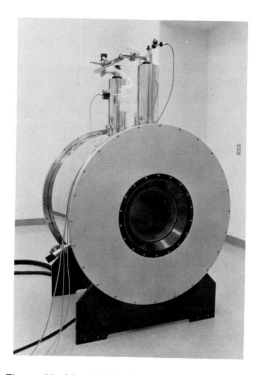

Figure 28–26   A 12-in. bore superconducting magnet

the net result would be loss of current and liquid helium. "Quench" is the term used to describe this disaster. There is a reason, therefore, for putting superconducting filaments in a copper matrix: the copper hopefully keeps the filaments from melting down during a quench. In addition, a disturbance in the fringing fields (the magnetic field outside the magnet that we cannot remove) can induce a quench of the magnet. Therefore, no large steel object should be moved around close to the magnet. Don't put these magnets close to elevators or parking lots. Although these two would probably not produce a quench, they would disturb the field and produce unreliable results. **Don't use steel rolling carts in the area. Don't use steel tools near the bore of the magnet.** They might well be sucked up into the bore. (This would be extremely dangerous, obviously, if there happened to be a patient in the magnet at the time.) Also, don't allow people with

pacemakers to wander freely about the area. The fringing fields could affect the pulse timing of the pacemaker. Finally, there is one other warning. **When a magnet undergoes a rapid quench, there is a tremendous amount of helium gas released in a very short time,** and this gas could make breathing difficult for patients. In an imaging system room, a large exhaust system must be available to remove the gas quickly.

Radio Frequency Coils

Now that the magnetic field, H, can be established, the next thing to do is to produce the varying H_1 field. Remember, H_1 must be perpendicular to H and must vary sinusoidally with the Larmor frequency. For H fields obtainable and gyromagnetic values that nuclei possess, the Larmor frequency will be somewhere in the radio frequency range (1–100 MHz). **The device that produces H_1 is called a radio frequency coil.**

There are several types of RF coils that may be used. Figure 28–27 shows representative coil configurations of two com-

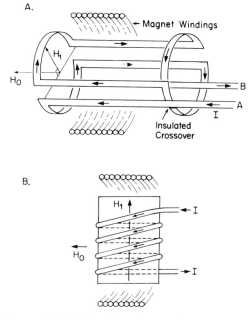

Figure 28–27   Configuration of RF coils

monly used types. The saddle-shaped coil is useful with supercon magnets because of similar geometry, and yet it gives perpendicular H and H_1 fields (Fig. 28–27A). With the saddle-shaped coil, the sample may still be inserted along the axis of the magnet. Normally the solenoidal coil is used with electromagnets, but the drawing here shows one in a supercon magnet (Fig. 28–27B). Note that the solenoidal RF coil is not along the axis of the magnet. For this configuration, the sample must be placed within the RF coil before the coil is inserted in the bore of the magnet. The solenoidal coil should give a better S:N ratio, but it is somewhat harder to use.

At this point, we should note that the RF coils so far have been used to produce the magnetic field, H_1. There is one other requirement: The NMR signal must be detected. The device should be one that detects low-energy signals at the Larmor frequency, which sounds like an RF coil, doesn't it? Indeed it is. Because we use a pulsed H_1 field, the H_1 RF coil may be used to detect the NMR signal during the time when it is not producing the H_1 field. It is only during this time that we can detect the NMR signal, however, so we can use one RF coil to produce the H_1 field and to detect the NMR signal. There may be times when we prefer to use two RF coils, one to produce H_1 and the other to detect the signal. If we do this, the two RF coils are normally placed in the magnetic field perpendicular to each other (and, of course, with H_1 still perpendicular to H).

Electronics

The job that the electronic devices must perform is to apply an RF voltage in pulsed sequence across the RF coil, detect the NMR signal (the free induction decay or spin-echo for the pulse sequence), and record or display the information in the desired form. With imaging, the electronics must also control the gradient coils (to be described later) and construct the image from the data.

Suppose we have a sample of interest within an RF coil, and both the sample and coil are within a magnetic field, H. If we knew the Larmor frequency, we could apply a single frequency to the RF coil to invoke the NMR signal, at least from those nuclei with a Larmor frequency equal to the one applied. There is the problem of local magnetic environment at each nucleus, which requires a slightly different Larmor frequency. To observe these slightly different Larmor frequencies, we must apply a range of frequencies to the RF coil (or, as in many physics experiments, slightly vary the magnetic field). Thus, we need a device to generate a sweep of RF frequencies about the Larmor frequency that we would have if there were no environmental effects. "Sweep" is really not the right word. If we apply a square wave pulse (such as that shown in Figure 28–12A for the FID), the pulse contains all the frequencies needed to excite the nuclei of interest. We cannot form a pulse at the Larmor frequency with only one frequency present, so we need a pulse generator with which we can vary the RF frequency to the Larmor frequency, fix the pulse width, and develop the pulse sequence. The pulse generator may not produce sufficient power, so we normally use an RF amplifier to feed the RF coil. The combined pulse generator and amplifier is sometimes called the "transmitter."

At the end of a pulse, we would like the RF coil to detect the NMR signal. Remember that the detection is accomplished by the decaying M vector inducing a current (voltage) at the Larmor frequency in the RF coil. We want the NMR signal to go into an RF amplifier that will not distort the signal. The NMR signal is considerably smaller than the input RF pulse. After the amplifier, there are several ways to proceed. Because we have described the Fourier transform method of producing the NMR spectrum, we will use that. If so, we need to digitize the signal and then use FT. The FT of the signal is what we would like to see displayed as the NMR information. Therefore, after the FT, we either display the signal or store it for later use. Figure 28–28 presents a basic block diagram of the NMR system.

But matters are hardly ever this simple. We must be able to keep track of or choose the phase of the RF pulse and the NMR signal. Furthermore, we use repetitive pulsing to improve the S:N ratio. A computer is not absolutely necessary, but most systems have one. Figure 28–29 shows the console for the 5-in. bore magnet, which has lots of knobs on it. This is representative of the control console for an NMR system that can measure the NMR signal for an entire small sample. (Things are not going to get any simpler, though, when we start imaging.)

NMR Spectrum

Figure 28–30 is a phosphorus (^{31}P) NMR spectrum of muscle in the human forearm. Dr. Ray L. Nunnally, of our Radiology Department, was kind enough to supply this spectrum with the following words:

A high-resolution phosphorus-31 NMR spectrum from the flexor carpi radialis and palmaris longus muscles of the human forearm. The peaks resolved are inorganic phosphate (P_i), phosphocreatine (PCr), and the α, β, and γ phosphorus atoms of adenosine triphosphate (ATP). PCr and ATP constitute the reserve and direct chemical species (respec-

tively) which yield energy to support cellular functions. This spectrum required two minutes of signal averaging using the standard pulse Fourier transform method. It was obtained on an Oxford Instruments 30-cm horizontal bore superconducting magnet operating at a field of 1.9 Tesla.

This is the same magnet shown in Figure 28–26, where it was called a 12-in. magnet.

NMR IMAGING TECHNIQUES

We have finally arrived at the point at which we can discuss imaging. The NMR systems and methods we have so far described have only been capable of viewing a sample as a whole and recording the NMR spectrum from the entire sample. With imaging we must be able to measure the NMR response from any selected point in the sample, and be aware of the position of the point in the sample. The point selection can be made if we can meet the **resonance condition ($\nu = \gamma H/2\pi$ or $\omega = \gamma H$)** at this point but at no other point in the sample. Or, perhaps, we might prefer to select more than one point. If we are skilled enough to meet the resonance condition at only one point, then it would not be hard to imagine that we could also know the location of the point. **The task in imaging is simply to do something with the applied field, H, so that the resonance will occur at only known points, and to record the resonance signal from those points.**

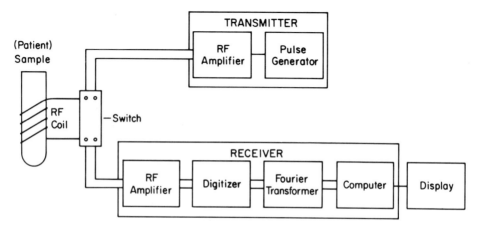

Figure 28–28   Schematic drawing of a nonimaging NMR system

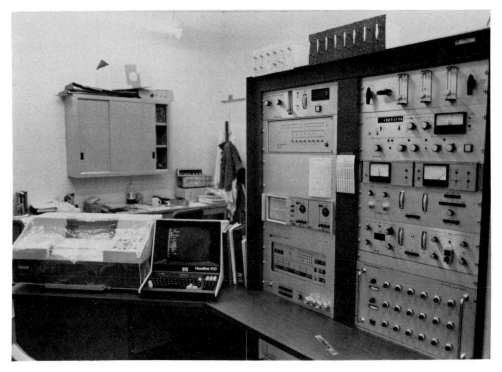

Figure 28–29 Console for a 5-in. bore supercon

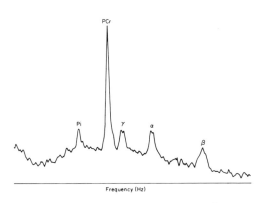

Figure 28–30 NMR spectrum for ^{31}P. (Courtesy of Dr. Ray L. Nunnally, University of Texas Health Science Center at Dallas, Radiology Department)

Once we have obtained resonance at only known positions, we can measure the NMR parameters for those positions. This means we can measure spin density (which relates to resonant nuclei density), spin-lattice relaxation time, T_1, or even spin-spin relaxation time, T_2. Perhaps the most common image obtained by NMR is the density of hydrogen across the sample. It is obtained by measuring the spin density of protons in the sample. It may be that we would rather know something about the variation of T_1 in the sample, so we would then measure T_1 at the resonant locations.

To complete an image, we must be able to move the resonance location throughout the entire sample. We know how to measure the NMR signal (FID or spin-echo from the pulse sequence). Now, if we could only vary the resonance throughout the sample, we would be ready to proceed. Several different techniques have been developed to move the resonance condition throughout the sample (and to keep track of the location of the resonance condition), and to collect information from all the points.

We cannot discuss all these methods, or even the details of any particular technique, but we can at least mention some of them. The various techniques can be grouped according to how much of the sample is measured at one time. Thus we have (1) point methods, (2) line methods, (3) plane methods, and (4) volume methods. Generally speaking, the point methods are the slowest, but give good resolution; the speed increases with increasing the amount of sample measured at one time (points 1–4). We feel that there hasn't been enough information gathered so far to dictate which method will be preferable for clinical imaging, so we will just have to wait. There appears to be a trend, however, toward the use of planar two-dimensional Fourier transforms, but we're not at all sure just where NMR imaging will fall in the radiologic scheme. We hardly feel it will replace the "tricorder" of Star Trek.

Point Methods

The most straightforward approach to imaging is to adjust the magnetic field, H, so that the resonance condition exists at only one point (or at least, in a small volume) in the patient. There have been two methods developed to produce the adjustment in the H field. The first is one in which the magnetic field is shaped (adjusted) by applying magnetic field gradients along all three coordinate axes (one of which, z, is along the H-field direction; the other two, x and y, are perpendicular to z and to each other). The gradients are applied by gradient coils that must be placed in the magnet. (In commercial imaging units the gradient coils will look like part of the magnet.) The coils are placed inside the magnet and make the effective bore of the magnet somewhat smaller. The gradient coils are constructed so that changing the currents through them will move the sensitive point (in which the resonance condition exists) throughout the sample volume.

The second sensitive point method employs alternating gradients. Here three orthogonal alternating gradients are applied throughout the sample volume. Each gradient is such that at one plane between the gradient coils the alternating (time-dependent) gradient is effectively zero; that is, the time-dependent field is zero. Because there are three such planes that are perpendicular, the intersection of these planes occurs at a point at which the field is not varying with time, but all other points in the sample are. Therefore, after application of the RF pulse, the NMR signal contains information that is composed of non-time-dependent (time-independent) information from the single point, and time-dependent information from all other points. Filtering the time-dependent information leaves only information from the point at which the field is not time-dependent. The time-independent point may be stepped through the sample by changing the input to the gradient coils.

The single-point methods, although slow, may be used to measure T_1 and chemical shifts. Another advantage is that the methods can be performed without a computer.

Line Methods

The line technique to be mentioned here is an extension of the last point method. Two perpendicular time-dependent magnetic field gradients are used to fix the resonance condition along a line (at which the two time-independent planes intersect). The distribution of spins along the resonance line is determined by applying a linear time-independent magnetic field gradient along the resonance line direction. The linear gradient varies the Larmor frequency of the spinning dipoles along the resonance line in a fashion that is linear with position along the line (see Fig. 28–21). The collected NMR signal is a composite FID of the spins along the resonance line plus all time-dependent signals from the rest of the sample. After the time-dependent signals are filtered out, the FT of the NMR signal gives the spin density at each Larmor frequency (and, therefore, at each position along the line).

The sensitive line (along which the resonance condition exists) may be moved throughout the sample volume by changing the ratio of currents in the two sets of gradient coils. The FT spectra may be displayed as varying intensity on a television monitor.

The line method is faster than the point methods because an entire line is read at one time. T_1, T_2, and chemical shift information, however, is harder to obtain. There are other line methods, but they all use gradient coils in some way to select the line along which the resonance condition is met.

Plane Methods

There are two plane methods that have been developed that we would like to discuss, for two reasons: 1) one method greatly resembles CT scanning, and 2) the other is the one most likely to be used in commercial imaging systems.

Suppose we have an object that we would like to image. In the plane method, we must first select the plane that we would like to image. Then we must be able to collect NMR information from each point in the plane and identify the unique point from which the NMR signal originated.

To illustrate the plane selection, we would like to place the object in the magnetic field, H. With a pair of properly designed gradient coils, we will add a magnetic gradient along the H-field direction. This gradient makes each plane along the H field have a different Larmor frequency. A drawing would be helpful, so Figure 28–31A shows the object as described. If the gradient coils have different currents, the field produced by the coils is not constant but varies along the length between the coils. In the illustration, the field caused by the gradient coils is He$_A$ at plane A, and so forth. Because H and He are parallel, they can be added to give the total magnetic field at a plane; the total net magnetic field at plane A is $H_A = H + He_A$. If we now irradiate the sample object with RF radiation at a frequency $\nu = \gamma H_B/2\pi$, we have the proper radiation for setting the resonance condition for those dipoles in plane B but not those in planes A and C. We have selected the plane at which resonance can occur. Any NMR signal we observed must come from plane B. Of course, if plane A were to be selected, all that would have to be done would be to change the frequency of the RF pulse. This procedure of plane selection is called selective radiation, and is used in both plane methods we are going to describe.

The thickness of the plane (at B) in which the dipoles find the resonance condition is determined by the field gradient, He, and by the spread of frequencies in the RF pulse. (Remember, any pulse will have more than one frequency.) We would like a large gradient and a single frequency to make the resonance plane thin. Of course, we accept tradeoffs in both. The RF pulse, however, may be contoured to some shape other than the square wave to reduce the number and amount of frequencies other than the desired Larmor frequency. Pulse shaping is normally done in imaging systems.

As a result, there is a plane at B that has the resonance condition. If the RF pulse were a 90° pulse, we would expect to see an NMR signal originating from all points in B. Suppose, though, that we apply a linear magnetic field gradient along a direction perpendicular to H (H is in the Z direction in Fig. 28–31A) that covers the entire volume of B. The nuclei in B will change their Larmor frequency and start precessing at different frequencies. The position of a nucleus along the linear gradient will determine its Larmor frequency, and all nuclei at that position along the gradient will have the same Larmor frequency. Consider Figure 28–31B. All nuclei with a given frequency produce an FID with that frequency. If we collect the NMR signal along the x direction, we get a composite FID composed of all the FIDs originating along the x direction, which looks like we have projected all the nuclei onto the x axis.

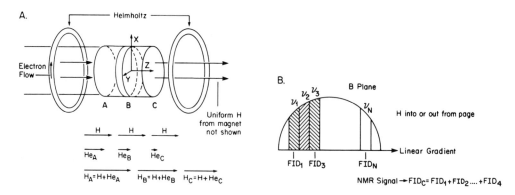

Figure 28–31 Plane methods of imaging use gradient fields

Also, if we use FT on the composite FID, we get a distribution of spins along the x direction. We have projected a plane onto a line, which is what we do in CT scanning. The next thing to do is to rotate the gradient (in the xy plane) and obtain another projection.

The image of the plane B can be reconstructed from these projections (if we collect enough of them, that is). This plane method of imaging looks exactly like CT scanning. The imaging method is called projection reconstruction zeugmatography (there's that word again). There are various modifications (selective radiation being one of them), but the concept of reconstruction by projection remains.

The next plane method employs two-dimensional FTs and phase information, as well as frequency information. First, select a plane by selective radiation of a 90° pulse (i.e., a linear magnetic gradient along H has already been applied). We now have a plane in the sample that is ready to be irradiated selectively. The RF pulse should be shaped to give the proper thickness of the slice of sample about the selected plane. Irradiate the sample with the 90° RF pulse of the proper frequency to fix the resonance condition in the selected plane. Note that at the end of the RF pulse, the free induction decay (FID) starts.

The object is to apply a linear gradient pulse perpendicular to H; call this the y direction (H is along z). This linear y-gra-

dient pulse is applied immediately at the beginning of the FID. The y-gradient pulse will cause the nuclei located at different y positions to precess at different Larmor frequencies. Therefore, the FID from each level along the y direction will have a different frequency. At the end of the y-gradient pulse, an x-gradient field is turned on. The purpose of the x gradient is to change the Larmor frequency of the FID along the x direction. The x-direction pulse is also called the read pulse, because the NMR signal is collected during this x-gradient pulse.

Figure 28–32 shows the gradient sequence as a function of time. Note the following, from top to bottom: a z gradient for plane selection; an RF-selective 90° pulse; a y gradient; and then an x gradient during which the NMR signal is collected. We would like to consider what happens to the FIDs during the y and x gradients. The illustration shows the plane at which the resonance condition will be fixed by the RF 90° pulse (Fig. 28–32). (In this drawing, the magnetic field H is perpendicular to the page.) Following the 90° pulse (note that the FID starts immediately), the y gradient changes the frequency of the FID, depending on the location along the y direction. **At the end of the y gradient, the FIDs are at different points in the decay curves which is critical to the imaging method.** We say that there is a phase dif-

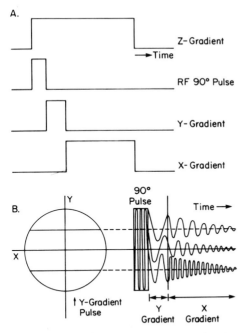

Figure 28–32 Gradient sequence for two-dimensional Fourier transform imaging

ference in the FIDs at the end of the y gradient.

Now the x gradient changes the FID frequency along the x direction, and produces a composite FID (a sample FID is shown in Figure 28–32) during the x gradient. This composite FID with the phase information is collected as the NMR signal. Note that the NMR signal is the sum of all the FIDs (of which we show only three) with their different phases (determined by the y gradient) and frequencies (determined by the x gradient). This signal is **Quadature-detected.** We will not describe this detection technique but, essentially, **it preserves the phase and frequency information from the NMR signal.** The information is digitized and stored in a computer until sufficient information is obtained to form an image of the selected plane. The phase and frequency are used to locate the xy position in the plane, and the FID amplitude is still used as a measure of the spin density of the nuclei.

The gradient sequence is repeated (nom-

inally, 180 times), with a small change in the y gradient for each sequence. This change is used to produce different values of the phase at the end of the y gradient. The change in the y gradient can be made simply by leaving the gradient on longer. A better method, however, is to change the strength of the y gradient for each pulse sequence.

When all information from each gradient sequence is stored in the computer, the computer is told to FT the data relative to the frequency (x direction) and relative to the phase (y direction). Therefore, the frequency and phase FT (with the FID amplitude) can give us the spin density profile in the xy plane. This is the image for the plane, and now we are ready to go to the next plane to make another image. The time required to collect the data from one plane is about 1 or 2 min, for a plane about 2 mm thick. T_1 measurements can be made, but require additional data.

Perhaps we can compare the NMR image to the image on a TV monitor. The TV image is composed of 512 horizontal lines, and each line is divided into 512 points (for a total of $512 \times 512 \cong 260,000$ points in each image). The y-gradient pulse (which produces phase difference information) might be thought of as a means of determining to which of the 512 horizontal lines the detected NMR signal belongs. After the signal is placed on the proper line, the x-gradient pulse (which produces frequency difference information) may be thought of as the means of assigning the signal to the correct point of the 512 along the line. (The amplitude of the FID could be compared to the brightness of the TV information at the point.) The difference from the TV analogy is that each "TV frame" of the NMR image is made up of the summation of about 180 images (i.e., the y gradient is varied 180 times per image).

Volume Methods

We will not describe any volume methods. They are only plane methods moved up to three dimensions, with an increase in computer capability.

HAZARDS

If we are going to use NMR as a diagnostic tool, we must place the patient within the magnetic field and irradiate the patient with RF pulses. There are three possible detrimental health effects that could be considered:

1. Effects of the constant field up to about 2 Tesla.
2. Effects caused by the RF irradiation.
3. Effects of rapidly changing magnetic field gradients.

So far, no short- or long-term detrimental effects have been observed from the fields and RF power used in NMR imaging.

We have already mentioned the dangers that exist around the apparatus. They are sufficiently important to note again. Do not have steel tools near the imaging apparatus. Be careful with patients who might have steel in their bodies (e.g., steel knee joints, hips, pins). Move such patients slowly around the magnets to prevent detrimental health effects to the magnets. Keep pacemakers away from any NMR unit. Have carts as free of steel as possible. Finally, have available a way to expel helium gas rapidly in large quantities in case of a rapid quench (for supercons). And, for electromagnets, take care not to let a patient come into contact with the field windings in the magnet or with the power leads to the magnet.

NMR IMAGE

Because we have gone through this topic of NMR, we can at least show you a state-of-the-art image (Fig. 28–33). It was made in a 0.35-Tesla supercon magnet by a spin-echo technique. (Notice we didn't discuss this technique.) The first echo was collected at 28 msec. A 1-sec cycle time was used, which allowed the data to be collected in 2 min.

You will probably see a few million NMR images before you're done. We hope our discussion has helped you to understand and interpret them.

ADDENDUM

In the material on NMR, we have used the symbol H to represent the applied magnetic field. Other discussions on NMR will sometimes use B to represent the magnetic field, which may be called the magnetic induction. These two symbols are used universally for H = magnetic field and B = magnetic induction. We feel the need for a few words on these two quantities.

A device such as a supercon does indeed produce a magnetic field, H. If we put some material in the magnetic field, however, the internal organization of the material may be changed so that the magnetic effects in the material are increased. That is, the magnetic field inside the material is larger than the magnetic field outside the material. We have induced an additional magnetic field (or we have, at least, increased the magnetic field) in the material. Therefore, we call the field inside the material the magnetic induction, B.

It is not hard to imagine that the magnetic induction in soft iron is greater than the magnetic induction in copper. In fact, we use soft iron in transformers simply to increase the magnetic field produced by the primary winding. The magnetic field, H, and the magnetic induction, B, are related very simply by $B = \mu H$, where μ is the magnetic permeability. It might be better to consider μ as the magnetic conductivity (because we have already discussed conductors). In a vacuum, which contains no material, $\mu = 1$ and $B = H$. In iron, μ can be as high as 1000. In air, $\mu = 1.0000004$. Consequently, we can discuss the magnetic field in the bore of a supercon, rather than the magnetic induction, with 0.00004% correctness. We doubt if we should worry too much about this error.

SUMMARY

Nuclear magnetic resonance (NMR) is a new modality for obtaining dynamic stud-

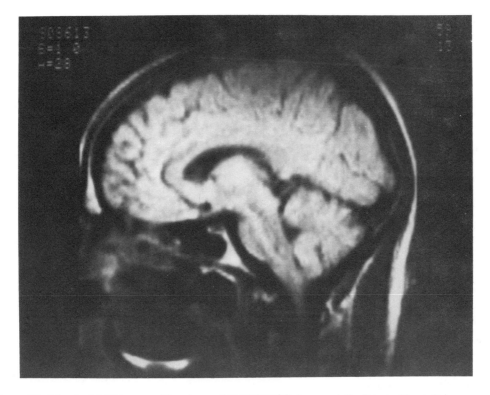

Figure 28–33 An NMR image. (Courtesy of DIASONICS, Inc. and Dr. Ray L. Nunnally)

ies of certain physiologic functions and for imaging proton density (and perhaps that of other nuclei) in the body. As the name suggests, NMR is the resonance transition between nuclear spin states of certain nuclei in an external magnetic field. As a prominent radiologist, R.H. Epstein, once said, "NMR is like sex: the first time you hear about it, you just can't believe it."

Only certain nuclei, those with a net spin angular momentum, can be observed by NMR techniques. The maximum observable spin angular momentum is given by $I\hbar$, where I is the "nuclear spin" and has a simple value for each elemental nucleus. Nuclei with $I = 0$ cannot be used in NMR studies. For most NMR studies, nuclei with $I = \frac{1}{2}$, including the proton, are investigated.

The spin angular momentum is important because it represents a spinning charge. A spinning charge will always produce a magnetic dipole moment (MDM, given the symbol μ), which makes the spinning charged nucleus behave like a tiny bar magnet. The MDM is a measure of the strength or size of the tiny magnet. The MDM is related to the spin angular momentum by

$$\mu = \gamma I\hbar \ (\gamma = \mu/I\hbar)$$

where γ is the gyromagnetic ratio. (The gyro part is $I\hbar$; the magnetic part is μ. Because μ is on top in the definition of γ, the ratio is sometimes called the magnetogyric ratio.) The gyromagnetic ratio has a unique value for each nuclear type.

If the tiny nuclear magnet is placed in a magnetic field, H, the tiny magnet will try to align itself along the magnetic field. Quantum physics rules prohibit exact alignment and, as a matter of fact, will allow only certain specified alignment orientations. There is a specific energy with each of these orientations. The nucleus may make a transition from one energy state to another by gaining or losing energy in an amount exactly equal to the energy difference between the two states. Whether there are two energy states ($I = \frac{1}{2}$), three energy states ($I = 1$), or more, the difference in energy that the nucleus must gain or lose is always $\Delta E = 2\mu H$. (Or, if you prefer, $\Delta E = \gamma \hbar H$.) NMR is nothing more than the induced transitions between spin states.

The inexact alignment in an H field of the tiny nuclear magnets causes the tiny magnets to precess about the magnetic field. The frequency of precession is called the Larmor frequency, and is given by

$$\nu_L = \gamma H / 2\pi$$

(If we consider $\Delta E = h\nu$, which represents a photon, the frequency of the photon is exactly equal to ν_L. This means that a nucleus, in order to go from a lower energy spin state to a higher energy spin state, must absorb energy equal to that of a photon with frequency ν_L.)

In a sample of observable size, there are a very large number of nuclei. For a nuclear type for which $I = \frac{1}{2}$, some nuclei are in the lower spin state and some in the higher state. At room temperature and in normal (available) magnetic fields, the number in each state is nearly the same, with about one nucleus per million more in the lower energy state. It is these "excess" nuclei that give an NMR signal.

We represent all these excess nuclei by a single quantity called the magnetization, M. It is easier to describe NMR signals in terms of M rather than of the excess individual nuclei (about 10^7 per mole). In a magnetic field, M will normally be exactly along H. It is the function of NMR to make M move away from H, and then to observe its return to alignment along H. (Remember, the nuclei are still changing spin states.)

The M vector is made to precess about a second field, H_1, that is effectively rotating about H (and perpendicular to H) at the Larmor frequency. The second field, H_1, is generated by applying an alternating voltage (alternating at the Larmor frequency) to an RF coil surrounding the sample. While H_1 is on, M will precess about H_1 at a frequency of $\gamma H_1 / 2\pi$. If H_1 is on long enough for M to rotate through $90°$, we have applied a $90°$ pulse; if M rotates through $180°$, we have a $180°$ pulse. When H_1 is turned off, M precesses about H and returns to its orientation along H. This motion of M, described as a beehive motion, induces a signal in the RF coil (again at the Larmor frequency). This induced signal is the NMR signal.

Following a $90°$ pulse, the signal induced in the RF coil is called the free induction decay (FID). M is free to return along H; it induces a signal in the RF coil that goes from a maximum value to zero (below noise, at least). The reduction in the signal is an exponential decay characterized by a decay time, T_2^*. T_2^* is determined by magnetic field inhomogeneities and by the dephasing of the nuclear spins.

The return of M along H following a $90°$ pulse is made up of two parts. The component of M along H grows from zero to some value while the component of M perpendicular to H (the transverse component) decays from some value to zero. Both are exponential functions characterized by two time constants called the relaxation times. T_1 is the time constant for the component along H, and is called the spin-lattice relaxation time. T_2 is the time constant for the transverse component, and is called the spin-spin relaxation time.

T_1 is determined by how quickly the nuclei can transfer energy to their surroundings (lattice) and return to the lower energy state. T_2 is determined by how quickly the nuclei can interact (transfer energy among themselves) to produce random distribution of the precessing nuclei about the H field. These are two NMR parameters that are of interest in describing the environment in which the nuclei are found. Nuclear spin densities are indicated by the amplitude of the FID.

The Larmor frequency is determined by the local magnetic field, and may vary from one environment to another for otherwise identical nuclei. NMR spectra are merely representations of identical nuclei that are found in slightly different magnetic fields because of local environmental effects.

For NMR imaging, the local magnetic fields are purposely varied in some prescribed fashion so that identical nuclei in different spatial locations will have different Larmor frequencies, thus producing FIDs with different Larmor frequencies. Imaging requires a measurement of the spin densities (amplitude of the FID with a particular Larmor frequency) and a method of relating the Larmor frequency to a spatial position.

The instrumentation for NMR requires a large magnet to produce the H field, radio frequency electronics to produce the RF pulse and to record the resulting NMR signal and, of course, sufficient electronics and computer power to store, manipulate, and display the NMR information.

NMR techniques seem to be safe, but there are some precautions that must be taken to ensure that patients are not damaged by the NMR instrumentation. In particular, the large magnetic fields are new to radiology and care must be taken with steel (iron) objects moving too close to the magnet. The field may produce irregularities in electronics implanted in the patient (e.g., a pacemaker). The effects of the RF pulse and gradient coils have not yet been determined.

It is likely that NMR will become a useful clinical tool. Certainly, further developments will be of great diagnostic interest.

REFERENCES

1. Bottomley, P.A.: NMR imaging techniques and applications: A review. Rev. Sci. Instrum., 59:1319, 1982.
2. Fullerton, G.D.: Basic concepts for nuclear magnetic resonance imaging. Magnet. Reson. Imag., 1:39, 1982.
3. Gore, J.C., Emery, E.W., Orr, J.S., and Doyle, F.H.: Medical nuclear magnetic resonance imaging. Invest. Radiol., 16:269, 1981.
4. Lauterbur, P.C.: Image formation by induced local interactions: Example employing nuclear magnetic resonance. Nature, 242:190, 1973.
5. McCullough, E.C., and Baker, H.L., Jr.: Nuclear magnetic resonance imaging. Radiol. Clin. North Am., 20:3, 1982.

INDEX

Page numbers in *italics* refer to figures; page numbers followed by 't' refer to tables.

505